Vascular and Interventional Radiology
Principles and Practice

 Thieme

Vascular and Interventional Radiology
Principles and Practice

Curtis W. Bakal, M.D., M.P.H.
Director, Vascular and Interventional Radiology
Beth Israel Medical Center
St. Luke's-Roosevelt Hospital Center
Long Island College Hospital
New York, New York
and
Professor of Radiology
Albert Einstein College of Medicine
New York, New York

James E. Silberzweig, M.D.
Associate Professor of Clinical Radiology
Albert Einstein College of Medicine
St. Luke's-Roosevelt Hospital Center
New York, New York

Jacob Cynamon, M.D.
Professor of Clinical Radiology
Albert Einstein College of Medicine
Montefiore Medical Center
New York, New York

Seymour Sprayregen, M.D.
Professor
Department of Radiology
Albert Einstein College of Medicine
Montefiore Medical Center
New York, New York

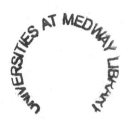

Thieme
New York • Stuttgart

Thieme Medical Publishers, Inc.
333 Seventh Ave.
New York, NY 10001

Editor: Kathleen P. Lyons
Editorial Assistant: Diane Sardini
Director, Production and Manufacturing: Anne Vinnicombe
Production Editor: Becky Dille
Marketing Director: Phyllis Gold
Sales Manager: Ross Lumpkin
Chief Financial Officer: Peter van Woerden
President: Brian D. Scanlan
Compositor: Northeastern Graphic Services, Inc.
Printer: Maple-Vail Book Manufacturing Group

Library of Congress Cataloging-in-Publication Data

Vascular and interventional radiology : principles and practices / Curtis W. Bakal ... [et al.].
    p.; cm.
  Includes bibliographical references and index.
  ISBN 0-86577-678-4 (alk. paper) – ISBN 3131079118 (alk. paper)
  1. Blood-vessels—Imaging. 2. Interventional radiology. I. Bakal, Curtis W.
  [DNLM: 1. Vascular Diseases—radiography. 2. Radiology, Interventional—methods.
WG 500 V33115 2002]
RC691.6.A53 V373 2002
616.1'30757—dc21
              2001058205

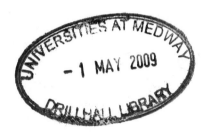
Printed in the United States of America
5 4 3 2 1
TMP ISBN 0-86577-678-4
GTV ISBN 3 13 107911 8

Contents

Contributors

Ramsey Abadir, M.D.
Horton Medical Center
Middletown, New York

Jacqueline Bello, M.D.
Director
Neuroradiololgy
and
Professor of Clinical Radiology
Albert Einstein College of Medicine
Montefiore Medical Center
New York, New York

Bruce Berkowitz, M.D.
Fort Collins Radiologic Associates
Fort Collins, Colorado

Steven E. Black, M.D.
Diagnostic Radiology Consultants
Chattanooga, Tennessee

Steven L. Dawson, M.D.
Head, GI Interventional Radiology
Department of Radiology
Massachusetts General Hospital
Boston, Massachusetts

Thomas J. DiBartholomeo, M.D.
Stamford Radiological Associates
Stamford, CT

Kevin W. Dickey, M.D.
Assistant Clinical Professor
Diagnostic Radiology
Yale University School of Medicine
and
Staff Interventional Radiologist
Hospital of St. Raphael
New Haven, Connecticut

Bernard G. Fish, M.D.
Associate Clinical Professor of Pediatric Cardiology
Section of Pediatric Cardiology
New York Medical College
Valhalla, New York

Andrei Frost, M.D.
Associate Professor of Clinical Radiology
Weiler Hospital
Albert Einstein College of Medicine
Montefiore Medical Center
New York, New York

Jeffrey D. Georgia, M.D.
Assistant Professor of Radiology
Uniformed Services University of Health Sciences
Department of Radiology
National Naval Medical Center
Bethesda, Maryland

Mark A. Greenberg, M.D.
Division of Cardiology
Montefiore Medical Center
New York, New York

Michael J. Hallisey, M.D.
Associate Professor of Medicine
University of Connecticut, Hartford Hospital
Connecticut Surgical Group
Hartford, Connecticut

Margaret E. Hansen, M.D.
CPO Radiology Associate
Dallas, Texas

Brad Hoppenfield, M.D.
Associated Radiologists of Singer Lake
Elmira Heights, New York

John A. Kaufman, M.D.
Professor
Dotter Interventional Institute
Oregon Health and Science University
Portland, Oregon

Andrew S. Kerr, M.D.
Department of Radiology
Metropolitan Hospital
New York, New York

Philip S. Lakritz, M.D.
Holmdel, New Jersey

Matthew A. Mauro, M.D.
Professor of Radiology and Surgery
Vice-Chairman, Department of Radiology
University of North Carolina School of Medicine
and
University of North Carolina Hospitals
Dept. of Radioloby
Chapel Hill, North Carolina

Steven G. Meranze, M.D.
Section Chief
Interventional Radiology
Vanderbilt University Medical Center
Nashville, Tennessee

Donald L. Miller, M.D.
Professor of Radiology
Uniformed Services
University of Health Sciences
National Naval Medical Center
Department of Radiology
Bethesda, Maryland

Timothy P. Murphy, M.D.
Associate Professor of Diagnostic Imaging
Rhode Island Hospital
and
Brown University School of Medicine
Providence, Rhode Island

Irene Osborn, M.D.
Department of Anesthesiology
Mount Sinai Hospital
New York, New York

Marlene Rackson, M.D.
Residency Program Director
Attending Radiologist
Beth Israel Medical Center
and
Assistant Professor of Radiology
Albert Einstein College of Medicine
Department of Radiology
New York, New York

Charles E. Ray, Jr., M.D.
Chief, Interventional Radiology
Denver Health Medical Center
and
Associate Professor of Radiology
University of Colorado Health Sciences Center
Denver, Colorado

Kenneth S. Rholl, M.D.
Chief, Interventional Radiology
INOVA Alexandria Hospital
Alexandria, Virginia
and
Associate Clinical Professor of Radiology
Department of Radiology
George Washington University

Anne C. Roberts, M.D.
Professor and Interim Chair
Department of Radiology
University of California at San Diego Medical Center/
Thomton Hospital
La Jolla, California

Melvin Rosenblatt, M.D.
New Rochelle, New York
and
Associate Professor
Yale University School of Medicine
Section of Vascular and Interventional Radiology
New Haven, Connecticut

Alla Rozenblit, M.D.
Associate Professor of Radiology
Department of Radiology
Albert Einstein College of Medicine
Montefiore Medical Center
New York, New York

Michael B. Rubin, M.D.
Department of Radiology
Sound Shore Medical Center
New Rochelle, New York
and
New Rochelle Radiology & MRI
New Rochelle, New York

J. Mark Ryan, M.D.
Duke University Medical Center
Department of Radiology
Durham, North Carolina

Alan H. Schoenfeld, M.S.
Department of Radiology
Montefiore Medical Center
New York, New York

Scott Segal, M.D.
Berkshire Medical Center
Pittsfield, MA

Randall W. Snyder III, M.D., M.A.
South Jersey Radiology Associates
Voorhees, New Jersey

Hugo Spindola-Franco, M.D.
Montefiore Medical Center
Albert Einstein College of Medicine
New York, New York

Keith M. Sterling, M.D.
Department of Radiology
Inova Alexandria Hospital
Alexandria, Virginia

Jonathan J. Trambert, M.D.
Clinical Director
Vascular and Interventional Radiology
Department of Radiology
Montefiore Medical Center
Weiler Hospital
and
Associate Professor of Radiology
Albert Einstein College of Medicine
Weiler Hospital
New York, New York

Samuel I. Wahl, M.D.
Irvington, New York

Arthur C. Waltman, M.D.
Director, Division of Vascular Radiology
Massachusetts General Hospital
Harvard Medical School
Boston, Massachusetts

Kenneth M. Zinn, M.D.
Radiology, Division of Interventional Radiology
Bridgeport Hospital/Advanced Radiology Consultants
Bridgeport, Connecticut

Foreword

Dr. Bakal has brought together contributors with a broad range of experience to create a text on a current spectrum of interventional procedures. As a discipline, we have had difficulty defining our interests and abilities. Some of the names offered include image-guided surgery, minimally-invasive medicine, and interventional radiology. All of them have strengths and weaknesses, confuse the public, and sometimes our professional colleagues. This text is the latest in an evolution, as with our discipline, from *Arteriography* edited by Herbert Abrams and *Interventional Radiology* edited by Christos Athanasoulis et al.

Through my 30 years in interventional radiology, I have had several startling experiences. One was the presentation of using arteriography to control bleeding from the gastrointestinal tract by Stanley Baum. It was this presentation that introduced me to the concept that a diagnostic method might also be the means to treat. Within a short span from the presentation patients who had been badly injured and were hemorrhaging to death from vascular injuries of the pelvis could be treated with embolization. Over the ensuing years, other momentous experiences and device improvements occurred expanding the usefulness of interventional radiology's practioners into many diseases and organ systems. Among these experiences are my being able to work with Andreas Gruntzig as he was developing balloon catheters for angioplasty of atherosclerotic lesions that eventually led to treatment for vessels from the head to the lower leg. Another was an opportunity to collaborate with Charles Dotter, who is the father of many of the current interventions from thrombolysis to TIPS and many catheters and devices.

Although there have been many other colleagues, too numerous to include here, with whom I have been associated and enjoyed their many contributions and personalities, I have really most appreciated those who trained in our department, including Dr. Bakal, and with whom I continue to maintain close friendships. Some of these colleagues are represented in this text and its wide scope is an example of the ingenuity and skill of the interventionalist. This text is an attempt to pull the many different therapies together in a format that allows one to gain the essence and approaches for these therapies without the overwhelming detail of history and materials.

This is text for where we are and, as I tell our students after introducing them to the Massachusetts General Hospital's Ether Dome and the images of medicine in the 19th century, that what we do now will also appear to be primitive in the future which is close. I look to a future where less invasive medicine is a better way to treat a patient than as Charles Dotter said "patients deserve to be treated better than a side of beef."

This text is the beginning and a first step.

Arthur C. Waltman, M.D.

Preface

This project grew out of a need for a book, covering the field of vascular and interventional radiology, that could be read in a month of evenings by radiology residents on a typical vascular and interventional radiology rotation. We wanted to give an overview of the field so that the reader could understand basic principles and approaches that were technical, clinical, and image-based. We did not want to be too encyclopedic, nor did we want to be only a list of differential diagnoses or a handbook. As this project moved forward, we realized that there are others who would benefit from a book of this nature: general radiologists, radiologic technologists, radiologic nurses, and VIR fellows early in their training.

To best achieve our goals, I felt that material covering generalized technical and imaging aspects should be grouped together at the beginning of the book, in Part I, allowing easy reference to the material. Part II would concentrate on the regional anatomy and the clinical and radiologic problems specific to that anatomy. Many of our chapters were written by our recent fellows or residents paired with a senior author. We asked each of them to write about the topic in a manner that would best help them at this stage of their career. No attempt was made to have all of the chapters conform to a single writing style or mode of organization. In a sense, the book is a collection of monographs covering virtually the entire spectrum of a growing and exciting field.

We hope that by reading this book, you will come to a better understanding of how diagnostic and interventional techniques can be applied to a broad spectrum of clinical problems.

Curt Bakal

Acknowledgments

We would like to thank the many colleagues in our departments who contributed ideas and advice.

Our assistants, Cynthia Caduhada, Cecilia Santos, and Eleanor Murphy, spent hours organizing, transcribing, and correcting text, references, and figure legends. At Thieme, Jane Pennington, Kathy Lyons, Diane Sardini, Anne Vinnicombe, and Becky Dille were crucial to seeing this project from start to publication.

To Pam and Matt, my points of light,
For their love and support.
Curtis W. Bakal

In memory of Mahboobeh Yashar.
James E. Silberzweig

To Aviva and Debora E. with love.
Jacob Cynamon

To Shoshana and Sharon with love.
Seymour Sprayregen

■ P A R T I ■

Basic Principles and Techniques

1

Vascular and Interventional Radiology
A Brief History

CURTIS W. BAKAL

Within months of Wilheim Roentgen's discovery of the x-ray in 1895, Lindenthal produced the first contrast-enhanced radiograph of the veins of the hand.[1,2] Clinical application of contrast angiography, however, would take more than two decades. From the 1920s through the 1950s, arteriography was performed infrequently—and by the translumbar approach. Vascular surgery was in its nascent stage, and diagnoses were made clinically without much diagnostic testing. For example, in 1923, Leriche described a group of young men with decreased or absent femoral pulses, bilateral claudication, and impotence, all on the basis of clinical findings and history. Leriche called this entity *aortitis terminalis* and suggested the possibility of surgical intervention.[3] Yet the diagnostic arteriogram as a routine clinical tool was years away.

In 1953, Seldinger described a transfemoral arterial access technique that used a puncture needle and guidewire, which allowed selective catheterization.[4] Coincidentally, the first use of a cloth vascular bypass graft also had just been reported.[5] During this decade, diagnostic arteriography of the cardiac and peripheral circulations was increasingly being used and refined. In the 1960s, radiologists began to develop "interventional" procedures. Many point to the landmark article that first described percutaneous transluminal angioplasty (PTA) by Dotter and Judkins as the birth of interventional radiology.[6,7] Dotter and Judkins summarized their article by suggesting that there would be "refinements of technique as well as further clarification" of the role of this attack on arteriosclerotic obstructions." The percutaneous transluminal treatment described in this article became a basis for an emerging class of minimally invasive therapies.

In 1974, the Society of Cardiovascular Radiology was founded with a membership of about 30 academic angiographers. In addition to diagnostic angiography, members of this society were beginning to expand their interventions: in addition to "Dottering" obstructive lesions, they were beginning to treat gastrointestinal bleeding and pelvic trauma by pharmacologic infusion or embolization.[8–13] Techniques for nonsurgical splenectomy and intravascular foreign body attraction soon were popularized.[14] The Society was later renamed the Society of Cardiovascular and Interventional Radiology.[15] Gruentzig and others refined the Dotter angioplasty technique by using an expandable balloon on a catheter shaft, which allowed smaller punctures to be made for arterial access and larger vessels to be dilated.[16,17] Real time ultrasound and computed tomography scanning allowed nonvascular percutaneous interventions to be developed and refined, notably intraabdominal abscess drainage.[18,19] This revolutionized the care of many patients with abdominal infections: Abdominal pus was no longer a surgical disease.

By 1985, small-vessel balloons and steerable guidewires became commercially available, allowing PTA of the infrapopliteal vessels.[20–23] Inferior vena cava filters, although still large in profile, were being placed by vascular and interventional radiologists as well as by surgical cut-down.[24] Within a few years, low osmolar contrast agents were to be commonly used for peripheral arteriography, increasing safety and patient comfort. Digital subtraction replaced cut film, and the multiplanar C-arm became standard in angiography and interventional radiology suites; these two technical advances allowed

diagnostic and interventional procedures to proceed more rapidly, eliminating the delays for processing cut films and for repositioning patients. The volume of studies that could be performed in a working day now could be expanded because the time per study was shortened; the interventional radiologists could expand their practices and push the envelope. The advent of smaller-profile catheters and hydrophilic guidewires allowed more expedient selection of smaller arteries for superselective embolization and infusion. The clinical use of thrombolytic agents began in the late 1980s for acute arterial and venous occlusions. Renal angioplasty became a first line technique.[25,26] The introduction of the vascular stent extended the range of lesions that could undergo successful angioplasty.[27,28]

By 1992, the Health Care Financing Administration developed a Medicare specialty designation for interventional radiology, and *interventional radiology* was defined in *Dorland's Illustrated Medical Dictionary* for the first time.[29] *The Journal of Vascular and Interventional Radiology*, born a few years earlier, was further defining the specialty.

By 1993, stent grafts made their appearance in the treatment of aneurysm disease and, to a lesser extent, occlusive disease. The transjugular intrahepatic portosystemic stent (TIPS), originally conceived in 1969, became a reality for treating the sequelae of portal hypertension.[30] By 1994, the subspecialty was recognized with accredited fellowships and a Certificate of Added Qualifications (CAQ) granted by the American Board of Radiology, officially recognizing its distinct status. Interventional radiologists had revolutionized the treatment of hemodialysis patients by using percutaneous, fluoroscopically guided techniques to enhance the longevity of hemodialysis catheters and arteriovenous fistulas and grafts.[31–33] Vascular and interventional radiologists were in the forefront of bringing peripheral vascular disease and abdominal aortic aneurysm screenings to their communities. Minimally invasive, nonsurgical treatment of symptomatic uterine fibroids by percutaneous embolization allowed the term *interventional radiologist* to escape from the medical community to the public's eye; by the year 2000, direct referral of patients to interventional radiologists by the Internet was becoming common.[33,34] New cutting-edge cancer treatments were being explored. Although magnetic resonance angiography and CTA had supplanted catheter-based diagnostic angiography in many areas of vascular diagnosis, the specialty grew substantially, predominantly becoming interventional in nature.

Membership in the SCVIR numbers more than 3,500. The Cardiovascular and Interventional Radiologic Society of Europe (CIRSE) in Zurich and the establishment of vascular interventional radiology societies in Central and Southern Asia and in South America confirms that interventional radiology is becoming a truly global subspecialty.

REFERENCES

1. Goodman PC. The new light: discovering and introduction; in a century of radiology. *Radiology*. Centennial American College of Radiology and Penn State College of Medicine Website. Available at: www.x-ray. hmc.psu.edu/rci/centennial.html. Accessed on October 16, 2000.

2. Trevert E. Something about x-rays for everybody: a review. In: Sprawls P, Petersen JE. *The X-Ray Century*, vol 2, no. 1. Lynn, MA: Bubier Publishing, 1896. Atlanta Emory University, Website. Available at: www.cc .emory.edu/X-RAYS/century.htm. Accessed on October 16, 2000.

3. Leriche R. Des oblitérations artérielles hautes (oblitération de la terminaison de l'aorte) comme cause des insuffisances circulatoires des membres inférieurs. *Bull Mem Soc Chir* 1923.

4. Seldinger S. Catheter replacement of the needle in percutaneous arteriography: a new technique. *Acta Radiol* 1953;139:368.

5. Vorhees AB Jr, Jaretzki A, Blakemore AH. The use of tubes construted from vinyon "N" cloth in bridging arterial defects: a preliminary report. *Ann Surg* 1952;135:332.

6. Dotter CT, Judkins MP. Transluminal treatment of arteriosclerotic obstruction: description of a new technique and a preliminary report of its application. *Circulation* 1964;30:654–670.

7. *SCVIR News.* 1997;10:10–12.

8. Baum S, Nusbaum M, Tumen HJ. Gastrointestinal bleeding. *Lancet* 1970;1:106–107.

9. Rosch J, Dotter CT, Brown MJ. Selective arterial embolization: a new method for control of acute gastrointestinal bleeding. *Radiology* 1972;102:303–306.

10. Baum S, Rosch J, Dotter CT, et al. Selective mesenteric arterial infusions in the management of massive diverticular hemorrhage. *N Engl J Med* 1973;288:1269–1272.

11. Ring EJ, Athanasoulis C, Waltman AC, Margolies MN, Baum S. Arteriographic management of hemorrhage following pelvic fracture. *Radiology* 1973;109:65–70.

12. Athanasoulis CA, Baum S, Waltman AC, Ring EJ, Imbembo A, Vander Salm TJ. Control of acute gastric mucosal hemorrhage: intra-arterial infusion of posterior pituitary extract. *N Engl J Med* 1974;290:597–603.

13. Waltman AC, Jang GC, Athanasoulis CA, Ring EJ, Baum S. Emergency gastrointestinal angiography. *Geriatrics* 1974;29:48–52.

14. Dotter CT, Rosch J, Bilbao MK. Transluminal extraction of catheter and guide fragments from the heart and great vessels: 29 collected cases *Am J Roentgenol* 1971;111:467–472.

15. *SCVIR News* 1997;10:10.

16. Gruentzig A, Hopff H. Perkutane Rekanalisation chronischer arterieller Veschulusse mit einem nuen Dilatationskatheter. *Dtsch Med Wochenschr* 1974;99:2502.

17. Wierny L, Plass R, Porstmann W. Long-term results in 100 consecutive patients treated by transluminal angioplasty. *Radiology* 1974; 112:543–548.

18. Gerzof SG, Robbins AH, Johnson WC, Birkett DH, Nabseth DC. Percutaneous catheter drainage of abdominal abscesses: a five-year experience. *N Engl J Med* 1981;305:653–657.

19. vanSonnenberg E, Ferrucci JT Jr, Mueller PR, Wittenberg J, Simeone JF. Percutaneous drainage of abscesses and fluid collections: technique, results, and applications. *Radiology* 1982; 142:1–10.

20. Schwarten DE, Cutcliff WB. Arterial occlusive disease below the knee: treatment with percutaneous transluminal angioplasty performed with low-profile catheters and steerable guide wires. *Radiology* 1988;169:71–74.

21. Brown KT, Schoenberg NY, Moore ED, Saddekni S. Percutaneous transluminal angioplasty of infrapopliteal vessels: preliminary results and technical considerations. *Radiology* 1988;169:75–78.

22. Casarella WJ. Percutaneous transluminal angioplasty below the

knee: new techniques, excellent results. *Radiology* 1988;169:271–272.

23. Bakal CW, Sprayregen S, Scheinbaum K, Cynamon J, Veith FJ. Percutaneous transluminal angioplasty of the infrapopliteal arteries: results in 53 patients. *AJR Am J Roentgenol* 1990;154:171–174.

24. Denny DF Jr, Dorfman GS, Cronan JJ, Greenwood LH, Morse SS, Yoselovitz M. Greenfield filter: percutaneous placement in 50 patients. *AJR Am J Roentgenol* 1988:150:427–429.

25. Tegtmeyer CJ, Sos TA. Techniques of renal angioplasty. *Radiology* 1986;161:577–586.

26. Martin LG, Casarella WJ, Gaylord GM. Azotemia caused by renal artery stenosis: treatment by percutaneous angioplasty. *AJR Am J Roentgenol* 1988;150:839–844.

27. Dotter CT, Buschmann RW, McKinney MK, Rosch J. Transluminal expandable nitinol coil stent grafting: preliminary report. *Radiology* 1983;147:259–260.

28. Palmaz JC, Laborde JC, Rivera FJ, Encarnacion CE, Lutz JD, Moss JG. Stenting of the iliac arteries with the Palmaz stent: experience from a multicenter trial. *Cardiovasc Intervent Radiol* 1992;15:291–297.

29. *SCVIR News.* 1998;11:11.

30. Rosch J, Hanafee W, Snow H, Barenfus M, Gray R. Transjugular intrahepatic portacaval shunt: an experimental work. *Am J Surg* 1971;121:588–592.

31. Mauro MA, Jacques PF. Radiologic placement of long term central venous catheters: a review. *J Vasc Interv Radiol* 1993;4:127–137.

32. Valji K, Bookstein JJ, Roberts AC, Ogleview SB, Pittman C, O'Neill MD. Pulse-spray pharmacomechanical thrombolysis of thrombosed hemodialysis access grafts: long term experience and comparison of original and current techniques. *AJR Am J Roentgenol* 1995;164:1495–1503.

33. Aruny JE, Lewis CA, Cardella JF, et al. Quality improvement guidelines for percutaneous management of the thrombosed or dysfunctional dialysis access: Standards of Practice Committee of the SCVIR. *J Vasc Interv Radiol* 1999;10:491–498.

34. Goodwin SC, Vedantham S, McLucas B, Forno AE, Perrella R. Preliminary experience with uterine artery embolization for uterine fibroids. *J Vasc Interv Radiol* 1997;8:517–526.

35. Spies JB, Warren EH, Mathias SD, Walsh SM, Roth AR, Pentecost MJ. Uterine fibroid embolization: measurement of health-related quality of life and after therapy. *J Vasc Interv Radiol* 1999;10(10):129–303.

2

Catheters and Guidewires

A. RAMSEY ABADIR AND JAMES E. SILBERZWEIG

■ Catheterization Techniques

Interventional radiology uses imaging technology to perform diagnostic and therapeutic procedures at target organs distant from a percutaneous access site. Virtually all interventional radiology techniques rely on a combination of needle, catheter, and guidewire systems. The basic principles of interventional radiology are remarkably similar across procedure types and organ systems. This chapter addresses the basic instrumentation and techniques used for percutaneous access, using arteriography as the prototype. Later chapters illustrate how the process can be adapted to manage a wide range of clinical situations.

The initial method used in diagnostic angiography was direct needle puncture with contrast injection into the arterial system. In 1953, Seldinger first described the combined use of a needle, guidewire, and catheter to access the arterial system for selective catheter angiography safely and without surgical exposure.[1] The Seldinger technique for catheter access consists of initial needle insertion into a blood vessel. Then a guidewire is placed through the needle and passed into the blood vessel lumen. The needle is "exchanged," leaving the guidewire in place, and finally a catheter is guided over the guidewire to the desired location. Initially, rubber urinary catheters were used; however, the emergence of plastics enabled the production of small-diameter, complex-shaped catheters. Seldinger's technique has remained relatively unchanged since its initial description for vascular access and has been adapted as a method to provide percutaneous access to nearly every organ system. The venous system, biliary tree, renal collecting system, peritoneal space, pleural space, and abscess cavities can be accessed using the Seldinger technique.

Vascular access

The basic steps for arterial access using the Seldinger technique are as follows: The skin is sterilized with a bactericidal solution, and the patient is draped to allow clean access to the puncture site. Bony landmarks and the abdomen are checked by use of fluoroscopy to ensure that the planned needle puncture is infrainguinal for femoral access and that there is no bowel contrast present that may potentially obscure the region to be examined. Local anesthetic is infiltrated, and a small dermatotomy is made with a no. 11 scalpel. The artery is palpated both proximally and distally to the puncture site, lining up the fingers along the vessel, and the needle is placed parallel to the artery and at an approximately 60-degree angle to the skin. The tip of the needle is place within the vessel using either a single- or double-wall technique (to be described later), at which point, strongly pulsatile blood return should be observed. If the observed blood return is weak, the needle might be only partially within the blood vessel, directed toward the side wall or a plaque, partially occluded with thrombus, within a vein, or within a branch arterial vessel; the needle must be repositioned or removed.

The needle is tipped downward to become more parallel to the vessel, and a guidewire then is placed through the needle into the lumen, thus securing access. The guidewire should pass easily into the vessel. Fluoroscopy is used to confirm guidewire position. If the guidewire

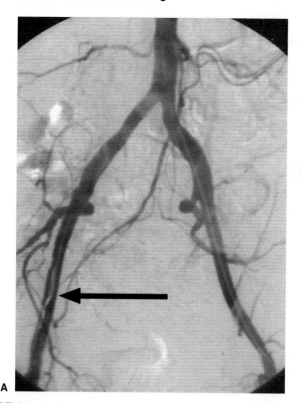
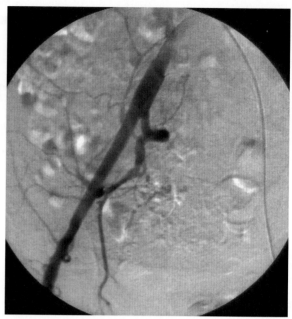

FIGURE 2-1. A: Iliac arteriogram from a left common femoral artery approach demonstrates an intimal dissection (*arrow*) caused by a previous right transfemoral catheterization. **B**: The dissection was "tacked down" by insertion of a Wallstent.

cannot pass easily, one of several circumstances may be occurring. The needle may be partially embedded in the vessel wall, the needle tip may be pointing at the side wall of the vessel, a branch vessel has been punctured, the vessel is extremely tortuous, or an atherosclerotic plaque or occlusion may be present. If the needle is partially buried, subintimal passage of the wire can occur, raising an intimal flap, which may be flow limiting or even occlusive (Fig. 2-1). If any resistance to wire passage is encountered, the wire should be removed. If pulsatile flow is still present, another attempt to pass the guidewire may be made, adjusting the needle to facilitate passage. A contrast injection may help to clarify the position of the needle tip. If these maneuvers are unsuccessful, the needle should be withdrawn and compression maintained at the access site for 5 to 10 minutes to avoid hematoma formation.

The needle is removed over the guidewire while manual pressure is maintained over the puncture site to prevent bleeding and hematoma formation. Clots that may have formed on the guidewire resulting from the needle removal should be wiped off using nonfriable gauze such as Telfa (Kendall Healthcare, Mansfield, MA, U.S.A.). A catheter now can be passed easily over the guidewire into the vessel, with tension being maintained on the guidewire to prevent catheter or guidewire kinking. The tapered catheter tip must closely approximate the size of

the guidewire so that the catheter tip does not catch on the vessel wall or kink the guidewire. The catheter can be advanced to the desired location, using the wire as a guide. The guidewire can be removed so that saline flush and contrast may be injected through the catheter. When the catheter is within the vessel and the guidewire is removed, heparinized saline must be flushed through the lumen approximately every 2 to 3 minutes to prevent formation of a clot within the catheter. Catheter flushing consists of aspiration of 3 to 5 mL of blood with a heparinized saline-filled 20-mL syringe, followed by injection of 5 to 10 mL of saline. The syringe tip is angled 45 degrees downward to allow the blood to settle in the dependent portion of the syringe and to prevent the introduction of air bubbles or reintroduction of blood. Double flushing, commonly used during cerebral angiography, consists of the aspiration of blood from one syringe followed by a heparinized saline flush using a second syringe.

Venous puncture is made in much the same way; however, there are slight differences. Single-wall and double-wall techniques may be used; however, suction must be applied because venous pressure is usually insufficient to drive blood through the needle.

Following completion of the procedure, the pulses distal to the catheter insertion site must be assessed before and after removal of the catheter. Occult emboli or pericatheter thrombosis may have occurred, necessitating thrombolysis. The catheter and guidewire need to be removed from the patient, ensuring minimal vessel trauma and little bleeding or hematoma formation.

Compression is maintained focally at the arterial puncture site, not the skin entry site, for 10 to 15 minutes in patients with a normal coagulation status. Coagulopathic patients, whether pathologic or iatrogenic, will require longer compression, as will sites that have had large catheters placed. The pulse should not be eliminated during manual compression, but no oozing should be observed. If no pulse is felt, the vessel may be occluded by overzealous compression or by compression that is not being applied over the artery. Devices (e.g., Femostop) have been designed that mechanically maintain compression once it is set up in the appropriate position. Percutaneous access closure devices have been developed recently and include collagen plugs deposited along the subcutaneous catheter tract and direct suture of the artery at the access site to aid in the suppression of bleeding.[2] Closure devices may be useful in anticoagulated patients or following removal of large-diameter catheters.

Access needles

Access needle diameter should be less than the catheter to be used; otherwise, the hole in the artery will be too large and blood will leak around the catheter. A 19-gauge needle is roughly the same size as a 4F catheter (19 gauge = 1/19 inch). The walls are made of thin steel to allow passage of guidewires of sufficient size. The proximal end is called the *hub* and has handles or a flange for better control. The tip of the needle may be blunt, with a sharp inner stylet, or it may be sharply beveled, with no inner stylet.

The method of access dictates the design of the needle. Seldinger's original double-wall technique uses a needle with a blunt hollow cannula into which a sharp, solid stylet is placed. Initially, the needle is placed through both walls of the vessel, and the stylet is removed. The blunt cannula tip is pulled back slowly until it enters the lumen and pulsatile blood return is seen. A wire then can be passed into the vessel (Fig. 2-2).

The one-wall technique employs a sharp, hollow, beveled needle with no inner stylet. The needle is inserted slowly until pulsatile blood return is seen (indicating an intraluminal position), and then the wire is passed through the needle. Only the more superficial wall of the vessel is crossed.

The choice of technique is primarily one of operator preference, but there are several technical considerations. The needle puncture in the far wall with the two-wall method might create a potential problem with bleeding, although this does not typically occur. The stylet punctures the wall, spreading the fibers rather than slic-

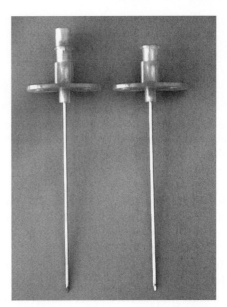

FIGURE 2-2. Access needles. Seldinger needle (*left*). One-wall needle (*right*).

ing them as with the single-wall needle. When the needle is removed, the elastic arterial wall tends to seal the defect. If thrombolysis is to be performed or the patient is coagulopathic, however, the one-wall approach may be preferred. Double-wall punctures in patients with aorto-bifemoral grafts (which usually are placed anterior to the native vessels) may enter the deep native vessel first on withdrawal of the needle, with good blood return seen.[3] The guidewire, however, will not pass through the diseased native arterial segment. A single-wall puncture is more likely to enter the graft first, enabling access to more proximal vessels. Similarly, when placing an inferior vena cava filter, the occasional femoral artery, which is immediately anterior to the vein, especially with low punctures, will be noted on the way in (by the presence of pulsatile return) before the vessel is accidentally dilated to the size needed to accommodate the filter. Single-wall needles are, by necessity, cutting needles, and they are helpful in scarred, postoperative groins. Even with a one-wall puncture, however, the pressure needed to enter the lumen may cause the vessel to collapse, with the net result of blood return being seen only after puncturing both walls and withdrawing the needle anyway.

The single-wall needle also is associated with several pitfalls. Because the needle is hollow, it may become occluded with tissue. Flushing is therefore recommended between passes. A more potentially serious problem is a result of the steep bevel that must be made to enable the needle to cut the arterial wall. A portion of the needle tip still may be within the vessel wall while the remainder of the needle tip is within the vessel lumen. Pulsatile blood return will be observed, but a wire passed with the needle in this position can be directed subintimally, thus causing

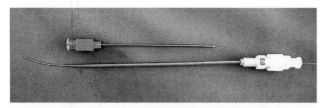

FIGURE 2-3. Micropuncture access set. Micropuncture needle, 21-gauge (*top*) coaxial dilators over an 0.018-inch guidewire (*bottom*).

a dissection of the vessel wall. When blood flow is seen, the needle should be repositioned (slightly withdrawn, rotated, or occasionally advanced) a millimeter or two to place the entire bevel within the lumen.

Specialty needles exist for various uses. Translumbar aortography is performed by using a long, hollow 18- or 19-gauge needle with a Teflon outer sheath. Biliary access is made with long, fine (21- or 22-gauge) needles. A Micropuncture access set (Cook, Bloomington, IN, U.S.A.) is available with a 21-gauge needle and a 0.018-inch guidewire (Fig. 2-3). The use of a small needle minimizes the risk of bleeding in the event multiple passes are required to obtain vascular access. The needle and guidewire are coupled with 4Fr or 5Fr coaxial dilators that allow the operator to place a standard 0.035-inch or 0.038-inch guidewire needed to pass a standard sized catheter into the lumen.

Sheaths and dilators

If large-diameter catheters are to be used, or if there is dense scar tissue or a tough synthetic graft is to be crossed, the use of graduated Teflon dilators may facilitate catheter passage. Dilators are short, stiff, thick-walled sections of catheter, available in a variety of sizes, with a long, tapered end that spread tissues more easily than a diagnostic catheter. Advancing a catheter over a stiffer wire also may facilitate passage of the catheter into the vessel and prevent guidewire kinking.

Vascular sheaths are used during cases that require multiple catheter manipulations and catheter exchanges. Sheaths should be used during complex manipulations, such as embolization; if the catheter tip becomes occluded, precluding passage of a guidewire, the catheter still can be removed via the sheath without losing vascular access. The use of a sheath decreases the friction on the catheter at the puncture site, allowing better transmission of the forces applied, and protects the groin and vessel from excessive trauma. Sheaths are also useful in patients with groin scarring from previous surgery, vascular bypass grafts, and obese patients.

Sheaths are constructed from short segments of thin-walled catheter material, often Teflon, and are sized according to the largest catheter they will accommodate.

For example a 5Fr sheath will accommodate a 5Fr catheter but is actually approximately 6.2 in outer diameter. They are placed into the vessel at the puncture site and left for the duration of the case, usually, so that all wires and catheters pass through them. A hemostasis valve is attached on the trailing end so that catheters and guidewires can be exchanged with minimal blood loss. A flushing sideport is provided and should be connected to a pressurized continuous saline flush whenever a nonocclusive catheter, guidewire, or nothing at all will be in the sheath for more than several minutes, as a large volume of clot may form in the lumen.

Insertion of a sheath is performed with a dilator in its lumen. If difficulty is encountered, a fluoroscopic check should be made to ensure the stiff dilator is following the wire into the vessel. The sheath should also be inspected to ensure that the thin leading edge has not become crimped by attempted insertions.

Vascular access sites

Femoral artery access

The femoral approach is generally favored for vascular work. The large caliber of the femoral vessels allows placement of relatively large-diameter catheters with a low risk of vessel thrombosis. The patient is placed in a supine position throughout the course of the examination. When properly performed, the puncture site can be effectively compressed against the femoral head following completion of the case.

In arteriography, the goal is to puncture the femoral artery below the inguinal ligament (which is attached superiorly to the anterior superior iliac spine and inferiorly to the pubic tubercle) but above the origin of the profunda femoral artery. Too low a puncture may increase the risk of pseudoaneurysm and arteriovenous fistula formation.[4,5] Puncture superior to the inguinal ligament exposes the patient to an increased risk of retroperitoneal hemorrhage.[6]

The inguinal crease is not always the appropriate location for a femoral puncture.[7] Especially in obese patients, the inguinal crease may be located far inferior to the actual inguinal ligament. Fluoroscopy of the femoral head should determine the puncture site; however, the actual inguinal ligament may bow as much as 3-cm inferior to the radiographically determined inguinal ligament.[8] The ligament is usually located 1.5-cm cephalad to the femoral head. In addition, the mid-femoral head is virtually always proximal to the bifurcation of the profunda femoral and superficial femoral arteries.[9] For retrograde punctures, the skin incision is therefore optimally placed over the lower margin of the femoral head, with the goal of entering the artery over the medial mid-femoral head. Antegrade arterial punctures should aim similarly but from the opposite direction. If the femoral vein is encountered, the needle should be withdrawn slowly because occasionally the artery overlies the vein. If the artery has not been crossed, withdrawing the needle nearly to its tip and redirecting the tip approximately one centimeter laterally usually will place the needle within the artery.

Pulseless femoral arteries may indicate aortoiliac occlusion and sometimes may preclude catheterization; however, a pulse might not be encountered in cases of severe aortoiliac artery stenosis, marked obesity, and hypotension. Techniques used to locate pulseless vessels include radiographic or anatomic landmarks, fluoroscopic visualization of mural calcifications, sonographic localization,[10] or contralateral puncture with wire placement in the desired vessel for localization.[11]

Upper-extremity access

When femoral access cannot be established secondary to occlusion of the femoral artery, iliac artery or aorta, or when it is technically advantageous to approach a vessel from above, an axillary or brachial puncture may be made. These sites are not routinely used because they are subject to an increased complication rate. One of the conditions often cited as a reason for an axillary puncture is the presence of femoral grafts. Studies comparing femoral graft puncture with axillary puncture, however, revealed a greater than fivefold increase in major complications with axillary access.[12] Prudence dictates that recently placed grafts, within 6 weeks or so, should be left undisturbed to avoid graft infection thorough fresh wounds.

The axillary artery puncture has a higher complication rate because of the local anatomy, which may result in both central and peripheral nervous system defects as well as local vascular lesions. It is more difficult to compress the axillary artery against the humeral head than it is to compress the femoral artery against the femoral head. The brachial plexus is immediately adjacent to the artery and is constrained by fascia. Direct injury to the brachial plexus may occur with direct needle puncture or with compression by hematoma formation. Damage to the femoral nerve during femoral artery puncture also can occur but happens with about one tenth the frequency.[13] The axillary artery is smaller than the femoral artery and is thus more susceptible to thrombosis after catheterization.

The brachial artery caliber is even smaller, and the increased risk of thrombosis dictates that it be approached with caution. The brachial artery has a poor collateral circulation, and brachial artery thrombosis puts the distal upper extremity at risk. The median nerve courses with the brachial artery, making it susceptible to injury. Major complications can be encountered in up to 2.9% of brachial artery catheterizations.[14]

If an axillary or brachial puncture is unavoidable, the techniques used are the same as for the femoral artery. No strict radiologic landmarks are used, and careful palpation is important. For axillary punctures, the arm is abducted 90 degrees or with the hand tucked under the patient's head to provide access and stretch the artery. The puncture is made in the lateral axillary fold as the artery crosses the humeral head here. High axillary punctures are to be avoided because compression is extremely difficult without the buttressing effect of the humerus. The brachial artery is punctured over the mid-humerus in the bicipital groove or at the antecupital fossa.

The left arm is chosen preferentially. A catheter placed through the right arm must cross all four of the cerebral vessel origins to reach the descending aorta, whereas only the left vertebral artery is encountered if the left arm is used. In elderly patients who have ectatic, atherosclerotic aortas, catheters and guidewires may preferentially enter the ascending aorta and cause unintentional left-sided heart catheterization. Although cardiac angiography is interesting, it is best done in a purposeful manner.

Translumbar access

One of the original access techniques used, although not often used currently, is translumbar aortography. The technique is used in cases where femoral and axillary access is unsuitable. The patient is positioned prone, and a long 18-gauge sheathed needle is advanced directly into the aorta from a left flank approach. The needle is withdrawn, leaving the sheath in place. After the procedure, the sheath is withdrawn, and the patient placed on his or her back with gauze underneath to tamponade external bleeding. Obviously, no compression can be applied to the site in this location; therefore, bleeding can be potentially disastrous. The hemorrhage is typically retroperitoneal, often resulting in a hematocrit drop of about 3%,[15] but it can progress and remain unrecognized until the patient becomes hemodynamically unstable.[16] The presence of coagulopathy is an absolute contraindication to translumbar aortography. Other potential complications include puncture of an abdominal aortic aneurysm; injury to the renal, splanchnic, or lumbar arteries; and even pneumothorax.

Both high and low translumbar punctures have been described, differing as to whether the aorta is entered below or above the renal and mesenteric vessels. Many institutions, if they perform translumbar aortography at all, use only the high approach to reduce the inadvertent puncture of an occluded or aneurysmal aorta. Preprocedural computed tomography or ultrasound can be helpful in this regard.

Some angiographers maintain that the risk of unrecognized hemorrhage precludes the exchange of catheters, excluding the performance of selective studies, or repositioning of the catheter once it has been placed. Several investigators, however, have used exchange and other techniques to achieve multiple studies from the translumbar approach.[15,17]

■ Guidewires

A guidewire appears deceptively simple. In fact, guidewires are highly specialized medical equipment whose properties interact with that of the catheter to produce a safe and accurate method of catheter placement. The basic characteristics of a guidewire include length, diameter, tip shape, core stiffness, taper, and coating.

Standard guidewires are 145 cm long, which allows easy insertion of catheters up to 100 cm long. Exchange guidewires are typically 260 cm long. The long length allows for removal of a catheter in its entirety from the body without dislodging the wire tip, which may be in a selective position. A new catheter can be placed then into exactly the same position as the prior catheter.

Except for several highly specialized guidewires, construction of most types of guidewires is similar. A tightly coiled stainless steel wire provides the body of the guidewire. The outer diameter of the coil is the width of the guidewire and usually is expressed in inches (0.018-inch, 0.035-inch, 0.038-inch). The standard diameter for guidewires used in diagnostic arteriography is 0.035 inches. Located centrally within the wire is a fine safety wire that is soldered to both the proximal and distal ends of the spring.[18] The safety wire helps prevent uncoiling of the spring if too much tensile force is applied.

A second thicker, stiffer wire, the *mandril core,* also is located within the central canal. The mandril is the prime determinant of a guidewire's overall stiffness. Guidewires range from soft to "coat hanger" stiffness. Almost all guidewires lead with a distance of nonstiffened spring to avoid trauma to the vessel walls. However, nearly all guidewires are stiff as they exit the tip of a catheter or a needle. The guidewire tip potentially can cause blood vessel wall injury if it is passed too forcefully.

The mandril core is tapered to allow a graduated transition from the stiff to the floppy sections of the wire. Both the length of the taper, usually expressed in 5-cm increments (normal, long taper, long-length taper), and the lengths of floppy wire are varied to produce wires with different characteristics. Long floppy segments are useful for gaining purchase in small tortuous vessels, whereas stiffer wires allow more controlled catheter manipulation. Movable core wires and variable stiffness wires have been manufactured to attempt to allow a single wire to have a variety of characteristics, but these models have limitations. A variant of the movable core wire is the steerable or tip-deflecting guidewire. The movable core is

fastened so that, when it is extended through the spring, the tip of the guidewire is displaced laterally. An example of how this may be used is to displace the tip of a catheter through the tricuspid and pulmonic valves in pulmonary angiography.

The leading tip can be straight, curved in a "J" configuration or angled. The J tip is often used because it is less traumatic, leading with a smooth curve rather than a straight tip, which can catch on atheromatous plaques and vessel origins. The curve is described by its radius, usually ranging from 1.5 mm to 15 mm, and chosen to match the size of the vessel. Large-diameter J-tipped wires also can be used to keep the wire tip out of branches with a smaller diameter than the J-shaped tip.

Most standard guidewires are coated with Teflon to allow easy travel of the catheter over them. Heparin-based coatings also have been used to reduce wire thrombogenicity. More recently, hydrophilic polymer coatings have been developed that, when wet, have an extremely low coefficient of friction. A hydrophilic-coated wire can be passed into small, tortuous vessels more easily and often is used to cross vessel occlusions. Hydrophilic-coated wires are available with straight and angled tips for selective catheterization.

Steerable guidewires are also available that can be used in combination with microcatheters for selective catheterization of small and tortuous branch vessels. The angiographer can angle the tips of these guidewires to facilitate selective catheterization. These guidewires are generally 0.014 inches to 0.018 inches in diameter.

The choice of guidewire is determined by several factors (Table 2-1). The catheter or needle to be used with the wire must have an end hole that will accommodate the guidewire diameter. It is unfortunate to have labored to place a wire in a difficult vessel and then realize that the catheter you need to use will not pass over that wire. The appropriate wire stiffness and taper must be selected. A floppy wire may be ideal to maneuver into the distal hepatic artery, but it might become hopelessly coiled in a tortuous, atherosclerotic iliac artery long before it gets there. Wires with insufficient stiffness also may not support passage of a catheter into a vessel, even though they are far out in the vessel. Conversely, a stiff wire passed through the tip of a shaped catheter just in a vessel origin is likely to deform the tip and flip it out of the vessel of interest. A wire with a long taper, however, can allow sufficient purchase to be obtained by the long floppy segment so that the stiff portion will follow. Obviously, this is where experience helps.

■ Catheters

Whether to deliver contrast, inflate a balloon, or pass a wire-based tool, such as a snare, the catheter is the con-

TABLE 2-1. Common Guidewires

Wire	Core Stiffness	Coatings	Tip	Features
Newton	Medium	Teflon	J 3–15-mm	All-purpose wire for navigating large to medium vessels, abscess cavities, etc. J tip is atraumatic and lumen seeking. Will not traverse small or tortuous vessels. Typically 0.035-in. to 0.038-in. diameter
Rosen	Stiff	Teflon	J 1.5 mm (short taper)	Useful for visceral artery exchanges where extra support needed, e.g., obese patients, tortuous vessels, stiff catheters. Typically, 175 cm to 180 cm long, 0.035-in. to 0.038-in. diameter
Bentson	Medium	Teflon	Straight with floppy tip	Very floppy, long straight tip good for crossing small, tortuous vessels or stenoses. Unless stiffer portion of wire placed into vessel of interest, may not be able to place catheter tip into selective position. 0.035-in. to 0.038-in. diameter
Amplatz	Very stiff	Teflon	Straight with relatively soft tip	May be used cautiously to guide large, stiff catheters such as angioplasty balloons, stents, or IVC filters, and for catheter exchanges. 0.035-in. to 0.038 in. diameter
Glidewire	Soft to stiff	Hydrophilic (extremely low coefficient of friction when wet)	Straight or angled	Extremely slippery wire used to pass occlusions, extremely small or tortuous vessels, or stenoses. Will easily dissect through vessel or other wall, so use with caution. 0.014-in. to 0.038-in. diameter
"Steerable"	Soft to stiff	Teflon, hydrophilic	Shapeable	Used with low-profile "tibial" balloons or coaxial catheters. 0.010-in. to 0.018-in. diameter, made of steel, platinum, or nitinol

VC, inferior vena cava

duit that allows the interventionalist to access a structure deep within the body (Table 2-2). Catheters are thus the most varied of the structures covered in this chapter because they have been adapted to perform a myriad of tasks, ranging from portosystemic shunts to draining abscesses. Highly specialized catheters are discussed in subsequent chapters.

In the not so distant past, a catheter was custom made for each patient. Creating a catheter consisted of selecting a roll of plastic tubing, cutting it to length, flaring one end to accept an injection hub, tapering the other end to fit the guidewire, and finally steaming various curves into the tip to access specific parts of the body.[19] Today preformed catheters are uniform in construction and available in almost any configuration. Catheters are constructed from a variety of materials, including polyethylene, nylon, Teflon, and polyurethane, with some radioopaque material incorporated in the wall. Polyethylene is easy to shape and is commonly used. Teflon is slippery and can be used for passing through scar or graft material. Nylon has good

TABLE 2-2. Common Catheters

Catheter	Types Available	Features
Straight	End hole, flush 3F to 7F	Basic catheter used to study vessel punctured or vessels with straight takeoffs
Pigtail	Flush, 3F to 8F	Large internal diameter, high flow capacity
Angled (Berenstein, Kumpe)	End hole, 3F to 7F	
Cobra family	End hole, side holes 3F to 7F	Visceral catheter: C1 for young patients with narrow aortas, C2 for patients over 50 yr of age
Headhunter family	End hole 3F to 7F	Designed for selective cervicocerebral artery catheterizations
Simmons (sidewinder), Sos Selective, Mikaelsson	End hole	Requires reformation in the aortic arch or aortic bifurcation
Neff, Omni Flush	4F, 5F	Simmons-pigtail hybrid: useful for crossing aortic bifurcation. Neff has side holes on leading curve for ease of injecting contralateral iliac artery. Omni Flush has sideholes on shaft

stiffness and torque-control characteristics. Some catheters incorporate a fine wire mesh (*braid*) in the wall to increase torque transmission to the tip.

Catheters are characterized by material, shape, outer diameter measured in French (1 mm = 3F), presence and number of side holes, length, maximal wire diameter accepted, and pressure rating. The most commonly used diagnostic catheters are 4Fr and 5Fr. The size influences the properties of the catheter, such as handling, maximal flow rate, and size of the hole made in the artery. Diagnostic catheters (3Fr) and coaxial microcatheters (2Fr to 3Fr), designed to fit into standard sized angiographic catheters or larger-diameter "guiding catheters," are used to access tortuous distal vessel branches or minimize access puncture size.[20,21]

The catheter is commonly divided into three parts: hub, shaft, and tip. The *hub* is on the trailing end and is where syringes and injectors can be attached and wires passed. The shaft provides length to the catheter to enable it to reach the target vessel. Catheter lengths are typically 65 cm for abdominal and pelvic arteriography and 90 to 100 cm for thoracic and carotid arteriography. The most common site for a catheter to fail during a power injection is at the junction of the hub and shaft because intraluminal pressure is highest there. Fortunately, this is external to the patient. The tip of the catheter is tapered to fit the guidewire and facilitate atraumatic percutaneous insertion.

Shape

Perhaps the most defining element of a catheter is its shape, as determined by the curves at its distal aspect. Some basic, all-purpose shapes are used in almost every case. Conversely, many catheters have been designed specifically to work for individual vessels.

High-volume, high-flow-rate studies in large vessels are best performed with pigtail catheters. The leading end of such a catheter is looped in a circle, and there are side holes on the distal straight shaft to evenly disperse contrast during injection. The pigtail shape resists catheter recoil, causing vessel injury, during high-flow contrast injection. (Pigtail shapes also are often used for drainage catheters because the distal circle helps prevent migration of the catheter. The side holes in drainage catheters are larger and are in the inner aspect of the pigtail curve to maintain patency as the drained space surrounding the catheter collapses. Additionally, during catheter exchange over a guidewire, the guidewire is less likely to exit a side hole located on the inner curvature of the loop.)

To catheterize a vessel selectively, the tip must be curved or angled in such a way as to engage the origin of the vessel of interest. Such catheters can be simple or complex, depending on the number of curves they contain. The primary curve is the curve closest to the catheter tip. Additional curves beyond the primary curve (secondary, tertiary) help to force the catheter tip deeper into the selected vessel once its origin has been engaged by contacting the opposite aortic wall. Additional curves also may help to stabilize the catheter against the aortic wall during contrast injection.

Simple shapes have only one or two curves, such as the hockeystick-shaped catheter (e.g., Berenstein, Kumpe). Some arteries, such as the celiac axis or internal iliac artery, have steeply angled origins and may be difficult to catheterize. Two solutions to this situation are to approach these arteries superiorly (from an axillary or brachial artery puncture) or to use a catheter that has a downward pointing tip. A downward pointing catheter tip from a femoral approach can be achieved by either inverting the curve of a traditional catheter on itself (e.g., making a Waltman loop from a braided cobra catheter) or by using a subset of complex catheters known as *recurvant catheters*. A Waltman loop can be created by catheterizing a branch vessel of the aorta, such as the renal artery. A guidewire then is positioned within the catheter so that the guidewire tip is at the origin of the branch vessel. Advancing the catheter and guidewire as a unit will form a loop in the aorta, drawing the tip out of the branch vessel. The tip is now directed inferiorly, ready for placement in a steeply angled vessel.[22]

Recurvant catheters have a trailing curve that turns the catheter 180 degrees back on itself, and the leading curve (*primary*) serves to engage the orifice of the vessel. Examples of these are the Simmons and Sos-Selective catheters (Fig. 2-4). The trailing curve must be reformed in a large vessel, such as the thoracic aorta or aortic bifurcation. Although a recurvant catheter may be used for abdomi-

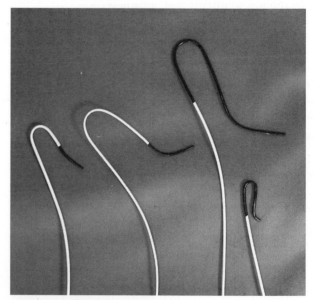

FIGURE 2-4. Recurvant selective catheters. Simmons 1, Simmons 2, Simmons 3, Sos selective (*left to right*).

nal visceral catherization, the catheter shaft must be long enough to reach the thoracic aorta to reform its trailing curve. The tip of the reformed catheter is brought superior to the origin of the intended vessel and drawn slowly down until the tip engages. An interesting point to note about looped catheters and recurvant shapes is that catheter manipulations now have the opposite effect that they normally do, inserting the catheter at the groin withdraws the tip from the vessel and pulling on it advances it further into the vessel.

Recurvant catheters need to be disengaged from their selective position before removal; otherwise, the vessel origin may be avulsed or dissected. In addition, recurvant catheters should have their curves opened by a guidewire before being removed from the patient.

Side holes

Catheters may have side holes in addition to the end hole to provide a larger surface area for contrast to exit the catheter (or for fluid to enter the catheter in the case of drainage catheters). A higher rate of contrast injection thus may be achieved (the taper of a catheter substantially reduces the diameter of the end hole compared with the remainder of the catheter lumen). In addition, a high-velocity jet, which potentially may damage the vessel, is not formed during forceful contrast injection, as may be the case with an end-hole catheter.

Flush catheters are designed for high-rate, high-volume injections. An example is the angiographic pigtail catheter that has side holes placed on the straight portion of the catheter, often several centimeters from the end, in a "flush" configuration (Fig. 2-5). The side holes serve to maximize the rate of contrast injection possible, center the catheter in the vessel, and minimize unwinding of the curved catheter tip. The number and size of holes are constrained by the need to maintain both the strength of the catheter and some output through the distal end. Flush catheters typically have 8 to 12 side holes. The lumen between the distal side hole and end of the catheter potentially can form clot if sufficient flow is not present during flushing.

Selective catheters, such as the cobra, are available as an end hole catheter or with two small sideholes immediately adjacent to the catheter tip. The presence of the side holes results in a diminished end hole jet during contrast delivery with a power injector and thereby decreases the risk of intimal injury.

Situations exist, however, where the use of an end-hole catheter is advantageous during selective catheterization. One or two side holes projecting into the parent vessel also may mask a situation in which the tip of the catheter is occlusive or buried in the vessel wall by allowing blood return. Rapid injection into such a "wedged" vessel, or into the wall, may precipitate vessel damage or rupture.

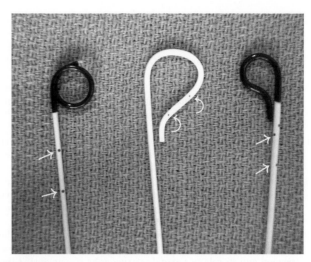

FIGURE 2-5. Flush catheters. Pigtail, Neff, Omni (*left to right*). The pigtail and omniflush catheters have small side holes on the distal catheter shaft to distribute the contrast and injection force evenly (*arrows*); the tip configuration serves predominantly as a stabilizer and blunt leading edge. The Neff catheter side holes (*curved arrows*) are on the short limb rather than on the shaft; the operator can pull the limb down the contralateral iliac artery for a slow selective injection rather than having to maneuver the catheter over the aortic bifurcation.

Side hole catheters should not be used for therapeutic embolization. The presence of a side hole increases the risk of entangling an embolization coil at the catheter tip. Use of side hole catheters is avoided in the coronary and cerebral circulation because of the increased risk of thrombus formation in the potentially stagnant blood in the side holes or tip with subsequent embolization.

■ Conclusion

In interventional radiology procedures, planning is imperative. If the basic aspects of the case are anticipated, unexpected situations can be handled in a rational fashion. Experience will provide a set of solutions to particular problems, but it does not substitute for a logical plan that avoids potential problems and equipment incompatibilities. If properly performed, a percutaneous intervention can provide valuable diagnostic information and effect a good therapeutic result with minimal risk.

REFERENCES

1. Seldinger SI. Catheter replacement of the needle in percutaneous angiography. *Acta Radiol* 1953;39:368–376.
2. Schrader R, Steinbacher S, Burger W, et al. Collagen application for sealing of arterial punctures in comparison to pressure dressings: a randomized trial. *Cathet Cardiovasc Diagn* 1992;27:298–302.
3. Eisenberg RL, Fiske CE, Hedgcock MW. Catheter angiography through aortofemoral grafts: inadvertent catheterization of the native iliac artery. *AJR Am J Roentgenol* 1979;32:852.

4. Kim D, Orron DE, Skillman JJ, et al. Role of superficial femoral artery puncture in the development of pseudoaneurysm and arteriovenous fistula complicating percutaneous transfemoral cardiac catheterization [Comment]. *Cathet Cardiovasc Diagn* 1992;126:327–328.

5. Altin RS, Flicker S, Naidech HJ. Pseudoaneurysm formation and arteriovenous fistula formation after femoral artery catheterization: association with low femoral punctures *AJR Am J Roentgenol* 1989;152:629–631.

6. Sreeram S, Lumsden AB, Miller JS, et al. Retroperitoneal hematoma following femoral artery catheterization: a serious and often fatal complication. *Ann Surg* 1990;4:328–333.

7. Lechner G, Jantsch H, Waneck R, et al. The relationship between the common femoral artery, the inguinal crease, and the inguinal ligament: a guide to accurate angiographic puncture. *Cardiovasc Intervent Radiol* 1988;11:165–169.

8. Rupp SB, Vogelzang RL, Nemcek AA, Jr. et al. Relationship of the inguinal ligament to pelvic radiographic landmarks: anatomic correlation and its role in femoral arteriography [Comment]. *J Vasc Interv Radiol* 1993;4:834.

9. Spijkboer AM, Scholten FG, Mali WP, et al. Antegrade puncture of the femoral artery: morphologic study. *Radiology* 1990;176:57–60.

10. Mozersky DJ, Olson RM, Coons HG, et al. Doppler controlled needle director: a useful adjunct to angiography. *Radiology* 1973;109:221–222.

11. Khangure MS, Chow KC, Christensen MA. Accurate and safe puncture of a pulseless femoral artery. *Radiology* 1982;144:927–928.

12. AbuRahma AF, Robinson PA, Boland JP. Safety of arteriography by direct puncture of a vascular prosthesis. *Am J Surg* 1992;164:233–236.

13. AbuRahma AF, Robinson PA, Boland JP, et al. Complications of arteriography in a recent series of 707 cases: factors effecting outcome. *Ann Vasc Surg* 1993;7:122–129.

14. Grollman JH Jr, Marcus R. Transbrachial arteriography: techniques and complications. *Cardiovasc Intervent Radiol* 1988;11:32–35.

15. Bakal CW, Friedland RJ, Sprayregen S, et al. Translumbar arch aortography: a retrospective controlled study of usefulness, technique, and safety. *Radiology* 1991;178:225–228.

16. Yandow D, Wojtowycz M, Alter A, et al. Detection of retroperitoneal hemorrhage after translumbar aortography by computerized tomography. *Angiology* 1980;31:655–659.

17. Quigley MJ, Sniderman KW, Yeung EY. Translumbar aortography: experience with a steerable pigtail catheter. *Can Assoc Radiol J* 1993;44:29–34.

18. Dotter CT, Judkins MP, Fische LH. Safety guide spring for percutaneous cardiovascular catheterization. *AJR Am J Roentgenol* 1966;98:957–960.

19. Baum S. Catheters and injectors. In: Abrams, H, ed. *Abrams' Angiography*, 2nd ed. Boston: Little, Brown and Company; 1971.

20. Wright KC, Wallace S, Charnsangavej C, et al. Flow-directed catheter for superselective arterial catheterization: an experimental evaluation. *Cardiovasc Intervent Radiol* 1986;9:54–56.

21. Reidy JF, Ludman C. The safety of outpatient arteriography using 3F catheters. *Br J Radiol* 1993;66:1048–1049.

22. Waltman AC, Courey WR, Athanasoulis C, et al. Technique for left gastric artery catheterization. *Radiology* 1973;109:732–734.

3

Filming and Injection Techniques

SAMUEL I. WAHL AND KENNETH M. ZINN

Selecting the proper filming technique and injection rate is critical in performing high-quality angiographic studies. Many variables must be considered, and each examination, or run must be tailored appropriately. The representative filming sequences and injection parameters provided herein are those typically used at our institutions, and they may need to be modified to suit the individual patient.

■ Image Acquisition

Currently, two basic filming techniques are used in angiography: conventional filmscreen imaging and digital subtraction angiography (DSA) imaging. Regardless of the techniques used, it is essential that a fluoroscopic or scout view of the area of interest be obtained at the start of the study, before any invasive manipulation is done. This is especially important in the abdomen, where retained barium from a recent computed tomography (CT) or gastrointestinal (GI) study could preclude obtaining an adequate examination. A scout film taken immediately after placing the patient on the table may also reveal an important element of an unknown clinical history. For example, we saw two patients in whom previously placed inferior vena cava filters were discovered on scout fluoroscopy when the patients were placed on the angiographic table for insertion of an inferior vena cava filter. In both cases, the patients were poor "historians," and they had incomplete medical charts. Furthermore, it is essential that overlapping vascular segments be separated by additional views when necessary to answer a clinical question and that multiple

views be obtained whenever critical information is needed (Figs. 3-1 and 3-2).

Film-screen angiography

Conventional film-screen imaging is often referred to as *cut-film imaging*. It has been largely replaced by digital acquisition techniques; however, it is of both historical and current interest because it is the basis on which the subsequent technology was derived. Cut-film arteriography uses cut sheets of film stacked or placed in a roll within a delivery magazine or cassette called a *rapid film changer*. Rapid film changers carry between 20 and 30 14 × 14-inch films. They operate at maximum filming rates of either four or six films per second (Puck, AOT-S; Siemens-Elema-Schonander, Inc., Elk Grove Village, IL, U.S.A.). The number of films per second and the duration of filming during an individual run are programmed into the system before each angiographic run. The most important consideration in determining the appropriate filming sequence is the rate of blood flow in the vessel(s) being studied as well as the particular pathology being investigated, with faster filming rates during the rapidly flowing arterial phase and slower filming during the capillary and venous phases. Filming near the contrast injection site generally mandates faster rates than filming downstream at a distance from the catheter. The goal is to maximize the diagnostic information obtained during each contrast injection without excessive contrast dose or exposure to the patient and without a waste of x-ray film or radiation.

Film or acquisition sequences

Filming sequences are stated as the number of films exposed per second for a specified duration of seconds. The

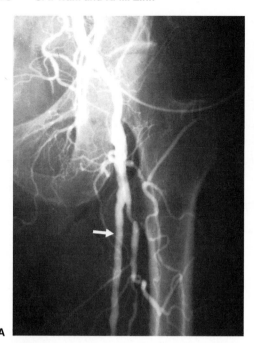
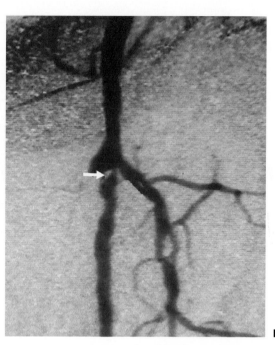

A   **B**

FIGURE 3-1. Multiple views are needed to uncover overlapped vessels in this 73-year-old man with critical ischemia and a failed left common femoral to above-knee vein-bypass graft. There is popliteal artery occlusion. The operating surgeon wishes to avoid the groin and is planning the proximal anastomosis from the proximal superficial femoral artery. (**A**) An anteroposterior (AP) view of the left femoral triangle and thigh. The arrow shows a patent proximal superficial femoral artery at the site of the proposed proximal anastomosis. (**B**) The oblique view demonstrates the occluded graft stump medially and the deep femoral artery laterally. The arrow highlights a tight stenosis at the origin of the superficial femoral artery, which was completely hidden in the AP view. This stenosis would result in compromised inflow into a graft placed distal to it and the graft would occlude. Ultimately, proximal anastomosis was placed at the common femoral artery as a result of this oblique angiogram.

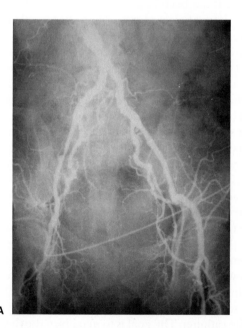
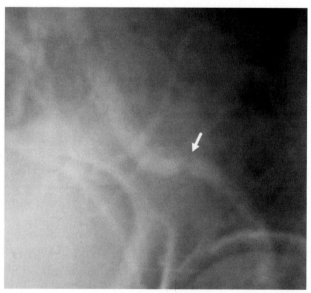

A   **B**

FIGURE 3-2. The angiogram and physical examination must correlate. (**A**) An anteroposterior (AP) pelvic angiogram, part of an aortofemoral runoff study. The patient has critical left lower-extremity ischemia, diffuse superficial femoropopliteal artery occlusive disease, and symmetric femoral pulses. Note the extensive significant disease in the right external iliac artery. (**B**) Right anterior oblique view of the left external iliac artery. The arrow highlights a significant lesion approximately 2 cm above the inguinal ligament, which was not seen in the AP view. Because the femoral pulses were palpated as symmetric, and there is extensive significant disease in the right external iliac artery, a hemodynamically significant lesion must be suspected somewhere in the left common external iliac artery, and multiple obliques are mandated until the etiology of the physical finding is found.

filming can be divided into segments, if so desired, to follow or parallel the blood flow. For example, a typical programmed run for a routine abdominal aortogram might be three films per second for 4 seconds and then one film per second for 8 seconds. This would expose a total of 20 films over approximately 12 seconds. In our institutions, we would express this particular film sequence as "3 for 4 and 1 for 8." Certain studies require that the filming continue well into the venous phase. For example, a typical filming sequence for selective superior mesentric arteriography for GI bleeding or superior mesenteric portography might be one film/per second for 10 seconds and then one film every other second until the film changer has exposed the entire magazine of film ("1 for 10, then 1/2 out"). Thus, the entire run would give a total of 20 films lasting for a total of 30 seconds, which is adequate for late venous visualization (Table 3-1).

Filming should be tailored to the patient and the anatomy. At one extreme, rapid flow through an arteriovenous fistula mandates a minimal framing rate of three frames per second; four to six frames per second may be needed. On the other hand, for imaging an aneurysm in a patient with low cardiac output, one exposure every second or every other second may suffice.

A scout film obtained prior to any contrast injection is used to verify proposed positioning and exposure technique. Scout films usually are obtained after any significant patient repositioning as well as at the start of any procedure.

The initial exposed film of the run is referred to as the *zero-second* film. This exposure is obtained just prior to contrast opacification. It provides a necessary baseline for dynamic evaluation of the film run and allows the radiologist to analyze the run for any contrast-related artifacts, for example, baseline calcium projected over an artery. Historically this film provided a "mask" for photographically subtracting out the bony background structures (after "polarizing" the film to reverse black and white) from the images so that only the vessels being studied are visualized. This process is called, for obvious reasons, *subtraction imaging*. Since the advent of DSA, photographic subtraction imaging is used infrequently, if ever; however, historically it provided the conceptual basis for DSA. Zero-second and scout films also serve as a baseline for dynamic evaluation of the run (e.g., to differentiate extravasated contrast from preexisting calcifications). This zero-second film differs from the scout film in that the zero film is included in the total filming run. In other words, it is the first of the sequence, whereas the scout film is obtained prior to the actual filmed run.

TABLE 3-1. Typical Filming and Flow Rates[a]

Study	Injection Rate	Filming	Projections	Comments
Aortic arch	40 mL total @ 20 mL/s	3/s × 4 s, 1/s × 8 s	30–45 RPO+ AP	Pigtail ~ 1.5 cm above valve
Thoracic aorta	60 mL total @ 30 mL/s	3/s × 4 s, 1/s × 8 s	45 RPO + AP	Include thoracic inlet to diaphragm
Abdominal aorta	40 mL total @ 20 mL/s or 30 mL total @ 15 mL/s	3/s × 4 s, 1/s × 8 s	AP or biplane filming	Catheter above celiac artery
Pelvic	30 mL total @ 15 mL/s	2/s × 3 s, 1/s × 8 s	AP	Oblique as needed; IPO will open iliac bifurcation
Internal iliac	25–40 mL total @ 2–4 mL/s	2/2 × 3 s, 1/s × 8 s	Ipsilateral PO	Ipsilateral ant. oblique with penis over contralateral thigh after intracavenous injection for impotence evaluation
Subclavian/axillary	12–20 mL total @ 3–4 mL/s	2–3/s × 4 s, 1/s × 6 s	AP	
Brachial	12 mL total @ 3 mL/s	1–2/s × 8 s	AP	Check for possible high brachial bifurcation at the axillary level; catheter placed in axillary artery
Radial/ulnar/hand	20–30 mL total @ 2–3 mL/s	1–2/s × 10–20 s	Hand supinated	Maximal vasodilation of extremity may be needed
Celiac	40–50 mL total @ 5–8 mL/s	2/s × 5 s, 1/s × 10 s	AP	
SMA	60 mL total @ 8 mL/s	1/s × 10 s, ½ s out	AP	Can use 30–60/mg intraarterial papaverine to enhance venous phase; film covers 30/s to ensure visualization of SMV-portal vein
IMA	15–20 mL total @ 2–3 mL/s	2/s × 5 s, 1/s × 10 s	AP	
Renal	12–15 mL total @ 4–8 mL/s	3/s × 3 s, 1/s × 6 s	AP or 30 IAO	For renal tumor evaluation, increase contrast volume and delay filming for visualization of renal vein
Selective pulmonary angiogram	40 mL total @ 20 mL/s	4/s × 4 s, 1/s × 4 s	AP and 45 IPO	Measure pulmonary artery pressure prior to contrast injection
IVC	60 mL total @ 30 mL/s	2/s × 3 s, 1/s × 8 s	AP	

AP, anteroposterior; IAO, ipsilateral anterior oblique; IMA, inferior mesenteric artery; IPO, ipsilateral posterior oblique; IVC, inferior vena cava; RPO, right posterior oblique; SMA, superior mesenteric artery; SMV, superior mesenteric vein.

[a] Flow rates and volumes are given for cut film or unsubtracted digital acquisition with full strength iodinated contrast material.

Digital subtraction angiography

Rather than exposing cut film at regular intervals, fluoro-scopically acquired images can be mapped sequentially into computer memory. The acquisition begins with "test shots," which are equivalent to scouts, obtained to see whether the angiographic unit's programmed exposure factors are correct. If the test shots are accepted, the actual acquisition series begins. As with conventional angiographic runs, a zero-second acquisition is obtained to act as the mask by slightly delaying the contrast injection during the acquisition. From this image, some or all the background structures can be digitally subtracted. Precontrast background information (the "zero" exposure, or "mask") can be subtracted out electronically from images obtained during contrast administration. Thus, underlying bone and soft tissue densities are subtracted out of each screen *pixel* (picture element) as contrast passes through the image. This markedly enhances contrast sensitivity. Nonsubtracted images always should be viewed along with the subtracted ones; in this manner, underlying bone or soft tissue artifacts can be accounted for (Fig. 3-3). Originally, intravenous injections were used to image the arterial circulation (intravenous digital subtraction angiography, or IV-DSA), but this still required a large amount of contrast, was subject to extensive motion artifact, and yielded only marginal spatial resolution; however, the use of intraarterial contrast injections (intraarterial digital subtraction arteriography, or IA-DSA) allowed the use of smaller volumes of iodine while retaining excellent contrast sensitivity; IA-DSA is also subject to less motion artifact. Over the last decade, technical advances have markedly improved spatial resolution as well.[1-3] Although decreased spatial resolution of DSA compared with film-screen arteriography still exists and can compromise the detailed evaluation of subtle small-vessel abnormalities, in clinical practice, the problem probably occurs infrequently. Thus, IA-DSA has replaced film-screen arteriography for most applications. The studies also can be interpreted directly from the computer monitor, thus eliminating the wait for processing a film run and significantly decreasing study time. Another advantage is that the images can be electronically post-processed to change the contrast and window level, integrate frames, and grade stenoses. Most angiographers prefer DSA to cut-film studies because the time required to complete the angiogram and the contrast load is significantly less than with DSA. Whereas spatial resolution is better than with cut films with DSA, DSA has a better chance of identifying extravasation (it is true that subtraction can be performed on cut films, but this is tedious and expensive). We have found that DSA induces copious artifacts when searching for a GI bleeding source (as a result of breathing and bowel motion), and we use high-resolution nonsubtracted digital acquisition in these settings with full-strength, low-osmolar contrast.

The superior contrast sensitivity of DSA allows considerable reduction in contrast density necessary to produce optimal images. Generally, the contrast agent can be di-

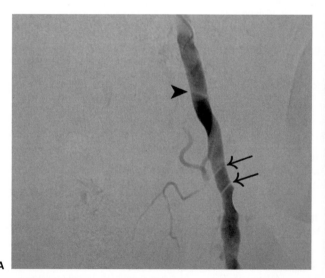

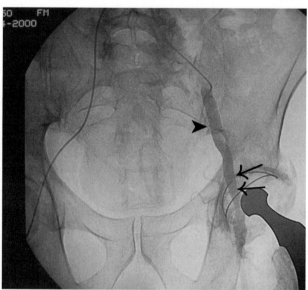

A

B

FIGURE 3-3. Comparison of the nonsubtracted and subtracted images is extremely important when interpreting digital subtraction arteriography. (**A**) Selective digital subtraction arteriogram of the left external iliac artery. The single arrowhead highlights a linear defect in more proximal external iliac artery, which might be interpreted as a guidewire-induced iatrogenic dissection. More distal defects (dual arrows) could be similarly interpreted. (**B**) The nonsubtracted image demonstrates that these are really substraction artifacts related to underlying bony cortex (arrowhead) and a hip prosthesis (dual arrows).

luted with saline by 25 to 50%. Injection rates can be reduced slightly compared with film-screen angiography, but total volumes can be reduced significantly. Moreover, one also has the option of using full-strength contrast in a nonsubtracted mode, which may be necessary for pulmonary arteriography, abdominal arteriography, and peripheral angiography, where bowel gas, respiration, or other patient movement causes motion artifact and pixel misregistration.

Digital "road mapping" is a helpful utility that aids in catheter negotiation through tortuous vessels and in other aspects of critical catheter placement. The operator leaves an overlay of the vasculature on the monitor from a previous contrast injection, which can be used as a map during the real-time fluoroscopic maneuvering of the catheter or guidewire.[3,4]

During the procedure, any fluoroscopic image can be saved or "grabbed" for future viewing. Also, the fluoroscopic image remains on the monitor and can be magnified without requiring additional fluoroscopy. Postprocessing adjustments always can be made to improve image quality. One new equipment option allows active rotation of the C-arm (up to 20 to 30 degrees/second) during contrast injection; this technique can obtain multiple projections during a single contrast run.

With all the advantages offered by DSA, only a few disadvantages are encountered. These stem primarily from sequential pixel malalignment resulting from patient, cardiac, respiratory, and bowel motion. The quality of DSA images is degraded significantly by motion, and this problem is particularly common with abdominal and pulmonary angiography. These problems, however, can be reduced by giving clear patient instructions and by using proper positioning and mild restraints. Postprocessing the acquisition by "pixel shifting" or selecting a new subtraction mask often eliminates motion-related degradation. Glucagon and abdominal compression also can be used before the study to decrease bowel activity. Current systems, however, allow high-quality, high-resolution nonsubtracted digital images to be obtained in 1024 × 1024 pixel matrices. Nonsubtracted digital images retain many of the benefits of subtracted studies, including decreased table time, and can be used where motion artifact significantly degrades the image; however, nonsubtracted digital images require contrast rates and volumes that approach those needed for cut-film arteriography.

The use of low osmolar contrast medium greatly reduces pulmonary irritation and therefore eliminates coughing during pulmonary angiography. By simply using a nonsubtracted mode, excellent pulmonary arterial visualization is accomplished, even in the presence of respiratory motion. With state-of-the-art digital systems, measures used to reduce bowel and respiratory motion are often unnecessary.

■ Aortofemoral Arteriography

Aortofemoral arteriography presents a special challenge to filming because the target vascular territory is considerably longer than conventional film or fluoroscopic field. The most basic approach would be to perform a separate series over each vascular segment, working proximally from the aorta down through the tibial and pedal arteries. This approach would require four or five separate film runs and contrast injections. More commonly used techniques for obtaining aortofemoral arteriograms generally employ a single programmed power injection and either table or image intensifier movement or special long film cassettes to acquire images in a single series. The more commonly used devices for aortofemoral arteriography are the stepping table and "bolus chasing." The long-leg changer (BC Medical Ltd., Montreal, Quebec, Canada), another such device, is no longer manufactured, but it is still in use.

A stepping table traditionally used a rapid film changer (Puck or AOT-S film changer 14 × 17-inch film) as the patient is moved in "steps" over several different stations, extending from the pelvis to the feet during a single contrast injection. A long-leg changer, on the other hand, is a ceiling-mounted x-ray tube that uses multiple (usually six) 14 × 51-inch film cassettes housed within a rotating film unit below the patient. The time interval between each cassette exposure can be tailored to the patient so as to ensure complete opacification from the distal aorta to the pedal vessels. Such large-field changers are advantageous for arteriography and venography of the lower extremities because the entire extremity can be evaluated on each exposure, and calculation of the timing for lower extremity arteriography is less crucial. The disadvantages are the need for an additional ceiling-mounted radiographic tube with a tube to a floor distance of between 87 and 110 inches and a maximum filming rate of one film every 2.5 to 3 seconds. Extremely long contrast columns (8 to 10 seconds) are imaged. Late-generation stepping tables can acquire images digitally.

Finally, new digital "bolus chasing" techniques are an alternative to both a traditional stepping table or a long-leg changer. With bolus chasing, the operator can control table movement manually while visualizing contrast opacification in real time. The operator then can alter the rate of the table movement to match the speed and position of the contrast bolus (i.e., bolus chasing), acquiring images longitudinally. Digital subtraction is accomplished by duplicating the table movement and frame rate after the contrast has dissipated to obtain a "mask." "Knee-arrival time" is computed by fluoroscopically observing a small test bolus of contrast arrive at the popliteal artery prior to the full injection; then it is used by the system's microprocessor to optimize the contrast injection rate and volume and to coordinate it with an appropriate acquisition sequence.

Opacification of extremities can be enhanced, if necessary, by inducing reactive hyperemia after the release of pressure cuffs from the calves, warming the extremity, or using vasodilators such as intraarterial nitroglycerin, tolazoline, or papaverine. Of these, transcatheter nitroglycerin, 200 µg, is preferred by some for augmenting visualization of the lower extremities.[1]

Spot films using 70-mm or 105-mm cameras are sometimes used in angiography, but the small size of the frames makes fine detail difficult to appreciate, and these are now considered "legacy" devices by many. Cineradiography is found primarily in cardiac angiography suites, but the high radiation doses and the cumbersome small-field film viewing make it insufficient for abdominal and extremity work. Most peripheral arteriograms do not require the extremely rapid frame rate necessary in cardiac angiography.

■ Flow Rates and Contrast Injectors

As stated previously, selecting the proper contrast flow rate for angiography is an extremely important part of a high-quality angiogram. Several programmable automated injection devices are commercially available that provide predictable and reproducible contrast volumes delivered at a specific flow rate for angiographic studies. For example, a routine (digital) abdominal aortogram may require a total contrast volume of 30 mL at a flow rate of 15 mL/second (i.e., a 2-second injection).

Power injectors must be programmed prior to each run, depending on the vascular territory being studied,

avoiding the inconsistent, unknown rates of hand injections. Furthermore, power injectors can deliver higher flow rates than hand injections. It is imperative that, prior to a power-injected run, a hand-delivered test injection be performed to ensure proper catheter position and to confirm the flow rate required.

The primary injection parameters programmed into the power injector prior to the run are the flow rate (mL/sec), the total contrast injection volume (mL), and the linear rise (Fig. 3-4). The flow rate is selected on the basis of vessel diameter and blood flow observed fluoroscopically with a hand injection. Total contrast volume depends on the desired column length and the size of the territory to be opacified. For example, a 1.5- to 2-second contrast column is sufficient to fill the field of a thoracic or abdominal aortogram. Image acquisition must be delayed so that at least one noncontrast zero-second image is acquired for a mask before the arrival of contrast in the field. When the area of interest is at the catheter injection site, the injection typically is delayed 0.5 to 1 second after the start of image acquisition. If imaging is remote from the site of injection, however, a variable delay in filming may be programmed to occur after the start of the contrast injection. For example, with a catheter injection in the common iliac artery and filming over the foot, a long filming delay (e.g., 7 to 10 seconds) can aid in extending the series to allow acquisition of a good foot arteriogram. A catheter-specific maximum pressure limit is set to avoid catheter rupture during power injection. (Note that pressure is not a primary parameter.) Pressure generated during injection is related to the viscosity of the contrast medium, the programmed flow rate, the catheter luminal diameter, and catheter material and length. For example, a typical nylon, 90-cm, 5F pigtail catheter might have a

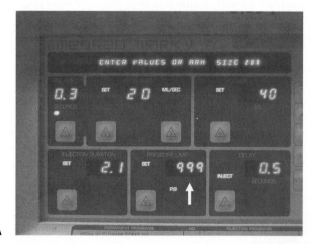

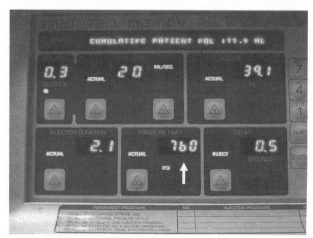

A   B

FIGURE 3-4. The injection settings for a flush aortogram are shown on the control panel from a Mark V power injector (Medrad, Inc., Pittsburgh, PA, U.S.A.). (**A**) The pressure limit is set 999 pounds per square inch (psi) just below the catheter pressure limit. (**B**) By using the "status function" button, the interventionalist can view the actual injection parameters after the run is completed. The arrow demonstrates that the combination of flow parameters, contrast viscosity, and catheter factors actually generated a pressure of 760, considerably less than the set pressure limit.

maximum pressure limit of 1050 pounds per square inch (psi). Excess pressure generally causes rupture at the catheter hub, where pressure is highest. At the set pressure limit, a power injector typically will terminate the injection so that rupture is avoided (Fig. 3-4).

Linear rise is an additional primary injection parameter. It is the time required from the onset of the injection (*zero flow*) to reach the maximum flow rate specified by the injector. Linear rise is used to avoid catheter recoil and should depend on the catheter type and position. A typical linear rise of 0.2 seconds is usually sufficient for multi-sidehole catheters during flush aortography. A longer linear rise (0.4 to 0.8 seconds) decreases the likelihood of catheter recoil (and selective vessel damage) and should be used during selective arteriography.* For example, if an end-hole catheter is selectively placed in a vessel, the sudden recoil produced by the maximum rate of injection without a gradual rise potentially could dislodge the catheter or, worse, damage the vessel. Nonselective flush catheters with sideholes may allow the use of a shorter linear rise (0.2 seconds) as the contrast is generally distributed equally in all directions from the multiple holes maintaining the catheter's position. Generally, selective catheters with sideholes should be used with medium to long linear rise times. Contrast injectors also usually include a contrast syringe heater to reduce contrast viscosity and to allow flow rates of up to 40 mL/sec.[5] The 4 to 5 Fr catheters commonly used today are subject to considerably more recoil for a given flow rate than the 6 to 7 French catheters that were common a few years ago; thus, we have tended to use longer linear rise times when in selective positions.

■ Contrast Agents

Our central tenet is to administer the minimal amount of contrast necessary to obtain complete diagnostic information or complete an interventional study. Increasing volumes may add additional risk to patients with poor cardiac output or renal failure. Low-osmolality contrast agents are preferred in most vascular and interventional radiology departments because they decrease patient discomfort and reduce the incidence of adverse side effects, such as contrast-induced renal failure compared with conventional, higher osmolar agents. They also appear to reduce minor contrast reactions, such as urticaria, nau-

sea, and vomiting. Although rare, severe and fatal reactions are not eliminated by using low-osmolar contrast agents. The efficacy of steroid prophylaxis with low osmolar contrast is controversial. Institution-specific protocols should be consulted and followed.[6–8]

The occurrence of clinically significant contrast-related renal dysfunction usually is associated with preexisting renal compromise. Advanced age and diabetes contribute to risk.[9] Patients with multiple myeloma may incur renal damage as a result of tubular precipitation in high-risk groups; so imaging examinations that do not require iodinated contrast material should be considered if they can give clinically useful data. It is essential that patients who are high risk for renal failure receive low osmolar contrast. Some angiographers use furosemide and mannitol infusions to maintain renal blood flow and prevent renal toxicity, but benefit from this protocol remains controversial.[10–13]

Full-strength iodinated contrast for angiography generally ranges from 300 to 370 mg/mL iodine. Dilute contrast for injection may be half to two-thirds strength when using digital acquisition. The newer contrast agents do not have anticoagulant properties typical of standard high-osmolar contrast; thus, it is essential that low-osmolar agents not be allowed to contact blood for long periods. Thus, care must be taken not to allow blood to dwell in power-injector syringes, tubing, or catheters prior to injection.

Despite the low incidence of contrast reactions using low-osmolar, iodinated contrast agents, the potential for problems in patients with a history of prior allergic reactions and in those with renal insufficiency remains. For this reason, carbon dioxide (CO_2) was developed as a viable alternative contrast agent.[14]

Carbon dioxide is a nonallergic, highly dissolvable gas that is excreted by the lungs, avoiding the nephrotoxicity of iodinated agents. By temporarily displacing blood, CO_2 decreases the radiographic density within the vessel lumen, essentially the opposite radiographic effect of traditional contrast agents. CO_2 can be used as an intravascular contrast agent for both diagnostic and interventional studies; however, because of its potential for neurotoxicity, it is not used for studies performed above the diaphragm. Special delivery techniques have been designed for CO_2 because it is colorless, and admixture with air can be fatal.[15] One must be careful to use small, controlled injection volumes and correct patient positioning to avoid gas trapping in nondependent structures such as the main pulmonary artery. The trapped gas can obstruct pulmonary blood flow, leading to cardiac failure. If the injection volume, duration, and interval are adequate, unlimited quantities of CO_2 can be used. CO_2 angiography has been used during TIPS (transjugular intrahepator portosystemic shunt) procedures with excellent results; however, its contrast resolution is inferior to

---

* This concept can be explained easily compared with sitting idle at a traffic light. When the light turns green, and you abruptly push your foot against the accelerator, a considerable amount of recoil will be placed on your head forcing it backwards; if you gradually depress the accelerator in a progressive linear fashion, however, much less recoil will be encountered.

iodinated agents, and it can cause discomfort during injection in a substantial minority of patients, interfering with study completion and adequacy.[15] CO_2 femoral arteriography may result in an incomplete distal study in up to 50 to 75% of patients.[16,17]

Because of the limitations of CO_2 as an alternative to iodinated contrast, interest has centered on utilizing gadolinium based agents (e.g., gadodiamide) for angiography. Gadodiamide has been used alone or in conjunction with conventional contrast or CO_2 for studies of the peripheral and renal arteries and the inferior vena cava. It appears to be equivalent to dilute iodinated contrast in its attenuation properties and may decrease the incidence of renal failure in at-risk patients.[18–21]

■ Conclusion

An understanding of the basic concepts of anatomy, physiology filming, and injection technique is key to obtaining a good diagnostic angiogram. Evolving digital technology has enabled the acquisition of diagnostic studies quickly and safely. Modification of standard techniques, judiciously applied, will serve to benefit patients and enhance the quality of the study.

REFERENCES

1. Cohen MI, Vogelzang RI. A comparison of techniques for improved visualization of the arteries of the distal lower extremity. *AJR Am J Roentgenol* 1986;147:1021–1024.
2. Crummy AB, Strother CM, Lieberman RP, et al. Digital video subtraction angiography for evaluation of peripheral vascular disease. *Radiology* 1981;141:33–37.
3. Crummy AB, Steighorst MF, Turski PA, et al. Digital subtraction angiography: current status and use of intra-arterial injection. *Radiology* 1982;145:303–307.
4. Katzen BT. Current status of digital angiography in vascular imaging. *Radio Clin North Am* 1995;33:1–14.
5. Kadir S. *Diagnostic Angiography.* Philadelphia: WB Saunders; 1986.
6. Katayama H, et al. Adverse reactions to ionic and nonionic contrast media: a report from the Japanese Committee on the Safety of Contrast Media. *Radiology* 1990;175:621–628.
7. Lasser EC, et al. Pretreatment with corticosteroids to alleviate reactions to intravenous contrast material. *N Engl J Med* 1987;317:845–849.
8. Lasser EC, Berry CC, Mishkin MM, et al. Pretreatment with cortecosteroids to prevent adverse reactions to nonionic contrast media. *AJR Am J Roentgenol* 1994;162:523–526.
9. Lautin EM, Freeman NJ, Schoenfeld AH, et al. Radiocontrast-associated renal dysfunction: incidence and risk factors. *AJR Am R Roentgenol* 1991;157:49–58.
10. Cruz C, Hricak H, Samhouri F, et al. Contrast media for angiography: effect on renal function. *Radiology* 1986;158:109–112.
11. Barrett BJ, Carlisle EJ. Metaanalysis of the relative nephrotoxicity of high-osmolality and low-osmolality iodinated contrast media. *Radiology* 1993;188:171–178.
12. Bettman MA. The evaluation of contrast-related renal failure. *Am J Roentgenol* 1991;157:66–68.
13. Golman K, Almen T. Contrast media-induced nephrotoxicity: survey and present state. *Invest Radiol* 1985;21:S92–S97.
14. Kerns SR, Hawkins IF. Carbon dioxide digital subtraction angiography: expanding applications and technical evolution. *AJR Am J Roentgenol* 1995;164:735–741.
15. Hawkins IF, Caridi JG, Kerns SR. Plastic bag delivery system for hand injection of carbon dioxide. *Am J Radiol* 995;165:1487–1489.
16. Diaz LP, Pabion IP, Garcia JA, Lopez M. Assessment of CO_2 arteriography in arterial occlusive disease of the lower extremities. *J Vasc Interv Radiol* 2000;1:163–169.
17. Rolland Y, Duvauferrier R, Lucas A, et al. Lower limb angiography: a prospective study comparing carbon dioxide with iodinated contrast material in 30 patients. *AJR Am J Roentgenol* 1998;171:333–337.
18. Kaufman JA, et al. Renal insufficiency: gadopentetate dimeglumine as a radiographic contrast agent during peripheral vascular interventional procedures. *Radiology* 1996;198:579–581.
19. Kaufman JA, et al. Gadolinium-based contrast agents as an alternative at vena cavography in patients with renal insufficiency: early experience. *Radiology* 1999;212:280–284.
20. Spinosa DJ, Angle JF, Hagspiel KD, Hartwell GD, Matsumoto AH. Lower extremity arteriography with use of iodinated contrast material or gadodiamide to supplement CO_2 angiography in patients with renal insufficiency. *J Vasc Interv Radiol* 1996;11:35–43.
21. Spinosa DJ, Matsumoto AH, Angle JF, Hagspiel KD. Use of gadopentetate dimeglumine as a contrast agent for percutaneous transluminal renal angioplasty and stent placement. *Kidney Int* 1998;53:503–507.

4

An Approach to Sedation and Monitoring

IRENE OSBORN AND RANDALL SNYDER

As the complexity and duration of diagnostic vascular and interventional procedures have increased, it has become more important to provide adequate comfort for the patient. Interventional radiologists must consider that patients are anxious about the procedure, will be in a supine position on a hard and generally uncomfortable procedure table, and are usually in a cold environment. Interventional radiologists also must address the pain or possibility of pain during the procedure. Monitoring the patient during the procedure, especially if conscious sedation is administered, and monitoring during recovery are essential. Patients must refrain from moving for much of the procedure, and cooperate in specific breath-holding maneuvers during some manipulations and during most image acquisitions. Thus, the role of sedation and monitoring is key.

Personnel attending to patients undergoing interventional procedures should have sufficient knowledge of the pharmacology, indications, and contraindications for relevant sedative agents and the ability to recognize and initiate treatment for any adverse reaction to those agents as well as have basic skills in emergency airway management and resuscitation. In addition to the supervising physician, the team should include a health professional whose primary job is monitoring the patient and who is available to the patient during the procedure and postprocedure recovery phase, until the patient has been transferred to appropriate recovery room personnel.[1]

Intravenous conscious sedation is a minimally depressed level of consciousness induced by the administration of pharmacologic agents, in which the patient retains conscious and independent ability to maintain a patent airway and to respond to physical and or verbal stimulation. Deep sedation is a controlled state of depressed consciousness or unconsciousness from which the patient is not easily aroused; it is accompanied by a partial or complete loss of protective reflexes, including the ability to maintain a patent airway independently and loss of appropriate response to physical stimulation or verbal command. During conscious sedation, a patient may start out anxious or agitated but will become tranquil, cooperative, and oriented; during the deepest level of conscious sedation, the patient may be somnolent, responding to commands only. When the patient enters a state of deep sedation, the patient may respond only to loud auditory stimuli or may exhibit sluggish or absent response to a loud stimulus or glabellar tap. Deep sedation is monitored under the care of an anesthesia, rather than a procedural, team.[2] General anesthesia is a controlled state of unconsciousness in which there is a loss of protective reflexes, including the ability to maintain a patent airway independently and to respond appropriately to physical stimulation or verbal command.

Before intravenous conscious sedation is instituted, a pertinent history and physical examination must be performed or they must be available from the day of the procedure. A specific allergic history is also necessary. An assessment of baseline vital signs, level of consciousness, motor function, electrocardiogram (ECG) and oximetry also should be done. In children, weight is needed to determine dose determination. During conscious sedation, intravenous access must be continually maintained. Monitoring of physiologic measurements should be performed and recorded at least every 15 minutes during the procedure and into the recovery phase. Physiologic parameters to be measured include level of consciousness, respiratory function, oximetry, blood pressure, and heart rate and rhythm. Supplemental oxygen and suction must be immediately available and a defibrillator with a crash cart that has backup emergency power also should be available immediately. These general principles apply to adults. Requirements for pediatric sedation and analgesia in children are somewhat more specific.[3]

■ Pharmacologic Agents

Widely used agents for anxiety in the interventional suite include the benzodiazepines midazolam (Versed) and diazepam (Valium). Lorazepam (Ativan) is another benzodiazepine that can be used for sedation. Like most other agents, benzodiazepines are usually administered intravenously. These anxiolytic agents are important components of intraprocedural sedation, but they can be used as the initial premedication soon after the patient has arrived in the angiography suite and consent has been obtained. Benzodiazepines provide anxiolysis and amnesia and have anticonvulsant properties; they are also reversible. These agents can cause respiratory depression and hypotension, and may interact with administered opioids (Table 4-1).

For analgesia, three commonly used opioids are morphine, meperidine (Demerol), and fentanyl. Opioids provide analgesia and sedation; they are reversible, but they may cause respiratory depression, nausea, and hypotension. Benzodiazepines and opioids may interact. Additional agents that may be useful include droperidol, a

major tranquilizer that supplements sedation and produces a calm appearance, but is not administered as a sole agent. Droperidol is useful for the prevention and treatment of nausea. Ketamine, administered intravenously over 2 to 3 minutes, may be used for additional analgesia. Ketamine may cause hallucinations and is generally given after benzodiazepines are first administered and the patient is reassured. Ketamine is a powerful analgesic that can be used in painful procedures such as percutaneous biliary drainage.

Reversal agents include flumazenil (Romazicon), which is used to reverse the effects of benzodiazepines, and naloxone (Narcan), which can reverse the effects of opioids.

■ Physiologic Monitoring: Vital Signs

Monitoring during conscious sedation by an independent observer who is trained in patient care and monitoring, such as a registered nurse or physician assistant, is mandatory.[1] Although physiologic monitoring is essential and required, it is not a substitute for direct patient observation. Patients undergoing conscious sedation should be quiet but easily arousable. Respiratory depression or apnea, hypotension, contrast reactions, and cardiac arrythmia and arrest can occur, and it is essential that the interventional radiologist be prepared to handle these potential adverse events. We also usually monitor patients undergoing procedures that do not use intravenous conscious sedation because patients may have comorbid conditions and because even benign procedures may engen-

TABLE 4-1. Commonly Used Agents for Conscious Sedation

Agent	Class/indication	Usual IV dosage	"Metabolism," common contraindications	Peak (min.)	Half life
Diazepam	Benzodiazepine: anxiolysis	5–10 mg (0.1 mg/kg)	Liver	30	21 h
Midazolam	Benzodiazepine: anxiolysis	2–5 mg (0.1 mg/kg) max	Liver Hypotension	10	2.5 h
Lorazepam	Benzodiazepine: anxiolysis	2.5 mg	Elderly		20 h duration of effect
Morphine sulfate	Opioid: analgesia	5–10 mg (0.15 mg/kg)	Liver Hypotension	20	3–4 h duration of effect
Meperidine	Opioid: analgesia	25–75 mg (1.0 – 1.5 mg/kg)	Liver Hypotension	20	2–4 h duration of effect
Fentanyl	Opioid: analgesia	1–2 microgram/kg	Liver CNS depressants ↑ intraocular pressure	5–10	2–4 h
Benadryl	Antihistamine	25–50 mg			
Naloxone	Reversal agent	0.1–0.2 mg	Hypertension	3	20 min.
Flumazenil	Reversal agent	0.2 – 1mg max		3–5	10 min. duration of effect
Ketamine	Analgesia	0.25 mg/kg	Increased intracranial pressure, Anxiety	5–7	2 h
Inapsine (Droperidol)	Anti-nausea agent	1.25–2.5 mg	Elderly debilitated pts.	20	4h

IV, intravenous

der physiologic responses (e.g., a peripherally inserted central catheter line in the right ventricle can induce an arrythmia).

The blood pressure may be taken manually, but, more commonly, automatic noninvasive arterial blood pressures are used. These automated devices also allow observation of the ECG, heart rate, respiratory rate, and pulse oximetry.

The width of the blood pressure cuff should be approximately 40% of the upper arm circumference, with the length approximately 80% of the arm circumference.[4] Falsely elevated blood pressures can be obtained with cuffs that are either too narrow or too loose.

The normal respiratory rate for adults is between 12 and 20 breaths per minute. Bradypnea may be associated with conscious sedation and analgesia and may signal oversedation. Tachypnea often is related to preprocedure anxiety, but it may have physiologic causes as well.

Pulse oximetry

Pulse oximetry uses spectrophotometry to measure changes in light absorption of blood. The pulse oximeter is an essential monitoring device that noninvasively measures arterial hemoglobin oxygen saturation (SaO_2), and pulse rate. Oxygen is highly bound to hemoglobin, and one hemoglobin module may bind zero to four molecules of oxygen.[5] For example, when four oxygen molecules are bound, the hemoglobin molecule is 100% saturated; when one is bound, it is 25% saturated. SaO_2 is the ratio of saturated hemoglobin to the total number of hemoglobin modules, and it is a fairly good reflection of arterial oxygenation. SaO_2 is directly related to the partial pressure of oxygen (PaO_2) via the well-known oxyhemoglobin dissociation curve. PaO_2 is a reflection of the amount of oxygen dissolved in the blood and normally ranges from 80 to 100 mm of mercury when pH and body temperature are normal. This is equivalent to an SaO_2 of 95 to 100%, the normal range seen on the pulse oximeter. Pulse oximetry is a reliable indicator of SaO_2 and has become the standard of care for patients receiving conscious sedation and analgesia. If the SaO_2 falls below 95%, immediate assessment of the patient's ventilation and status should be performed. Pulse oximetry provides an indication of early hypoxemia. Because procedural positioning or even draping of the patient may make it difficult to observe the patient's ventilatory status, it is an essential tool in providing uninterrupted continuous monitoring of the patient.

Capnography allows monitoring end expiratory carbon dioxide and can be used for early detection of hypoventilation and airway obstruction. Its use is becoming increasingly encouraged for monitoring patients undergoing conscious sedation.

Electrocardiogram

The final, but by far the most important, monitoring parameter is the ECG. We monitor the ECG in virtually *all* patients undergoing vascular and interventional procedures, even those performed without conscious sedation. A procedure should not be started until an adequate tracing is obtained. ECG monitoring requires the proper placement of at least two sensing electrodes and a third ground or reference electrode. Because the ECG is a small (1 mV) electrical signal, its measurement is susceptible to electrical interference from other sources, especially power cords, electrocautery, and patient motion. It is important that electrodes have adequate contact gel and be applied to clean, dry skin.

The most commonly monitored lead is lead II because the P wave is easily seen and has the greatest voltage in this lead. This orientation allows enhanced detection of dysrhythmias as well as diagnosis of inferior wall ischemia. Lead V5 is monitored for the detection of myocardial ischemia because the bulk of left ventricular myocardium lies beneath it. If only a three-lead system is available, a modified V5 lead can be obtained by placing the right arm lead under the right clavicle, the left arm lead in the V5 position, and the left leg lead in its usual position while monitoring lead I.[6]

A preprocedural rhythm strip should be obtained as standard protocol so that any potential change in rhythm or ST segment that is appreciated can be compared with a baseline later. If the patient has significant cardiac disease, a five-lead system may be used which will provide 80 to 96% sensitivity for the detection of intraprocedural cardiac events. Lead II alone has a sensitivity of only 18 to 33%. Prompt treatment of dysrhythmias or tachyarrhythmias is often necessary in the interventional suite. A working knowledge of ACLS may be helpful in these situations.

■ American Society of Anesthesiologist Classification

In 1940 the American Society of Anesthesiologists (ASA) developed a physical status classification for patients receiving anesthesia and surgery to standardize physical and clinical status for statistical analysis and outcomes research for hospital records (Table 4-2). This classification was further modified by Dripps et al in 1961, and it remains the standard classification used by anesthesiologists and others to characterize the patients' physical status preprocedurally or preoperatively.[7] Although it was not intended as such, the ASA physical status classification has since been shown to correlate well with the perioperative mortality rate.

TABLE 4-2. Physical Status Classification of the American Society of Anesthesiologists*

Class[a]	Description	Mortality rate (%)
1	Healthy patient	0.06–0.08
2	Mild systemic disease	0.27–0.4
3	Severe systemic disease, not incapacitating	1.8–4.3
4	Severe systemic disease that is a constant threat to life	7.8–23
5	Moribund, not expected to live 24 h irrespective of operation	9.4–51

[a]Refs: 7, 8
** An E is added to ASA status to designate an emergency operation.

Underlying disease is only one of many factors that contribute to perioperative complications. ASA physical status classification is a useful tool in planning anesthetic management and level of intraprocedural monitoring and it can be used by the interventionalist to categorize potential procedural risk.[8] In some institutions, ASA classification is used as criterion for calling an anesthesia consultation for procedural management in interventional radiology.

Patients receiving intravenous conscious sedation should recover in an area where continuous monitoring and resuscitative equipment are available. Patients should be monitored to full recovery by a return to baseline mental status and vital signs. Many institutions utilize an objective scoring system, such as the Aldrete or modified Aldrete score.[9,10] The Aldrete system scores patients from 0 to 2 on five parameters: activity, respiration, circulation (blood pressure), consciousness, and skin color. Return to physiologic baseline or an adequate pre-set score on these parameters is required for discharge from the procedure area (intensive monitoring, phase I) to a less intensive recovery area (phase II). Additional discharge criteria from the phase II area may include the ability to tolerate the fluids taken orally, minimal or absent nausea or vomiting, lack of dizziness when sitting, a complete

return to the baseline level of consciousness, absence of pain, and ability to urinate.[4] If short-acting sedation agents have been used, some patients may be discharged from this area in as little as 1 hour, but other procedural factors may mandate longer observation (e.g., the presence of an arterial puncture site or the need to watch for bleeding after deep organ biopsy). When short-acting reversal agents are used during the procedure, it is essential to observe the patient for a sufficient time to allow observation of the reemerging effects of the longer-acting agonists; this is typically 2 hours if short-acting benzodiazepines and opioids have been used. Patients should be cautioned not to drive or operate heavy machinery for at least 24 hours after the administration of analgesic sedative agents. Patients should not be sent home with pain that cannot be controlled with oral analgesics, and they should have 24 hour emergency contacts and written postoperative instructions before discharge.

REFERENCES

1. American College of Radiology. Standard for use of intravenous conscious sedation. *1998 ACR Standards*. Reston, VA: ACR; 1998
2. Ramsey MAE, Savage TM, Simpson TRJ, Goodwin R. Controlled sedation with alphaxalone-alphadolone. *BMJ* 1974;2:656–659.
3. American College of Radiology. Standard for pediatric sedation/analgesia. *1998 ACR Standards*. Reston, VA: ACR, 1998.
4. Watson DS. *Conscious Sedation/Analgesia*. St. Louis: Mosby; 1998.
5. Westmiller SW, Hoffman LA, Wiseman M. Understanding transtracheal oxygen delivery. *Nursing* 1989; 12:43–47.
6. Morgan GE, Mikhail MS. *Clinical Anesthesiology*. Norwalk: Appleton & Lange; 1992.
7. Dripps RD, Lamont A, Eckenhoff JE. The role of anesthesia in surgical mortality. *JAMA* 1961;178:261.
8. Muravchick S. *The Anesthetic Plan: From Physiologic Principles to Clinical Strategies*. St. Louis: Mosby Year Book; 1991.
9. Aldrete JA, Kroulik D. A postanesthetic recovery score. *Anesth Analg* 1970;49(6):924–934.
10. Aldrete JA. Modifications to the postanesthesia score for use in ambulatory surgery. *J Perianesth Nurs* 1998;13(3):148–155.

5

Magnetic Resonance and Computed Tomographic Angiography

JOHN A. KAUFMAN

The choice of an imaging modality for patients with vascular disease is no longer straightforward. Conventional angiography has benefited greatly from the development of safer contrast agents, sophisticated catheters and guidewires, and digitally enhanced image acquisition. Innovations in cross-sectional imaging technology, however, have resulted in a number of less invasive vascular imaging modalities. It is now conceivable that in a single institution the following menu could exist for vascular imaging: film-screen angiography, intraarterial digital subtraction angiography (IADSA), intravenous DSA (IVDSA), magnetic resonance angiography (MRA), computed tomographic angiography (CTA), duplex and color-flow ultrasound, contrast enhanced ultrasound, transesophageal/transluminal ultrasound, three-dimensional ultrasound, intravascular ultrasound, and isotope angiography. How does one choose the correct test, or is there such a thing? This chapter focuses on two of these modalities: CTA and MRA and when each should be used.

The ideal vascular imaging modality would be rapid, accurate, painless, risk free, applicable to all patients, easy to interpret, and inexpensive. Because of its proven accuracy and wide acceptance by clinicians, traditional angiography is the standard against which all new modalities must be compared. Traditional angiography provides reliable diagnostic images and is applicable to large numbers of patients, but it is associated with some degree of discomfort and risk.[1] MRA and CTA hold promise as noninvasive imaging modalities that can provide accurate angiographic information quickly in large numbers of patients. Both modalities have different strengths and weaknesses, which in many cases are complementary.[2] The clinical evaluation and application of MRA and CTA

are ongoing, yet there is no doubt that these techniques will have important roles in vascular imaging in the future.

■ Basic Techniques

MR imaging/MRA

Principles of MR imaging

One need only understand that MR imaging (MRI) is based on the detection of radiofrequency signals emitted by protons spinning within a powerful magnetic field. In the bore of an MR scanner, protons in tissue preferentially align the axes of their spins with the magnetic field (*longitudinal magnetization*). By applying a radiofrequency pulse to the protons, the spins can be deflected momentarily, or "tipped," out of alignment with the magnetic field, in a plane perpendicular to the magnetic field (*transverse magnetization*). The degree of deflection is determined by characteristics of the radiofrequency pulse and is described as the flip angle. As the protons realign with the magnetic field (*relaxation*), a signal (*echo*) is created. Images are created that emphasize the vectors of the longitudinal (*T1*) or transverse (*T2*) relaxation of the spins as they realign. In general, short echo times reflect the longitudinal magnetization (*T1 weighted*), and long echo times the transverse magnetization (*T2 weighted*). By varying how often and how forcefully the protons are tipped, as well as when the echo is sampled, the same tissue may appear alternatively bright or dark. The complex behavior of protons in magnetic fields provides the basis for the wide variety of pulse sequences and imaging strategies available in MRI.

MRI technology

Most first-generation of MR scanners were constructed using a central tunnel or bore lined with coiled superconducting wires. Generally, the higher the field strength (measured in Tesla [T], and ranging from 0.3 to 1.5 T for most clinical scanners), the larger the actual scanner and the higher the signal-to-noise ratio in the images. Although these scanners remain in active clinical use, newer "open" magnet designs are becoming available. These scanners offer the practical advantages of accommodating larger patients than the older devices as well as presenting a less confined scanning environment to claustrophobic patients. Of great interest to vascular and interventional radiologists is the possibility of performing MR-guided procedures in magnets with open designs that permit access to the patient during scan acquisition. Sophisticated targeting and device tracking technology is required in this environment, and special equipment construction is necessary for working within the strong magnetic field. Nevertheless, this technology offers great promise, particularly in patients in whom pathologic processes can be imaged only by using MRI.[3]

Principles of MRA

One of the most common non-contrast enhanced applications of MRI in vascular and interventional radiology is MRA. Early in the clinical application of MRI, it was noted that flowing blood sometimes appeared bright on images of the brain and body. The brightness of the blood suggested that angiographic information could be obtained without catheterization and injection of iodinated contrast agents. In a landmark article in *Science* in 1985, Wedeen and co-workers published the first true angiographic images created using MR techniques.[4] The initial clinical applications of MRA were in the intracranial arterial circulation and the extracranial carotid arteries. Now MRA is performed in all areas of the body, with the most common nonneurological applications being lower-extremity arteries and veins, the abdominal aorta, the renal arteries, the portal veins, and the thoracic aorta.[5–14]

The two most common MRA techniques are time-of-flight (TOF) and phase-contrast (PC) MRA. Both techniques can be used to acquire data on a slice-by-slice basis [two-dimensional (2-D)] or as a volume acquisition [three-dimensional (3-D)]. In general, thinner images can be obtained using 3-D techniques, but signal-to-noise is better in 2-D images. Acquisitions also may be cardiac gated, so that images are obtained at the same level throughout the cardiac cycle or at different levels at the same point in the cardiac cycle. Images obtained at one level throughout the cardiac cycle can be displayed in a

movie loop (*cine*), which is useful in situations such as evaluting cardiac valvular competence. Gating to obtain images at multiple levels at the same point in the cardiac cycle minimizes pulsatility artifact and signal loss in multiphasic flow.

TOF/MRA

The most widely available MRA technique for body applications is TOF MRA. With this technique, stationary tissues are subjected to multiple and frequent radiofrequency pulses; so the spins do not have time to realign (*relax*) with the magnetic field, resulting in saturation of the tissues and only a weak signal. Blood that flows into the area being imaged contains spins that have not yet been subjected to the radiofrequency pulses. These fresh, or unsaturated, spins emit a strong signal when they first enter the area being imaged and thus appear bright (Fig. 5-1). If the blood is exposed to the radiofrequency pulses for any length of time, however, it will become saturated and indistinguishable from the surrounding stationary tissues. This problem is particularly troublesome when using 3-D or volume imaging or when vessels are in the plane of a 2-D slice (Fig. 5-2).

Flow from all directions into a slice or volume will be visualized during MRA unless measures are taken to select flow in the direction of interest. With TOF MRA this visualization usually can be accomplished by saturating the spins in unwanted blood with radiofrequency pulses before they enter the area being imaged. These radiofrequency pulses are applied in a broad presaturation slab positioned outside the area of interest (Fig. 5-3). For example, with 2-D TOF MRA of the lower extremity arteries, source images are acquired in the axial plane; to

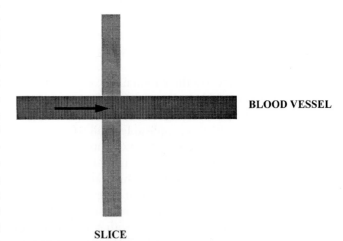

BLOOD VESSEL

SLICE

FIGURE 5-1. Schematic diagram of time-of-flight magnetic resonance angiography. Signal from background tissues is suppressed by repetitive radiofrequency pulses. Signal is emitted from the fresh spins in blood as it enters the imaging volume or slice.

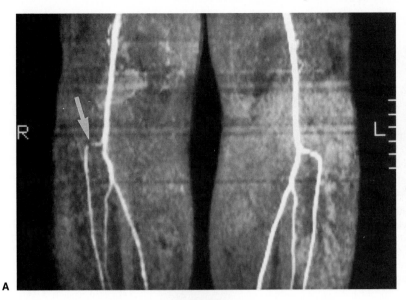

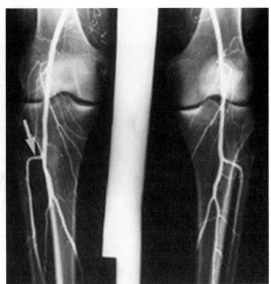

A

B

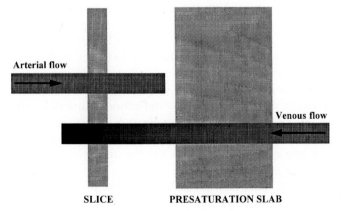

C

SLICE

FIGURE 5-2. Saturation of signal from in-plane flow. **A:** Coronal maximum intensity projection of a two-dimensional time-of-flight magnetic resonance angiogram of the popliteal arteries and proximal tibial arteries. The source images were acquired in the axial plane. There is loss of signal in the horizontal (in-plane) portion of the right anterior tibial artery origin (*arrow*), which could be due to either a stenosis or artifactual signal loss. **B:** Conventional angiogram of the same patient shows that this artery is normal (*arrow*). **C:** Schematic diagram illustrating saturation of in-plane flow.

Arterial flow

Venous flow

SLICE   PRESATURATION SLAB

FIGURE 5-3. Saturation slabs are critical in time-of-flight imaging to eliminate unwanted signal from flowing blood. In this schematic, arterial blood entering the slice from the left contains fresh spins that can be imaged. The spins in venous blood are saturated when they pass through a saturation slab outside of the imaging slice, so that no signal is emitted when they enter the slice.

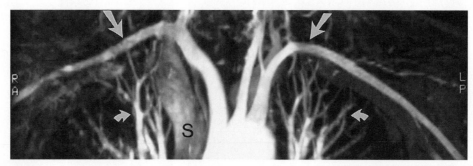

FIGURE 5-4. Gadolinium-enhanced, three-dimensional magnetic resonance angiogram of a normal aortic arch. Note that the subclavian artery flow (*arrows*), which reverses direction within the imaging volume, does not become saturated, and retains excellent signal because of the gadolinium. The pulmonary arteries and veins (*curved arrows*) are visible within the chest. The superior vena cava (S) is faintly seen as a result of rapid shunting of gadolinium through the cerebral circulation and enhancement of the jugular veins and subsequently the superior vena cava.

eliminate signal from the veins, a presaturation slab is placed inferior to the slice of interest (i.e., toward the feet), thus saturating spins in the venous blood before they flow into the slice. To obtain a 2-D TOF MR venogram of the lower extremities, the presaturation slab is repositioned superior (i.e., toward the head) to the slice of interest to saturate the spins in the arterial blood before they flow into the slice. Care must be taken when imaging tortuous vessels, however, as they may loop into the presaturation slab and appear occluded on the MRA.

Flowing blood produces the brightest signal when the spins all move at the same velocity, in the same direction, and perpendicular to the plane of image acquisition. Unfortunately, blood flow is complex in vivo as a result of such diverse factors as shear along the vessel wall; changes in velocity and acceleration resulting from cardiac activity, elastic recoil of arterial walls, and stenoses; and turbulence caused by tortuosity of blood vessels, aneurysms, or stenoses. Each of these factors results in some loss of signal from blood with all MRA techniques. Strategies to reduce this signal loss include techniques such as flow compensation and cardiac gating, but all incur a time penalty.

Gadolinium-enhanced MRA

One of the most effective strategies to increase intravascular signal with TOF sequences is the addition of an MR contrast agent, such as gadolinium, as described by Prince.[15] This agent has been applied most successfully to 3-D acquisitions, although it can be used with 2-D imaging as well. Gadolinium-based contrast agents act to shorten the T1 of blood and tissues. In conventional MRI, a dose of 0.1 mmol/kg (0.2 mL/kg) is administered intravenously before the patient is placed in the scanner to evaluate the soft tissues. For vascular imaging, a relatively large volume of gadolinium contrast (up to 0.4 mmol/kg, or 0.8 mL/kg) is injected rapidly during the acquisition of a 3-D volume. The arteries are preferentially enhanced, much in the same fashion that arteries are visualized during rapid venous injection of iodinated contrast agents with IVDSA. This technique eliminates loss of signal resulting from slow, turbulent, or in-plane flow.[15] Large fields of view can be covered without signal loss in blood that remains within the imaging volume (Fig. 5-4). This technique has become widely used in body MRA.

PC MRA

PC MRA is both more complex and less widely available than TOF sequences because the demands on scanner hardware, particularly gradient coils, are greater with PC than with TOF MRA. The fundamental principles of PC MRA are that gradients vary in strength within the magnetic field, and the phase of a spin will vary in proportion to the strength and duration of an applied magnetic gradient (Fig. 5-5). If equal and opposite gradients are applied, a spin that remains stationary will deflect in an equal and opposite manner. When the vectors of these opposite and equal deflections are subtracted, the net value (or *phase shift*) is zero. When a moving spin is exposed to the same equal and opposite gradients, the spinning proton moves to a physically different place within the magnet during the time between application of the gradients. The strength of the gradients varies depending on their location within the magnetic field. As a result, the vectors of the deflections caused by the gradients are opposite but not equal. Subtraction of these two opposite but unequal vectors results in a measurable net phase shift, which then can be displayed as signal, whereas stationary background tissues with a net phase shift of "0" have no signal. The larger the phase shift (the greater the distance that the spin moves or the larger the

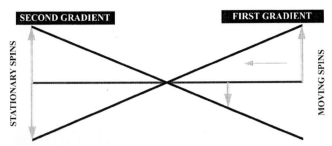

FIGURE 5-5. Schematic drawing of the principle of phase-contrast angiography. When stationary spins are exposed to equal and opposite gradient pulses, the deflections of the spins are equal and opposite; therefore, there is no net signal. When the same gradient pulses are applied to a moving spin, the deflections are opposite but not equal because of variation in gradient strength within the magnet. Therefore, a net signal is created that can be imaged. (After Dumoulin CL, Souza SP, Pelc NJ. Phase sensitive flow imaging. In: Gottschalk A, ed. *Magnetic Resonance Angiography: Concepts and Applications.* Potchen EJ, Siebert JE, Haacke EM, St Louis: Mosby, 1993).

applied gradient), the stronger the signal. PC MRA is by definition a purely subtractive technique in that only moving spins will be visualized, with no need to saturate background tissues as in TOF techniques.

The direction of flow is an important consideration in PC MRA because phase shifts occur only in the direction of the phase encoding gradient. Blood flow in most areas of the body is complex, rather than unidirectional. Consider the right renal artery, which arises from a slightly anterior location on the abdominal aorta, curves posteriorly behind the inferior vena cava, and then curves inferiorly toward the renal hilum. Imaging only right-to-left flow in this artery would result in incomplete visualization of the proximal and distal portions of the vessel. By acquiring phase shifts in all three directions (right to left, superior to inferior, and anterior to posterior), a complete study of the vessel can be performed (Fig. 5-6). Unfortunately, one pair of gradients is required per direction to create phase shifts. With each set of gradients used, the time required to perform the study increases. Fortunately, flow in three directions can be imaged with four, rather than six, gradients using a technique known as Hadamard multiplexing. Nevertheless, the time required to complete a PC acquisition is long relative to TOF MRA.

One of the most critical elements of PC MRA is the velocity of the blood flow to be imaged. The goal of PC imaging is to maximize the phase shifts in flowing spins (large shifts result in brighter-appearing flow in the final images). Phase shift is directly proportional to several constants (such as the strength of the magnetic field) and to the variables of velocity of the spins and the amplitude of the gradients. Thus, larger gradients are required to im-

age slow flow and smaller gradients to image faster flow. The parameter that describes this relationship is *velocity encoding* (V_{enc}), usually calibrated in centimeters per second. For example, normal main renal artery flow is approximately 100 cm/sec; so one would select a V_{enc} slightly higher than the expected flow (perhaps 110 cm/sec) to optimize visualization of flow in this portion of the vessel. Flow at other velocities (such as in the peripheral intrarenal arteries) will not image as well. Furthermore, if the flow is slower than expected, perhaps because of severe occlusive disease in the artery or poor cardiac output, imaging at a high V_{enc} will result in poor visualization of the main renal artery flow. Currently, there is no widely available method for quickly determining which V_{enc} will result in the best image for a particular vessel in a particular patient. This limitation of PC MRA is one of the major impediments to more widespread application of this technique.

The information acquired during PC MRA can be processed in several ways. The most common technique is *phase difference,* in which phase shifts are assigned a pixel value and color based on the value of the subtracted phase angle (Fig. 5-7). The intensity of the pixel reflects the size of the phase shift, with the most intense pixels representing flow closest to the value of the V_{enc}. Directional information can be provided easily by displaying the pixels as either black or white; spins moving in the direction of the velocity gradients appear white, and those moving in the opposite direction appear black. Spins moving in a direction at right angles to the velocity gradients have no signal. A common artifact is the abrupt transition of one pixel color to another that occurs when the velocity of flow exceeds the V_{enc}, termed *aliasing,* and is easily recognized by the irregular interface between the two colors caused by the pixel edges (Fig. 5-8).

Limitations

All MRA techniques are subject to certain limitations. Patients with pacemakers, intraocular or intraaural metallic foreign bodies, or claustrophobia cannot undergo imaging. Most MR units carefully screen patients with both a questionnaire and a brief interview with the technologist before scanning. Patients who are hemodynamically unstable require careful monitoring during scanning using specialized equipment that is compatible with strong magnetic fields. Turbulent flow (such as immediately distal to a stenosis) is difficult to image with non-gadolinium-enhanced techniques, as the spins are extremely disorganized in orientation and appear as areas of signal loss. Lastly, uncooperative patients or those with dementia may not be able to remain still during image acquisition, introducing motion artifacts that can render a study uninterpretable.

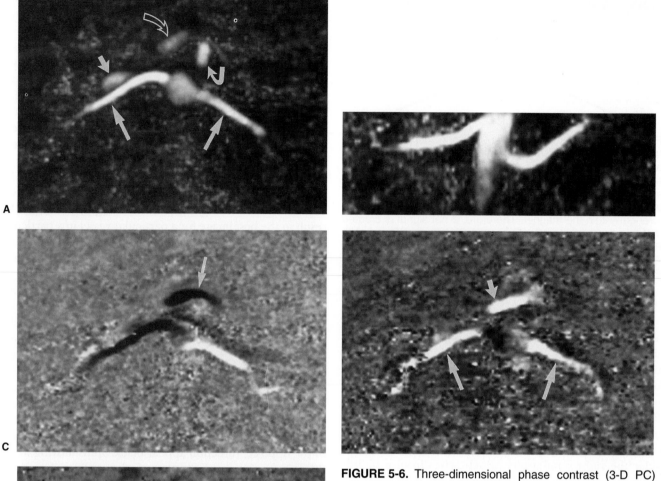

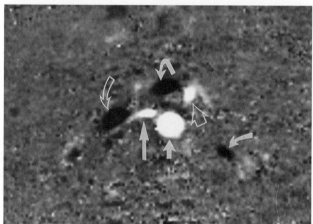

FIGURE 5-6. Three-dimensional phase contrast (3-D PC) magnetic resonance angiogram of the renal arteries of a normal volunteer illustrating the directional information produced by PC imaging. Velocity encoding was 100 cm/sec for this study, and flow in all three directions was imaged. **A:** Axial maximum intensity projection (MIP) of the speed images (all flow is white). Notice the anterior-to-posterior course of the renal arteries (*large straight arrows*). The inferior vena cava (IVC) (*small straight arrow*) is anterior to the right renal artery. The superior mesenteric artery (SMA) (*solid curved arrow*) and the superior mesenteric vein (SMV) (*open curved arrow*) are anterior to the aorta. The splenic vein can be seen anterior to the SMA. Note also the absence of any anatomic detail in the background. **B:** Coronal MIP of the same images. Notice the slightly caudal course of the right renal artery and the cranial course of the left renal artery. The tapered appearance of the distal aorta is due to loss of signal from saturation of spins within the 3-D imaging volume. **C:** Axial image showing right-to-left flow. The flow in the left renal artery is white (blood flows from the aorta to the left), whereas flow in the right renal artery is black (blood flows from the aorta to the right). Notice how the aorta and SMA are not well visualized. Why is flow in the splenic vein (*arrow*) black? **D:** Axial image showing anterior-to-posterior flow. The renal arteries (*large arrows*) are white because flow is posterior toward the kidneys (refer to A). The SMV (*small arrow*) is also white because it has a slighly posterior trajectory toward the portal vein. Again, notice how the aorta and SMA are not well seen. **E:** Axial image showing superior to inferior flow. Using the preceding four images, explain why the aorta (*short straight arrow*), SMA (*open straight arrow*), and proximal right renal artery (*long straight arrow*) are white, whereas the distal left renal artery (*curved arrow*), SMV (*tightly curved arrow*), and IVC (*open curved arrow*) are black.

a value that is an average of both. There is no way to separate these two structures retrospectively using current postprocessing techniques.

A major determinant of the value assigned to a voxel are its dimensions. If an image is constructed of voxels that are too large, small objects may get "lost" (partial volume averaging). The dimensions of voxels are determined by the field of view of an image, the slice thickness, and the matrix size. For example, in a 3-D MRA with a 20-cm field of view, a slice thickness of 2 mm, and a 256 × 256 matrix, the effective voxel size will be 0.8 × 0.8 × 2.0 mm. Because these voxels are rectangular, the highest resolution images will be obtained when viewing the data set from the angle that presents the voxels on end. When voxels are true cubes, they are considered isotropic and can be viewed with equal resolution from any angle. One of the objectives in MRA and CTA is to create source images that are composed of the smallest pixels and voxels possible while maintaining adequate signal-to-noise ratios (the smaller the voxel, the greater the impact of background noise). Matrices of 512 × 512 are routinely available with CTA, whereas 256 × 256 is more typical for MRA.

The most common technique for image postprocessing is maximum intensity projection (MIP), in which the highest value voxels within a stack of 2-D images or a 3-D volume are projected as a single image in any plane (Fig. 5-12). Multiple images can be created with incremental degrees of rotation around any axis. Restricted MIPs can be created easily by limiting the amount of the source data set to be projected. The chief advantage of this technique is that the low-intensity background structures are not projected, which results in images that are pleasing to view because of a very high signal-to-noise ratio. This is also the chief disadvantage of the technique, because subtle abnormalities present on source images may not appear on the final projection.[27]

A simple postprocessing technique that retains all the data present in source images is *reformatting*, a technique that essentially reslices the source data in different planes from the original acquisition. For example, a stack of axial images can be reformatted into images in the coronal or sagittal plane, or a curved reformat can be used to trace the path of a renal artery as it arises from the aorta and travels through the retroperitoneum (Fig. 5-13). The integrity of the source data is preserved while the structure of interest is depicted from the most advantageous angle. A major limitation of this technique is the extreme dependence on operator input to maintain accuracy: Appropriate selection of viewing planes or curves is essential for accurate diagnosis. Furthermore, reformatted images can only be one pixel or voxel thick, thus limiting the amount of data that can be displayed.

Segmentation techniques divide the image data sets into flow and nonflow groups, or "segments," using a number of different strategies. In *thresholding*, one of the most widely available methods of segmentation, an operator can set a threshold value below which all data are discarded. Other techniques include region-growing (*seed*) algorithms, in which the user defines a starting point within a vessel, and adjacent voxels are tested automatically for inclusion or exclusion. Segmentation techniques permit modification of large data sets to include only pertinent information. As with MIPs, insensitivity to subtle abnormalities is a major limitation unless these techniques are performed carefully.

3-D rendering techniques provide the most dramatic displays of MRA and CTA data. This form of postprocessing imparts a "real" appearance to the vessels in that they seem to have both volume and depth (Fig. 5-14). Spatial relationships are self-evident, rather than deduced. Colorization schemes can be superimposed on the images to emphasize various structures. The two most common displays are *surface* or *volume rendering*. The former is a representation of the vascular data as a shell, and the latter presents the data as a solid object. These post-processing techniques usually are performed on independent workstations equipped with fast processors using proprietary software. Data sets must be edited heavily when using segmentation techniques and excision of unwanted portions of the images to produce satisfactory 3-D renderings.[28] In addition, the actual source images must have good contrast between vascular structures and background tissues. For these reasons, all 3-D renderings must be viewed with care before rendering a diagnosis, because important information can be omitted at several stages during creation of the final images. A fundamental rule of MRA and CTA is that the source images always must be reviewed whenever a questionable finding is present on any type of postprocessed image.

■ Specific Applications

Lower-extremity arteries

Peripheral arterial occlusive disease is a common problem in developed countries. The evaluation of patients with claudication, rest pain, or tissue loss begins with an accurate history, a careful physical examination, and noninvasive tests, such as pulse-volume recordings. Before any intervention, accurate morphologic information about the lower-extremity arteries is required. Conventional angiography is the "gold standard" method for acquiring these data, despite its invasive nature. Among the noninvasive techniques, MRA is particularly suited to evaluation of lower-extremity occlusive disease. In some centers, MRA has become the primary means of imaging these patients.[5]

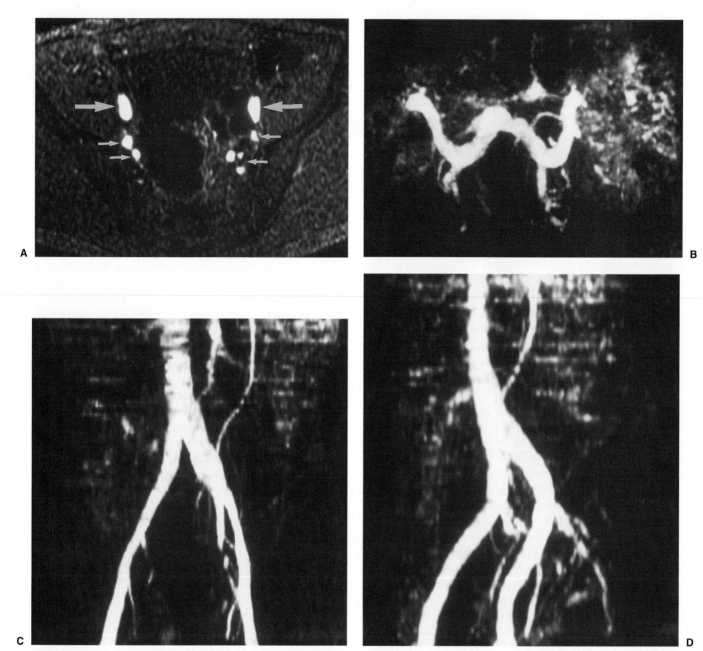

FIGURE 5-12. Maximum intensity projection (MIP) display of a two-dimensional time-of-flight magnetic resonance (MR) venogram of the pelvis. **A:** Axial slice from the source MR venogram shows the external iliac veins (*large arrows*) and branches of the external iliac veins (*small arrows*). Note the excellent background signal suppression. **B:** Axial projection of a MIP of the entire stack of axial slices. The vague area of increased signal in the upper right of the image is due to bowel motion. **C:** Coronal projection of a MIP of the entire stack of slices creates a display of the data that looks like a venogram. **D:** Right posterior oblique projection of the MIP of the entire stack of slices shows the 3-dimensional relationships that can be demonstrated with this technique. (*Continued*)

MRA

Flow in the normal peripheral muscular arteries is pulsatile, with a triphasic wave form (rapid forward flow with systole, a brief period of retrograde flow as the aortic valve closes, and then slow forward flow during diastole). In the presence of occlusive disease, flow becomes slow and nonpulsatile. This type of flow is ideal for imaging with 2-D TOF sequences. Most lower-extremity MRA protocols are based in part on 2-D TOF techniques, with image acquisition in the axial plane, and an inferior saturation band to mask venous flow. Imaging acquisition in the axial plane is used because flow in most of the peripheral arterial segments will be perpendicular to the slice and thus have maximal flow-related enhancement. Two

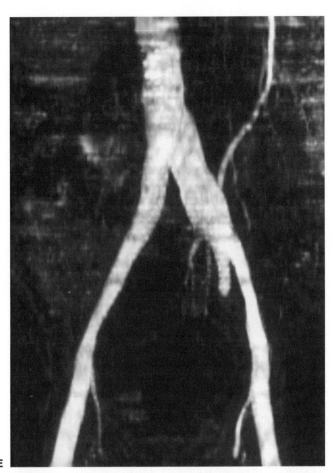

E

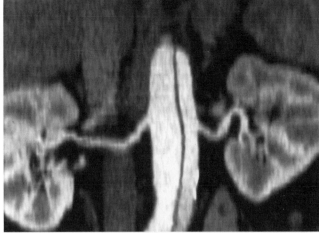

A

Path of tracing for curved coronal reformat

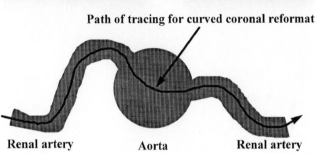

Renal artery   Aorta   Renal artery

Axial Slice   B

FIGURE 5-12. (*Continued*) E: Restricted coronal MIP of the central 4 cm of each slice improves the appearance of the final image by eliminating much of the background noise. Note that the internal iliac veins are truncated because they are excluded from the MIP.

FIGURE 5-13. Curved coronal reformation of the renal arteries from a computed tomographic angiogram of a patient with an aortic dissection. **A:** This coronal image, which is 1 pixel thick, was created by tracing the course of the renal arteries through the retroperitoneum from the axial source images. This explains why the aorta appears truncated at the top of the image. **B:** Schematic showing how the curved coronal reformat is proscribed from the axial source image.

areas where this is not true, and thus where in-plane saturation is difficult, are tortuous iliac arteries in the pelvis and the origin of the anterior tibial artery. Typical slice thicknesses are 1.5 to 3.0 mm, with the highest-resolution images obtained when imaging with thin slices, high matrices, and small fields of view. Recently, gadolinium-enhanced 3-D acquisitions of the aorta, pelvis, and thighs have replaced 2-D TOF as the primary imaging technique. 2-D TOF remains important for imaging the tibial and pedal vessels. The pelvis and thigh usually can be imaged in the body coil, but the lower extremities must be imaged in either the extremity or the head coil to achieve consistent diagnostic results (Fig. 5-15). The average study requires 1 to 2 hours to image from the toes to the aortic bifurcation.

One of the chief advantages of MRA in imaging distal vessels is that extremely slow flow beyond occlusions is detected easily using this technique, but it is sometimes difficult to demonstrate with conventional angiography if collateral formation is poor (Fig. 5-16). Although results

vary among institutions, depending on the specifics of both the MR and the conventional angiographic techniques, there is no doubt that MRA is an excellent method for imaging the pedal vessels in the presence of extensive proximal occlusive disease.[5] A major disadvantage of MRA is that it is sometimes difficult to determine the quality of the vessel, as calcium is not seen on these images. Retrograde flow below an occlusion is frequently saturated by the inferior saturation band in 2-D TOF imaging, thus making an occlusion appear longer than it actually is.

The pelvic arteries can be difficult to image accurately by using 2-D TOF techniques if the vessels are tortuous or aneurysmal. Contrast-enhanced MRA using rapid injection of gadolinium chelates during acquisition of a 3-D TOF sequence has largely resolved this issue (Fig. 5-17). Pitfalls of this technique include difficulty with timing of contrast injections when ultrafast acquisitions are used.

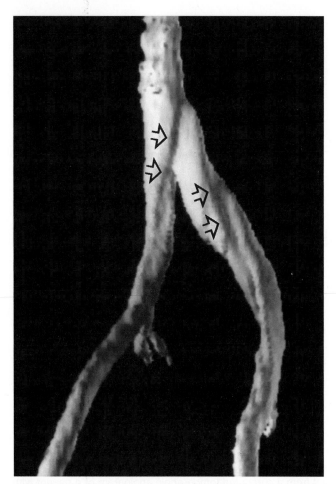

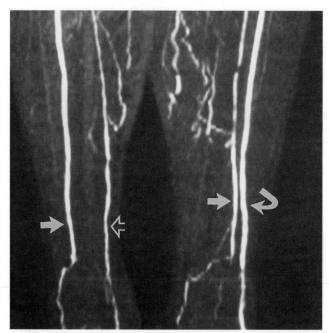

FIGURE 5-15. Coronal maximum intensity projection of a two-dimensional time-of-flight magnetic resonance angiogram of the tibial arteries in a patient with occlusion of the external iliac, femoral, and popliteal arteries bilaterally. Performed in the head coil, both legs were imaged at the same time. On the patient's right, the peroneal (*solid arrow*) and posterior tibial (*open arrow*) arteries are patent. On the patient's left, the peroneal (*solid arrow*) and anterior tibial (*curved arrow*) arteries are patent. Multiple small collateral vessels are present in the medial calf bilaterally.

FIGURE 5-14. Shaded surface display of the two-dimensional time-of-flight pelvic magnetic resonance venogram from Figure 5-12. Note that the three-dimensional display allows appreciation of such details as the impression on the inferior vena cava and iliac veins by the common iliac arteries (*arrows*).

In addition to occlusive disease, other uses of lower-extremity MRA include evaluation of tibial vessels before plastic reconstructive procedures, staging of vascular malformations and tumors, and diagnosis of popliteal artery entrapment by anomalous muscular or tendonous structures.

Limitations

There are many limitations of MRA of the lower extremities; careful patient selection is therefore important to avoid unnecessary examinations. Patients who are uncooperative, subject to frequent involuntary movements, or claustrophobic, or who have metallic joint prostheses in the extremity of interest should not undergo MRA because the studies undoubtedly will be inadequate or incomplete. MRA does not have the image resolution to detect subtle intimal irregularities or to distinguish between atherosclerosis and other types of occlusive disease such as arteritis. Patients who will clearly require a catheter-based intervention based on history, physical examination, and noninvasive studies, should proceed directly to angiography if access to MR scanners is limited. Lastly, patients with traumatized or acutely ischemic, threatened limbs should not be studied with MRA because valuable time may be lost if the study is inadequate or a catheter-based intervention is needed.

CTA

The role of CTA in the evaluation of peripheral vascular occlusive disease is dependent on the anatomic area that must be imaged. CTA of the infrainguinal runoff is subject to the same limitations as conventional contrast angiography: Vessels distal to severe proximal occlusive disease are difficult to opacify with contrast. In general, this is not a good modality for studying diseased infrapopliteal and pedal arteries. CTA is an excellent modality for evaluation of the pelvic and femoropopliteal arteries, because there is no degradation of the images as a result of tortuousity or the presence of aneurysms. In addition, there is little movement of retroperitoneal structures in the pelvis with respiration compared with the abdomen, so breath-holding is less of an issue. In many cases, pelvic CTA is combined with a study of the abdominal aorta.

High-quality pelvic CT angiograms can be obtained using injection of contrast (60% iodine) at 3 to 5 mL/sec, 5 mm collimation, and a pitch of 1 to 2. An appropriate delay should be used, preferably calculated from a test bolus of 20 mL and sequential acquisition of slices at the aortic bifurcation over 20 to 30 secs. Bowel contrast should be avoided, as high density barium or gastrografin interferes with subsequent image postprocessing. Diagnostic lower-extremity studies from the inguinal ligament to the midcalf can be acquired using a 5-mm collimation, a pitch of 1,200 mL of contrast injected at 2 to 3 mL/sec, and two 60-sec. spirals.[21] It should be kept in mind that the average conventional bilateral lower-extremity angiogram requires 70 to 100 mL of contrast.

An advantage of CTA over MRA in the peripheral vessels is that the study is always performed with contrast, so that pulsatility, turbulence, and retrograde or in-plane flow do not degrade image quality. For example, cross-femoral grafts are imaged easily by CTA.

Limitations

Major limitations of CTA are the large amount of iodinated contrast required, and the difficulty of grading the degree of stenosis in the presence of heavy vascular calcification.

Lower-extremity veins and the inferior vena cava

MR venography

Blood flow in veins is, as a rule, slower and less pulsatile than flow in adjacent arteries. Most MRA techniques favor blood flow with these exact characteristics. Indeed, MR venography has proved a highly accurate means of evaluation of the lower-extremity and pelvic veins and the inferior vena cava. In most studies, the sensitivity and specificity for detection of lower-extremity deep venous thrombosis with MR venography exceed 90%.[8]

The indications for MR venography include detection of thrombus; evaluation of anomalous lower-extremity venous drainage, such as Klippel-Trenauny disease; and presurgical evaluation of venous anatomy in patients with suspected intracaval extension of renal cell carcinoma. In most institutions, lower-extremity ultrasound is the study of choice (on both the basis of cost and availability) for detection of infrainguinal deep venous thrombosis, and MR venography is useful for documenting pelvic extent or origin of thrombus, as this anatomic region is an important "blind spot" for ultrasound (Fig. 5-18).

The most commonly applied technique for MR venography is 2-D TOF, because of its sensitivity to slow flow and its ability to cover large anatomic areas.[8] To select venous flow, the saturation band is placed over the arterial inflow (superior if axial slices are used). Thicker slices are used with MR venography than with MRA, because the detection of thrombus does not require the same resolution in all planes as grading of stenoses. The thicker slices also permit more anatomic coverage in less time. Other than increased slice thickness and repositioning the saturation band, little modification is required of arterial 2-D TOF sequences; however, anatomic T1-weighted images are an important part of pelvic and abdominal MR venography with which to exclude the presence of extrinsic compression of venous structures by masses.

CT venography

The indications for CT evaluation of the lower extremity and pelvic veins, and the inferior vena cava are the same as MR venography. CT is a highly accurate means of evaluating the pelvic veins and inferior vena cava for patency and involvement by masses. An advantage of CT of the veins in the pelvis and abdomen is the acquisition of useful cross-sectional anatomic information about extravascular structures. A major limitation is the demand placed on the tube by the large area (ankles to inferior vena cava) that must be covered in patients with suspected thromboembolic disease.

Lower-extremity CT venography can be performed by direct injection of contrast into the extremity under evaluation. Dilute contrast injected at a low rate (Omni 300 or equivalent diluted 1:5 with normal saline and injected at 2 mL/sec), with a 35-sec. delay, 10-mm collimation, and a pitch of 2 will permit examination of the lower extremity from the ankle to the inferior vena cava (17). Although initial results are promising, the indications for extremity CT venography have yet to be determined. In certain situations, the cross-sectional images obtained with CT venography may be essential to resolve complex anatomic relationships, an extrinsic lesion with mass effect on a vein, or to characterize an intravascular process.

The pelvic veins and inferior vena cava also can be imaged by infusion of contrast into a peripheral upper extremity vein. Contrast is injected at a lower rate than for CTA (2–3 mL/sec), and a delay sufficient to allow venous enhancement is used. Scanning too soon will result in differential opacification of the vena cava at the level of the renal veins, which may lead to interpretive errors. The thickness of the collimation will vary with the desired degree of coverage, but 5 mm should be adequate for most cases. Similarly, the pitch will vary from 1 to 2 based on the amount of coverage required. Breath-holding is necessary for optimal helical CT studies of the inferior vena cava.

Abdominal aorta and visceral branches

The primary indications for MRA and CTA of the abdominal aorta and its visceral branches are preoperative staging of aortic aneurysms or occlusions, diagnosis of

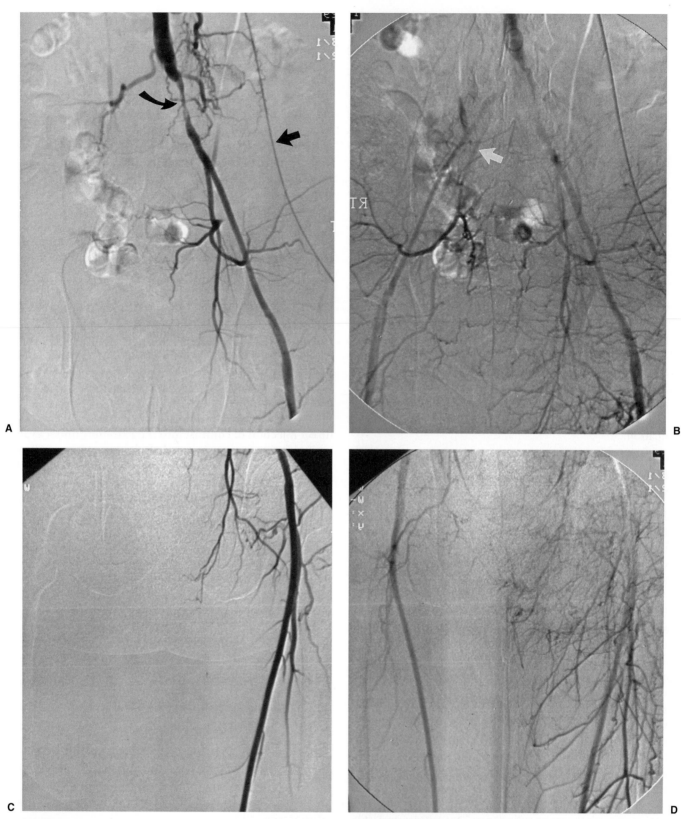

FIGURE 5-16. Comparison of conventional angiography and two-dimensional time-of-flight (2-D TOF) magnetic resonance (MR) angiography in a patient with severe aortoiliac occlusive disease and absent femoral pulses. **A:** Digital subtraction angiogram (DSA) of the pelvis. The study was performed by translumbar puncture of the upper abdominal aorta (*straight arrow* = catheter). Note the severe left common iliac artery stenosis (*curved arrow*) and occlusion of the right common iliac artery. **B:** Delayed image from the same injection shows reconstitution of the right external iliac artery via the right hypogastric artery (*arrow*). **C:** Early image from DSA of the femoral arteries in the same patient shows opacification of vessels on the left but not the right. **D:** Late image from the same injection as C shows delayed faint opacification of the femoral vessels on the right. (*Continued*)

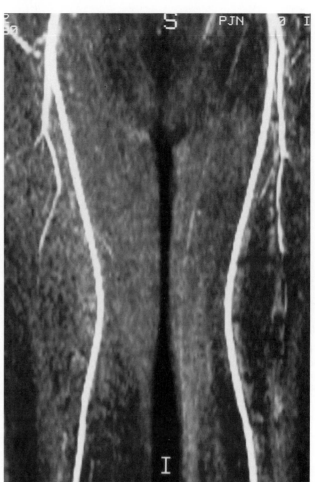

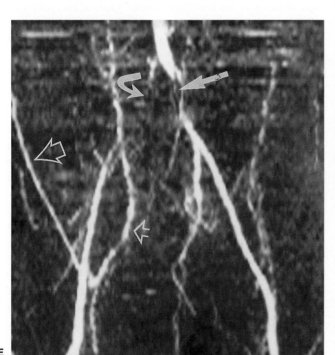

E   F

FIGURE 5-16. (*Continued*) E: Coronal maximum intensity projection (MIP) of the 2-D TOF MR angiogram of the same patient shows severe stenosis of the left common iliac artery (*straight arrow*) and occlusion of the right common iliac artery (*curved arrow*). Note the visualization of flow in the right iliac-circumflex artery (*large open arrow*) and right inferior epigastric artery (*small open arrow*) but not on the left. These vessels are seen because they act as collaterals to the right leg in this patient with right common iliac artery occlusion. F: Coronal MIP of the 2-D TOF MR angiogram of the same patient shows excellent bilateral visualization of vessels.

renal artery stenosis, and evaluation of abdominal extension of aortic dissection.[9,11,12,15,19,29] Additional indications include evaluation of renal artery anatomy in transplant donors, diagnosis of mesenteric ischemia resulting from proximal superior mesenteric artery occlusion, and depiction of hepatic artery anatomy in potential liver transplant recipients.[16,25] Neither study should be obtained for suspected acute rupture of an abdominal aortic aneurysm, as this diagnosis can be made most expeditiously by a noncontrast CT scan of the abdomen (the presence of an abdominal aortic aneurysm and high attenuation blood in the retroperitoneum or peritoneum).

MRA and CTA are reported to be highly accurate in the evaluation of the abdominal aorta and its branches, although large prospective comparative studies are lacking.[11–13,15,16,23,25] The image resolution of both techniques is less than that of conventional angiography; so it

is not uncommon to miss small accessory renal arteries or subtle intimal abnormalities. MRA does not require iodinated contrast (and therefore can be used with impunity in patients with renal failure or contrast allergies), but it can be difficult to obtain because the number of MR scanners is limited. CTA is more readily available and easier to perform than MRA but it requires large volumes of iodinated contrast (sometimes in excess of that used for conventional angiography).

MRA

A complete MR examination of the abdominal aorta and its branches requires both anatomic T1-weighted images and flow-sensitive sequences.[11] The anatomic sequences are essential for evaluation of vessel morphology and the solid organs. Occasionally, important coincidental pa-

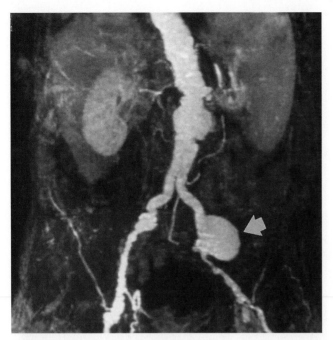

FIGURE 5-17. Coronal maximum intensity projection of a gadolinium enhanced three-dimensional magnetic resonance angiogram of the aorta and pelvis in patient with a prior aorto-biliac graft. A large left iliac artery anastomatic pseudoaneurysm (*arrow*) is clearly demonstrated. Note the absence of signal loss in this aneurysm.

thology such as renal carcinomas may be detected. Because background signal is suppressed in MRA, aneurysms lined with mural thrombus may be easily overlooked on flow sequences.

MRA of the abdominal aorta can be performed with both TOF or PC sequences;[11,12] however, imaging of the whole abdominal aorta can be time consuming and requires large fields of view in which loss of signal as a result of saturation can be troublesome. Gadolinium-enhanced 3-D MRA obviates many of the limitations of standard TOF and PC sequences in the abdomen.[15] This technique permits image acquisition in the coronal plane, with fields of view large enough to cover the area from the diaphragm to the inguinal ligament (Fig. 5-17). This is important in evaluation of aortic aneurysms or dissections, because detection of both the proximal and the distal extent of these lesions is crucial for management. With ultrafast pulse sequences, gadolinium-enhanced abdominal MRAs can be obtained in a single breath-hold.[21]

MRA of the renal and visceral arteries is a much more focused examination than aortic studies. Usually, a T1-weighted sequence is used to localize the vessels of interest (we find the sagittal plane is best). Whenever possible, flow sequences are constructed with thin slices (1.5–2.0 mm), high-resolution matrices (256 × 256 or 512 × 512), and a plane of acquisition that will maximize the likeli-

hood of including the entire vessel of interest. The most widely used sequence is gadolinium-enhanced 3-D MRA (Fig. 5-19) in the coronal plane. In general, the highest accuracy of MRA is for proximal atherosclerotic disease of the renal and visceral arteries.

Determination of the clinical importance of a renal artery stenosis can be difficult, particularly when the lesion appears to be less than severe. One of the potential advantages of MRA is that quantitative measurements of flow can be used as adjuncts to angiographic images in questionable cases.[30]

CTA

CTA of the abdominal aorta and its visceral branches provides information about vascular structures and adjacent organs with a single acquisition. In addition, vascular calcification is readily visible on CTA source images, but invisible on MR angiograms. This can be either a help or a hindrance, because visualization of calcification may aid in planning interventions, but it may obscure the origins of small vessels.[19,23] A crucial prerequisite for high-quality studies is the patient's ability to suspend respiration for 20 to 40 sec., because the visceral vessels move with normal breathing. As always, careful attention must be given to the delay between contrast injection and initiation of the scan. For patients with normal renal function, CTA is an excellent modality for evaluation of the abdominal arteries (Fig. 5-20).

Studies of the abdominal aorta usually are designed to use thin (3 mm) collimation at the level of the renal and proximal visceral arteries, and thicker (5–7 mm) collimation for the infrarenal aorta through the external iliac arteries.[29] In most patients, it is not possible to scan the abdominal aorta and iliac arteries with 3-mm collimation in a single breath-hold (even with a pitch of 2, this would require a scan of 1.5–2 min.). Some scanners are capable of variable pitch and collimation, whereas others require interruption of the scan in the mid-abdomen to change parameters. Contrast (60% iodine) should be injected at a rate of 3 to 5 mL/sec for a total volume of 120 to 150 mL.

When the focus of the study is evaluation of the renal and visceral branches of the aorta, extended anatomic coverage is less important. In general, the pelvic arteries do not need to be included in these acquisitions. Therefore, these studies can be tailored to maximize small-vessel detail with collimations of 3 mm and a pitch of 1 to 1.5.[19,23,25,29] Dense opacification with contrast is necessary to provide adequate visualization of the distal portions of vessels. If possible, contrast (60% iodine) should be injected at a rate of 5 mL/sec for a total volume of 120 to 150 mL. An important pitfall of renal and visceral CTA is densely calcified atherosclerotic plaque, which can make grading of degree of luminal stenosis difficult.

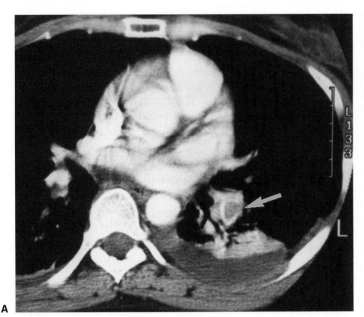 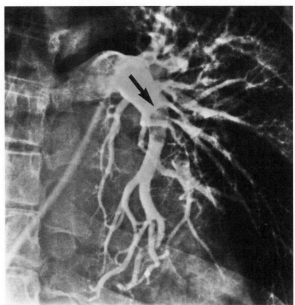

FIGURE 5-23. Diagnosis of pulmonary embolism by computed tomographic (CT) angiography. **A:** Axial slice from a CT angiogram shows an intraluminal filling defect (*arrow*) in the left lower lobe pulmonary artery. Note that there is also partial left lower lobe atelectasis and a left pleural effusion. **B:** Conventional selective left pulmonary angiogram on the same patient confirms the large embolus (*arrow*) in the left lower lobe pulmonary artery.

false-positive readings because of their proximity to interlobar pulmonary arteries, and interpretation in areas of pulmonary atelectasis or consolidation can be difficult.[22,35] Postprocessing such as oblique sagittal reformations or MIPs may help clarify questionable findings. A major advantage of helical CT for pulmonary embolism is that alternative thoracic pathology may be discovered that explains the patient's symptoms. Typical helical CT protocols for pulmonary embolism use injection rates of 3 to 5 mL/sec for 150 mL and lower concentrations of iodine to avoid streak artifact from dense opacification of the superior vena cava.[22] Other parameters include 3- to 5-mm collimation, a pitch of 1 to 1.7, and a 10- to 15-sec. delay, depending on the patient's hemodynamic status. Breath-holding is essential to minimize motion artifact.

Thoracic veins

Occlusion of the central veins of the chest can occur as a result of extrinsic compression by malignancy or inflammatory processes, invasion by tumor, or iatrogenic causes such as central venous access catheters or pacemakers. Patients may present with swelling localized to one arm when the occlusion is limited to the subclavian/brachiocephalic veins or facial swelling when the superior vena cava is involved. Although ultrasound is useful for the axillary, subclavian, and jugular veins, it cannot visualize the more central thoracic veins. Conventional upper-extremity venography is an excellent modality for evaluation of the patency of the peripheral and central veins,

but it provides no information about structures extrinsic to the veins. MRI and CT of the chest can provide both flow and anatomic information.

MR venography

The most widely used MR venographic technique for the thoracic veins is 2-D TOF, because of the sensitivity of the pulse sequence for slow flow and the short acquisition times.[14] Gadolinium-enhanced 3-D acquisitions show great promise in evaluation of the thoracic veins. Images can be acquired in any plane, although the axial and coronal planes are generally preferred. Relative to arterial studies, the slices for thoracic venography can be thick (2–4 mm), as the goal of the study is to image the large venous structures. Conventional T1-weighted images in the axial and coronal planes are important to permit evaluation of the perivascular tissues.

CT venography

CT evaluation of central venous occlusion provides information about both vascular patency and adjacent soft tissues with one acquisition but may require contrast injection into both upper extremities for complete evaluation. Dilute contrast (30%) should be used to minimize streak artifacts, and injection rates should be lower than for arterial studies (1–2 mL/sec for 80 mL). The base of the neck should be included in the area scanned to evaluate the patency of the jugular veins. Collimation of 5 to 7 mm, a pitch of 1 to 1.5, and a delay of 20 to 30 is sufficient for most patients.

Extracranial carotid arteries

Accurate imaging of the extracranial carotid arteries is a major priority in the management of patients at risk for, or with symptoms of, cerebrovascular disease. The importance of carotid artery imaging has been emphasized by recent studies suggesting that aggressive surgical treatment of internal carotid stenoses of 60 to 70% or greater reduction in diameter prevents stroke.[36,37] Although carotid noninvasive studies (CNIS) with duplex colorflow ultrasound are the most widely available and cost efficient means of carotid artery evaluation, MRA and CTA have major roles in carotid imaging. MRA and CTA may be used to confirm the results of CNIS or as a primary means of imaging the carotids in patients already undergoing MR or CT evaluation for cerebral ischemia. In many institutions conventional carotid angiography is now performed only to resolve disagreements between CNIS and MRA or CTA.

MRA

MRA of the carotids is one of the most widely accepted applications of this technique.[38] The carotid arteries are superficial, reliable in location, and subject to a limited range of pathology (primarily occlusive disease or dissection). These characteristics allow imaging with specialized coils designed to capitalize on the proximity of the carotid arteries to the anterior tissues of the neck. Typically, the "workhorse" sequence of carotid MRA is 2-D TOF (1.5-mm slices, with a superior saturation band to eliminate venous signal). Imaging of the carotid arteries from the level of the thoracic inlet to the petrous portion of the carotid is quick (7–9 mins.) using 2-D TOF MRA. Numerous studies have shown a 75 to 95% agreement between MRA and conventional angiography, and surgery can be performed safely on the basis of concordant high-quality CNIS and MR angiograms.[39]

There are several limitations to 2-D TOF MRA of the extracranial carotid and vertebral circulation. The general tendency to overestimate the degree of stenosis is a concern in situations in which surgery may be decided purely on the severity of the stenosis.[27] In general, a focal area of signal loss is indicative of a 70% or greater reduction in luminal diameter; however, extremely slow flow in an otherwise patent vessel (such as distal to a critical internal carotid artery stenosis) will appear as a complete occlusion due to saturation. Lastly, the superior saturation band will mask reversed arterial flow such as in the vertebral artery in the presence of a severe subclavian artery origin occlusive disease.[40]

Alternative MRI strategies of the carotid arteries include 3-D TOF and PC sequences, as well as gadolinium-enhanced 3-D TOF. The thinner partitions used with 3-D sequences reduce signal loss in areas of turbulence and improve the characterization of lesions. The amount of anatomic coverage is limited with non-contrast 3-D acquisitions because of long acquisition times and saturation of flow in large volumes. Strategies for increasing the area imaged include multiple overlapping thin 3-D TOF slabs and the use of gadolinium contrast agents. Gadolinium-enhanced 3-D studies are immune to signal loss from slow or turbulent flow and therefore permit more accurate grading of lesions. When reversal of flow in an artery is suspected as the cause of signal loss on a 2-D TOF study, a single 2-D PC slice with a V_{enc} of 40 to 80 cm/sec and flow encoding in the superior-inferior direction can be used to confirm the diagnosis.

CTA

Evaluation of the carotid arteries with CTA is quick and simple because of the limited number of imaging strategies available with CT (contrast enhancement) and the small area of anatomic coverage (the neck). In comparison to MRA, there is no signal loss in areas of slow or turbulent flow vascular, and calcification is readily apparent. The latter may be a helpful feature when planning carotid surgery.

A collimation of 1 to 3 mm with a pitch of 1 usually provides excellent images. Contrast should be injected at 2 to 3 mL/sec for a total of 100 to 120 mL. A delay of 1220 secs. is adequate if a timing bolus is not used. Swallowing should be suspended for the duration of the 30- to 60-second scan.[29]

Although the results of early comparative studies (conventional angiography versus CTA) were mixed, the simplicity of this technique has resulted in widespread clinical implementation.[41] This technique is particularly valuable when flow is extremely slow, as vessel patency still can be demonstrated. In patients with renal insufficiency or contrast allergies, an alternative imaging modality such as MRA should be considered.

■ Conclusion

MRA and CTA have the potential to assume many of the diagnostic functions of conventional angiography. Much work is required to determine and validate the best applications of these two techniques. MRA is the least invasive and will be particularly valuable in the imaging of patients who have renal failure and contrast allergies. CTA is easier and likely to be more accessible (many more practices have CT scanners than MR scanners), but it will always require radiation and iodinated contrast. A working knowledge of both techniques is important for all persons interested in the care of patients with vascular diseases.

REFERENCES

1. Egglin TK, O'Moore PV, Feinstein AR, et al. Complications of peripheral arteriography: a new system to identify patients at increased risk. *J Vasc Surg* 1995;22:787–794.

2. Mistretta CA. Relative characteristics of MR angiography and competing vascular imaging modalities. *J Magn Reson Imaging* 1993;3: 685–698.

3. Jolesz FA, Blumenfeld SM. Interventional uses of magnetic resonance imaging. *Magn Reson Q* 1994;10:85–96.

4. Wedeen VJ, Meuli RA, Edelman RR, et al. Projectile imaging of pulsatile flow with magnetic resonance. *Science* 1985;230:946–948.

5. Baum RA, Rutter CM, Sunshine JH, et al. Multicenter trial to evaluate vascular magnetic resonance angiography of the lower extremity. *JAMA* 1995;274:875–880.

6. Finn J, Kane R, Edelman R, et al. Imaging of the portal venous system in patients with cirrhosis: MR angiography vs duplex doppler sonography. *AJR Am J Roentgenol* 1993;161:989–994.

7. Drutman J, Gyorke A, Davis WL, et al. Evaluation of subclavian steal with two-dimensional phase contrast and two-dimensional time-of-flight MR angiography. *Am J Neuroradiol* 1994;15:1642–1645.

8. Carpenter JP, Holland GA, Baum RA, et al. Magnetic resonance venography for the detection of deep venous thrombosis: comparison with contrast venography and duplex Doppler ultrasonography. *J Vasc Surg* 1993;18:734–741.

9. Fellner C, Strotzer M, Geissler A, et al. Renal arteries: evaluation with optimized 2D and 3D time-of-flight MR angiography. *Radiology* 1995;196:681–687.

10. Finn JP, Zisk JHS, Edelman RR, et al. Central venous occlusion: MR angiography. *Radiology* 1993;187:245–251.

11. Kaufman JA, Geller SC, Petersen MJ, et al. MR imaging (including MR angiography) of abdominal aortic aneurysms: comparison with conventional angiography. *AJR Am J Roentgenol* 1994;163:203–210.

12. Kim D, Edelman RR, Kent KC, et al. Abdominal aorta and renal artery stenosis: evaluation with MR angiography. *Radiology* 1990;174:727–731.

13. Krebs TL, Daly B, Wong JJ, et al. Vascular complications of pancreatic transplantation: MR evaluation. *Radiology* 1995;196:793–798.

14. Rose SC, Gomes AS, Yoon HC. MR angiography for mapping potential central venous access sites in patients with advanced venous occlusive disease. *Am J Roentgenol* 1996;166:1181–1187.

15. Prince MR. Gadolinium-enhanced MR aortography. *Radiology* 1994;191:155–164.

16. Alfrey EJ, Rubin GD, Kuo PC, et al. The use of spiral computed tomography in the evaluation of living donors for kidney transplantation. *Transplantation* 1995;59:643–645.

17. Baldt MM, Zontsich T, Stumpflen A, et al. Deep venous thrombosis of the lower extremity: efficacy of spiral CT venography compared with conventional venography in diagnosis. *Radiology* 1996;200: 423–428.

18. Brink JA, Lim JT, Wang G, et al. Technical optimization of spiral CT for depiction of renal artery stenosis: in vitro analysis. *Radiology* 1995;194:157–163.

19. Galanski M, Prokop M, Chavan A, et al. Renal artery stenoses: spiral CT angiography. *Radiology* 1993;189:185–192.

20. Gavant ML, Menke PG, Fabian T, et al. Blunt traumatic aortic rupture: detection with helical CT of the chest. *Radiology* 1995;197:125–133.

21. Lawrence JA, Kim D, Kent KC, et al. Lower extremity spiral CT angiography versus catheter angiography. *Radiology* 1995;194: 903–908.

22. Remy-Jardin M, Remy J, Deschildre F, et al. Diagnosis of pulmonary embolism with spiral CT: comparison with pulmonary angiography and scintigraphy. *Radiology* 1996;200:699–706.

23. Rubin GD, Walker PJ, Napel S, et al. Spiral CT of renal artery stenosis: comparison of three-dimensional rendering techniques. *Radiology* 1994;190:181–189.

24. Sostman HD, Layish DT, Tapson VF, et al. Prospective comparison of helical CT and MR imaging in clinically suspected acute pulmonary embolism. *J Magn Reson Imaging* 1996;6:275–281.

25. Winter TC III, Freeny PC, Nhgiem HV, et al. Hepatic arterial anatomy in transplantation candidates: evaluation with three-dimensional CT arteriograms. *Radiology* 1995;195:363–370.

26. Zeman RK, Berman PM, Silverman PM, et al. Diagnosis of aortic dissection: value of helical CT with multiplanar reformation and three-dimensional rendering. *AJR Am J Roentgenol* 1995;164:1375–1380.

27. Anderson CM, Saloner D, Tsuruda JS, et al. Artifacts in maximum-intensity-projection display of MR angiograms. *Am J Roentgenol* 1990;154:623–629.

28. Leung DA, McKinnon GC, Davis CP, et al. Breath-hold, contrast-enhanced, three-dimensional MR angiography. *Radiology* 1996; 201:569–571.

29. Stehling MK, Lawrence JA, Weintraub JL, et al. CT angiography: expanded clinical applications. *Am J Roentgenol* 1994;163: 947–955.

30. Laissey JP, Faraggi M, Lebtahi R, et al. Functional evaluation of normal and ischemic kidney by means of gadolinium-DOTA enhanced TurboFLASH MR imaging: a preliminary comparison with ^{99}Tc-MAG3 dynamic scintigraphy. *Magn Reson Imaging* 1994;12: 13–19.

31. Rodgers PM, Ward J, Baudouin CJ, et al. Dynamic contrast-enhanced MR imaging of the portal venous system: comparison with x-ray angiography. *Radiology* 1994;191:741–745.

32. Hartnell GG, Finn JP, Zennie M, et al. MR imaging of the thoracic aorta: comparison of spin-echo, angiographic, and breath-hold techniques. *Radiology* 1994;191:697–704.

33. Nienaber CA, von Kodolitsch Y, Nicolas V, et al. The diagnosis of thoracic aortic dissection by noninvasive imaging procedures. *N Engl J Med* 1993;328:1–9.

34. Krinsky G, Rofsky N, Flyer M, et al. Gadolinium-enhanced three dimensional MR angiography of acquired arch vessel disease. *AJR Am J Roentgenol* 1996;167:981–987.

35. Gefter WB, Hatabu H, Holland GA, et al. Pulmonary thromboembolism: recent developments in diagnosis with CT and MR imaging. *Radiology* 1995;197:561–574.

36. Executive Committee for the Asymptomatic Carotid Atherosclerosis Study. Endarterectomy for asymptomatic carotid artery stenosis. *JAMA* 1995;273:1421–1428.

37. Ferguson GG. Current status of prospective, randomized trials of symptomatic carotid bifurcation disease. *Semin Vasc Surg* 1995; 8:46–54.

38. Patel MR, Kuntz KM, Klufas RA, et al. Preoperative assessment of the carotid bifurcation: can magnetic resonance imaging and duplex ultrasonography replace contrast angiography? *Stroke* 1995; 26:1753–1758.

39. Lustgarten JH, Solomon RA, Quest DO, et al. Carotid endarterectomy after noninvasive evaluation by duplex ultrasonography and magnetic resonance angiography. *Neurosurgery* 1994;34:612–618.

40. Drutman J, Gyorke A, Davis WL, et al. Evaluation of subclavian steal with two-dimensional phase contrast and two-dimensional time-of-flight MR angiography. *Am J Neuroradiol* 1994;15: 1642–1645.

41. Link J, Brossman J, Grabener M, et al. Spiral CT angiography and selective digital subtraction angiography of internal carotid artery stenosis. *Am J Neuroradial* 1996;17:89–94.

6
▪▪▪

Clinical and Noninvasive Evaluation of Peripheral Vascular Disease

KENNETH S. RHOLL and KEITH M. STERLING

Evolution in technology surrounding vascular disease has resulted in increased treatment options for persons afflicted with peripheral vascular disease (PVD). Decreased morbidity and mortality associated with newer procedures have led to broadening of the indications for the treatment of these patients. Additionally, recent innovations in vascular imaging have enhanced the ability to detect vascular disease using less invasive techniques. Despite these advances, optimal care of the patient with PVD still requires a balanced approach between conservative therapy and more invasive procedures. Maintaining this balance necessitates an ongoing process of evaluation of the disease process and its effects on the patient. The importance of the clinical evaluation cannot be overstated. In many cases, the clinical presentation may be straightforward and a tentative diagnosis made on the basis of a directed history and physical examination. In others, however, the diagnosis may be less certain. Objective data supplied by the noninvasive vascular laboratory can be of great use in evaluating patients with suspected PVD, not only documenting the presence of disease but also providing information about the location, severity, and etiology of the disease process. Conversely, data supplied by the noninvasive vascular laboratory should be viewed in the context of the clinical presentation. Only then can appropriate decisions regarding therapeutic options be made.

Evaluation of the patient with PVD requires an understanding of the pathophysiology and natural history of the disease. PVD is a disease of the aging population. Its frequency increases rapidly with age, from 3 to 5% in patients under 60 years of age to more than 20% in patients over 75 years of age.[1–5] Many patients decrease their activity level with advancing age; therefore most

cases of PVD in the general population are not symptomatic and pose no threat to the patient. An estimated four of five patients with demonstrable PVD are asymptomatic.[3–4] Other patients with PVD present with varying clinical manifestations, intermittent claudication being the most frequent presenting symptom. It is important to realize that PVD generally runs a benign course: 75% of patients will stabilize (60%) or improve (15%) their clinical status without intervention following their initial presentation.[6] Fewer than 25% will have significant clinical progression. Amputation is infrequent: Only 5 to 6% of patients progress to this point over a 10-year period.[6–7] Patients who smoke cigarettes and who have diabetes have a greater risk. Long-term follow-up of these patients reveals an amputation rate of 20% or greater.[1,8] With regular exercise and risk-factor control, however, most patients will demonstrate significant improvement.[9–12] A study of patients undergoing a supervised exercise program established not only clinical improvement but also evidence of significant metabolic improvement after 12 weeks.[9]

The risk factors for PVD are well known: hypertension, smoking, diabetes mellitus, abnormal cholesterol levels, obesity, and a strong family history.[1,3–5] Men are at higher risk than women, although this difference is reduced with advancing age. The presence of concomitant vascular disease in other organ systems cannot be ignored. Increased morbidity and mortality among patients with intermittent claudication are well documented.[1–3,5–6,8,13–17] One third of patients with claudication die within 10 years of their presenting symptoms, and two thirds of these patients will have experienced a major cardiovascular event. A review of patients undergoing treatment for PVD reveals a mortality rate even higher than the general population with claudication: 5-year mortality rates are 25 to 40% and 10-year rates, 50 to 75%.[1,3,5,8,13] The vast majority of these deaths are secondary to atherosclerotic heart disease. In one study of patients who underwent vascular surgery, all 14 patients with diabetes mellitus and coronary artery disease died within 5 years.[18] Similarly, in a second study, all patients with diabetes mellitus who had undergone aortofemoral reconstruction died within 5 years of surgery.[19] Clearly, although intermittent claudication itself is generally benign, the associated ramifications are markedly increased morbidity and mortality compared with the general population, in large part as a result of the effects of atherosclerotic disease on other organ systems, mainly the coronary and cerebral vasculature. Risk-factor modification should be a significant part, if not the mainstay, of any therapeutic regimen. Attempts to modify risk factors should be initiated, beginning with patient evaluation.

■ Clinical Evaluation

Evaluation of the patient with suspected PVD should begin with a directed history and physical examination. Much can be determined simply by listening to the patient's description symtoms. Relevant details such as onset (gradual versus acute), character, location, and aggravating and relieving factors should be sought. Combining the clinical history with findings extracted during physical examination will aid in determining the nature and extent of the disease process.

History

Intermittent claudication, reported by about 70% of patients at initial presentation, is the most frequent complaint of patients with PVD.[2–5] *Claudication* (from the Latin word claudicatio, meaning *to limp*) is defined as muscular pain brought on by exercise and relieved by rest. Onset is predictable in terms of the activity level required to produce the symptoms. Similarly, the symptoms rapidly resolve with rest of the extremity. There is generally no relation to position of the extremity. The discomfort itself tends to be described by patients as a "cramping" pain in the body of the muscle; however, the perception may vary from patient to patient. The quality of discomfort may range from a sharp searing or stabbing pain to an aching discomfort. Others complain of numbness, heaviness, fatigue, or weakness. Vasculogenic claudication must be differentiated from other states, such as neurogenic claudication and arthritis.[20] Neurogenic claudication or pseudoclaudication may be associated with spinal stenosis. Therefore, there is generally less predictability regarding onset with exercise. Interestingly,

although these patients may be limited in their ability to ambulate, they may experience no limitation with alternative forms of exercise, such as an exercise bicycle, because of the postural changes associated with the alternative exercises. Additionally, in contradistinction to vascular claudication, relief frequently is delayed following cessation of exercise and may require additional change in position.[20] Unfortunately, because both of these diseases are increasingly common with advancing age, they may coexist. Similarly, arthritic complaints, usually joint centered, may be confused with claudication. Onset may occur after rather than during exercise, and relief is delayed and often positional. The noninvasive vascular laboratory with exercise testing can be extremely useful in differentiating true vascular claudication from other conditions.

Claudication characteristically develops in the muscles of the calf, although other sites may be involved. In part this relates to the heavy dependence on the calf muscles during walking, frequently the only source of significant exercise in the aging population. Distribution of disease also plays a significant role. Although younger patients affected by PVD frequently present with an aortoiliac distribution, the femoropopliteal system more frequently is involved in the older population.[4,21] In fact, multisegment disease is common in patients who have PVD symptoms. Because the effects of disease on perfusion are hemodynamically cumulative as one progresses distally in the arterial tree, it is reasonable that the calf muscles are frequently the site of most significant ischemia when walking. Other sites of claudication occasionally dominate. Young women frequently present with lesions involving the distal aorta and its bifurcation.[22] With proximal disease, patients may complain of symptoms involving the buttocks or thighs.[21] Similarly, men with disease in this distribution may experience erectile dysfunction. Conversely, foot claudication may be the presenting symptom in patients with isolated distal vessel disease, such as Buerger's disease.[23,24] Unusual character or distribution of symptoms may be the cause of significant delay in diagnosis and treatment.[21]

As the degree of ischemia worsens, the limitations imposed on the patient increase, and symptoms may occur at rest. Ischemic rest pain occurs when perfusion of the extremity is inadequate to meet the basic metabolic needs of the tissues.[25] Because perfusion status is extremely tenous at this point, small changes in perfusion brought about by positional changes may either alleviate or aggravate symptoms. The patient may describe the need to hang the distal extremity over the edge of the bed at night for symptomatic relief provided by the gravitational advantage in perfusion. Frequently, the patient may need to get up at night to "walk off" the pain, seemingly a contradiction. Minor trauma to the extremity with this level of impaired perfusion may result in tissue breakdown or cutaneous ulceration. A small cut or blister that is generally an innocuous event in the otherwise healthy patient may become a limb-threatening lesion. Similarly, with significant ischemia, cellulitis can progress rapidly despite adequate antimicrobial treatment. Revascularization of these extremities is critical to long-term limb salvage and, depending on the clinical situation, should not be delayed. Further decrease in perfusion invariably will lead to tissue loss. Although tissue damage at this point may be irreversible, limb salvage still can be attained with revascularization and wound care.

Symptoms of chronic limb ischemia generally have an insidious onset, although patients frequently relate the onset to some event in their lives. As might be expected, patients presenting with rest pain usually relate a long history of worsening claudication before, seeking medical help. Ischemia, however, may present in an acute fashion, often with abrupt onset of severe pain in the calf or foot. Depending on the severity of the ischemia, the patient may complain of paresthesias or numbness rather than pain or describe sudden onset of coolness and discoloration with either cyanosis or pallor. Motor function also may be impaired; the patient may be unable to move the foot or toes. Generally, the symptoms are so sudden and severe that medical attention is sought immediately. If there is delay in presentation, however, the acute, severe symptoms may subside to some degree because collateral beds gradually supply some reperfusion to the affected limb. Alternatively, without improved perfusion, clinical status may deteriorate rapidly, with tissue breakdown and the development of gangrenous changes.

Acute ischemia may be secondary to an embolic or thrombotic event. Emboli can occur anywhere in the arterial tree but frequently lodge at sites of arterial division where vessel caliber is reduced suddenly. Large emboli may adhere to the aortic bifurcation, affecting both lower extremities. The common femoral bifurcation and the popliteal trifurcation are two additional frequent sites of emboli, each presenting with a different distribution of ischemia. Occasionally, microembolization will occur to the most distal vascular beds. The sudden appearance of one or more painful, discolored toes in the presence of palpable pedal pulses, called the *"blue toe syndrome,"* is characteristic of atheroembolization to the digital arteries (Fig. 6-1).[26] In general, this condition is thought to represent embolization from a proximal ulcerated atherosclerotic lesion. Depending on the severity of the proximal lesion, there may be an antecedent history of claudication. Occasionally, a similar presentation occurs secondary to a proximal critical stenosis without demonstrable ulceration. Presumably, small thromboemboli account for the distal arterial occlusions. A thorough history may reveal prior episodes of distal embolization. Even in the presence of palpable pulses, distal embolization warrants further investigation of the source of em-

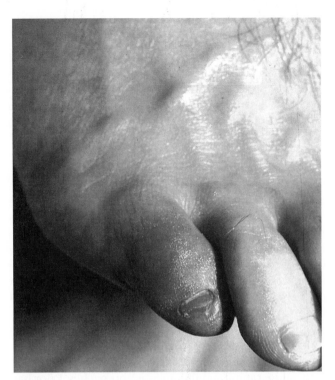

FIGURE 6-1. A 48-year-old man presented with the acute onset of a painful discolored fifth toe. A focally ischemic digit in the face of normal pulses is characteristic of the "blue toe syndrome." Note the normal cutaneous features, hair distribution and venous distention indicating lack of chronic ischemia.

boli. Many of the inciting lesions are treatable by percutaneous techniques.

Thrombosis as a cause of acute ischemia may involve native vessels or bypass grafts. If there is thrombosis of a vessel with preexisting stenosis, careful questioning frequently will yield a preceding history of claudication. The differentiation of in situ thrombosis of a diseased vessel from embolic occlusion of an otherwise healthy vessel carries different prognostic and therapeutic implications. Thrombectomy is much less likely to be successful if the underlying vessel is diseased; thrombolysis and angioplasty may represent an attractive alternative. In addition to stenotic disease, aneurysmal disease is particularly susceptible to sudden thrombosis and or embolization.[27,28] Acute ischemia secondary to popliteal artery thrombosis should lead to an investigation of the underlying artery (as well as the contralateral artery) to exclude aneurysmal disease. A similar picture may be encountered with popliteal entrapment with or without associated aneurysm formation. Again, examination of the contralateral extremity is crucial, because the disease is frequently bilateral. Bypass grafts frequently fail without prior clinical symptoms, and a history of claudication may not be encountered. Routine graft surveillance is therefore thought to be warranted to avoid the consequences of graft failure.[29,30]

Further interrogation regarding the involvement of vascular disease in other organ systems should be undertaken. As previously noted, cardiovascular and cerebrovascular events account for most of the mortality in this patient population. The presence of significant disease involving these organ systems may alter the therapeutic approach to the patient. Risk factors should be elucidated, and initial efforts at risk-factor modification begun. Family history is important not only for its prognostic value, but it also occasionally aids in determining the source of disease. A family history of thrombotic events may suggest a hypercoagulable state, although this is found infrequently. These events more often involve the venous system but occasionally result in arterial emboli or thrombosis, particularly following instrumentation, such as arterial catheterization or vascular surgery. Surgical history, particularly as it pertains to the vascular system, should be outlined in detail. Prior grafts may alter significantly both diagnostic and therapeutic approaches. Unusual graft anatomy or occlusive disease can interfere with angiographic and therapeutic approaches. Prior harvesting of the saphenous vein may limit surgical alternatives.

Current medications, particularly those with vascular effects, such as anticoagulants and vasoconstricting agents, should be recorded. Drug interactions and side effects are not infrequent and may have consequences for therapeutic endeavors. Specific inquiry must be made regarding certain drugs (e.g., nicotine patches) because often the patient does not perceive these agents as being medication

Physical examination

With the clinical history in mind, a directed physical examination should be performed to evaluate the patient's vascular status. The investigation should include a basic cardiovascular examination as well as an evaluation of the possible effects of vascular disease on the extremities. Auscultatation of the heart is performed to exclude arrhythmias such as atrial fibrillation and significant murmurs. The carotid arteries, abdomen, and pelvis, including the femoral arteries, are auscultated for the presence of bruits. A thorough assessment of peripheral pulses by palpation includes both upper and lower extremities. Pulses should be recorded as absent, diminished, normal, or hyperdynamic bilaterally. If a pulse is absent by palpation, its presence should be ascertained by using a handheld Doppler device. Although the dorsalis pedis pulse may be absent by palpation in up to 12% of the normal population, absence of the posterior tibial pulse is a strong indicator of disease.[4] The presence of significant soft tissue edema or open ulceration may confound the

process of palpation; again, Doppler evaluation may be necessary. Palpation also should be used to investigate possible aneurysmal disease at common sites of formation including the abdominal aorta, common femoral arteries, and popliteal arteries (the most frequently ignored site). Blood pressures obtained from both upper extremities should be recorded as part of the vascular examination.

Inspection of the extremities is performed to evaluate for signs of acute and chronic arterial insufficiency. In addition to pulse evaluation, this should encompass inspection of the quality of the skin, the distribution of hair on the extremities, cutaneous temperature, capillary refill and neuromuscular function, each as it relates to the presence of vascular disease. Chronic arterial insufficiency leads to trophic skin changes with thin, shiny skin, particularly in the pretibial region.[11] Loss of normal hair distribution occurs from the distal calf and dorsum of the foot. Nails may become thickened and brittle. With increasing severity of chronic ischemia, dependent rubor may be present owing to relatively fixed vasodilation in the distal arteriolar and capillary beds. With the patient in a sitting or erect position, the foot and distal calf are ruborous, whereas in the supine position, particularly with the extremity elevated, the extremity appears pale. Temperature changes, which are more pronounced in the acutely ischemic limb, may be present in chronic ischemia, particularly if the limb is left without the thermal protection of a sock or blanket for a brief period. Comparison of proximal to distal and side-to-side is made. Capillary refill is evaluated by applying gentle pressure to the skin or nail bed, followed by release and observation of the return of the normal pinkish color. Capillary refill, normally 1 to 2 seconds, becomes increasingly delayed with the severity of the ischemia. As ischemia progresses and the limb becomes threatened, sensory and muscular function are affected. These changes are generally most pronounced in acute, severe ischemia. With chronic ischemia, muscle mass begins to atrophy, accounting for much of the weakness encountered. Finally, inspection should include a thorough evaluation of skin integrity. Tissue breakdown, ulceration, and frank gangrene may occur with severe ischemia. Ulceration tends to occur at pressure points in the distal extremities, including the regions around the malleoli, heels, heads of the metatarsals, and toes. Frequently undetected without careful inspection are lesions between the toes. Detection of tissue breakdown is extremely important because these lesions, untreated, may become infected and life threatening. Ischemic ulcerations tend to be dry, punched-out lesions with well defined borders (Fig. 6-2). Usually little erythema is found unless infection is present. These ulcerations should be differentiated from venous ulcers, which tend to be weeping, indurated lesions around the distal calves (Fig. 6-3). Associated cutaneous changes of venous

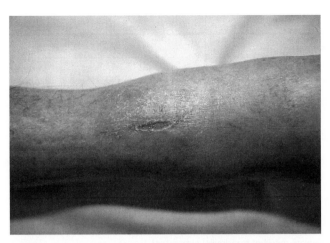

FIGURE 6-2. A 68-year-old woman presented with a chronic ulcerated lesion along the anterior aspect of her shin. The lesion is well defined, dry and shows little associated erythema. The surrounding skin is atrophic with a paucity of hair. Although unusual in position, the lesion is characteristic of an ischemic ulcer.

stasis are frequently present with brawny edema and brownish discoloration of the skin. Dilated superficial varicosities also may be in the region of a venous ulcer.

The physical examination in acute limb ischemia may be quite different from that of chronic disease. Initially, pulses are severely diminished to absent because collaterals have had little time to form. The underlying skin and hair distribution are frequently normal, although in the case of acute graft occlusion, the stigmata of chronic disease may have previously developed. Color change may be pronounced, with the distal ischemic portion of the extremity having a blanched or marbled appearance in the more severe cases. Differential temperature of the

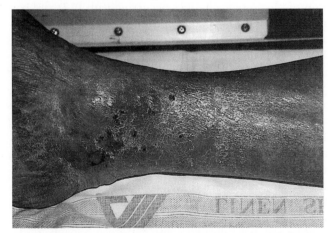

FIGURE 6-3. A 58-year-old black man presented with chronic cutaneous ulceration around the medial malleolus. The reddish brown discoloration of the skin and the distribution around the ankle are typical of chronic venous stasis changes.

affected extremity is usually pronounced. The level of temperature change should be recorded as well as marked on the extremity. As the ischemic process evolves, a well-defined line of demarcation develops between the perfused proximal extremity and the ischemic distal portion. As collateral perfusion increases following the acute episode, this line of demarcation tends to move distally. Capillary refill may be markedly delayed or absent. Evaluation of motor and sensory function is critical in these patients because it aids in the determination of limb viability. Sensory changes range from none to complete anesthesia. Patients with threatened but reversible ischemia frequently note dysethesia or paresthesia of the affected extremity. The presence of diabetes may confuse the issue because peripheral neuropathy is frequently present.[31] Comparison with the contralateral extremity should be performed in all patients but is particularly useful when an underlying neuropathy is present. Similarly, muscle function ranges from normal to paralysis; weakness is a sign of the threatened limb. Generally, tissue breakdown is not present at initial presentation owing to the acuity of the process. Without revascularization, however, the threatened to irreversible limb may progress rapidly to frank gangrenous changes. When present, these changes may represent a contraindication to revascularization, particularly if infection is present, owing to the milieu of toxic substances that may be released from the affected limb.

To provide consistency in the evaluation and reporting of the ischemic limb, a system of grading extremities has been developed for both acute and chronic limb ischemia (Table 6-1) using clinical findings and objective criteria that may be provided by the vascular laboratory.[32–35] In addition to prognostic implications, therapeutic decisions can be made consistently using these standardized categories. For instance, percutaneous thrombolytic treatment of the acutely threatened limb may be appropriate in many cases. If the clinical status of the extremity declines rapidly, with loss of sensory and motor function, there is frequently insufficient time for thrombolytic agents to restore perfusion, and surgical revascularization may be more appropriate. The goal of the clinical evaluation of the patient is to document the vascular status of the patient, providing a basis for any therapeutic decision, whether conservative or invasive.

Noninvasive Vascular Testing

Although the importance of the clinical evaluation cannot be overstated, objective data supplied by the noninvasive vascular laboratory can be of great use in the evaluation of patients with suspected PVD, not only documenting the presence of disease but also providing information as to the location, severity, and etiology of the disease process. For instance, there may be a paucity of physical findings in

TABLE 6-1. Clinical categories of limb ischemia (31–35)

Acute limb ischemia

Category	Description	Capillary refill	Motor impairment	Sensory impairment	Arterial Doppler	Venous Doppler
Viable	Not immediately threatened	Intact	None	None	Audible, ankle pressure > 30 mm Hg	Audible
Threatened	Salvageable if promptly treated	Intact, slow	Mild	Mild	Inaudible	Audible
Irreversible	Major tissue loss, amputation required regardless of treatment	Absent (marbling)	Profound, paralysis (rigor)	Profound, anesthetic	Inaudible	Inaudible

Chronic limb ischemia

Grade	Category	Clinical description	Objective criteria
	0	Asymptomatic; no hemodynamically significant lesion	Normal result of treadmill[a]/ stress test
I	1	Mild claudication	Treadmill completed, postexercise AP >50 mm Hg but>25 mm Hg below normal
	2	Moderate claudication	Symptoms between categories 1 and 3
	3	Severe claudication	Treadmill test cannot be completed, postexercise AP<50 mm Hg
II	4	Ischemic rest pain	Resting AP ≤40mm Hg, flat or barely pulsatile metatarsal plethysmography, toe pressure <30 mm Hg
III	5	Minor tissue loss, nonhealing ulcer, focal gangrene with diffuse pedal edema	Resting AP ≤ to 60 mm Hg, ankle or metatarsal plethysmography flat or barely pulsatile, toe pressure <40 mm Hg
	6	Major tissue loss, extending above transmetatarsal level, functional foot not salvageable	Same as for category 5

a Treadmill at 2 mph with a 12% grade for 5 min. AP = Ankle pressure.

many patients with intermittent claudication. The absence of peripheral pulses is an unreliable finding. Patients with high levels of activity may be severely limited despite the presence of palpable peripheral pulses on resting examination. Therefore, a diagnosis of intermittent claudication is sometimes difficult, with history and physical examination having false-positive and false-negative rates in the range of 44% and 19%, respectively.[36] The noninvasive laboratory can provide objective data regarding the presence or absence of disease in patients whose complaints suggest claudication. Frequently, the ability of the noninvasive vascular laboratory to provide correlation of the disease process with the patient's symptomatology is of equal importance, especially in patients whose clinical presentation may not fit the classical description of vascular disease. The information provided is therefore vital to the success of any management, whether conservative or invasive.

In addition to the evaluation of the patient with suspected intermittent claudication, indications for noninvasive vascular testing include documentation of disease in the severely ischemic extremity, nonhealing ulcers, assessment of potential wound or amputation healing, vasospastic disorders, entrapment syndromes, trauma, and evaluation of other lower-extremity complaints. Before any intervention is undertaken, an initial evaluation can be invaluable in procedural planning, serving also as a baseline against which the results of the intervention can be gauged. The vascular noninvasive examination is extremely useful in monitoring the status of the disease process, documenting the stability or progression of disease, and allowing correlation with changes in the patient's clinical status. Traditionally, the most important task of the noninvasive laboratory has been documentation of physiologic changes occurring with PVD and correlation of this information with the patient's symptomatology.[37] More recently, however, noninvasive testing has been performed for anatomic mapping, possibly eliminating the contrast angiogram for certain patients.[38,39] Vascular testing, therefore, may be divided into examinations that provide primarily physiologic information and those that provide primarily anatomic information. Because it is not cost effective to perform every modality available in the noninvasive laboratory on every patient, consideration should be given to the desired information, using modalities that can provide this information best and most efficiently. If intervention is considered, most patients will proceed to angiography, and anatomic testing may be redundant. Physiologic testing, by evaluating the overall perfusion of the extremity, may be more useful in allowing one to decide whether intervention is indeed warranted. When specific anatomic questions are present, anatomic testing such as duplex imaging or magnetic resonance angiography (MRA) may provide this information. The expansion of the modalities available in vascular testing allows tailoring of the examination to fit the needs of the clinician and patient.

Ankle brachial indices

Measurement of arterial blood pressures at the ankle with comparison branchial pressure constitutes the simplest noninvasive screening test for PVD. Ankle brachial indices (ABIs) are determined by measuring the systolic pressure from both the dorsalis pedis and the posterior tibial arteries at each ankle and dividing by the higher of the two brachial pressures. In normal subjects, the ABIs should be approximately 1.0, with values of less than 0.95 suggesting the presence of vascular disease.[33,37,40,41] The degree of depression of the ABI correlates fairly well with the severity of the disease. Although there is significant variability, ABIs in the range of 0.75 to 0.9 correspond to mild, often single-segment (e.g., aortoiliac or femoropopliteal) disease. Patients, if active, may experience symptoms of mild claudication. ABIs in the range of 0.5 to 0.75 are indicative of moderate ischemia; two arterial segments are frequently involved. Depending on the level of activity, the clinical picture may range from asymptomatic to fairly severe claudication. ABIs below 0.5 usually indicate multisegment disease (frequently with multiple occlusions) and generally are associated with severe claudication that may approach rest pain. Below 0.3, ischemia is severe and tissue breakdown is likely. Absolute ankle pressures of less than 50 mm Hg also are associated with severe ischemia and likely tissue breakdown.[33,40] Measurement of ABIs represents a simple, reproducible screening test for arterial disease, requiring only minimal equipment, namely a handheld Doppler unit and a sphygmomanometer. A significant drawback to ABIs is the insensitivity of the technique to mild disease. An active person may have normal resting ABIs but may develop limiting ischemia with exercise. Moreover, pressures may be artificially elevated in patients with calcific, noncompliant vessels, as is frequently seen in diabetic patients with medial sclerosis. ABIs greater than 1.0 are commonly seen in diabetic patients despite fairly severe ischemia demonstrable by other techniques.[31,37] The presence of bilateral upper-extremity arterial disease may also result in artificially elevated ABIs. Finally, other than laterality, there is no anatomic information provided. Despite these limitations, determination of ABIs should be part of any physical examination for PVD.

Segmental limb pressures

Determination of segmental limb pressures (SLP) in the lower extremities adds some anatomic information to that provided by ABIs. Initially, ankle pressures are measured for both the posterior tibial and the dorsalis pedis arteries. The stronger pulse (higher systolic pressure) then is used for determination of SLPs. Measurements then are performed using a series of blood-pressure cuffs along both lower extremities. In the three-cuff technique, cuffs are placed at the midthigh, calf, and ankle levels; with the four cuff technique, the thigh is divided into high-thigh and low-thigh measurements. Systolic pressures are determined as the cuffs are sequentially inflated and deflated at each level while monitoring the stronger pedal pulse distally. Cuffs appropriate to the size of the extremity should be used to avoid artificially high measurements in large extremities. Although ideally, using larger cuffs for the thighs, the artifactual elevation of pressures measured by cuff would be avoided and SLPs in a patient without PVD all would be equivalent to the brachial pressure, thigh pressures tend to be overestimated by at least 30 mm Hg, particularly in patients with a more obese body habitus.[37,40] Intraarterial pressure measurements have demonstrated that actual systolic arterial pressure in the iliac and femoral arteries is about equal to branchial pressures. Familiarity with the body habitus of the patient being examined and the equipment and cuffs used in the laboratory is therefore critical. With this knowledge, appropriate compensation for this artifact can be made and the potential error in diagnosis avoided. SLPs are compared from proximal to distal in each extremity as well as from side to side. In general, a segmental drop in pressure between any two segments of greater than 20 to 30 mm Hg is indicative of stenotic disease in the underlying segment.[37,40] Similarly, a difference of greater than 15 to 20 mm Hg from side to side suggests significant disease at or above the cuff in the extremity with the lower measurement. Advantages of SLPs include limited equipment requirements and an element of anatomic specificity in the detection of disease. Similar to the determination of ABIs, however, medial sclerosis again can result in artificial elevation of pressure measurements. In diabetic patients, in whom healing potential is frequently the greatest concern, measurement of toe pressures may aid in this concern. Because digital arteries are generally less affected by medial sclerosis and therefore the measurement of pressure more accurate. In general an absolute toe pressure of greater than 50 mm Hg and a toe brachial index of 0.6 or greater is normal. Absolute toe pressure of at least 30 mm Hg is ordinarily required for healing.[37,42] Another significant disadvantage of SLPs is the inability to differentiate an occlusion from a stenosis. Although occlusive disease generally results in a larger pressure reduction than stenotic disease, collateral circulation may diminish this differential. This determination may be critical in a patient with intermittent claudication who may be a candidate for percutaneous revascularization but may not meet the criteria for a surgical procedure. Despite these limitations, deter-

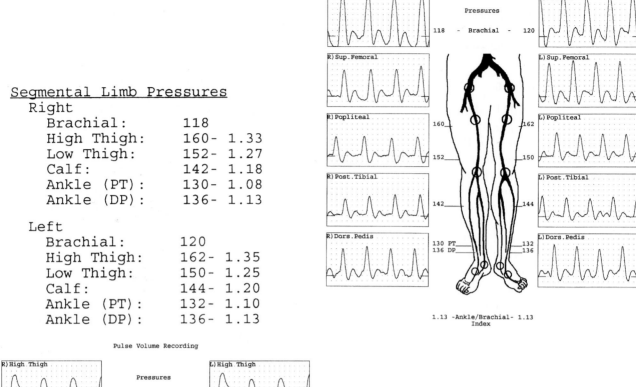

Segmental Limb Pressures

Right
Brachial:	118	
High Thigh:	160-	1.33
Low Thigh:	152-	1.27
Calf:	142-	1.18
Ankle (PT):	130-	1.08
Ankle (DP):	136-	1.13

Left
Brachial:	120	
High Thigh:	162-	1.35
Low Thigh:	150-	1.25
Calf:	144-	1.20
Ankle (PT):	132-	1.10
Ankle (DP):	136-	1.13

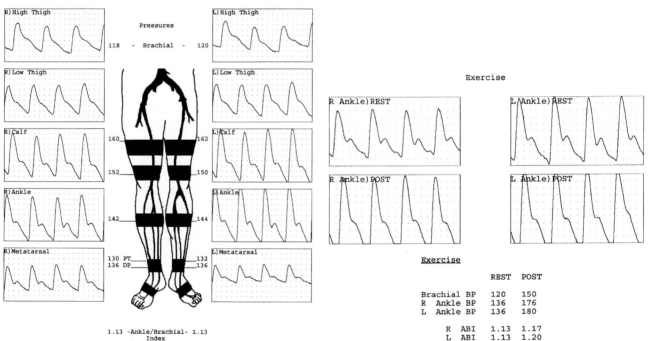

FIGURE 6-4. Physiologic noninvasive arterial examination from a 62-year-old man presenting with complaints of bilateral calf aching when walking. **A:** Resting segmental limb pressures are normal bilaterally with ankle brachial indices (ABIs) greater than 1.0. Note the side-to-side symmetrically and the gradual decline from high thigh to ankle. **B:** Doppler waveform analysis is also normal with triphasic waveforms throughout both lower extremeties. **C:** Resting volume plethysmography recordings demonstrate normal perfussion throughout the lower exremeties. Note the progression in amplitude from the high thigh to the calf. Side to side, there is symmetry with normal morphology throughout the lower extremities. **D:** The patient was exercised on a treadmil with a 12% grade at 2.0 miles hour for 5 min. He noted aching in the calves during the latter part of the exercise protocol and during the recovery period. Following exercise, there was maintenance of normal ABIs with simultaneous rise in ankle and brachial pressures. Plethysmographic tracings obtained at the ankle demonstrated a normal increase in perfusion following exercise with continued normal waveform morphology. There was no evidence of exercise induced ischemia; the symptoms were therefore not secondary to arterial insufficiency. PT-posterior tibia; DP-dorsal pedis BP-blood pressure.

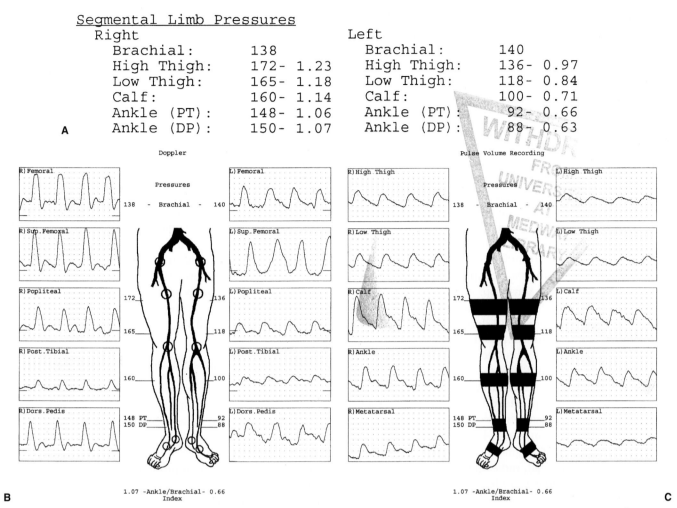

FIGURE 6-5. Physiologic nonivasive testing in an obese 48-year-old woman complaining of cramping pain in the left calf when walking more than 100 yards. She also noted occasional buttock discomfort when climbing stairs. The examination indicates the pressure of severe obstruction in the left iliac arterial system. **A.** Resting segmented limb pressures demonstrate a significant decrease in the left high thigh pressure when compared to the right. No additional significant gradients are present on the left. Examination on the right is normal with an ABI greater than 1.0. **B:** Doppler waveforms analysis is markedly abnormal throughout the left lower extremity. The left common femoral artery waveform is broad and monophasic. Note that further degradation below the common femoral artery may be difficult to detect. On the right there is degradation of the posterior tibial artery waveform which may indicate disease in this vessel. The remaining waveforms show no significant abnormality. **C:** Resting volume plethysmography recordings are dramatically degraded in the left thigh indicative of significant inflow obstruction. Distal to this there remains a normal progression in amplitude to the calf suggesting that the femoral popliteal system is intact. Note the diminutive amplitude of the thigh waveforms on the right. This is frequently seen in obese patients with a relatively low muscle mass. PT-posterior tibia; DP-dorsal pedis.

mination of SLPs remains a simple, reproducible means of quantifying PVD and its effects on the perfusion status of the extremities (Figs. 6-4A and 6-5A).

Doppler waveform analysis

Frequently performed in conjunction with SLPs, Doppler waveform analysis (DWA) represents another of the traditional techniques for the evaluation of vascular disease. Assessing the changes that occur in the directional Doppler waveform can provide additional information regarding the location and severity of PVD. Although directional Doppler waveform information is part of more sophisticated duplex Doppler techniques, the information can be obtained with simpler, less expensive continuous wave (CW) Doppler instrumentation. Using a CW Doppler probe aligned longitudinally with the long axis and at about 45 degrees to the transverse axis, directional Doppler waveforms are obtained at multiple levels where the arteries are superficial, typically including the common femoral, popliteal, posterior tibial, and dorsalis pedis arteries. Waveforms also can be obtained from the superficial femoral artery (SFA) and peroneal artery, although the depth and position adjacent to other arteries make these results somewhat less reliable. The normal resting peripheral arterial waveform has a triphasic morphology, which is indicative of a high-resistance distal vascular bed (Fig. 6-6). There is a sharp systolic upstroke indicating flow in an antegrade direction, followed by a sharp downstroke and brief reversal of flow early in diastole. The third phase is that of a gradually decreasing antegrade flow through the remainder of diastole. With increasing disease proximal to the site of insonation, there is degradation of the triphasic waveform, initially becoming biphasic and then monophasic, with loss of the retrograde component of flow (Fig. 6-6b).[11,37,43] Because blood must flow through a stenosis, or through collateral circulation around an occlusion, the waveform becomes broader and systolic upstroke more gradual. The amplitude of the waveform also is decreased with disease proximal to the site of insonation. Because gain settings, probe frequency, and depth of the vessel cause variation in the absolute amplitude of the Doppler waveforms, with consistent technique, comparison is still useful from side-to-side and level-to-level.

Generally, the information provided by DWA is used in conjunction with that provided by other modalities such as SLPs and plethysmographic techniques to quantify and localize disease. For instance, in a patient in whom a significant gradient in segmental pressures is noted between the thigh and calf, indicating femoropopliteal disease, relatively normal Doppler waveforms obtained in the SFA and popliteal artery would strongly suggest that the offending lesion resides in the distal popliteal artery or its trifurcation. Conversely, if no SFA signal can be obtained and a monophasic popliteal signal is detected, an SFA occlusion is likely present. The information produced by DWA is therefore complementary; however,

DWA may be affected by several artifacts. The technique is technologist dependent, requiring careful alignment of the Doppler probe with the vessel. In the obese patient, in whom the inguinal crease is frequently well below the femral bifurcation, examination through the inguinal crease will result in insonation of the SFA or profunda femoral artery (PFA) rather than the common femoral artery, which may lead to an errant diagnosis of inflow disease. Vessel misidentification also may occur in the thigh when a muscular branch of the PFA is mistakenly identified as the SFA. Similarly, in the distal calf, anterior tibial and peroneal arteries are in close proximity, and misidentification may occur. Another potential source of error is the presence of plaque in the artery at the site of insonation, particularly if the plaque is densely calcified. Finally, DWA is less useful in multisegment disease. Further changes in the Doppler waveform from distal vessel disease become extremely subtle when significant proximal disease is present causing an already degraded waveform (Figs. 6-4B and 6-5B).

Plethysmographic techniques

Current plethysmographic techniques as they relate to noninvasive vascular testing include volume plethysmography and photoplethysmography (PPG).[11,34,37,40,43] Strain-gauge plethysmography, which provides information similar to these techniques, is used less frequently owing to the additional equipment requirements and its cumbersome nature. Plethysmographic techniques are somewhat unique in the their primary function is the evaluation of the actual perfusion of the extremity regardless of the route of blood delivery. Whereas most modalities are directed at determining the condition of the underlying arterial tree, plethysmographic techniques evaluate the effect of the disease process on the extremity. These techniques are therefore uniquely suited for correlation of symptoms with the physiologic effects of disease as well as for the prediction of wound healing. The information provided is complementary to that provided by other noninvasive techniques

Volume plethysmographic recordings (VPRs), also known as pulse-volume recordings (PVRs), and segmental limb plethysmography are performed by using a multiple cuff technique similar to that of SLPs and therefore are frequently obtained concurrently.[37,40,43] The technique requires a specialized piece of equipment for standardized cuff inflation and recording changes in extremity volume as measured by the cuffs. With the patient supine, the cuffs are sequentially inflated to a standardized pressure, usually in the range of 60 mm Hg. The cuffs remain connected to the VPR instrument, which then records the change in the size of the extremity with each cardiac cycle. This change represents the blood flow into and out of that segment of the extremity. This process is repeated at each

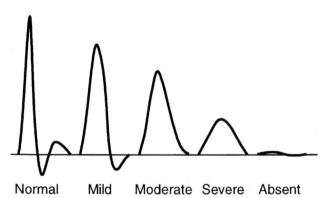

Normal   Mild   Moderate   Severe   Absent

FIGURE 6-6. Diagrammatic representation of Doppler waveform morphology. The waveform on the left illustrates a normal triphasic waveform seen at rest in the peripheral arteries. With mild disease proximal to the point of insonation, the signal becomes biphasic. With progressive proximal disease, there is further degradation of the waveform.

of the three or four levels (depending on which technique is chosen) in both extremities. A metatarsal cuff may be added detect the further effects of distal vessel disease. Transmetatarsal waveforms may be especially valuable in foot claudicators and in evaluating the healing potential of distal cutaneous lesions or planned surgery or amputation.

PPG represents a technique of evaluating perfusion at the cutaneous level.[37,42,43] Using photoelectric cells affixed to the skin with double-stick tape, variation in the blood content of the underlying tissues is recorded. Although not true plethysmographic tracings, the resultant recordings closely resemble those of other plethysmographic techniques and are evaluated in a similar fashion. Generally, PPG is performed to evaluate the presence of pulsatile flow in the digits, although cutaneous measurements can be made at other sites of interest. Healing potential, particularly in the case of cutaneous ulceration, can be estimated rapidly. Most commercially available plethysmographic instruments include the capability of performing PPGs with little additional cost or equipment.

The normal arterial plethysmographic tracing, either VPR or PPG is characterized by a steep anacrotic limb with a sharp crest followed by a steep concave catacrotic limb (Fig. 6-7).[37,43] The normal catacrotic limb is characterized further by presence of a reflected diastolic wave in its midportion. Because the VPR relates to the inflow and outflow of blood from the segment being studied, the amplitude depends on the relative proportion of vascularized tissue underlying the cuff. In the extremity, muscle accounts for the tissue with the greatest relative perfusion, whereas fat and bone have little effect on the recording. Therefore, the amplitude of the VPR depends on the relative muscle mass underlying the cuff. The proximal thigh in most persons contains significant amounts of fat, with relative muscle mass increasing from the thigh to the calf. The ankle and metatarsal regions are low in fat and composed mostly of bone. VPRs, therefore, tend to increase in amplitude from the thigh to the calf, and then to decrease in amplitude from the calf to the ankle and metatarsal regions. The contour of the waveform, however, should remain relatively constant. Additionally, symmetry normally should be maintained from side to side. Abnormalities secondary to PVD include a decrease in the slope of the anacrotic limb, rounding and delay in the crest, decreased rate of decline in the catacrotic limb with the slope becoming flat to convex, and loss of the reflected diastolic wave (see Fig. 6-7). Additionally, loss of the normal progression in amplitude from thigh to calf may indicate intervening disease. Side-to-side asymmetry also may be an indication of disease in the limb with decreased relative amplitude. Remembering that abnormalities in VPRs are related to perfusion, abnormal VPRs may be categorized as demonstrating mild, moderate, or severe underlying ischemia.[37,40,43] Because perfusion of any segment of limb relates to the status of the inflow vessels to that segment, some anatomic information is gained regarding the location of the disease (Figs. 6-4C and 6-5C). For instance, normally the upper thigh depends on the aortoiliac segment, common femoral artery, and PFA; and occlusive disease in any of these segments will degrade VPRs obtained in the upper thigh. The SFA, however, contributes little to the supply of the upper thigh. Abnormalities involving the SFA would be not be expected to result in an abnormal VPR at this level. VPRs obtained at the calf level, however, are extremely dependent on the SFA and popliteal artery. Occlusive disease in this segment would be expected to have a profound effect on the calf VPR, whereas the thigh VPR would be preserved. It should be remembered that the quality of the VPR depends on all sources of perfusion, including the normal arterial pathways, collateral arterial pathways, and bypass grafts. In the normal situation, the PFA would be expected to contribute little to the perfusion of the calf, but with an SFA occlusion the calf may become totally dependent on the PFA and its collateral supply. Therefore, when interpreting VPRs, a comprehensive knowledge of arterial anatomy and potential collateral pathways is mandatory. Additionally, familiarity with the patient and prior surgical and percutaneous vascular procedures is imperative. PPGs are interpreted in a fashion similar to VPRs. The tracings indicate perfusion of the underlying tissue regardless of the proximal anatomy. Typically, abnormalities are characterized as mild, moderate, or severe and related to ischemia of the underlying tissue.[37,42,43]

Usually, VPRs are performed in concert with other noninvasive modalities, such as SLPs, resulting in a basic segmental map of occlusive disease and its physiologic effects on the patient. VPRs are unaffected by noncompressible arteries and are therefore particularly useful in patients who have diabetes or chronic renal failure. Addi-

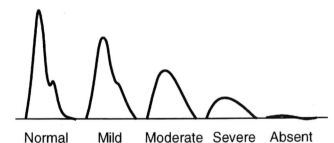

Normal   Mild   Moderate Severe Absent

FIGURE 6-7. Diagrammatic representation of volume plethysmography recording (VPR) morphology. The waveform on the left illustrates a normal VPR waveform with sharp upstroke during the anacrotic phase and a normal catacrotic phase with a prominent reflected diastolic wave. With progressive inflow disease, the waveform becomes increasingly degraded with decreased amplitude, broadening of the waveform, and decreased amplitude.

tionally, the performance of VPRs depends less on technique and therefore are less susceptible to the artifacts seen in DWA. VPRs require a cooperative patient because motion artifact will severely degrade the quality of the tracings. Additionally, analogous to SLPs and DWA, VPRs do no distinguish reliably between stenotic and occlusive disease; in this respect, the strength of VPRs is also a weakness. Depending on the extent of the collateral circulation, at rest, a patient with significant occlusive disease may have relatively normal VPRs. In these patients, exercise testing will provide valuable clinical and physiologic information.

Exercise testing

Physiologic testing with SLPs, DWA, and plethysmographic techniques have the advantage of segmental localization and quantification of disease while simultaneously evaluating the relative effects of the disease on perfusion of the extremities. In patients with a characteristic clinical presentation and moderate to advanced disease, the resting evaluation frequently will be adequate for diagnosis and treatment planning. In patients with atypical presentations or in patients with less advanced disease who are symptomatic only with exertion, exercise testing allows a more thorough evaluation, with the opportunity to correlate the patient's symptoms with physiologic changes that occur with exercise.[37,40] Because the presence of vascular disease and the presence of lower-extremity symptoms are not necessarily related, exercise testing provides the vital link between the presentation and the disease. Exercise testing, therefore, should be performed in anyone with exertional symptoms and a normal to near-normal resting evaluation and in patients whose clinical presentation does not correspond to the findings on resting evaluation.

Many forms of exercise testing are available to the vascular laboratory. Walking on a treadmill generally best simulates most patients, inciting activity while allowing for some quantification of exertion (Fig. 6-8). A standard examination typically includes walking on a treadmill with a mild grade (10–12 degrees) at 1.5 to 2.0 miles per hour for 5 min. Depending on the activity level required to produce symptoms, the rigor of the test may be increased or decreased appropriately and recorded. If the treadmill is poorly tolerated, the patient may be ambulated in the hallway until symptoms occur. Other forms of exercise, such as heel lifts, can produce the physiologic changes of exercise induced ischemia. Relating the patient's symptoms to his or her presenting complaints may be less reliable, however.

Finally, postocclusive reactive hyperemia may be induced to simulate the physiologic changes of exercise. With this technique, a blood pressure cuff is placed at the thigh or calf level and inflated to suprasystolic pressure

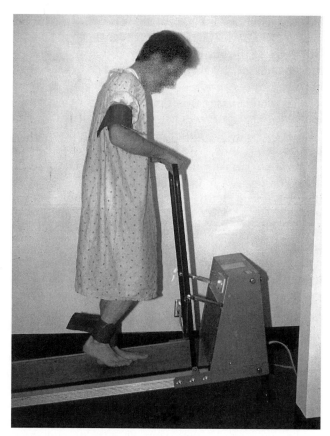

FIGURE 6-8. A standardized treadmill test represents a quantifiable, reproductive means of duplicating the physiologic conditions that produce most patients exercise-related complaints. The patient is monitored for symptoms during and after exercise. The blood pressure cuffs are left in place allowing for rapid measurement of ankle brachial indices and volume plethysmography recordings following exercise.

for several minutes. When the cuff is deflated, the underlying ischemic muscle is vasodilated and the changes of exercise simulated. This technique may be useful in patients unable to undergo standard treadmill testing, such as amputees; arthritic patients; or patients with significant cardiopulmonary, neurologic, or other conditions that limit their ability to comply with a treadmill test. The inflation of a limb cuff to suprasystolic levels, however, is frequently poorly tolerated. During exercise testing, the onset and quality of the patient's symptoms are recorded in addition to the level of activity. Following exercise, repeat ankle and brachial pressure measurements are made as expeditiously as possible. Some laboratories also perform repeat VPRs at the ankle level. Delayed measurements may be obtained to document recovery of the extremities as well. Simultaneously, the resolution of any symptoms that occurred with the exercise testing should be noted.

The normal response to exercise is maintenance or increase in brachial and ankle pressure.[37,40] ABIs should remain at approximately 1.0. The normal plethys-mographic response is that of increased amplitude with maintenance of a normal contour (see Fig. 6-4D). The increased amplitude is a result of increased perfusion of the exercised muscle. A reduction in the absolute ankle pressure, a decrease in the postexercise ABI, and degradation of the VPRs are abnormal responses. An abnormal exercise response correlating to the production of symptoms in a patient is a strong indicator of symptomatic vascular disease. A patient with pseudoclaudication, however, should not demonstrate an abnormal exercise response despite developing symptoms during exercise. Another form of abnormal treadmill exercise response is a significant decrease in brachial pressure, which may indicate silent myocardial ischemia and cardiac dysfunction. Should this occur, the patient should be monitored and the appropriate health care personnel notified. Contraindications to exercise testing include evidence of ongoing myocardial ischemia, severe respiratory disease, or physical disability that make exercise testing impractical. Nonetheless, few patients are unable to undergo some form of exercise testing. This technique should be used in all patients who experience exertional symptoms, but no clear correlation can be made between the findings on resting evaluation and the presentation. In patients with relatively normal resting examinations, exercise testing may not only document the disease process but also serve as the only means to document the results of therapy serving as a baseline study for future examinations. Despite the many advantages of physiologic noninvasive vascular testing, the lack of anatomic specificity continues to be its major drawback. For this reason and others, interest in vascular ultrasound for the diagnosis of vascular disease is growing.

Vascular ultrasound

With continued development in duplex ultrasound technology, vascular ultrasound has asserted itself as a primary modality in noninvasive vascular testing. The initial sonographic techniques with B-mode imaging and articulated arm scanners were poorly suited for vascular testing.[29,30,38,44-52] Resolution was poor, and although plaque occasionally was detected, there was no reliable means of quantification. Additionally, the techniques were so cumbersome that it was impractical to interrogate more than a focal segment of artery. Real-time gray-scale imaging with high-frequency transducers improved resolution considerably. Plaque could be detected and characterized as homogeneous, heterogeneous, or calcific; however, disease still could not be quantified adequately. The addition of gated Doppler technology to the ultrasound scanner, now known as *duplex ultrasonography,* resulted in the ability to detect plaque and, to some extent, measure its effect on blood flow in the vessel. More recently, color

Doppler technology has been added to most instruments used for vascular diagnosis. Although the color map itself does not quantify disease adequately, and indeed may obscure plaque if not used appropriately, it is extremely useful in surveying the arterial tree, identifying those segments where additional gated Doppler interrogation is necessary. This combination of technology has made vascular ultrasound a practical, reliable technique for the evaluation of vascular disease.

Protocols for peripheral arterial vascular ultrasound differ widely. The most rigorous examination is evaluation of the entire arterial tree from the abdominal ultrasound to the ankle bilaterally. A strong case can be made to include the aortoiliac segment because of the relative high frequency of stenotic and aneurysmal disease in these patients.[27-28,37,44-45] Similarly, knowledge of the runoff vessels in the calf has prognostic implications for any revascularization procedure undertaken more proximally. Many laboratories confine their evaluation to the femoropopliteal segment because interrogation of the entire arterial tree can be extremely cumbersome and protracted. Because inflow is extremely important, these protocols rely on indirect information obtained at the femoral level to predict the quality of the aortoiliac segment. Although a more thorough examination is preferred, the examination can be tailored to the specific information that is being sought. The limitations of vascular ultrasound must be understood clearly to avoid both false-positive and false-negative diagnoses, particularly when performing less than a complete examination.[46,52]

The technique of peripheral vascular ultrasound involves visual evaluation of the entire segment using grayscale technique, with or without color Doppler imaging, and segmental gated Doppler interrogation. The gray-scale evaluation should include evaluation for vascular abonormalities, such as plaque and aneurysmal disease, as well as other soft tissue abnormalities and recording representative images. The gated Doppler interrogation should encompass normal segments as well as regions of abnormality for morphological and hemodynamic comparisons. Evaluation of the femoral artery segment at a minimum should include measurements from the common femoral artery and the proximal, mild, and distal SFA, in addition to measurements from the abnormality identified.

The addition of real-time color Doppler can aid the technologist in directing the gated Doppler examination to specific regions of interest by detecting disturbances in the normal flow patterns (Fig. 6-9). An angle of 60 degrees or less should be used for evaluation of Doppler waveforms because angles of greater than 60 degrees result in significant error in velocity calculation. Only with consistent meticulous technique will reliable results be obtained. At each site, interrogated Doppler spectral

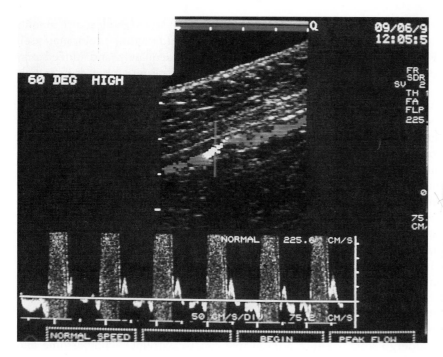

FIGURE 6-9. Color duplex imaging performed in the femoropopliteal arterial system of this 72-year-old man revealed a focal flow disturbance in the color map. Gated Doppler performed in the region revealed a peak systolic velocity in excess of 200 cm/sec. Measurement of the adjacent "normal" vessel demonstrated a PSV of 65 cm/sec. Angiography subsequently confirmed a moderately severe stenosis at the site.

waveforms should be recorded with measurement of peak systolic velocity (PSV). Finally, although focal abnormalities can be well characterized by vascular ultrasound little information is available regarding the physiologic effect of the disease on the patient. The Intersocietal Commission for the Accreditation of Vascular Laboratories (ICAVL) requires that some physiologic testing be done concomitantly with vascular ultrasound; at a minimum, ABIs are required.

Interpretation of vascular ultrasound combines the criteria used in DWA with an evaluation of PSVs.[38,44–47] Similar to DWA performed with CW Doppler, waveforms obtained by the gated Doppler technique in peripheral arteries at rest normally should have a triphasic pattern with steep systolic upstroke, an initial rapid diastolic downstroke with brief reversal of flow, followed by a gradually declining antegrade diastolic flow. Loss of this normal triphasic waveform is a strong predictor of proximal disease.[38] The degree of waveform degradation correlates to the severity of the disease proximal to the site of interrogation. Alteration of Doppler waveforms most commonly are used to grade disease in the aortoiliac system but may be useful in detecting obstructive disease throughout the arterial tree. For studies limited to the femoropopliteal segments, this may be the only indicator of proximal inflow disease; its importance therefore cannot be overstated. Loss of the reverse component of flow also may be encountered in Doppler waveforms just before a high-grade stenosis or occlusion.[37,44,45] This event should not be mistaken for poststenotic Doppler change because the systolic upstroke in the preocclusive lesion remains quite steep, and there is very poor diastolic antegrade flow ow-

ing to the high resistance of the distal lesion. Doppler waveforms within stenotic lesions will demonstrate increasing frequency shift (velocity), spectral broadening with filling of the normal clear window under the systolic peak, and loss of the reverse component of flow.[38,44,45,47]

PSV criteria most frequently are used to grade stenotic lesions in the femoropopliteal segments. Absolute velocities as well as comparison with normal adjacent segments are the basis of most commonly used criteria.[38,44–48] A PSV of greater than 200 cm/sec or a doubling of the PSV within a lesion is indicative of a stenosis of at least 50% severity (Fig. 6-9). A PSV of 400 cm/sec or greater or a quadrupling of PSV indicates a severity of 75% or greater. Although use of these criteria provides a simple means of grading stenoses in the femoropopliteal system, disease in either inflow or outflow may affect its accuracy.[4,8] Absolute PSV in particular will be reduced, with proximal occlusive disease resulting in false-negative studies. Although the use of PSV ratios may overcome this limitation, a "normal" adjacent segment may not be available for comparison.

The greatest advantage of duplex evaluation of the peripheral arteries is the ability to localize and characterize the disease process. Differentiation of an occlusion from a stenosis has clear significance when considering therapeutic options for PVD. Similarly, determining the length of an occlusion may influence therapeutic decisions. Besides being able to localize a lesion, the quality of the surrounding vessel can be assessed differentiating focal from diffuse disease. Finally, detection of associated abnormalities such as aneurysmal disease, pseudoaneurysms, and arteriovenous fistulae represents a significant advantage of the technique. Limitations are largely those associated with ultrasound in general. Obesity and bowel gas can limit the ability to visualize the aortoiliac segments significantly. Densely calcific plaque also may obscure regions of interest, especially in patients with diffuse disease.

Recently, the use of duplex imaging for graft surveillance has become more popular.[48–51] Peripheral bypass grafts may occlude without warning, such as preocclusive claudication. Traditional physiologic techniques may not detect graft abnormalities soon enough to avoid occlusion.[48] Routine surveillance with duplex imaging has been used to detect abnormalities in grafts so that repair can be effected before graft thrombosis occurs. Techniques of graft surveillance vary but generally include Doppler interrogation of the entire graft and its anastomoses. Measurement of a midgraft PSV in a "normal" segment provides a reproducible means of assessing flow within the graft, which is easily compared longitudinally in time. In addition to this measurement, a combination of color Doppler and gated Doppler can be used to detect focal abnormalities typically occuring at the anastomoses or, in the case of vein grafts, in the region of venous valves. A midgraft PSV of 45 cm/sec is frequently used as the cutoff value; values below this suggest impending graft failure. In addition to focal graft stenoses, however, graft diameter and outflow resistance play a significant role in determining the midgraft PSV.[49] Interval decrease in the midgraft PSV has been used as an indicator of graft dysfunction. Because of the variability in midgraft velocities, interrogation of the entire graft searching for focal graft abnormalities has been advocated. Using criteria similar to that for native arteries, a doubling of PSV at the site of abnormality compared to the adjacent "normal" segment indicates a significant stenosis of at least 50% severity.[49–52] Because most vein-graft failures occur within the first year, some researchers have advocated initial surveillance of the entire graft to detect the early failing graft, followed by less rigorous, intermittent midgraft evaluation.

■ Conclusions

Despite the increasing awareness of atherosclerotic vascular disease in the coronary and cerebral vasculature, the diagnosis of PVD frequently eludes clinicians. With its typically insidiousonset, the symptoms of PVD frequently are ignored or ascribed to the natural aging process. In the past, physicians have been reluctant to treat patients with PVD because of the relative morbidity and mortality associated with traditional revascularization procedures. Many clinicians may be unaware of newer, less invasive revascularization techniques that have safely and effectively expanded the indications for treatment of PVD. Although many patients will stabilize or improve with con-

servative measures after initial presentation, others will progress in their disease and require more aggressive therapy. Optimal care of patients with PVD requires timely, accurate diagnosis, starting with an appropriate history and physical examination. In advanced disease, these may be adequate to establish the diagnosis of PVD. Frequently, however, the diagnosis is not clear and the extent of disease is not readily apparent. The vascular laboratory therefore serves as an excellent resource in the diagnosis and management of vascular disease. As a screening modality, the vascular laboratory is cost effective in differentiating which patients intervention may be warranted from those who need only conservative management, thereby avoiding unnecessary diagnostic angiography. Similarly, the vascular laboratory aids in pretreatment planning in patients who will undergo angiography and percutaneous or surgical revascularization. Follow-up of PVD and revascularization procedures is also greatly facilitated, identifying patients who may be failing conservative management or who may need additional intervention. New technologies have added greatly to the armamentarium available to the vascular laboratory. The vascular clinician must choose the modality that will provide the most useful information in a cost-effective manner. In general, the most important task of the noninvasive laboratory remains not only the documentation of the presence and extent of disease but also the correlation of this information with the patient's symptoms. Many patients have atypical presentations that may require modification of the "standard" examination. A thorough understanding of the strengths and weaknesses of each of the noninvasive modalities is necessary for appropriate testing. Furthermore, only by combining the clinical evaluation with noninvasive testing can appropriate interpretation and diagnosis be made.

References

1. Vogt MT, Wolfson SK, Kuller LH. Lower extremity arterial disease and the aging process: a review. *J Clin Epidemiol* 1992;45:529–542.
2. Kannel WB, Skinner JJ, Schwartz MJ, Shurtleff D. Intermittent claudication: incidence in the Framingham Study. *Circulation* 1970;41:875–883.
3. McDaniel MD, Cronenwett JL. Basic data related to the natural history of intermittent claudication. *Ann Vasc Surg* 1989;3:273–277.
4. Criqui MH, Fronek A, Barrett-Connor E, et al. The prevalence of peripheral arterial disease in a defined population. *Circulation* 1985;71:510–515.
5. Hertzer NR. The natural history of peripheral vascular disease: implications for its management. *Circulation* 1991;(Suppl I) 83:I-12–I-19.
6. Cronenwett JL, Warner KG, Zelenock GB et al: Intermittent claudication: current results of nonoperative management. *Arch Surg* 1984;119:430–436.
7. Imparato AM, Kim G, Davidson T, Crowley JG. Intermittent claudication: its natural course. *Surgery* 1975;78:795–799.
8. Peabody CN, Kannel WB, McNamara PM. Intermittent claudication: surgical significance. *Arch Surg* 1974;109:693–697.

9. Hiatt WR, Regensteiner JG, Hargarten MS, et al. Benefit of exercise conditioning for patients with peripheral arterial disease. *Circulation* 1990;81:602–609.

10. Veith FJ, Gupta SK, Wengerter KR, et al. Impact of nonoperative therapy on the clinical management of peripheral arterial disease. *Circulation* 1991;83(Suppl I):I-137–I-142.

11. Mannick JA. Evaluation of chronic lower extremity ischemia. *N Engl J Med* 1983;309:841–843.

12. Lundgren F, Dahllof A, Lundholm K, et al. Intermittent claudication-surgical reconstruction or physical training. *Ann Surg* 1989;209:346–355.

13. Coffman JD. Intermittent claudication: not so benign. *Am Heart* 1986;112:1127–1128.

14. Criqui MH, Coughlin SS, Fronek A. Non-invasively diagnosed peripheral arterial disease as a predictor of mortality: results from a prospective population-based study. *Circulation* 1985;72:768–773.

15. Dormandy J, Mahir M, Ascady G, et al. Fate of the patient with chronic leg ischemia. *J Cardiovasc Surg* 1989;30:50–57.

16. Kannel WB, McGee DL. Update on some epidemiologic features of intermittent claudication. *J Am Geriar Soc* 1985;33:13–18.

17. Newman AB, Sutton-Tyrell K, Vogt MT, Kuller LH. Morbidity and mortality in hypertensive adults with a low ankle/arm blood pressure index. *JAMA* 1993;270:487–489.

18. Malone JM, Moore WS, Goldstone J. Life expectancy following aortofemoral arterial grafting. *Surgery* 1977;81:551–555.

19. DeWeese JA, Rob CG. Autogenous venous grafts ten years later. *Surgery* 1977;82:755–784.

20. Goodreau JJ, Creasy JK, Flanigan P, et al. Rational approach to the differentiation of vascular and neurogenic claudication. *Surgery* 1978;84:749–757.

21. Sise MJ, Shackford SR, Rowley WR, Pistone FJ. Claudication in young adults: a frequently delayed diagnosis. *J Vasc Surg* 1989;10:68–74.

22. Cronenwett J, Davis J, Gooch J, et al. Aortoiliac occlusive disease in women. *Surgery* 1980;88:775–784.

23. McKusick VA, Harris WS, Ottesen OE, et al. Buerger's disease: a distinct clinical and pathological entity. *JAMA* 1962;181:5–9.

24. Goodman RM, Elian B, Mozes M, et al. Buerger's disease in Israel. *Am J Med* 1965;39:601–615.

25. Coffman JD. Intermittent claudication and rest pain: physiologic concepts and therapeutic approaches. *Progr Cardiovasc Dis* 1979;22:53–72.

26. Brewer ML, Kinnison ML, Perler BA, White RI. Blue toe syndrome: treatment with anticoagulants and delayed percutaneous transluminal angioplasty. *Radiology* 1988;166:31–36.

27. Vermilion BD, Kimmins SA, Pace WG, Evans WE. A review of one hundred forty-seven popliteal aneurysms with long-term follow-up. *Surgery* 1981;90:1009–1014.

28. Dawson I, van Bockel JH, Brand R, Terpstra JL. Popliteal artery aneurysms: long-term follow-up of aneurysmal disease and results of surgical treatment. *J Vasc Surg* 1991;13:398–407.

29. Erickson CA, Towne JB, Seabrook GR, et al. Ongoing vascular laboratory surveillance is essential to maximize long-term in situ saphenous vein bypass patency. *J Vasc Surg* 1996; 23:18–27.

30. Turnipseed WD, Acher CW. Postoperative surveillance: an effective means of detecting correctable lesions that threaten graft patency. *Arch Surg* 1985;120:324–328.

31. Treiman RL. Peripheral vascular disease in diabetic patients: evaluation and treatment. *Mt Sinai J Med* 1987;54:241–244.

32. Rutherford RB, Flanigan DP, Gupta SK, et al. Suggested standards for reports dealing with lower extremity ischemia. *J Vasc Surg* 1986;4:80–94.

33. Rutherford RB, Becker GJ. Standards for evaluating and reporting the results of surgical and percutaneous therapy for peripheral arterial disease. *J Vasc Intervent Radiol* 1991;2:169–174.

34. Ahn SS, Rutherford RB, Becker GJ, Comerota AJ, et al. Reporting standards for lower extremity arterial endovascular procedures. *J Vasc Surg* 1993;17:1103–1107.

35. Rutherford RB. Standards for evaluating results of interventional therapy for peripheral vascular disease. *Circulation* 1991;83(Suppl I):I-6–I-11.

36. Marinelli MR, Beach KW, Glass MJ, et al. Noninvasive testing vs. clinical evaluation of arterial disease: a prospective study. *JAMA* 1979;241:2031–2034.

37. Bernstein EF. *Vascular Diagnosis*, 4th ed. St. Louis: Mosby, 1993;169–641.

38. Cossman DV, Ellison JE, Wagner WH, et al. Comparison of contrast angiography to arterial mapping with color-flow duplex imaging in the lower extremities. *Surgery* 1989;10:522–529.

39. Yucel EK, Dumoulin CL, Waltman AC. MR angiography of lower-extremity arterial disease: preliminary experience *J Magn Reson Imaging* 1992;2:303–309.

40. Raines JK, Darling RC, Buth J, et al. Vascular laboratory criteria for the management of peripheral vascular disease of the lower extremities. *Surgery* 1976;79:21–29.

41. Applegate WB. Ankle/arm blood pressure index: a useful test for clinical practice. *JAMA* 1993;270:497–498.

42. Barnes RW, Thornhill B, Nix L, et al. Predictions of amputation wound healing: role of Doppler ultrasound and digital photoplethysmography. *Arch Surg* 1981;116:80–83.

43. Barnes RW. Noninvasive diagnostic assessment of peripheral vascular disease. *Circulation* 1991;83(Suppl I):I-20–I-27.

44. Moneta GL, Strandness DE. Peripheral arterial duplex scanning. *J Clin Ultrasound* 1987;15:645–651.

45. Kohler TR, Nance DR, Cramer MM, et al. Duplex scanning for diagnosis of aortoiliac and femoropopliteal disease: a prospective study. *Circulation* 1987;76:1074–1080.

46. Polak JF, Karmel MI, Meyerovitz MF. Accuracy of color Doppler flow mapping for evaluation of the severity of femoropopliteal arterial disease: a prospective study. *J Vasc Intervent Radiol* 1991;2:471–479.

47. Edwards JM, Coldwell DM, Goldman ML, Strandness DE. The role of duplex scanning in the selection of patients for transluminal angioplasty. *J Vasc Surg* 1991;13:69–74.

48. Allard L, Cloutier G, Durand L, et al. Limitations of ultrasonic duplex scanning for diagnosing lower limb arterial stenoses in the presence of adjacent segment disease. *J Vasc Surg* 1994;19:650–657.

49. Green RM, McNamara J, Ouriel K, Deweese JA. Comparison of infrainguinal graft surveillance techniques. *J Vasc Surg* 1990;11:207–215.

50. Belkin M, Raftery KB, Mackey WC. A prospective study of the determinants of vein graft flow velocity: implications for surveillance. *J Vasc Surg* 1994;19:259–267.

51. Mills JL, Bandyk DF, Gahtan V, Esses GE. The origin of infrainguinal graft stenosis: a prospective study based on duplex surveillance. *J Vasc Surg* 1995;21:16–25.

52. Dalsing MC, Cikrit DF, Lalka SG, et al. Femorodistal vein grafts: the utility of graft surveillance criteria. *J Vasc Surg* 1995;21:127–134.

7

Vascular Recanalization Techniques

BRAD M. HOPPENFELD AND JACOB CYNAMON

This chapter is an overview of the techniques of percutaneous intervention for recanalizing stenotic or occluded vessels. The indications and results for peripheral vascular, renal vascular, and venous intervention are discussed in subsequent chapters.

As early as 1964, Dotter and Judkins reported on the use of coaxial catheters to restore flow to a gangrenous extremity.[1] In 1974, Gruentzig and Hopff introduced a double-lumen balloon catheter that revolutionized the field of interventional radiology.[2] Stents, which were introduced in the late 1980s, helped to improve the results obtained with angioplasty alone. A suboptimal angioplasty now can be converted to a successful procedure with the placement of a stent. Acutely thrombosed vessels can be treated with the judicious use of thrombolytic agents. Lesions uncovered after clot dissolution can be treated with balloon angioplasty. These recanalization techniques can be used immediately after the diagnostic arteriogram either via the same percutaneous access used for the diagnostic arteriogram or through a second access site, thus simplifying the procedure.

Diagnostic arteriography should be performed only after a complete vascular workup, including noninvasive testing. Patients should have clear indications for revascularization, which include rest pain, nonhealing ulcers, gangrene, or severe claudication failing attempts at conservative therapy (i.e., smoking cessation and a consistent exercise program).[3–5]

When treating patients with peripheral vascular disease, we choose to access the vascular system, when possible, through the common femoral artery contralateral to the symptomatic extremity. This approach facilitates angioplasty or thrombolysis using the original puncture and does not preclude performing a second percutaneous puncture of the symptomatic extremity once the pathology is defined. The Seldinger technique, using either a double-wall or single-wall needle, is used to enter the common femoral artery. It is extremely important to enter the common femoral artery below the inguinal ligament and above its bifurcation to limit complications such as retroperitoneal hematomas, pseudoaneurysms, and arteriovenous fistulae.[6,7] Using fluoroscopy, the common femoral artery is entered in its course over the lower half of the femoral head. The inferior epigastric artery and the deep circumflex iliac artery are good anatomic landmarks for the position of the inguinal ligament because these vessels arise off of the most distal aspect of the external iliac artery. If a prior angiogram is available, it should be reviewed to note the position of these vessels. It is safe to assume, however, that the inguinal ligament does not dip below the midfemoral head in almost all cases. It is important to puncture the common femoral artery over the midfemoral head. Too high a puncture may lead to retroperitoneal hematomas secondary to an inability to achieve adequate compression, and too low a puncture may lead to an arteriovenous fistula because the artery and vein tend to overlie each other in this region.

When treating peripheral vascular disease, a bilateral femoral arteriogram is performed from the level of the renal arteries to the feet. Appropriate oblique views of the pelvis and groin must be obtained to exclude lesions at the bifurcations of the common iliac artery and common femoral artery. When evaluating the angiogram, one

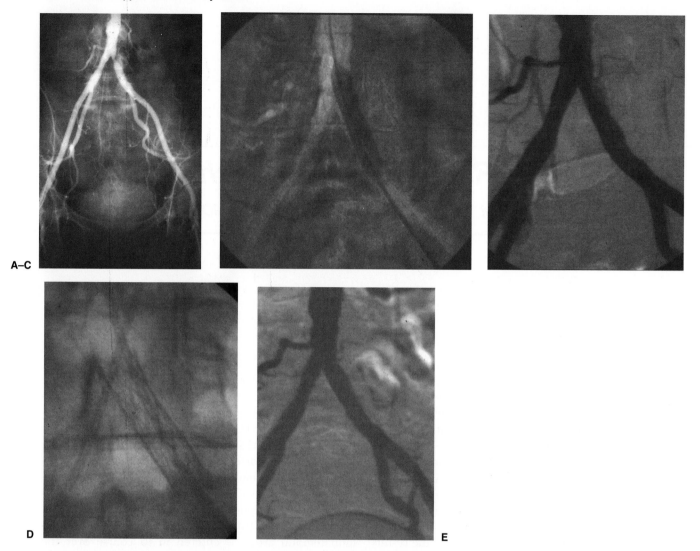

FIGURE 7-1. A 45-year-old man, a smoker presented with half block claudication on the left. **(A)** Angiogram via the right common femoral artery demonstrates a focal moderate to severe stenosis at the origin of the left common iliac artery. A left common femoral artery puncture is performed, and pressures obtained above and below the lesion demonstrate a 40-mm mercury gradient. **(B)** Percutaneous angioplasty is performed with an 8 mm × 4 cm balloon via the left common femoral artery approach. **(C)** Postpercutaneous transluminal angiography demonstrates a residual defect with persistent pressure gradient. **(D)** A Palmaz P294 stent (Cordis, Johnson & Johnson Corp.,) is deployed across the lesion. **(E)** Poststenting angiogram demonstrates resolution of the lesion. No further pressure gradient is observed.

must take into consideration the patient's history, physical examination, and noninvasive studies. If the angiogram does not correlate with these studies, additional views must be obtained to uncover lesions that may not be clearly evident on the original arteriogram.

Percutaneous transluminal angioplasty for peripheral atherosclerotic disease is best performed on short focal stenoses or occlusions in large vessels. Lesions longer than 10 cm are considered less likely to have good initial and long-term results.[8,9] With the use of stents, however, even long lesions in the aortoiliac distribution can be treated successfully.[10] Results in the femoropopliteal distribution are less rewarding; however, when dealing with shorter lesions, results are acceptable. Even tibial vessels

can be treated with angioplasty; however, these vessels should be treated only for limb-salvage indications. When treating occlusions, one must be convinced that the occlusion is chronic. If the occlusion is relatively acute, the incidence of embolization resulting from a clot may be high. Therefore, if an occlusion is suspected to be less than 6 weeks old, a primary angioplasty without prior thrombolysis probably should not be performed.

■ Aortoiliac Angioplasty

If an aortic or iliac lesion is identified or suspected, pressures must be obtained above and below the lesion to

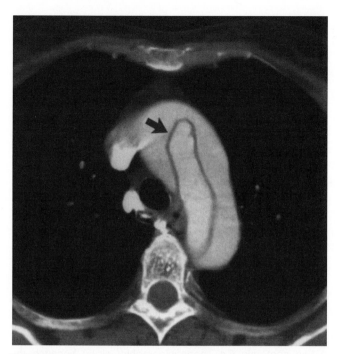

FIGURE 5-22. Axial image at the level of the aortic arch from the same contrast enhanced computed tomographic angiogram of a type I aortic dissection seen in Fig. 5-11. The intimal flap (*arrow*) is clearly visible because of the contrast-enhanced blood in the surrounding lumen. Postprocessed images are not necessary to make the diagnosis of dissection.

native technique for aortic imaging) for detection of great vessel origin injuries and arch vessel anomalies such as replacement of the left vertebral artery to the aortic arch are unknown.

To image the entire thoracic aorta, a collimation of 3 to 7 mm with a pitch of 1 to 2 is necessary.[27] A collimation of 7 mm may seem relatively thick, but it is important to remember that the thoracic aorta and the great vessels are large vascular structures. Cardiac pulsatility is an important source of artifacts on axial source images as well, particularly in the region of the aortic root. Crescentic linear artifacts can occur that may be confused with dissection flaps.

Contrast (60% iodine) injection rates should be 3 to 5 mL/sec for a total of 100 to 150 mL.[25,27] Although injection of contrast via an arm vein is typical, it may introduce streak artifacts from intense opacification of the brachiocephalic veins and superior vena cava. In most cases, it is not time efficient in an unstable patient to try to find a suitable injection site in the lower extremities, and the streak artifact is not severe enough to warrant such a maneuver. A slightly shorter delay may be required than for abdominal CTA but timing boluses should be used whenever possible. Breath-holding is necessary for optimum imaging.

Pulmonary arteries

An accurate, safe, and quick noninvasive technique to diagnose pulmonary artery thromboembolism would be a major advance in patient care. Pulmonary embolism is one of the most feared entities in clinical practice, and yet it remains frequently an elusive diagnosis. Although the morbidity of pulmonary angiography is in actuality low, many clinicians are reluctant to pursue imaging beyond ventilation/perfusion (V/Q) scans. One of the limitations of V/Q scans is that the results of scans for pulmonary embolism are expressed as a probability, rather than a binary "yes"or "no" result. The promise of cross-sectional angiographic techniques is that a more definitive diagnosis will be rendered.[35]

MRA
MRA of the pulmonary arteries is challenging because patients are frequently ill, the characteristics of flow are complex in the pulmonary vasculature, and emboli vary in size from several centimeters to several millimeters. Excellent preliminary results have been reported with a number of techniques, including 2-D TOF, 2-D PC, and 3-D gadolinium-enhanced sequences.[35] The most widely used sequences are 3-D gadolinium-enhanced, with or without breath-holding. An important advantage of MRA in pulmonary embolism is that the lower extremities and pelvis can be screened for DVT with MR venography at the same time. A major limitation is that detection of small peripheral emboli is poor with MRA. In general, pulmonary artery MRA as a clinical tool remains available at only a limited number of institutions.[35]

CTA
Helical CTA for pulmonary embolism has been embraced enthusiastically because of the simplicity of the technique and the wide availability of helical CT scanners. Central emboli are detected with a greater than 95% sensitivity and specificity, although the sensitivity for small peripheral emboli is much lower.[22] Given this limitation, the unresolved question becomes, What represents a clinically "significant" pulmonary embolism? If one accepts that all pulmonary emboli are important, whether peripheral or central, massive or small, then pulmonary angiography should be considered in patients with negative helical scans. CT for pulmonary embolism has a potential role as a first line imaging test for patients with suspected pulmonary embolism and normal renal function. This modality will not be appropriate for patients with tenuous or compromised renal function.

As with CTA of the thoracic aorta, the axial images are frequently diagnostic in helical CTA of the pulmonary arteries. The diagnostic feature of pulmonary embolus is an intraluminal filling defect within a pulmonary artery (Fig. 5-23). Interbronchial lymph nodes can result in

advantage of CT is that the arterial phase can be imaged with an initial scan using a 20-sec. delay. In addition, information about the periportal soft tissues can be obtained at the same time, and the direction of portal flow has no impact on venous opacification. The latter is also a disadvantage, as direction of flow cannot be determined from CT data.

Thoracic aorta

The thoracic aorta is subject to a wide range of pathology, including aneurysm formation, dissection, arteritis, traumatic transection, and congenital lesions such as coarctation. The most appropriate imaging modality for a specific patient depends on the suspected diagnosis, the clinical status of the patient, and the information needed to make a management decision. For example, an unstable patient with a suspected ruptured thoracic aortic aneurysm may be imaged initially with a noncontrast CT scan of the chest; if an aneurysm is detected and blood is present in the mediastinum or pleural cavity, no further workup may be necessary. At the other end of the spectrum, a stable patient who is being monitored for a known dissection can be imaged with MR or contrast-enhanced CT. In general, MRI has no role in the patient with a suspected acute traumatic aortic transection.

MRA

Most MRI of the thoracic aorta can be accomplished using T1-weighted images in multiple planes (axial, coronal, sagittal, sagittal-oblique).[32] Nonangiographic sequences have a greater than 95% sensitivity and specificity for detection of aortic dissection (Fig. 5-21), and the multiplanar acquisitions allow accurate determination of the relationship between the left subclavian artery and pathologic processes such as dissections and descending aortic aneurysms.[33] Cardiac gating and respiratory compensation should be used to maximize image quality.

MRA sequences are most useful in the thoracic aorta to confirm flow in dissections or to diagnose occlusive disease of the great vessel origins. For example, flow in a false lumen in a dissection may be so slow that it appears gray on T1-weighted images. To distinguish between a patent or thrombosed false lumen, a flow sensitive sequence is required. Cardiac gated axial 2-D PC sequences with a V_{enc} set to detect slow flow (40 cm/sec) with flow encoding in the superior-inferior direction can answer the question quickly. For occlusive disease of the great vessel origins, 2-D and 3-D TOF, as well as 3-D PC sequences, all have been employed with success. One of the challenges of thoracic aortic MRA is that flow is multidirectional and, in the presence of aneurysms or dissections, slow and turbulent. Dynamic gadolinium contrast-

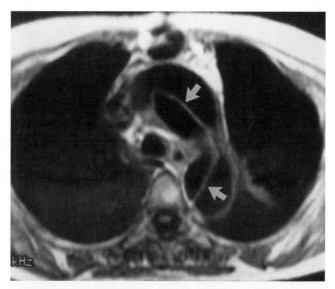

FIGURE 5-21. Axial T1-weighted image from just below the aortic arch in a patient with a type I aortic dissection. The dissection flap (*arrows*) is seen in the lumens of both the ascending and the descending aorta. The flap is readily visible in this anatomic (i.e., nonangiographic) study because the flowing blood in the aorta exits the slice before it can be imaged, and thus it appears black.

enhanced 3-D techniques are useful in these cases because there is no loss of signal resulting from slow or complex directional flow.[34]

CTA

Helical acquisition of thoracic aortic CT scans allows imaging from the thoracic inlet to the diaphragm in 20 to 40 secs. Furthermore, when imaging an unstable patient, intensive care equipment such as monitors, respirators, and infusion pumps is safe to use in the scanner room. For these reasons, helical CT is the preferred modality for unstable patients with suspected acute thoracic aortic pathology. As with MRI, most diagnoses can be arrived at from the axial source images. Multiplanar reconstructions usually supplement, rather than supplant, the axial source images.

Contrast-enhanced CT has a greater than 95% sensitivity and specificity for aortic dissection and transection.[25,27] The diagnosis of dissection requires demonstration of blood (flowing or thrombosed) on both sides of an intimal flap (Fig. 5-22). In many centers, no further imaging of dissections is obtained if the CT is of high quality. Traumatic aortic transection is implied from the presence of a mediastinal hematoma adjacent to the aortic arch, although pseudoaneurysms may be visualized on contrast-enhanced studies. Stable patients with positive CT scans should undergo angiography to confirm and localize the injury, because the sensitivities and specificities of CT (or transesophageal echo [TEE], an alter-

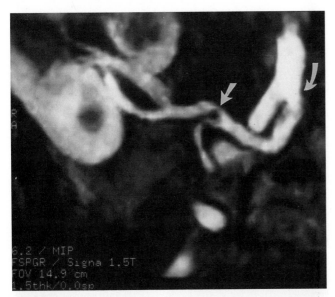

FIGURE 5-19. Oblique restricted maximum-intensity projection of a gadolinium-enhanced three-dimensional time-of-flight magnetic resonance angiogram of a transplanted kidney located in the right pelvis. There is moderate narrowing of the renal artery anastomosis with the right hypogastric artery (*straight arrow*). The origin of the hypogastric artery is patent (*curved arrow*).

Portal, splenic, and mesenteric veins

Imaging of the portal venous system is performed most commonly for patency, involvement by malignant tu-

mors, or evidence of portal hypertension. Results with both MR and CT portal venography have been excellent;[6,25] however, it is important to keep in mind that duplex color-flow ultrasound is an inexpensive and rapid alternate method of assessing the portal venous system.

MR venography

The portal venous system is well suited to imaging with MR techniques because portal blood flow is slow and nonpulsatile. The entire portal venous system can be imaged quickly with 2-D TOF, 2-D PC, and 3-D gadolinium-enhanced sequences, particularly when acquired in the coronal plane. With PC sequences the V_{enc} should be between 10 and 30 cm/sec. The direction of flow in the portal vein (important in patients with suspected portal hypertension) can be determined from display of PC images with directional encoding or with saturation bands in TOF sequences.[6] Excellent results also have been reported with gadolinium contrast-enhanced techniques.[31]

CT venography

Portal venous imaging with helical CT scanners requires a longer delay than arterial imaging, frequently as long as 60 sec. Contrast (60% iodine) is injected at a rate of 2 to 4 mL/sec, for a total volume of 100 to 150 mL. Scanning should begin caudal and progress cephalad, as this is the same direction as flow within the mesenteric veins. Breath-holding is necessary to minimize motion artifact. A major

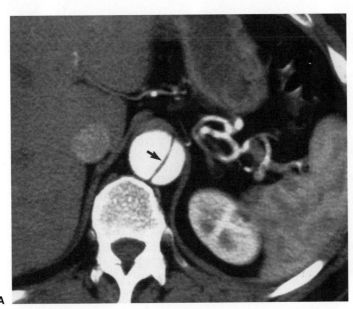

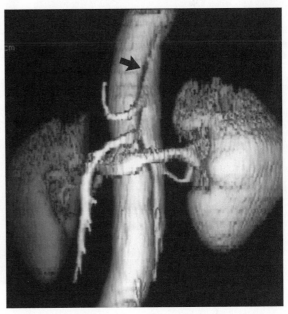

A   B

FIGURE 5-20. Computed tomographic (CT) angiogram of a patient with a type III aortic dissection. **A:** Axial source image above the level of the celiac artery shows contrast-enhanced flow on both sides of an intimal flap (*arrow*) in the abdominal aorta. This finding is diagnostic of dissection. **B:** Shaded surface display of the CT angiogram. The relationship of the dissection flap (*arrow*) to the abdominal vessels is clearly demonstrated. The flap appears as a cleft in the contrast column because of the postprocessing algorithm used to create the surface display.

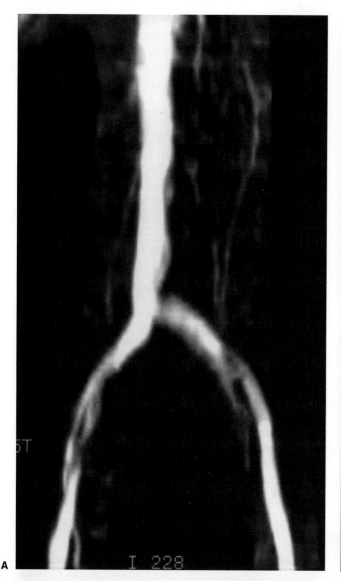

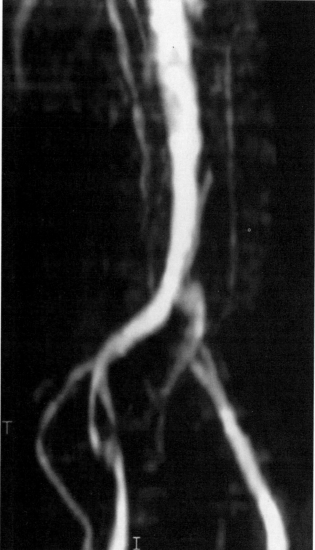

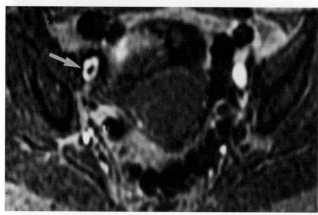

FIGURE 5-18. Magnetic resonance (MR) venogram of the pelvis in a patient with suspected right lower-extremity deep vein thrombosis but a normal ultrasound examination. **A:** Coronal maximum intensity projection (MIP) of a two-dimensional time-of-flight (2-D TOF) MR venogram. What do you think? **B:** Right anterior oblique MIP of the same study. Now what is your diagnosis? **C:** Axial source image from the 2-D TOF MR venogram shows an intraluminal filling defect in the right external iliac vein (*arrow*) consistent with thrombus. Note that the thrombus is completely surrounded by a bright signal (i.e., flow), explaining why the thrombus is so hard to see in the coronal projection. This case underscores the importance of reviewing source images to evaluate suspicious findings.

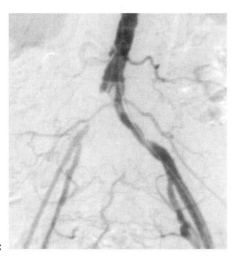
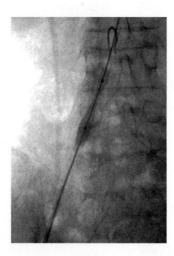
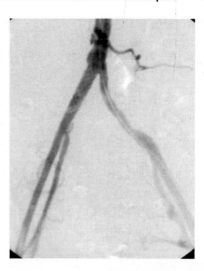

A–C

FIGURE 7-2. An 82-year-old woman presented with severe claudication of the right lower extremity. **(A)** Diagnostic arteriogram from the left common femoral artery demonstrates an occlusion of the right common iliac artery. **(B)** A retrograde puncture of the right common femoral artery was performed, and a guidewire was passed across the lesion. The lesion was primarily stented with a Palmaz P394 stent (Cordis, Johnson & Johnson Corp.). **(C)** Postangioplasty and stenting angiogram demonstrates the recanalized right common iliac artery. Note that the right external iliac artery has an enlarged caliber as a result of increased arterial flow.

document its hemodynamic significance. Any resting gradient is considered significant. If no resting gradient is present, a vasodilator such as 60 mg of papaverine or 100 to 200 µg of nitroglycerin should be administered intraarterially distal to the lesion in question. A peak systolic gradient of greater than 10 mm of mercury is considered significant.[11] When the outflow is markedly obstructed (such as in the presence of both superficial femoral artery and profunda femoral artery disease), there may not be a demonstrable gradient, despite the presence of a high-grade stenosis. These lesions should be identified and treated. If a bypass is performed below a significant

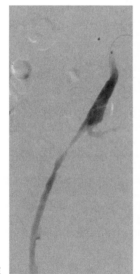
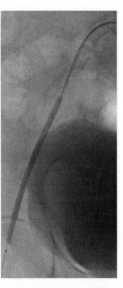
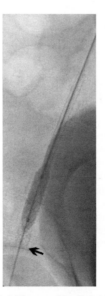
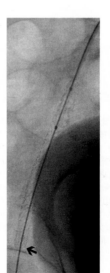
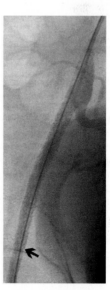

A–E

FIGURE 7-3. A 78-year-old man presented with a failing right femoral to distal bypass graft. **(A)** Initial arteriogram was performed from the left common femoral artery, a Sos Omni flush catheter (Angiodynamics) was advanced into the right common iliac artery, where a selective right iliac angiogram demonstrates a long external iliac stenosis. **(B)** An up and over Balkin contralateral 7 Fr sheath (Cook Group Company) was advanced into the right common iliac artery from the initial left common femoral artery puncture. A guidewire is advanced beyond the lesion and a 4 mm × 10 cm balloon was used to deliver a 78-mm-long IntraStent (Intratherapeutics) across the lesion. **(C)** The stent is opened further with a 7 mm × 2 cm balloon. **(D)** There is no foreshortening with this balloon-expandable stent. **(E)** Poststenting angiogram demonstrates resolution of the lesion.

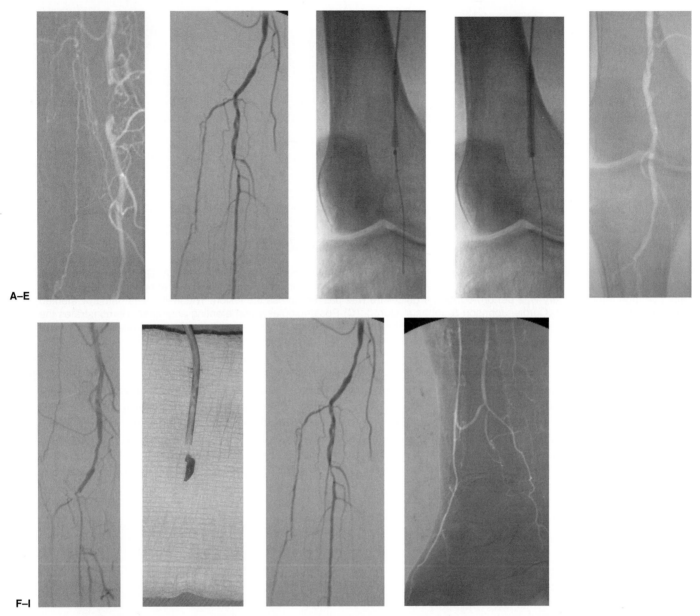

A–E

F–I

FIGURE 7-4. An 83-year-old man with diabetes presented with a nonhealing ulcer of the right heel. (**A**) A short-segment occlusion of the popliteal artery is identified on the initial arteriogram performed via the left common femoral artery. A right common femoral antegrade puncture is performed to treat the lesion, and this digital image of the lesion is acquired. (**B**) Arteriogram of the distal runoff demonstrates occlusions of the midportion of the anterior tibial and of the posterior tibial arteries. The tibial–peroneal trunk is patent, and there is mild disease at the origin of the peroneal artery. (**C**) Angioplasty of the popliteal lesion is performed with a 4 mm × 4 cm balloon. (**D**) The balloon is brought to full profile. (**E**) Postangioplasty angiogram demonstrates resolution of the popliteal occlusion, but the distal runoff appears obstructed. (**F**) Occlusion of the anterior tibial artery and tibial–peroneal trunk is noted in the runoff evaluation. A 6 Fr guiding catheter is advanced over the guidewire to the site of occlusion. (**G**) Aspiration thromboembolectomy is performed with the guiding catheter, and the embolus is removed. The catheter and aspirated embolus are displayed on the gauze pad. (**H and I**) Postaspiration angiogram demonstrates recovery of the original runoff.

lesion, the bypass may be compromised as a result of inadequate flow. Iliac angioplasty and stent placement can be performed around the aortic bifurcation using the puncture site of the diagnostic arteriogram. In many circumstances, we choose to puncture the ipsilateral common femoral artery in a retrograde fashion. This approach allows for simultaneous arterial pressure measurements above and below the lesion and facilitates accurate straight-line stent placement at the origin of the common iliac artery, if necessary (Fig. 7-1).

All interventions should be performed through a vascular sheath. The sheath usually facilitates the interven-

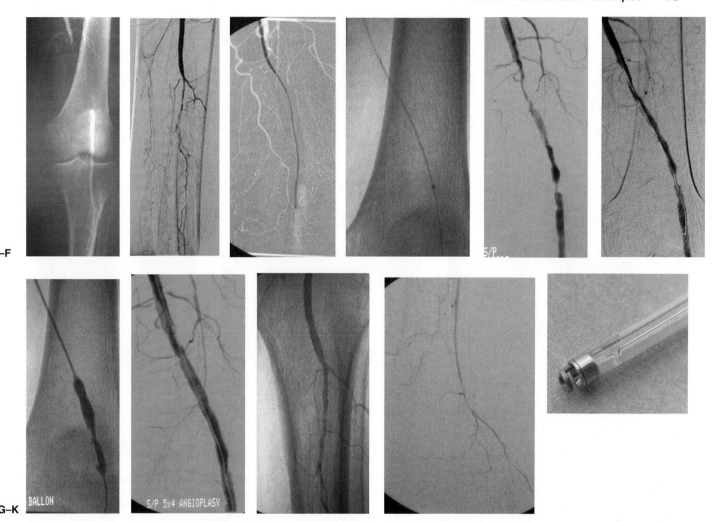

FIGURE 7-5. A 68-year-old man presented with new-onset rest pain in the right lower extremity. **(A)** Diagnostic angiogram is performed from the right common femoral artery, demonstrating occlusion of the left popliteal artery. **(B)** Significant three-vessel tibial disease is noted with reconstitution of the distal anterior tibial artery. **(C)** An up and over Balkin contralateral 5.5 Fr sheath (Cook Group Company) was advanced into the external iliac artery. A 5 Fr Berenstein catheter (Angiodynamics) was advanced over a Bentson guidewire (Angiodynamics, Inc.) into the popliteal artery, and a Possis Angiojet device (Possis Medical) was passed over a V-18 control wire (Boston Scientific) across the occlusion. **(D)** Closeup of the Possis Angiojet removing thrombus. **(E)** Post-Possis angiogram demonstrates a channel and underlying lesions. At this point, the patient became asymptomatic. Two hours of thrombolysis with rt-PA was performed at 2 mg/hour drip into the superficial femoral artery to dissolve any residual clot that may not have been removed by the Possis device. **(F)** Significant improvement was noted following thrombolysis. **(G)** An angioplasty of the stenotic lesion was performed with a 5 mm × 4 cm balloon. **(H)** Postangioplasty angiogram demonstrates a good result. **(I)** The infrapopliteal angiogram is unchanged. **(J)** There is reconstitution of the distal anterior tibial and dorsalis pedis arteries. **(K)** Photograph of the Possis Angiojet's Halo catheter.

tion by allowing for rapid catheter exchange, easier post-procedure angiographic evaluation, and decreased patient discomfort in the groin; it is associated with a lower incidence of complications. All patients are routinely pretreated with aspirin as an antiplatelet agent. Although many physicians use intraprocedural anticoagulation with heparin, its value is unconfirmed, and excessive use of heparin may lead to a higher incidence of local complications such as hematomas and pseudoaneurysms. With the current advances of endoluminal closure devices, full anticoagulation is less problematic. Ideally, tight stenotic lesions should be crossed using road mapping. The best guidewire catheter combination to cross the stenosis depends on the lesion and the operator.

Long lesions, external iliac artery lesions, and occlusions also can be treated. The optimal percutaneous therapy for iliac occlusions has not yet been determined. These lesions have been treated with initial lysis and subsequent angioplasty or stenting of the underlying lesions. Other successful treatments include primary stenting of iliac occlusions[12–15] (Fig. 7-2). The response to

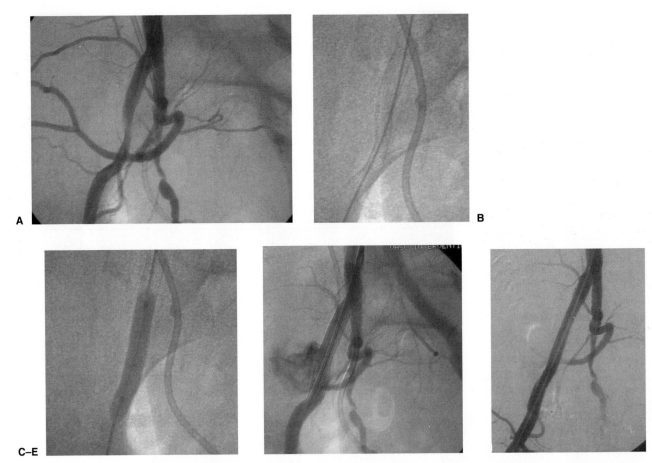

FIGURE 7-6. A 57-year-old woman with metastatic cervical cancer, postradiation therapy, presented with claudication progressing to rest pain in the right lower extremity. **(A)** Diagnostic arteriogram performed from the right common femoral artery demonstrates a significant lesion across the right external iliac artery. A significant pressure gradient is identified. **(B)** A 7 × 60 mm Smart Stent (Cordis, Johnson & Johnson Corp.) is deployed across the lesion. Following angioplasty, rupture of the iliac artery is suspected from the patient's continued pain and confirmed with angiography. **(C)** The balloon is inflated across the rupture to control the bleeding. **(D)** Bleeding continues despite prolonged balloon inflation. **(E)** A covered stent is deployed, the rupture is controlled (as demonstrated in the poststenting angiogram), and the iliac lesion is resolved.

balloon angioplasty of longer lesions is often less than ideal. Suboptimal angioplasty or an occlusive dissection is not uncommon; therefore, many interventional radiologists would recommend stenting these lesions primarily (Fig. 7-3). A balloon-expandable stent (e.g., Palmaz-Schatz, Cordis, Johnson & Johnson Corp., New Brunswick, NJ, U.S.A.) (see Fig. 7-1B) an IntraStent (Intratherapeutics, St. Paul, MN, U.S.A.) (see Fig. 7-3) or a self-expanding stent such as the Wallstent (Boston Scientific Corp., San Ramon, CA, U.S.A) or Smart Stent (see Fig. 7-17D) (Cordis, Johnson & Johnson Corp., New Brunswick, NJ, U.S.A.) (see Fig. 7-17D) can be placed. Suboptimal angioplasty of ideal lesions also can be managed by placing a stent (see Fig. 7-1). After intervention, pressures should be obtained again to assess hemodynamically the adequacy of the intervention.[11,16–18]

Most complications of angioplasty can be managed nonoperatively. The most common complication is a hematoma, usually self-limited at the puncture site. Pseudoaneurysms can be treated definitively by using ultrasound-guided compression or percutaneous thrombin injection. In situ thrombosis or distal embolization during or after angioplasty can be treated with intra-arterial thrombolytics, with suction thromboembolectomy using a guiding catheter (Fig. 7-4), or with the Possis Angiojet device (Possis Medical, Minneapolis, MN, U.S.A.). Obstructing flaps can be stented. Iliac rupture is a feared complication because these patients may require surgery to prevent exsanguination. Iliac rupture is suggested by the presence of continued pain after the angioplasty balloon is deflated and the presence of free extravasation of contrast after angioplasty. The angioplasty balloon should be immediately reinflated across the lesion to tamponade the rupture. The patient then can be considered for transfer to the operating room for repair of the vessel; alternatively, a covered stent (if available) can be delivered via the femoral access to exclude the rupture (Fig. 7-6).

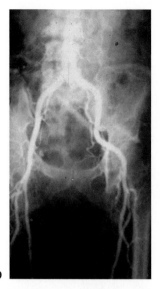
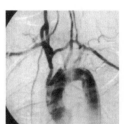
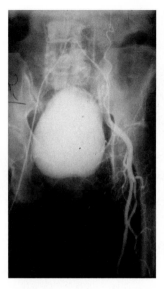
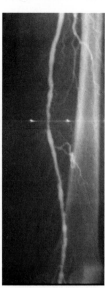

A–D

FIGURE 7-7. A 70-year-old woman, a smoker with diabetes, presented with a nonhealing ulcer of the left foot. **(A)** Long-leg cut-film film angiogram demonstrates a steep bifurcation of the aorta. **(B)** Mild to moderate disease is present in the superficial femoral artery and popliteal artery, with a severe (99%) stenosis of the proximal popliteal artery in the adductor canal. **(C)** Despite the steep bifurcation, a second puncture is avoided, and an up and over Balkin contralateral 5.5 Fr sheath (Cook Group Company) was advanced into the left common iliac artery. A guidewire is advanced beyond the lesion, and a 5 mm × 3 cm balloon angioplasty is performed. **(D)** Postdilatation angiogram demonstrates an adequate result.

■ Superficial Femoral and Popliteal Artery Intervention

Stenoses or occlusions of the superficial femoral artery and popliteal artery up to 10 cm long are considered amenable to balloon angioplasty. These lesions can be approached from the contralateral extremity by using the common femoral artery access created during the diagnostic arteriogram (Fig. 7-7). Using an "over-the-corner" sheath markedly facilitates the advancement of balloon catheters across lesions using the contralateral approach.

Alternatively, an antegrade puncture can be performed. An antegrade puncture can be technically challenging, especially in obese patients. Again, one must be careful to enter the common femoral artery (CFA) at the midfemoral head, below the inguinal ligament and above its bifurcation (Fig. 7-8). The guidewire then must be selectively advanced into the superficial femoral artery (SFA). Several techniques have been developed to redirect the wire that preferentially advances into the profunda femoral artery (PFA): After documenting that the entry point is into the CFA, the needle can be redirected to the contralateral wall and the wire readvanced; alternatively, the floppy tip of a moveable core wire can be advanced into the profunda and allowed to herniate into the SFA. Another method is to exchange the needle for a directional catheter and retract it under fluoroscopy to redirect a wire into the SFA. A fourth method is to exchange the needle for a 4 French dilator, place a 0.018-inch guidewire into the PFA, and withdraw the dilator into the CFA; then, using road mapping, a second 0.018-inch guidewire is advanced through the dilator, directing it into the SFA; finally, a dilator with a sidehole proximal to the endhole (Cope-Saddekni SFA Access dilator, Cook Group, Bloomington, IN, U.S.A.) can be advanced into the PFA and retracted until a wire can be advanced through the sidehole and into the SFA. After the wire is in place in the SFA, a vascular sheath is introduced. Most physicians anticoagulate patients during the procedure to prevent thrombus formation resulting from partially obstructed flow, catheter manipulations, or balloon inflation.

Using road mapping, a directional catheter and floppy guidewire (the choice of guidewire and catheter is operator and lesion dependent), the lesion is crossed. The catheter then is exchanged for a balloon of appropriate size and length. Alternatively, the angioplasty balloon can be used with an appropriate guidewire primarily to cross the lesion, thereby saving a catheter exchange. The postangioplasty result is evaluated by a repeat angiogram while maintaining a guidewire across the angioplasty site. Less than a 30% residual stenosis without embolic complication constitutes a successful result. Embolic complications can be managed with thrombolysis or suction aspiration (see Fig. 7-4). If there is an obstructing flap or a residual stenosis, a prolonged dilatation can be attempted to improve this initial result or to tack down the flap. Alternatively, stents can be used to bridge obstructing flaps postangioplasty; however, the long-term patency of femoropopliteal stents is not well documented.

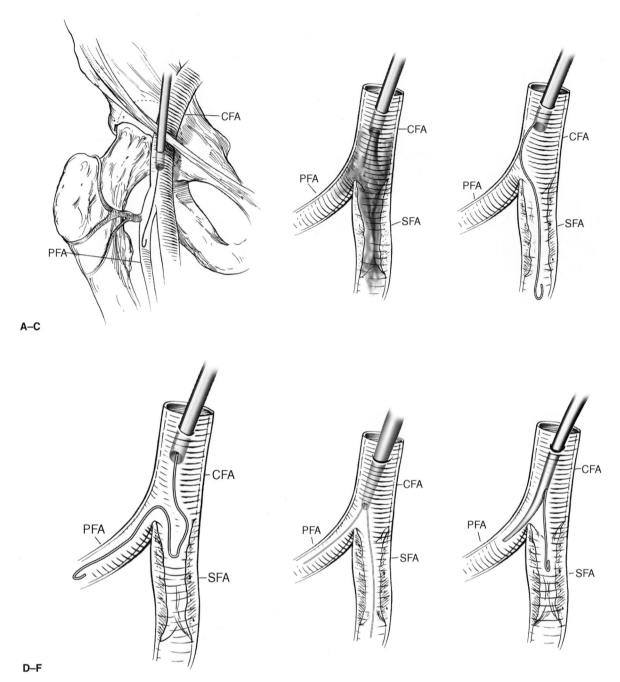

A–C

D–F

FIGURE 7-8. (A) Diagram of antegrade puncture of the common femoral artery over the midfemoral head. **(B)** Demonstration of redirection of the needle tip by injecting contrast to identify the superficial femoral artery from the profunda. **(C)** Demonstration of redirection of the guidewire into the superficial femoral artery (SFA) through the needle. **(D)** Demonstration of redirection of the guidewire by herniation of the wire into the SFA. **(E)** Demonstration of using a 4 Fr dilator with two 0.018-inch guidewires, one in the profunda, while the dilator is retracted and the second wire is passed down the SFA. **(F)** Demonstration of Saddekni dilator (Cope-Saddekni SFA access dilator: Cook Group) redirecting the wire into the SFA.

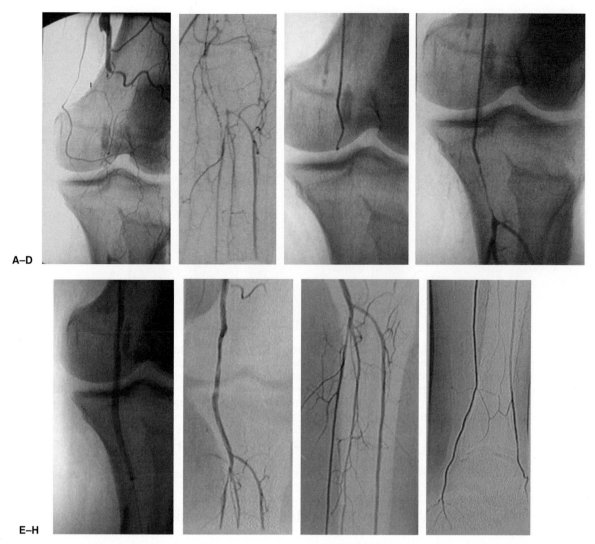

A–D

E–H

FIGURE 7-9. An 85-year-old diabetic man presented with a nonhealing right heel ulcer. (**A**) Diagnostic angiogram is performed from the left common femoral artery demonstrating a long right popliteal artery occlusion. Note the large collateral immediately above the popliteal occlusion. (**B**) Note the reconstitution of the distal popliteal at the trifurcation. (**C**) A 5 Fr Berenstein catheter is brought to the "nubbin" of the lesion and a Bentson guidewire is used to enter the subintimal plane of the vessel. The catheter and guidewire are advanced into the subintimal plane. (**D**) The catheter and wire reenter into the true lumen of the popliteal artery and an angiogram is performed to demonstrate reentry. (**E**) A 4 mm × 10 cm balloon angioplasty is performed. (**F–H**) Post angioplasty arteriogram demonstrates the smooth subintimal space and the straight-line flow into the tibial vessels, continuing to the foot.

Although long SFA lesions typically are not treated percutaneously, Bolia[18a] described subintimal angioplasty as an alternative to bypass or routine angioplasty. This procedure requires a subintimal passage of a guidewire at the proximal end of a lesion and reentry into the native lumen at or distal to the diseased segment (Fig. 7-9). The subintimal space is usually a smooth, nonthrombogenic surface. If the inflow and outflow are sufficient, a good long-term response can be expected. This work needs to be corroborated by other investigators.

■ Infrapopliteal Angioplasty

The availability of low-profile balloon catheters that can be delivered through a 4 or 5 Fr sheath and thinner, steerable guidewires has made tibial angioplasty technically feasible; the results have shown it to be quite durable.[19] The indications for infrapopliteal angioplasty are primarily limb salvage. These patients require straight-line flow to the foot by at least one of the three tibial vessels. The challenge in these patients is to reestablish straight-line flow.

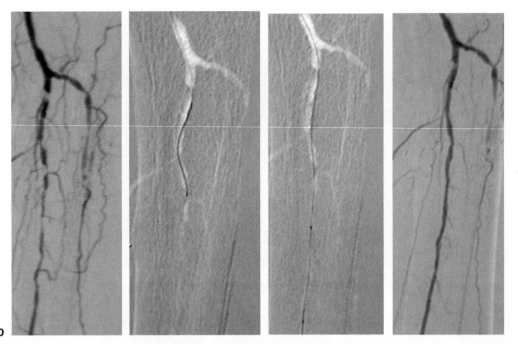

A–D

FIGURE 7-10. A 78-year-old woman with a history of posterior wall myocardial infarction, status post four-vessel coronary artery bypass graft with 25% ejection fraction presented with a 2-month history of a nonhealing vein donor site in the left lower extremity. **(A)** Diagnostic angiogram is performed from the right common femoral artery. Although it is mildly diseased, there are no focal stenoses identified above the left popliteal artery. Occlusion of the left anterior tibial and posterior tibial arteries with severely diseased peroneal artery is identified. **(B)** An antegrade puncture of the left common femoral artery is performed, and a 4 Fr sheath is advanced into the superficial femoral artery SFA. A V-18 control wire (Boston Scientific) is advanced into the peroneal artery and across the multiple peroneal stenoses. **(C)** A low-profile 2.5 mm × 4 cm balloon is used to angioplasty the peroneal stenoses, as well as the tibial–peroneal trunk. **(D)** Postangioplasty angiogram demonstrates significantly improved distal runoff.

Infrapopliteal angioplasty generally should be performed by an antegrade puncture of the ipsilateral CFA. Our patients are routinely given an antiplatelet agent (aspirin) prior to the angioplasty. The patient should be anticoagulated systemically throughout the entire procedure to prevent clot formation in the tibial vessels during catheter manipulation and prolonged angioplasty. The lesions should be crossed using road mapping. A 0.018-inch platinum-tipped guidewire or glidewire (Terumo, Tokyo, Japan) should be used to cross the stenosis or occlusions, allowing a low-profile angioplasty balloon to be used (Fig. 7-10). As opposed to femoral angioplasty, where the use of vasodilators may be helpful but nonessential, vasodilators in the tibial distribution are extremely helpful to avoid spasm in these small vessels. We routinely use 100 to 200 µg of nitroglycerin in bolus form.

The presence of long SFA occlusive disease requiring bypass and focal tibial lesions is not uncommon. An approach to be considered in this group of patients is an above knee bypass and an intraoperative angioplasty of the tibial vessels. This combined approach can save limbs while preserving the vein and reducing the morbidity associated with a distal bypass.

■ Renal Artery Angioplasty

The workup for patients with suspected renal vascular hypertension or progressive azotemia is discussed elsewhere. If a renal artery stenosis is suspected, an arteriogram should be performed. Typically, the arteriogram is performed from a femoral approach with anteroposterior (AP) and multiple obliques so as to evaluate adequately the osteal segment and the more peripheral segments and intrarenal segments of the renal arteries. If a renal artery stenosis is identified, a renal angioplasty should be considered.[20–30] Before embarking on any renal intervention, a bailout option should be identified so that if there is a noncorrectable injury to the renal artery, an appropriate surgical repair can be performed. Because many surgeons choose to bypass the renal artery off the celiac axis, it would be prudent to perform either a lateral aortogram to evaluate the origin of the celiac axis or to measure pressures in the celiac artery to reveal any hemodynamically significant proximal celiac artery stenosis. Judicious use of vasodilators, such as intraarterial nitroglycerin, should be used throughout the case to limit or prevent the degree of spasm in the renal arteries. The patient should be fully heparinized throughout the procedure.

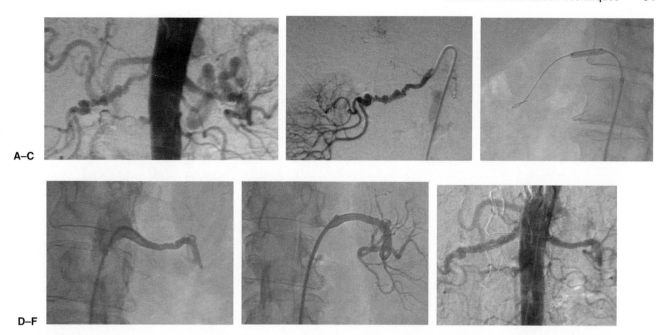

A–C

D–F

FIGURE 7-11. A 32-year-old woman presented with persistent hypertension, unable to control on three medications. **(A)** Flush aortogram is performed through an Omni Flush catheter (Angiodynamics) from the right common femoral approach. Bilateral renal artery lesions are identified, consistent with fibromuscular dysplasia. **(B)** A selective right renal angiogram is performed using a Sos Omni Selective catheter (Angiodynamics), demonstrating fibromuscular dysplasia (FMD) throughout the renal artery. **(C)** A marker sheath is advanced to the level of the renal orifices. A V-18 control wire (Boston Scientific) is advanced into the renal artery and across the multiple lesions. Angioplasty is performed with a 5 mm × 2 cm balloon across the lesions. **(D)** After achieving good results in the right renal artery, a 5 Fr Sos Omni selective catheter is advanced into the left renal orifice, and a selective angiogram is performed. Multiple distal lesions are identified consistent with FMD disease. **(E)** The V-18 control wire is advanced across the left renal artery lesions, and angioplasty is again performed with the 5 mm × 3 cm balloon. **(F)** Postbilateral angioplasty angiogram demonstrates excellent results in both renal arteries.

The existing diagnostic catheter should be changed to a 5 Fr sheath. Before the renal artery evaluation is begun, the appropriate oblique that demonstrates the renal artery orifice must be determined. This may involve cranial–caudal angulation in addition to lateral rotation in a tortuous aorta. We choose to catheterize the renal arteries using a short sidewinder catheter such as a Sos-Omni catheter (Angiodynamics, Queensbury, NY, U.S.A.) and a platinum-tipped, tapered guidewire, such as a TAD II (Mallinckrodt, St. Louis, MO, U.S.A.). After the wire crosses the lesion, the catheter is pulled down, which causes the tip to advance beyond the lesion. The guidewire is advanced farther into the renal artery. The catheter is removed, leaving the guidewire in place. The balloon is advanced over the guidewire, and the dilatation can be performed (Fig. 7-11). The patient should be fully anticoagulated during the entire procedure. A postangioplasty angiogram must be performed while the guidewire is still in place. This can be done via a second 3 or 4 Fr catheter in the same sheath. Alternatively, a multisidehole catheter can be placed over the existing guidewire, and an injection via a Tuohy–Borst adapter can be performed around the guidewire. Finally, a second catheter can be placed from the other groin for the follow-up angiogram. Arterial pressure across the lesion before and after the procedure may be helpful in assessing the degree of improvement in the vessel after balloon angioplasty. Resistant osteal lesions or obstructing dissections can be treated with a renal artery stent, which should be placed while in the oblique orientation previously determined to demonstrate the renal orifice best. An 8 Fr guiding catheter or a long 7 Fr sheath is placed across the lesion. Typically, a short balloon-expandable stent (i.e., P154) can be advanced into position across the lesion. The guiding catheter or sheath is retracted, and contrast is injected through the guiding catheter or sheath to document the location of the stent in reference to the lesion. The stent position then can be adjusted and deployed with precision. The postdeployment position can again be determined by injection through the guiding catheter or sheath. Renal spasm can be treated with additional doses of intraarterial nitroglycerin. Thrombosis of the renal artery can be treated with a thrombolytic agent. Distal embolization also can be treated with a thrombolytic infusion or suction thromboembolectomy using a guiding catheter or the Possis Angiojet. The most feared complication is that of renal arterial rupture. The patient may experience continued pain after balloon deflation.

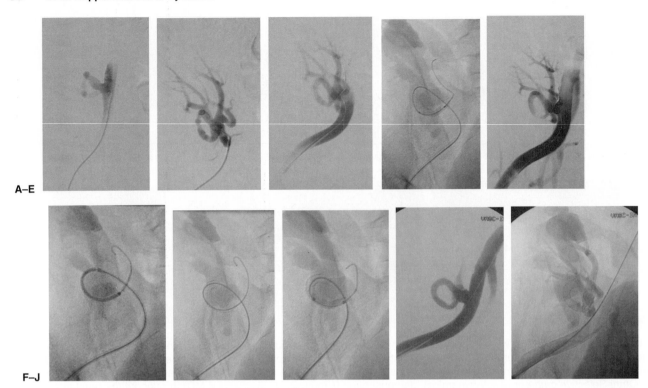

FIGURE 7-12. A 32-year-old man with hypertension, poorly controlled on three medications, and renal failure presented with a failing renal transplant. The transplant artery continued to demonstrate increased flow velocities on duplex ultrasound despite two attempts at surgical correction. (**A**) Renal transplant artery is identified off the right external iliac artery (from a right common femoral artery retrograde approach). (**B**) Selective renal transplant arteriogram demonstrates the looping course of the transplant artery. Multiple lesions were noted, including a distal kink in the artery. (**C**) Post 4 mm × 2 cm balloon angioplasty arteriogram demonstrates resolution of the dysplastic appearing lesions but no change in the distal kink. (**D**) A prolonged 5 mm × 2 cm balloon inflation was performed at the distal lesion. (**E**) Elevated intrarenal pressures and a residual angiographic lesion confirm a persistent stenosis. (**F**) A 7 × 40 mm Smart Stent (Cordis, Johnson & Johnson Corp.) was deployed across the lesion as well as across the adequately dilated portion of the renal artery. (**G**) The Smart Stent demonstrates a kink at the same region. (**H**) The Stent then is expanded with the 5 mm × 2 cm balloon. (**I**) Good angiographic result is obtained with no pressure gradient. (**J**) Unsubtracted view of the post stent arteriogram demonstrating the appearance of the Smart Stent in this tortuous renal artery. The blood pressure management improved with the patient using only one medication. Renal function also improved with the blood creatinine level decreasing to 1.6 mg/dL.

In addition, extravasation of contrast during the postprocedure angiogram may be seen. If a renal artery rupture is noted, the balloon should be reinflated immediately across the renal artery rupture to tamponade the vessel. The patient then is brought to the operating room for repair of the vessel; alternatively, a covered stent can be placed to exclude the rupture from circulation. The results of renal angioplasty are discussed later in this book.

If an obstructing flap occurs during renal angioplasty or if elastic recoil prevents the renal artery from being adequately dilated, a stent can be placed in the renal artery to salvage an otherwise failed angioplasty (Fig. 7-12). Renal stents probably should not be placed in vessels smaller than 6 mm because the long-term results are poor. Care must be taken to position the stent appropriately in the renal artery. In an osteal lesion, the stent should protrude into the aorta by a millimeter or two to ensure that the osteal lesion is totally covered.

Angioplasty or stenting of the subclavian artery, the carotid arteries, and the mesenteric vessels all have been performed (Fig. 7-13). The techniques are similar to angioplasty and stenting elsewhere as described here; however, a thorough understanding of the anatomy and physiology of the region being treated is necessary to treat appropriately and successfully the symptomatic lesions.

■ Techniques for Thrombolysis

Acute and subacute occlusions of native arteries and bypass grafts can be treated using a fibrinolytic agent. The indications and contraindications and results are discussed in subsequent chapters.

Urokinase was the agent of choice for most interventional radiologists because of its known dosing efficacy

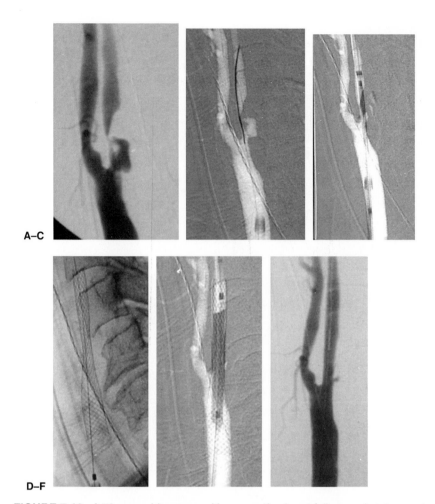

A–C

D–F

FIGURE 7-13. A 79-year-old woman with congestive heart failure and status post myocardial infarction, a poor operative risk for conventional surgery, presents with a history of right hemispheric transient ischemic attacks. **(A)** Arteriogram performed from the right common femoral artery demonstrates an ulcerated stenosis of the right internal carotid artery. **(B)** A guiding catheter is advanced into the right common carotid artery and an 0.018-inch platinum-tipped guidewire is used to cross the lesion. **(C)** The lesion is predilated with a 4-mm balloon, and an 8 × 40 mm Wallstent (Boston Scientific Corp.) is advanced across the lesion. **(D)** The Wallstent is deployed across the lesion. **(E)** The Wallstent is postdilated with a 6 mm × 4 cm balloon. **(F)** Poststent angiogram demonstrates no significant residual stenosis of the internal carotid artery with a small residual ulcer present.

(80 to 120,000 U/hour) and acceptable complication rate. All the lytic agents work by activating the body's endogenous lytic enzyme, plasmin. Plasmin will degrade fibrin plugs. If a systemic lytic state is reached, any site of vascular injury may bleed. Therefore, rather than use systemic, intravenous lysis, interventional radiologists have advanced the concept of direct lytic infusion into the thrombus. Because urokinase is not currently available, other lytic agents are being used and evaluated: Alteplase (r-tPA, recombinant tissue plasminogen activator, Genentech, Carmel, NY, U.S.A.) at 0.5 to 1 mg/hour and Retavase (r-Reteplase, recombinant plasminogen activator, Centocor, Inc., Malvern, PA, U.S.A.) at 0.5 to 1 unit/hour are being used with good results.[31–37]

The diagnostic angiogram usually is performed via the asymptomatic extremity. After the occlusion is identified

and the decision to treat with lysis is made, it can be performed via the original puncture or via a direct puncture of the CFA of the affected extremity. Iliac occlusions invariably are treated around the bifurcation, whereas SFA or infrapopliteal artery occlusion can be treated with either approach. The advantage of using the original puncture is that an additional puncture on the side requiring lysis is not performed, thereby reducing the incidence of bleeding from a puncture site. The disadvantage is that any follow-up therapy such as angioplasty, aspiration, or stenting in the popliteal or tibial vessels may be more difficult.

The next step is to advance a catheter into the occluded native artery or bypass graft (Figs. 7-14 and 7-15). It is best to advance a catheter with multiple sideholes where the end hole either is occluded by a valve, as in

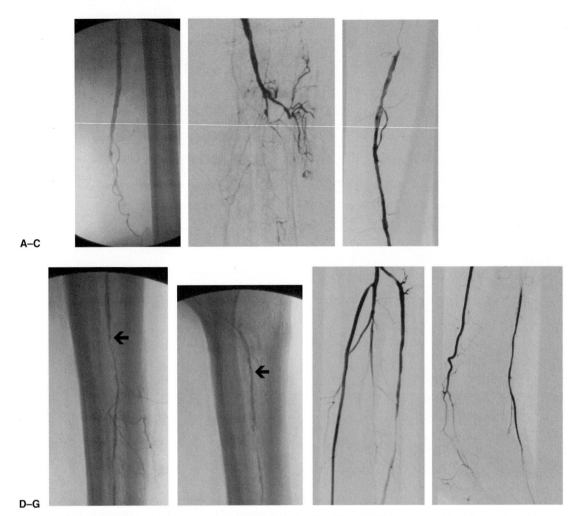

A–C

D–G

FIGURE 7-14. A 65-year-old man, a smoker, presented with a 2-week history of progressive ischemia and rest pain in the left calf and foot. (**A**) Angiogram performed from the right common femoral artery demonstrates severe stenosis of the popliteal artery at the adductor canal. (**B**) Occlusions are identified in all three tibial vessels. (**C**) A Balkin Contralateral 5.5 Fr sheath (Cook Group Company), was advanced into the external iliac artery, and the popliteal stenosis is angioplastied with a 4 mm × 4 cm balloon. (**D**) A SP catheter (Medi-tech, Boston Scientific Corp.) is advanced into the posterior tibial artery and the artery is laced with a total of 120,000 U of urokinase. (**E**) The SP catheter (Medi-tech, Boston Scientific Corp.) then is advanced into the anterior tibial artery and tibial–peroneal trunk, lacing each of these in turn (a total of 250,000 U of urokinase was used). An overnight thrombolytic drip of 120,000 U/h of urokinase is begun through a Berenstein catheter (Angiodynamics) positioned in the popliteal artery. (**F**). Postthrombolysis arteriogram clearly demonstrates improvement in the tibial runoff. (**G**) Both the posterior tibial and anterior tibial arteries again provide flow into the foot.

the Cragg catheter (MTI,) or a multi-side hole catheter that is occluded with a tip occluding wire (Angiodynamics, Cook), or a routine guidewire, causing most of the infusion to exit the side holes in a relatively even distribution. The catheter should be positioned so that the proximal side hole is at or close to the top of the clot and the distal side hole is just proximal to the end of the clot. A coaxial system (a multi-side hole catheter with an infusion wire coaxially in the catheter) may be required to achieve these levels of infusion. A typical infusion rate of urokinase would be a total of 240,000 U/hour for the first 4 hours and then reduced to between 80,000 and 120,000 U/hour for the duration of

therapy. Alternatively, r-tPA 0.5 mg to 1 mg/hour can be used. Occasionally, a higher dose of 1 to 2 mg/hour will be used over a short period and then reduced to the lower 0.5 to 1 mg/hour range for overnight infusions. Concomitant heparin should be used sparingly to reduce the incidence of pericatheter thrombosis. We typically give a bolus of 2000 U of heparin to the patient, followed by a heparin infusion of 500 U/hour. The partial prothrombin time (PTT) is monitored closely and should be less than twice the normal value (this corresponds to a 40 to 70 range at our institution). Care should be taken not to over-anticoagulate the patient because the incidence of bleeding, including groin he-

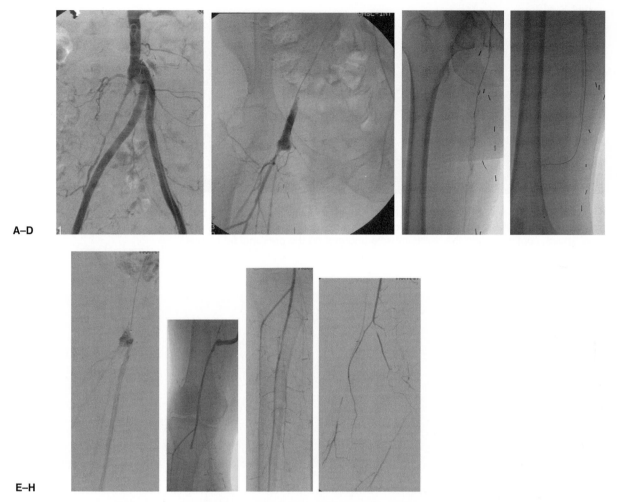

A–D

E–H

FIGURE 7-15. A 43-year-old woman with a patent aortobifemoral bypass graft and occluded femoral to popliteal bypass graft presented with an acute history of right limb ischemia involving both sensory and motor loss from the midcalf to the foot. (**A**) Diagnostic arteriogram is performed from the left common femoral artery, demonstrating the patent aortobifemoral bypass graft. (**B**) The femoral-to-popliteal graft hood is opacified, but the graft is occluded. (**C**) A Berenstein catheter was passed into the graft. (**D**) An SP catheter (Medi-tech, Boston Scientific Corp.) then was advanced through the graft, into the distal graft, and the graft was laced with 250,000 U of urokinase. (**E**) An overnight drip of urokinase was begun at 120,000 Units/hour. (**F**) Postthrombolysis arteriogram demonstrates patent graft with residual thrombus in the peroneal artery. An SP catheter (Medi-tech, Boston Scientific Corp.) then was directed into the peroneal artery and was laced with 250,000 U of urokinase. Then a urokinase drip was begun from the level of the popliteal artery at 80,000 U/hour. (**G**) The patient was brought back to the angiosuite that afternoon. Postthrombolysis angiogram demonstrates dissolution of the peroneal thrombus. (**H**) Straight-line flow into the foot is restored.

matoma, retroperitoneal hematoma, and intracerebral hemorrhage, may increase with excessive anticoagulation combined with a lytic agent (Fig. 7-16).

Follow-up arteriography should be performed as necessary and when practical. When a case is started in the morning, we typically restudy the patient late in the afternoon. If the case was started in the afternoon, we restudy the patient the next morning. During the follow-up evaluation, the catheter position can be adjusted to optimize the lytic effect.

Often patients experience increased pain during the lysis, which may be due to lysis and embolization of small clots. With continued infusion, these episodes are usually

self-limited and often resolve completely. If the pain and ischemia persist, a repeat angiogram is warranted. If emboli are identified, the catheter or an injectable guidewire can be advanced to the emboli to continue thrombolysis, "chasing" the emboli down the leg, lacing the vessels with thrombolytics, and continuing the infusion until the emboli dissolve (see Fig. 7-17). When the clot is lysed, a search should be done for an underlying lesion that may have caused the graft to clot or the native artery to occlude. If a lesion is found, it should be corrected by angioplasty, stent placement, or surgery, whichever is considered appropriate based on the lesion identified (Fig. 7-18).

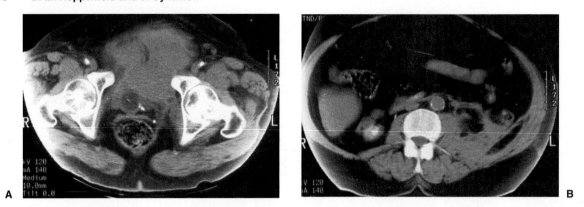

FIGURE 7-16. Hematomas are not uncommon when treating with lysis; occasionally, they can be quite large. (**A**) Computed tomography scan of the pelvis demonstrates blood in the anterior abdominal wall. (**B**) The hematoma extended up the retroperitoneal space, continuing into the psoas muscle and around the perirenal fat planes.

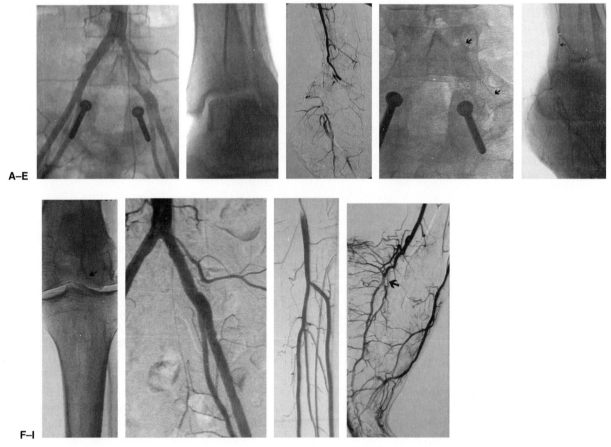

FIGURE 7-17. A 44-year-old woman presented to the emergency room with acute right foot ischemia, blue toes, and rest pain. She is several years status post lower back surgery, having had pedicle screws placed from an anterior approach. (**A**) Diagnostic arteriogram is performed via the right common femoral artery. A complex, irregular lesion is identified in the left common iliac artery. It is postulated that this may have been an iatrogenic injury from the patient's previous back surgery. (**B**) Occlusions of the distal anterior tibial artery. (**C**) Occlusions of the posterior tibial artery are noted. Most likely, these occlusions were responsible for the patient's acute limb ischemia and postulated to be emboli off the common iliac lesion. (**D**) An 8 × 40-mm Smart Stent (Cordis, Johnson & Johnson Corp.) was placed across the common iliac lesion. (**E**) The posterior tibial and anterior tibial arteries were laced with 2.5 mg of rt-PA through an SP catheter (Medi-tech, Boston Scientific Corp., Watertown, MA). (**F**) A Berenstein catheter (Angiodynamics) was left in the popliteal artery, and an overnight drip of 1 mg/hour rt-PA was begun. (**G**) Follow-up angiogram demonstrates resolution of the common iliac lesion. (**H**) After 15 hours of thrombolysis, there is normal three-vessel runoff from the popliteal artery. (**I**) There is reconstitution of the posterior tibial, dorsalis pedis, and plantar arteries, with minimal residual thrombus in the most distal aspect of the posterior tibial artery. The patient was pain free with a warm foot.

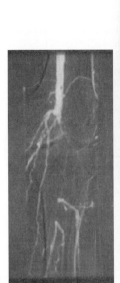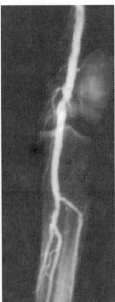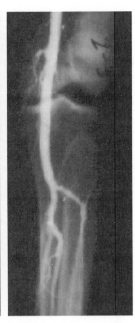

A–C

FIGURE 7-18. A 57-year-old man presented with acute rest pain and mild sensory loss in the left foot. **(A)** Diagnostic arteriogram is performed from the right common femoral artery, and a popliteal occlusion is identified. An Up and Over Balkin Contralateral 5.5 Fr sheath (Cook Group Company) was advanced into the left external iliac artery, and a Berenstein catheter was advanced to the level of the popliteal occlusion. The occlusion was crossed with a Bentson guidewire. An infusion catheter was placed within the popliteal occlusion, and an overnight urokinase drip was begun at 120,000 U/hour. **(B)** Postthrombolysis arteriogram demonstrates dissolution of the popliteal and tibial thrombus and identifies the underlying lesion of the popliteal artery. A 5 mm × 2 cm balloon angioplasty was performed of the popliteal stenosis. **(C)** Post angioplasty arteriogram demonstrates resolution of the lesion and return of straight-line flow into the tibial vessels and to the foot.

REFERENCES

1. Dotter CT, Judkins MP. Transluminal treatment of arteriosclerotic obstruction: description of a new technique and a preliminary report of its application. *Circulation* 1964;30:654.
2. Gruentzig A, Hopff H. Perkutane rekanalization chronischer Arterieller: Verschlusses miteinem nellen dilatation-katheter Modification de Dotterchinik. *Dtsch Med Wochenschr* 1974;9:2502.
3. Darcy MD. Lower extremity arteriography: current approach and techniques. *Radiology* 1991;178:615–621.
4. Standards of Practice Committee of the Society of Cardiovascular and Interventional Radiology. Standards for diagnostic arteriography in adults. *J Vasc Inter Radiol* 1993;4:385.
5. Motarjeme A, Gordon GI, Bodenhagen K. Thrombolysis and angioplasty of chronic iliac artery occlusions. *J Vasc Interv Radiol* 1995;6:66s–72s.
6. Casteneda-Zuniga WR, Formanek A, Tadavarthy M, et al. The mechanism of balloon angioplasty. *Radiology* 1980;135:565–571.
7. Waugh JR, Sacharias N. Arteriographic complications in the DSA era. *Radiology* 1992;182–243.
8. Becker GL, Katzen BT, Dake MD. Non-coronary angioplasty. *Radiology* 1989;170:921–940.
9. Pentecost MJ, Criqui MH, Dorros G, et al. Guidelines for peripheral percutaneous transluminal angioplasty of the abdominal aorta and lower extremity vessels. *Circulation* 1994;89:511.
10. Henry M, Amor M, Ethevenot G, et al. Palmaz stent placement in iliac and femoropopliteal arteries: primary and secondary patency in 310 patients with 2–4 year follow-up. *Radiology* 1995;197:167.
11. Tetterroo E, Van Engelen AD, Spithoven JH, et al. Stent placement after iliac angioplasty: comparison of hemodynamic and angiographic criteria. *Radiology* 1996;201:155.
12. Dyet JF, Gaines PA, Nicholson AA, et al. Treatment of chronic iliac artery occlusions by means of percutaneous endovascular stent placement. *J Vasc Interv Radiol* 1997;8:349–353.
13. Reyes R, Maynar M, Lopera J, et al. Treatment of chronic iliac artery occlusions with guide wire recanalization and primary stent placement. *J Vasc Interv Radiol* 1997;8:1049.
14. Sullivan TM, Childs MB, Bacharach JM, et al. Percutaneous transluminal angioplasty and primary stenting of the iliac arteries in 288 patients. *J Vasc Surg* 1997;25:829–839.
15. Vorwek D, Guenther RW, Schuermann K, et al. Primary stent placement for chronic iliac artery occlusions: follow-up results in 103 patients. *Radiology* 1995;194:745.
16. Martin EC, Katzen BT, Benenati JF, et al. Multicenter Trial of the Wallstent in the iliac and femoral arteries. *J Vasc Interv Radiol* 1995;6:843–849.
17. Palmaz JC, Laborde JC, Rivera FJ, et al. Stenting of the iliac arteries with the Palmaz Stent: experience from a multicenter trial. *Cardiovasc Interv Radiol* 1992;15:291–297.
18. Palmaz JC, Sibbitt RR, Reuter SR, et al. Expandable intraluminal graft: preliminary study. *Radiology* 1985;156:73–77.
18a. Bolia A. Percutaneous intentional extraluminal (subitimal) recanalization of crural arteries. *Eur J Radiol* 1998;28:199–204.
19. Bakal CW, Cynamon J, Sprayregen S. Infrapopliteal percutaneous transluminal angioplasty: what we know. *Radiology* 1996;200:36.
20. Brawn LA, Ramsey LE. Is improvement real with percutaneous transluminal angioplasty in the management of renovascular hypertension? *Lancet* 1987;2:1313–1316.
21. Derkx F, Schalekamp M. Renal artery stenosis and hypertension. *Lancet* 1994;344:237–239.
22. Dorros G, Prince C, Mathiak L. Stenting of a renal artery stenosis achieves better relief of the obstructive lesion than balloon angioplasty. *Cathet Cardiovasc Diagn* 1993;29:191–198.
23. Dorros G, Jaff M, Jain A, et al. Follow-up of primary Palmaz-Schatz

stent placement for atherosclerotic renal artery stenosis. *Am J Cardiol* 1195;75:1051–1055.

24. Cicutok P, McLean G, Oleaga J. Renal artery stenosis: anatomic classification for percutaneous angioplasty. *AJR Am J Roentgenol* 1981;137:599–601.

25. Gruentzig A, Kuhlman V, Vetter W. Treatment of renovascular hypertension with percutaneous transluminal dilatation of a renal artery. *Lancet* 1978;1:801–802.

26. Palmaz JC, Kopp DT, Hayashi H, et al. Normal and stenotic renal arteries: experimental balloon-expandable intraluminal stenting. *Radiology* 1987;164:705–708.

27. Sos TA, Pickering TG, Sniderman K, et al. Percutaneous transluminal renal angioplasty in renovascular hypertension due to atheroma or fibromuscular dysplasia. *N Engl J Med* 1983;309:274–279.

28. Soulen MDC. Renal angioplasty: underutilized or overvalued? *Radiology* 1994;193:19–21.

29. Tegtmeyer CJ, Brown J, Ayers CA, et al. Percutaneous transluminal angioplasty for the treatment of renovascular hypertension. *JAMA* 1981;246:2068–2070.

30. White CJ, Ramee SR, Collins TG, et al. Renal artery stent placement. *J Endovasc Surg* 1998;5:71–77.

31. Andaz S, Shields DA, Scurr JH, et al. Thrombolysis in acute lower limb ischemia. *Eur J Vasc Surg* 1993;7:595–603.

32. Bero CJ, Cardella JF, Reddy K, et al. Recombinant tissue plasminogen activator for the treatment of lower extremity peripheral vascular occlusive disease. *J Vasc Interv Radiol* 1995;6:571–577.

33. Ouriel K, Shortell CK, Azodo MW, et al. Acute peripheral arterial occlusion: predictors of success in catheter directed thrombolytic therapy. *Radiology* 1994;93:561–566.

34. Ouriel K. Surgery vs. thrombolytic therapy in the management of peripheral arterial occlusion. *J Vasc Interv Radiol* 1995;6:48s–54s.

35. Ouriel K, Veith FJ, Sasahara AA. Thrombolysis or peripheral arterial surgery (TOPAS): phase I results. *J Vasc Surg* 1996;23:64–73.

36. Rauber K, Heidinger KS, Kemkes-Matthes B. Coagulation alterations due to local fibrinolytic therapy with recombinant tissue plasminogen activator (rt-PA) in patients with peripheral arterial occlusive disease. *Cardiovasc Interv Radiol* 1997;20:169–173.

37. Semba CP, Murphy TP, Bakal CW, et al. Thrombolytic therapy with use of Alteplase (rt-PA) in peripheral arterial occlusive disease: review of the clinical literature. *J Vasc Interv Radiol* 2000;11: 149–161.

8

General Principles of Embolization and Chemoembolization

CHARLES E. RAY JR. and ARTHUR C. WALTMAN

Transcatheter embolization is a frequently performed procedure that can be used for myriad clinical indications. Whether used to stop active bleeding, as palliative therapy for benign or malignant lesions, as a form of organ ablation, or in combination with chemotherapy as primary oradjunctive therapy for malignancies, embolization procedures are becoming more common in both large medical centers and community practice settings.

This chapter outlines general principles of embolic and chemoembolic therapy, with particular attention to the techniques used and to which clinical entities may benefit from such catheter directed therapy.

■ Technique

Delivery systems

Depending on the size of the vessel or vessels to be embolized and the embolic agent to be used the two general types of delivery methods are *selective catheter* and *coaxial catheter* systems. Selective catheterization usually is performed with preformed curved catheters ranging from 5 to 7 Fr in diameter. Techniques used in selective catheterization are discussed in other chapters; most commercially available tapered end-hole catheters are sufficient for embolization procedures. The advent of coaxial systems has allowed superselective catheterization with minimal risk to the selected vessel. Many systems, such as the Tracker-325 system (Target Therapeutics, San Jose, CA), consist of a 3 Fr catheter with a large inner lumen diameter that allows delivery of sizable embolic materials such as Gelfoam pledgets (Upjohn, Kalamazoo, MI), or microcoils,

which do not appreciably risk occluding the catheter. By using a coaxial system, the operator may catheterize the vessel of choice virtually without regard to vessel size, thus significantly decreasing the risk of both nontarget embolization and damage to the underlying vessel.

Balloon-occlusion catheters (BOCs) are useful for embolization procedures, particularly when alcohol is used as the embolic agent (see later). BOCs are compliant balloons designed to conform to the shape of the vessel in which they are inflated, in contrast to angioplasty balloons, which are designed to produce a significant radial force intended to fracture a plaque. Angioplasty balloons should not be used as BOCs, because of the notable potential risk of dissection of the vessel in which the balloon is inflated.

When large particles such as Gelfoam pledgets are used for embolization, care must be taken to use a selective catheter or coaxial system with an inner diameter and taper large enough to prevent occlusion of the catheter by the embolic material. A catheter with an end-hle only also should be used to prevent inadvertent nontarget embolization through a catheter side hole. In addition, if an adhesive material such as cyanoacrylate is used, the glue must be mixed with tantalum powder for radiopacity and the delivery catheter must be flushed with dextrose solution, because exposure of the glue to ionic compounds causes instant polymerization and catheter occlusion.

Embolic agents

The number of embolic agents has increased significantly recently; however, it must be kept in mind that a combined approach using multiple agents is often most useful.

To choose the embolic agent needed, the anticipated end result of the embolization procedure must be understood. For instance, embolization for bleeding from a posttraumatic pseudoaneurysm has a different goal from embolization/ablation of a renal tumor preoperatively. Similarly, embolization for bleeding from a renal tumor has a purpose different from that of preoperative embolization of the same pathology. Large embolic agents such as coils and Gelfoam pledgets may be used for embolization of large vessels in organs with abundant collateral supply, such as the stomach or liver, in which proximal vessels can be occluded safely without risk of tissue infarction due to the extenssive collateral network. Large agents may be also used in tissues with an end-organ vascular supply in which the entire blood supply to the area of interest is to be occluded; however, large agents should not be used in vessels in which future embolization or transcatheter therapy is anticipated. By occlusion of the only vascular supply to a region, future selective catherization will be precluded by occluding the sole vascular access to the pathology. In contrast to large agents, liquid agents such as alcohol or glue will embolize to the most distal vascular supply and cause infarction by occluding the smallest arterioles supplying a lesion. Because collateral supply occurs at a site proximal to the embolization, liquid embolization is effective in destroying tissue even when there is significant parasitization or collaterization of blood supply from an adjacent source; however, it should not be used unless cell death and necrosis are the desired end results.

A second characteristics that must be considered when choosing an embolic agent is the desired degree of permanence of the occlusion. In particular, some materials are biodegradable, and recanalization of the embolized vessel should be anticipated. Most vessels embolized with Gelfoam pledgets and powder will recanalize within 2 to 3 weeks.[1] Starch microspheres represent another biodegradable agent with an in vivo half-life of 20 to 30 min.[2] Angiography 1 week after cross-linked collagen embolization of the hepatic artery reveals a normal hepatic arterial system and more complete return within 3 months.[3] Autologous blood clots, a fourth degradable agent, that are currently used infrequently because of the ready availability of other agents.

Polyvinyl alcohol (PVA) particles are a commonly used permanent agent, with sizes ranging from approximately 50 to 2800 μm. Embolization with PVA particles usually causes a permanent occlusion of vessels that corresponds to the size of the particles used. Other materials that have been used experimentally or in clinical trials include polylactic acid microspheres,[4] ethylene vinylacetate copolymer particles dissolved in polyvinyl alcohol,[5] and human dura mater.[6]

Embolization with particulate agents is considered complete when slowing of flow, not complete statis, is visualized. Because all arteries will tend to "back thrombose" to the previous bifurcation point when a distal occlusion is encountered, excessive embolization will decrease outflow enough that the entire feeding artery may thrombose. Fluoroscopically noted reflux is another indicator that the embolization procedure should be stopped.

■ Use of embolization in Clinical settings

Nonneoplastic

Active bleeding

Hemorrhage is a clinical setting in which transcatheter embolotherapy may prove useful. Embolization of active bleeding almost always provides a less invasive form of patient management than surgical alternatives, and in certain clinical settings, such as postradiation or postsurgical fields, it may prove to be the only viable alternative because of the difficulty of surgery in such an operative field. Active bleeding may be caused by a number of etiologies, including inflammation, neoplasm, trauma, and congenital or developmental abnormalities. Once again, the desired end result of the embolization and the degree of permanence required are essential factors in determining the embolic agent of choice.

Because bleeding caused by inflammation is usually a temporary situation (i.e., over time and with appropriate medical management, the artery will likely stop bleeding), a temporary embolic occlusion is usually sufficient. In such cases, embolotherapy is a temporizing procedure performed to allow coagulation or healing to occur within the vessel. In addition, because inflammatory etiologies may cause further bleeding within the same organ later, a temporary occlusion is desired so that future embolizations may be performed if needed. Finally, because the desired end result is not organ ablation or cell death but rather cessation of bleeding and tissue preservation, distal embolic agents, such as liquid or small particles, are usually contraindicated in inflammatory causes of hemorrhage.

Two inflammatory etiologies in which embolotherapy has proven efficacious include gastrointestinal (GI) and pulmonary hemorrhage. Transcatheter embolization of GI bleeding is documented best in the setting of benign causes, such as peptic ulcer disease, erosive gastritis, and Mallory-Weiss tears. In the case of peptic ulcer disease, most patients undergo endoscopy with an attempt at sclerotherapy; however, in patients in whom sclerotherapy fails or with recurrent bleeding after initial medical and endoscopic therapy, patients may be referred for angiography and possible embolotherapy. In addition, unstable patients who have massive upper GI bleeding may benefit from emergent embolotherapy preceding, or in lieu of, surgical therapies.[7] Embolic agents used in the treatment of peptic ulcer bleeding have included Gelfoam pledgets, stainless steel coils, PVA particles, glue, and autologous clots.[7–9] Occlusion of the more distal vasculature with agents such as glue prevents the formation peripheral collateral blood supply, thereby predisposing the embolized tissue to infection and increasing the risk of postembolization ischemic complications such as fibrosis and duodenal stenosis.[8] Central occlusion with larger agents, such as coil occlusion of the gastroduodenal artery, allows collateral vessels to supply the distal tissue and precludes tissue infarction without compromising success of the embolization procedure.[8] Gelfoam pledgets are the most commonly used agent; however, because temporary occlusion may or may not be sufficient, permanent central occlusion with coils is another possible therapeutic alternative.[7–9] In the setting of massive upper GI bleeding without angiographic evidence of a bleeding site, embolization of the left gastric artery with Gelfoam pledgets or coils decrease the risk of recurrent GI bleeding (0% versus 50%).[10] Embolization of the left gastric artery without angiographic documentation of bleeding can be justified because approximately 85% of gastric hemorrhage is caused by a lesion supplied by the left gastric artery.[11]

Embolotherapy for GI bleeding from benign causes other than peptic ulcer disease also has been successful. One study demonstrated technical success in all patients treated with emergent Gelfoam pledget and coil embolotherapy for active small intestinal hemorrhage; five of six (83%) patients survived hospitalization.[9] Similar success rates have been noted in other studies for pathology as varied as jejunal ulcers, pseudoaneurysms, and Meckel's diverticulum.[12]

Transcatheter embolotherapy in the treatment of hemoptysis also has proved efficacious.[13,14] Because of the dual vascular supply to the lungs, the likelihood of postembolization tissue infarction is low, even with use of distal embolic agents such as PVA particles or liquid agents. Most pulmonary hemorrhages resulting from benign causes arise from the bronchial circulation; embolotherapy, therefore, typically is performed through the systemic circulation rather than the pulmonary arteries. There is great variability in the number and origins of the bronchial arteries; 43% of patients demonstrate a common trunk supplying the left and right bronchial arteries, and most patients demonstrate two or three bronchial arteries in total.[15] Although they are small in the normal setting, the bronchial arteries become significantly enlarged in the setting of chronic inflammatory disease. Concurrent with bronchial artery enlargement, systemic-to-pulmonary artery communications develop, exposing the pulmonary arterial bed to greatly elevated pressures and causing rupture of the pulmonary arteries into con-

tiguous airways.[16] It is therefore from these pulmonary arteries that bleeding arises; however, pressure in the pulmonary arteries normalizes after the bronchial arteries are embolized, causing cessation of bleeding. Although rare, bleeding arising directly from the pulmonary circulation can be seen with Rasmussen aneurysms or pulmonary arteriovenous malformations (AVMs).[17]

If embolotherapy of the bronchial artery is being considered, caution should be exercised because of the potential origin of anterior spinal artery branches from the bronchial circulation. Contributions to the anterior spinal artery from the right bronchial artery are seen in approximately 5% of patients, whereas contributions from the left bronchial artery are decidedly rare.[14] Branches supplying the anterior spinal artery are angiographically visualized by a characteristic "hairpin" course that is anterior to the vertebral column; the artery then descends or ascends in the midline. Although embolization procedures can be performed with coaxial catheterization of the bronchial artery beyond the origin of the spinal branches, the possibility of severe cord compromise must be considered before such a procedure is undertaken. Experimental evidence suggests that particles larger than 250 μm are too large to enter small spinal feeders[18] and therefore may be used safely in bronchial artery embolization. Some authors advocate that spinal cord infarction is a potential rather than real possibility, with reported cases of transverse myelitis occurring before the advent of nonionic contrast media.[19]

Benign disease processes that cause bronchial arterial bleeding include infectious causes such as tuberculosis and aspergillosis and noninfectious inflammatory causes such as bronchiectasis, pulmonary sarcoid, and cystic fibrosis.[14,17] Chronic inflammatory processes can cause significant recruitment of collateral vessels from the subclavian, axillary, internal mammary, intercostal, and phrenic arteries.[20] In the setting of persistent or recurrent hemoptysis following successful bronchial artery embolization, repeat diagnostic angiography as well as embolotherapy of other potential collateral vessels should be undertaken. Some authors advocate bronchial artery embolization as a preemptive therapy in patients with cystic fibrosis before they develop potentially massive hemoptysis.[21] The embolic material of choice in patients with enlarged bronchial vessels and chronic inflammatory processes is PVA particles larger than 250 μm but not large enough to occlude the vasculature at the proximal artery level. These agents embolize distal enough to preclude significant collateral vessel recruitment while allowing repeat embolotherapy to be performed if needed. Larger permanent agents such as coils are contraindicated because repeat embolotherapy will be difficult, if not impossible, because of the proximal vessel occlusion. Success rates for hemostasis following bronchial artery embolization range from 77% to 91%.[13–15,17] The success rates do

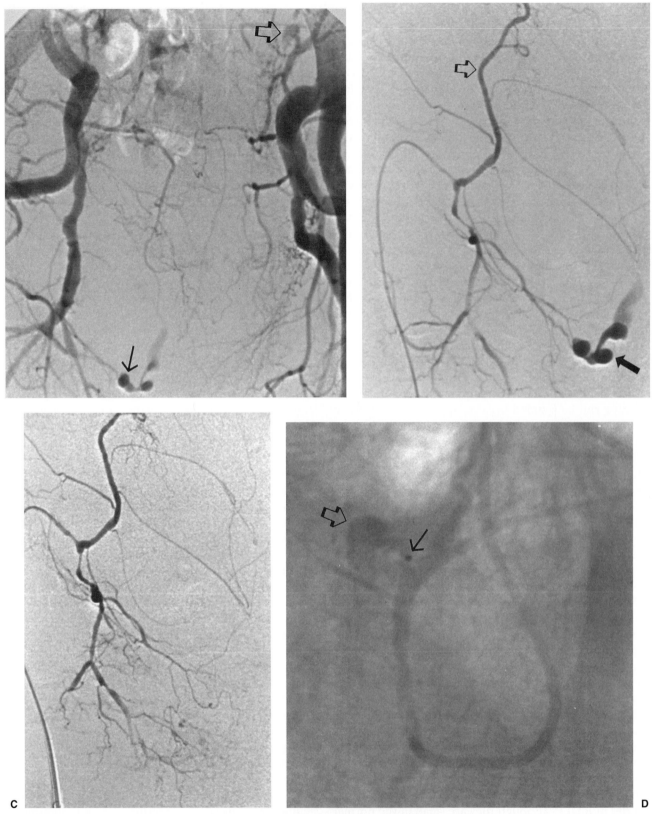

FIGURE 8-1. A 68-year-old man who fell from a ladder, and sustained multiple pelvic and femoral fractures. **A:** Anteroposterior digital subtraction angiogram of the pelvis demonstrating contrast extravasation (*arrow*) arising from the right external pudendal artery and traumatic pseudoaneurysm arising from the left iliolumbar artery (*open arrow*). **B:** Selective injection of the right external pudendal artery demonstrating contrast extravasation (*arrow*) arising from a branch vessel. Note the replaced inferior epigastric artery arising from the external pudendal (*open arrow*). A 3 Fr coaxial catheter was placed distal to the inferior epigastric artery origin for gelfoam embolization. **C:** Selective injection of the right external pudendal artery and embolization with Gelfoam pledgets using a coaxial catheter system demonstrating complete cessation of contrast extravasation. Flow to the inferior epigastric artery is preserved by using the coaxial system. **D:** Selective injection of the left iliolumbar artery demonstrating the pseudoaneurysm (*open arrow*). *Arrow* denotes tip of 3 Fr coaxial catheter. (*Continued*)

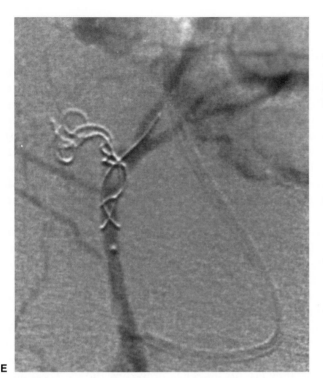

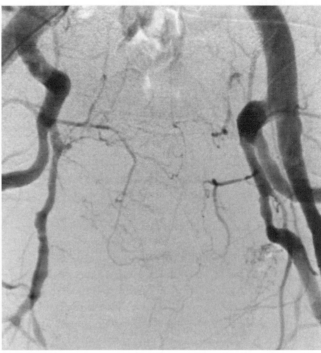

E

F

FIGURE 8-1. (*Continued*) E. Selective injection of the left iliolumbar artery showing embolization with Gelfoam pledgets and coils and demonstrating complete occlusion of the traumatic pseudoaneurysm. **F:** Final postprocedure angiogram demonstrating complete cessation of contrast extravasation and occlusion of the pseudoaneurysm noted in (A).

not appear to differ significantly among the various inflammatory causes.

Trauma

In addition to inflammatory causes of bleeding, embolization may be used in patients presenting with hemorrhage following trauma; However, in the setting of trauma the underlying nature of the vessels as well as the desired endpoint differ greatly from those seen in the setting of chronic inflammatory disease. In most instances, posttraumatic bleeding involves previously healthy vessels that undergo acute changes such as transection or pseudoaneurysm formation; temporizing measures are frequently all that are required to allow the vessel to undergo the healing process or to stabilize the patient preoperatively. Because of these differences, the embolic agents differ from those seen with hemorrhage from chronic inflammatory diseases.

Hemorrhage associated with pelvic fractures is one of the most frequent traumatic settings in which embolotherapy is used. Fractures in which the constraining ligaments of the pelvis are damaged are most likely to cause severe hemorrhage; placement of an external orthopedic fixation device stabilizes the pelvis in addition to stopping venous, osseous, and minor arterial hemorrhage.[22] External fixation devices, therefore, are recommended in patients who are hemodynamically stable and in whom ar-

teriography and embolotherapy are not considered immediately necessary for patient survival. In patients in whom persistent bleeding is suspected following external fixation, diagnostic angiography is necessary to exclude an arterial source of hemorrhage. It is estimated that approximately 7% to 11% of patients with pelvic fractures will require embolization.[22]

The most common sources of arterial hemorrhage following pelvic trauma are branches of the internal iliac arteries (Fig. 8-1). Cut-film angiography is the preferred method for initial diagnostic angiography done because of the presence of bowel motion artifact in the pelvis during digital subtraction angiography (DSA), although DSA may be sufficient in patients who are hemodynamically unstable and in whom time is crucial. It is recommended that distal aortogram be done before selective catheterization of the internal iliac arterie is performed because of the possibility of concomitant arterial damage to other vessels,[22,23] followed by selective angiography of both internal iliac arteries. In most cases, temporary occlusion to stop active extravasation is sufficient, because arterial spasm, thrombosis, and possibly arterial repair will occur once the patient is hemodynamically stable. Because of the rich collateral network within the pelvis, tissue infarction is an uncommon complication of embolization with large agents. Although coils have been used with success, permanent occlusion usually is not considered necessary,[23,24] and Gelfoam pledgets are the embolic material of choice.[22] Preemptive embolization of arterial branches that are transected but not actively bleeding, as evidenced angiographically by complete occlusion secondary to spasm, is advocated by some authors because the likelihood of delayed hemorrhage is significant in this setting.[22] Finally, many trauma patients are hypothermic and therefore coagulopathic, delaying clot formation and possibly allowing retrograde collaterals to open and bleed.[25]

Posttraumatic hemorrhage also can be visualized in other organ systems such as the kidney,[24] spleen,[17,26] and liver.[24] Organ preservation is often the goal in such patients, and superselective catheterization and embolotherapy in a hemodynamically stable patient are warranted. In unstable patients, however, proximal occlusion may be the most timely and effective therapy. In the setting of active bleeding from the spleen following blunt trauma, proximal coil occlusion of the splenic artery obviated laparotomy in 94% of patients, and splenic salvage was achieved in 97% of patients.[26] Iatrogenic trauma, including complications arising during diagnostic angiography, also may be amenable to transcatheter embolotherapy.[27]

Arteriovenous malformations

Vascular malformations represent vascular abnormalities that can be characterized best by the appearance of the endothelial cells at histologic examination.[28] AVMs, as opposed to hemangiomas, demonstrate normal endothelial cells and mast cells that tend to grow over time; histologically, multiple arteriovenous communications, are present representing the nidus of the malformation, with multiple feeding arteries and draining veins. Conversely, arteriovenous fistulae (AVFs) represent a single communication between a feeding artery and a draining vein, usually occurring in larger vessels than those seen with AVMs.

AVMs are a clinically difficult entity, often requiring several surgical procedures that may or may not be curative. AVMs can be divided into primarily *arterial malformations*, demonstrating high-flow and arteriovenous shunting, and primarily *venous malformations*, demonstrating phleboliths and slow flow.[29] Unless the nidus is embolized, AVMs will continue to recur and grow over time; in addition, several niduses may be encountered. Embolotherapy is directed against the nidus rather than the feeding arteries because embolization of the feeding vessels will occlude flow only temporarily and will stimulate collateral flow to the AVM. Because the targeted vessels are small, embolization agents include small particles or, most frequently, liquid agents such as glue or alcohol (Fig. 8-2).[17,30-32] In patients with predominantly venous malformations, or in those with lesions than are anatomically difficult to treat by transcatheter arterial embolization, direct puncture and alcohol instillation on the venous side of the malformation have proved efficacious.[33]

AVFs constitute a distinct histopathological entity with both a single feeding artery and a single draining vein. Because of this single, relatively large communication, and because preservation of the feeding artery is a primary goal, larger embolic agents such as coils are most efficacious when placed directly into the fistula itself;[17,30,34] if the fistula cannot be entered directly, the fistula may be sandwiched by placing coils into the feeding artery proximal and distal to the fistula, thus essentially isolating the fistula and preventing flow into it so that it may thrombose. Although this method may be effective, it can be used only when the feeding artery can be sacrificed completely without risk to organs distal to the fistula.

Pulmonary AVMs have a variety of histologic subtypes, the most common type involving a single feeding artery and a single draining vein, therefore representing a fistula rather than a malformation. Whereas embolization with detachable balloons acheived great success in the past, they are no longer approved by the v.s. Food and Drug Administration (FDA), nor are they or commercially available.[35] Glue has been used as an embolic agent although care must be taken to ensure that deposition occurs only in the fistula itself because downstream embolization could have severe consequences.[30]

Organ ablation

Embolization procedures for organ ablation for benign etiologies include splenic embolization in the treatment of hypersplenism[36–38] and renal embolization in end-stage kidney disease for the management of hypertension and nephrotic syndrome.[17,39] Splenic embolization can be performed either as definitive therapy for hypersplenism[37,38] or as a preoperative procedure.[36] When used as definitive therapy, it is recommended that 10% to 20% of the splenic arterial supply be spared to prevent infection from encapsulated organisms.[17,37,38] Because proximal occlusion of the main splenic artery may compromise pancreatic supply or collaterals may reconstitute the splenic artery from the short gastric branches,[36] embolization of the intraparenchymal splenic artery branches or arterioles is recommended. Embolic agents have included Gelfoam pledgets,[37,38] PVA particles,[40] and Silastic spheres.[41] While initial technical success rates approach 100%,[37] platelet counts may decrease again within 6 month, indicating recurrent hypersplenism,[42] and up to 23% of patients may require further intervention.[43] When used as adjunctive therapy before splenectomy to decrease the amount of blood loss at surgery, embolization can be performed safely with gelatin sponge particles, PVA particles, coils, or a combination of these agents.[36]

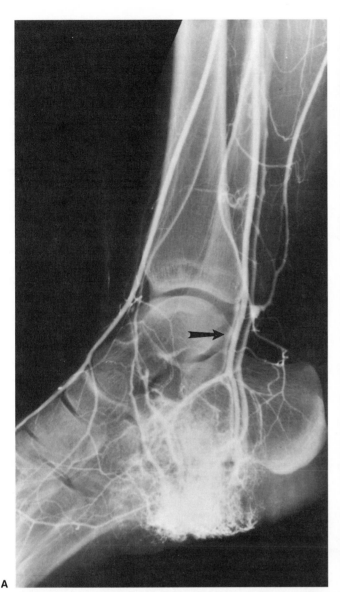
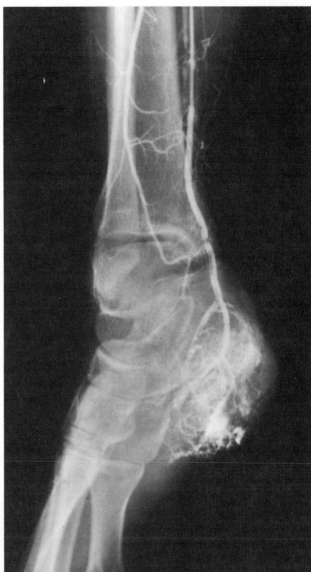

A   B

FIGURE. 8-2 A 20-year-old woman with a pulsatile, painful heel mass. **A:** Diagnostic angiography with the catheter placed above the popliteal artery trifurcation demonstrates a hypervascular heel mass with large feeding branches arising from the posterior tibial artery. Notice the early draining posterior tibial vein (*arrow*) indicating significant arteriovenous shunting. **B:** Angiography performed with the catheter in the tibioperoneal trunk following embolization with small polyvinyl particles. Note the decreased vascularity and the lack of early draining veins postembolization.

Renal ablation procedures may be used in patients with end-stage renal disease who are on dialysis or who are postrenal transplantation in order to prevent renovascular hypertension or nephrotic syndrome arising from the native kidneys.[17,39] The desired end result for "catheter nephrectomy" is complete organ necrosis and ablation; the embolic agents of choice are therfore liquid agents, such as alcohol, with or without concomitant permanent large-vessel occlusion with coils.[17,39] If accessory renal arteries are present, they all must be embolized to allow complete renal infarction. In addition, arteries arising from the renal artery such as the inferior adrenal, infe-

rior phrenic, and ureteral branches should be recognized and spared if possible.[39]

Neoplastic

sterile embolization

Embolization of tumors may be performed as an adjunct to other therapies such as systemic chemotherapy or surgery, as definitive therapy for the treatment of certain benign neoplasms, as palliative therapy for complications of neoplasms, or in combination with chemotherapy as chemoembolization. Sterile embolization procedures include those in which there is no combination of the embolic agent with chemotherapeutic or immunologic medications (Fig. 8-3).

Sterile embolization for complications arising from primary or metastatic neoplasms may prove helpful. Hemorrhage caused by neoplasms may be treated in the same manner as bleeding from benign sources discussed above with some modifications. In particular, hemoptysis arising from lung carcinoma may arise from the pulmonary as well as the systemic circulation; pulmonary angiography is therefore necessary in the absence of a bleeding source on the bronchial angiogram. Regardless of the organ involved, care must be taken to avoid permanent central vascular occlusion, such as with coils, because many tumors are likely to rebleed over time, and vascular access to the tumor must remain uncompromised. Hypervascular tumors, such as renal cell carcinoma or carcinnoid, are more likely to respond to embolotherapy because of the large amount of neovascularity. Occasionally, hepatic tumors parasitize blood supply from other vessels, which also may require embolization.[44]

Palliative therapy may be provided by tumor embolization. Tumors causing symptoms by their proximity, size, or hormonal activity may respond to embolotherapy. Hepatic arterial embolotherapy, using Gelfoam pledgets, Gelfoam powder, or PVA particles, has proved efficacious for symptomatic relief in patients with hormone-secreting tumors metastatic to the liver, with clinical or laboratory response rates ranging from 69% to 100%.[45–47] In-

creased survival rates in patients with metastatic carcinoid undergoing sterile embolization[46] and sterile embolization of other primary or secondary liver neoplasms have demonstrated increased survival rates.[48] Doppler ultrasound of the liver before and after embolization may be helpful in determining residual or recurrent disease.[49] Embolotherapy also has proved efficacious for control of tumor-induced hypoglycemia in patients who have fibrosarcoma.[50]

In some benign settings, embolization may be considered a curative procedure rather than an adjunct. Uflacker demonstrated cures in two patients by using arterial embolization as the sole treatment for benign insulinomas of the pancreas.[51]

Embolotherapy also can be used as a preoperative procedure to decrease the amount of blood loss at surgery. The goal of embolization in these patients is decreased blood flow rather than infarction and cell death; therefore, for patients scheduled for embolization close to the time of surgery, larger agents such as colis have been used to decrease the major blood supply to tumors because collateral flow is unlikely to develop prior to taking the patient to the operating room. A potential disadvantage to large vessel embolization is the possibility of distal embolization into an aortic branch due to manipulations performed during the operative procedure. Gelfoam pledgets or large PVA particles may also be used. Although liquid embolic agents may be helpful,[52] they are not used commonly because of the in-

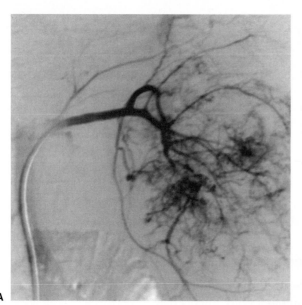
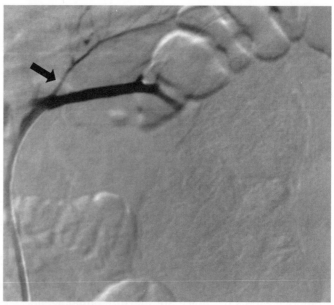

FIGURE. 8-3 A 22-year-old woman who had undergone removal of the right kidney for childhood Wilm's tumor who had develop left-sided Wilm's as an adult tumor. Preoperative embolization was performed to decrease blood loss at surgery. **A:** Selective digital subtraction angiogram of the left kidney demonstrating solitary left renal artery with neovascular changes compatible with Wilm's tumor. **B:** Selective left renal angiogram showing embolization with Gelfoam pledgets and absolute alcohol and demonstrating complete cessation of flow to the kidney. Note the preserved flow in the superior capsular and inferior adrenal branches (*arrow*).

creased risk and time required when using liquid embolic agents.

Chemoembolization

Chemoembolization combines the effects of locoregional chemotherapy and embolization during the same procedure to obtain a synergistic effect of both therapies. The liver is the most common organ to undergo chemoembolization because of the high prevalence of disease and dual vascular supply to the organ. Whereas the normal liver derives its blood supply largely from the portal vein, in the setting of hepatic malignancy approximately 90% of the blood supply to the tumor arises from the hepatic artery,[53] allowing most of the chemoembolic agent to be delivered to the tumor rather than to normal parenchyma during hepatic artery chemoembolization (HACE). Perhaps surprisingly, even in the setting of portal venous obstruction,

HACE, may be performed without significant risk of hepatic infarction (Fig. 8-4).[54]

Chemoembolization of hepatic malignancies is reserved for surgically unresectable lesions. It should be considered adjunctive or palliative therapy, although scattered cases of cure have been reported.[55] In addition, HACE is a multistage procedure, with patients undergoing embolization every 8 to 12 weeks for the duration of their disease or until hepatic insufficiency develops. The risks of HACE increase greatly with worsening liver dysfunction,[56–59] and the risk and benefits of repeat procedures should be weighed. Alternative therapies such as systemic or locoregional chemotherapy, percutaneous alcohol ablation, or cryosurgery are other options that may be considered for the same patient population as those undergoing HACE. Cryosurgery requires an open surgical procedure, and both percutaneous alcohol ablation

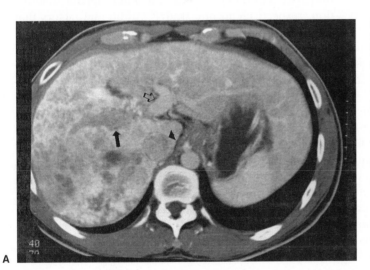

A

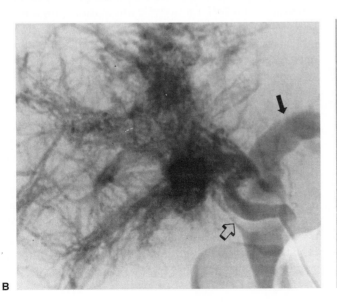

B

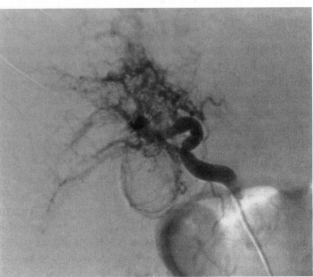

C

FIGURE 8-4. A 33-year-old man with hepatocellular carcinoma and portal vein invasion was referred for chemoembolization. **A:** Contrast-enhanced computed tomography scan of the liver demonstrated diffuse neoplastic involvement of the right hepatic lobe with tumor thrombus occluding the right portal vein (*arrow*). The left portal vein remains patent (*open arrow*) and supplies an enlarged left hepatic lobe. Tumor thrombus is also noted in the inferior vena cava (*arrowhead*). **B:** Selective digital subtraction angiogram of the right hepatic artery demonstrating diffuse neovascularity involving the distribution of the markedly enlarged right hepatic artery. Note the early visualization of the left portal vein (*arrowhead*) due to rapid arteriovenous shunting; tumor thrombus is visualized again in the right portal vein (*open arrow*). **C:** Selective angiogram of the right hepatic artery showing chemoembolization with Gelfoam and Adriamycin/mitomycin C/cisplatin slurry. There is marked diminution of neovascularity within the right hepatic lobe and no evidence for significant arteriovenous shunting, determined by nonvisualization of the left portal vein as demonstrated in (B).

and cryosurgery are limited by the number and size of hepatic lesions. Systemic and locoregional infusion chemotherapy requires doses of chemotherapy exceeding those used for HACE with added side effects for the patient. Only HACE combines the ischemic effects of embolization with locoregional delivery of chemotherapy to the hepatic malignancies.

Chemoembolization may be performed as an adjunct to surgery.[60] Increased survival rates in patients with recurrent hepatocellular carcinoma were found in those who underwent HACE after partial hepatectomy (42% versus 18% at 3-year follow-up).[60] A 3-year survival rate of 77% was found in patients with initially inoperable hepatotomas who underwent HACE and subsequently were determined to be operative candidates.[61]

The technique used for HACE varies widely according to the institution where the procedure is undertaken. A coaxial system frequently is used to increase delivery of the chemoembolic mixture to the area of greatest interest; in patients with diffuse disease, chemoembolization may be performed in either the proper hepatic artery or in both the right and left hepatic arteries selectively. Embolizing one lobe per procedure in patients with diffuse disease may decrease the likelihood of hepatic insufficiency.

Because tissue necrosis and cell death are the anticipated end results of the procedure, distal embolic agents are used. Gelfoam powder and small PVA particles are the most commonly used embolic agents,[58–62] because liquid sclerosing agents may cause biliary sclerosis or necrosis of normal hepatic parenchyma. Proximal embolic materials, in particular coils, are to be avoided because repeat chemoembolization is the rule rather than the exception and vascular access to the tumor must be maintained. Lipiodol also is used frequently either in isolation or in combination with other embolic agents; lipiodol by itself has an affinity for hepatomas and presumably will increase the amount of chemoembolic agent delivered to the hepatoma compared with normal surrounding tissue.[57–64] The chemotherapeutic agent may be delivered first, followed by embolization, or it may be mixed into a slurry with the embolic agent itself. The latter protocol is preferred at our institutions, because delivery of the chemotherapeutic agent before embolization decreases the amount of the agent trapped with the tumor as a result of persistent arterial flow flushing the chemotherapeutic agent from the hepatic artery into the systemic circulation before arterial occlusion at embolization.

Protocols for the chemotherapy agents used vary widely from institution to institution. The most commonly used agents include Adriamycin,[57,59] cisplatin,[57,61,63] mitomycin C,[60,62] and 5-fluorouracil.[65] The chemotherapeutic agent used should vary depending on the type of hepatic malignancy; in other words, different agents given systemically, are used for hepatoma metastatic colon carcinoma, and metastatic carcinoid, and similar agents should be considered for locoregional therapy such as chemoembolization. Consultation with medical oncologists proves helpful when deciding on the appropriate drug regimen.

Results for patients undergoing HACE depend on the type of malignancy being treated. The tumors that have been investigated most extensively include hepatocellular carcinoma (HCC). metastatic endocrine tumors, and metastatic colorectal carcinoma. Hepatocellular carcinoma response rates vary with the protocol used, the size and histologic type of tumor, and the degree of underlying hepatic insufficiency. Regarding the degree of insufficiency, patients with more severe underlying liver disease tend to have decreased survival compared with patients whose hepatocyte function is relatively normal before HACE is performed.[58,59] The 2-year survival rates of patients with HCC treated by HACE were 49% 29%, and 9% for patients with Pugh's class A, B, and C hepatic dysfunction, respectively in one study.[59] Additional factors that are poor prognostic indicators include tumor type and extension, portal vein involvement, tumor area, and presence of ascites and icterus;[66] other studies have shown no prognostic significance to tumor type and portal vein involvement.[56] Most studies demonstrate a 2-year survival for HCC treated with HACE of between 33% and 38%,[57,63,65] although survival rates of up to 92% at 2-years have been reported in patients with HCC with a diameter smaller than 4 cm.[58] A recent European study, however, demonstrated no significant increase in the survival rates for patients with HCC undergoing HACE, although this study has major methodological shortcomings.[63]

Chemoembolization of metastatic endocrine tumors gives perhaps the best results of all liver malignancies.[46,52,65,68–70] In this patient population, it is estimated that because of diffuse involvement of the liver fewer than 10% of all patients are surgical candidates.[68] Response rates vary from 70% 100%[46,68,70] when using symptomatic relief as the endpoint, whereas biologic response, as evidenced by decreased levels of hormonal breakdown products, is seen in 57% to 100% of patients.[65,68,69] Carcinoid syndrome appears to respond somewhat more favorably to HACE than to other hormonally active metastatic tumors.[69]

Benefits from chemoembolization of metastatic colon carcinoma are less apparent. Response rates, measured by a decrease in the size of tumors on follow-up imaging studies or a decrease in the serum carcinoembryonic antigen levels, range from 33 to 87%.[55,70,71] One study demonstrated complete disappearance of liver metastases in 17% of patients, although these results have not been duplicated.[55] Survival rates in patients who undergo HACE are comparable to those in patients who undergo systemic chemotherapy.[72]

Adjunctive therapy is of paramount importance in the HACE patient population. Anticipated side effects of HACE include right upper quadrant pain, fevers, nausea, and transiently elevated liver enzymes.[57,61,63–65] Pain is frequently severe enough to warrant narcotic therapy and should be anticipated by both physician and patient. Nausea usually can be controlled by antiemetic medication such as granisetron or compazine. Liver enzymes almost invariably will elevate immediately following the procedure as a result of hepatocyte death; however, persistently elevated enzymes beyond 3 weeks may indicate hepatic infarction, and repeat HACE may be contraindicated.[57,63]

Infection following HACE is relatively uncommon, with sepsis occuring in fewer than 1% of patients.[73] Because hepatic abscess formation can be a relatively severe side effect, broad-spectrum antibiotic coverage is given immediately before and for 24 hours after the procedure. Fever following the procedure is relatively common and may indicate drug effect or tumor lysis rather than infection; however, a persistently elevated fever may indicate abscess formation and cross-sectional imaging of the liver should be performed. The imaging results must be interpreted carefully because gas may be visualized in the tumor or parenchyma following embolization as a result of the injection of air trapped by the embolic particles themselves. Persistent or increased amounts of gas on follow-up imaging studies should increase the suspicion of infection.

REFERENCES

1. Van Allen RJ, Pentecost MJ. Transcatheter control of hemorrhage in the cancer patient. Semin Intervent Radiol 1992;9:38–44.
2. Ball ABS. Regional chemotherapy for colorectal hepatic metastases using degradable starch microspheres: a review. Acta Oncol 1991; 30:309–313.
3. Daniels JR, Kerlan RK, Dodds L et al. Peripheral hepatic arterial embolization with crosslinked collagen fibers. Invest Radiol 1987; 22:126–131.
4. Ichihara T, Sakamoto K, Mori K, et al. Transcatheter arterial chemoembolization therapy for hepatocellular carcinoma using polylactic acid microspheres containing aclarubicin hydrochloride. Cancer Res 1989;49:4357–4362.
5. Kinoshita A, Yamada K, Ito M, et al. Ethylene vinylacetate copolymerparticles dissolved polyvinyl alcohol (2,000-mer) solution as an embolic material for vascular anomalies:a preliminary study. Intervent Neuroradiol 1994;36:65–68.
6. Maton PN, Camilleri M. Griffin G, et al. Role of hepatic arterial embolisation in the carcinoid syndrome. BMJ 1983;287:932–935.
7. Okazaki M, Higashihara H, Ono H, et al. Embolotherapy of massive duodenal hemorrhage. Gastrointest Radiol 1992;17:319–323.
8. Lang E. Transcatheter embolization in management of hemorrhage from duodenal ulcer: long-term results and complications. Radiology 1992;182:703–707.
9. Okazaki M, Furui S, Higashihara H, et al. Emergent embolotherapy of small intestine hemorrhage. Gastrointest Radiol 1992;17:223–228.
10. Lang EV, Picus D, Marx MV, et al. Massive upper gastrointestinal hemorrhage with normal findings on arteriography: value of prophylactic embolization of the left gastric artery. AJR Am J Roentgenol 1992;158:547–549.
11. Kelemouridis V, Athanasoulis CA, Waltman AC. Gastric bleeding sites: an angiographic study. Radiology 1983;149:643–648.
12. Okazaki M, Higashihara H, Koganemaru F, et al. Emergent embolization for control of massive hemorrhage from a splanchnic artery with a new coaxial catheter system. Acta Radiol 1992;33:57–62.
13. Zhang J, Cui Z, Wang M, et al. Bronchial arteriography and transcatheter embolization in the management of hemoptysis. Cardiovasc Intervent Radiol 1994;17:276–279.
14. Mauro MA, Jaques PF, Morris S. Bronchial artery embolization for control of hemoptysis. Sem Intervent Radiol 1992;9:45–51.
15. Uflacker R, Kaemmerer A, Picon PD, et al. Bronchial artery embolization in the management of hemoptysis: technical aspects and long term results. Radiology 1985;157:637–644.
16. Stoll JF, Bettman MA. Bronchial artery embolization to control hemoptysis: a review. Cardiovasc Intervent Radiol 1988;11:263–269.
17. Keller FS. Embolization in the chest, abdomen and pelvis. In: Mueller PR, vanSonnenberg E, Becker GJ, eds. Syllabus: a diagnostic categorical course in interventional radiology, Oak Brook: Radiological Society of North America 1991:205–212.
18. Boushy SF, Helgason AH, North LB. Occlusion of the bronchial arteries by glass microspheres. Am Rev Respir Dis 1971;103:249–263.
19. Feigelson HH, Ravin HA. Transverse myelitis following selective bronchial arteriography. Radiology 1965;85:663–665.
20. Keller FS, Rosch J, Loflin TG, et al. Non-bronchial systemic collateral arteries: significance in percutaneous embolotherapy for hemoptysis. Radiology 1987;164:687–692.
21. Cohen AM, Doershuk CF, Stein RC. Bronchial artery embolization to control hemoptysis in cystic fibrosis. Radiology 1990;175:401–405.
22. Ben-Menachem Y, Coldwell DM, Young JWR, et al. Hemorrhage associated with pelvic fractures: causes, diagnosis and emergent management. AJR Am J Roentgenol 1991;157:1005–1014.
23. Katz MD, Teitelbaum GP, Pentecost MJ. Diagnostic arteriography and therapeutic transcatheter embolization for post-traumatic pelvic hemorrhage. Semin Intervent Radiol 1992;9:4–12.
24. Ben-Menachem Y. Embolotherapy in trauma. In: Mueller Pr, vanSonnenberg E, Becker GJ, eds. Syllabus: a categorical course in interventional radiology, Oak Brook: Radiological Society of North America, 1991:213–218.
25. Ben-Menachem Y, Handel SF, Ray RD, et al. Embolization procedures in trauma: the pelvis. Semin Intervent Radiol 1985;2:158–181.
26. Sclafani SJA, Weisberg A, Scalea TM, et al. Blunt splenic injuries: nonsurgical treatment with CT, arteriography, and transcatheter arterial embolization of the splenic artery. Radiology 1991;181:189–196.
27. Chung JW, Park JH, Han JK, et al. Perforation of the gastroduodenal artery induced by steerable guidewires in two cases: treatment of hemorrhage by embolization. Cardiovasc Intervent Radiol 1994; 7:41–43.
28. Finn MC, Glowacki J, Mulliken JB. Congenital vascular lesions: clinical applications of a new classification. J Pediatr Surg 1983; 18:894–900.
29. Coldwell DM, Stokes KR, Yakes WF. Embolotherapy: agents, clinical applications, and techniques. Radiographics 1994;14:623–643.
30. Burrows PE, Fellows KE. Techniques for management of pediatric vascular anomalies. In: Cope C, ed. Current techniques in interventional radiology. Philadelphia: Current Medicine, 1995:11–28.
31. Yakes WF, Luethke JM, Parker SH, et al. Ethanol embolization of vascular malformations. Radiographics 1990;10:787–796.
32. Rao VRK, Mandalam KR, Gupta AK, et al. Dissolution of isobutyl

2-cyanoacrylate on long-term follow-up. AJNR Am J Neuroradiol 1989;10:135–141.

33. Gomes AS. Embolization therapy of congenital arteriovenous malformations: use of alternate approaches. Radiology 1994;190:191–198.

34. Nakamura T, Isobe Y, Ueno E, et al. Successful arterial embolization of arteriovenous fistula in the portal circulation. Gastrointest Radiol 1992;17:324–326.

35. White RI, Lynch-Nyhan AL, Terry P, et al. Pulmonary arteriovenous malformations: techniques and long-term outcome of embolotherapy. Radiology 1988;169:663–669.

36. Hickman MP, Lucas D, Novak Z, et al. Preoperative embolization of the spleen in children with hypersplenism. J Vase Interv Radiol 1992;3:647–652.

37. Spigos DG, Jonasson O, Mozes M, et al. Partial splenic embolization in the treatment of hypersplenism. AJR Am J Roentgenol 1979;132:777–782.

38. Kumpe DA. Partial splenic embolization in children with hypersplenism. In: LaBerge JM, Durham JD, eds. Portal hypertension: options for diagnosis and treatment. San Francisco: Society of Cardiovascular and Interventional Radiology, 1995;205–226.

39. Borge MA, Jaques PF, Mauro M, et al. Percutaneous renal ablation in children with end-stage renal disease. J Vase Intervent Radiol 1992;3:467–474.

40. Casteneda-Zuniga WR, Hammerschmidt DE, Sanchez R, et al. Nonsurgical splenectomy. Am J Roentgenol 1977;129:805–811.

41. Guilford WB, Scatliff JH. Transcatheter embolization of the spleen for control of splenic hemorrhage and in situ splenectomy: an experimental study using silicone spheres. Radiology 1976;119:549–553.

42. Yoshika H, Kuroda C, Shinichi H, et al. Splenic embolization for hypersplenism using steel coils. Am J Roentgenol 1985;144:1269–1274.

43. Brandt C, Rothbarth L, Kumpe D, et al. Splenic embolization in children: long-term efficacy. J Pediatr Surg 1989;24:642–645.

44. Macaulay SE. Internal mammary artery embolization for hepatic tumors. Cardiovasc Intervent Radiol 1995;18:20–24.

45. Marlink RG, Lokich JJ, Robins JR, et al. Hepatic arterial embolization for metastatic hormonesecreting tumors: technique, effectiveness, and complications. Cancer 1990;65:2227–2232.

46. Mitty HA, Warner RRP, Newman LH, et al. Control of carcinoid syndrome with hepatic artery embolization. Radiology 1985;155:623–626.

47. Maton PN, Cannlleri M, Griffin G, et al. Role of hepatic arterial embolization in the carcinoid syndrome. BMJ 1983;287:932–935.

48. Chuang VP, Wallace S. Hepatic artery embolization in the treatment of hepatic neoplasms. Radiology 1981;140:51–58.

49. Tanaka K, Inoue S, Numata K, et al. Color Doppler sonography of hepatocellular carcinoma before and after treatment by transcatheter arterial embolization. AJR Am J Radiol 1992;158:541–546.

50. Lengle SJ, Hecht ST, Link DP, et al. Palliative embolization of fibrosarcoma for control of tumor-induced hypoglycemia. Cardiovasc Intervent Radiol 1995;18:255–258.

51. Uflacker R. Arterial embolization as definitive treatment for benign insulinoma of the pancreas. J Vase Intervent Radiol 1992;3:639–646.

52. Winkelbauer FW, Niederle B, Graf O, et al. Malignant insulinoma: permanent hepatic artery embolization of liver metastases—preliminary results. Cardiovasc Intervent Radiol 1995;18:353–359.

53. Sigurdson ER, Ridge JA, Kemeny N, et al. Tumor and liver drug uptake following hepatic artery and portal vein infusion. J Clin Oncol 1987;5:1836–1840.

54. Pentecost MJ, Daniels JR, Teitelbaum GP, et al. Hepatic chemoembolization: safety with portal vein thrombosis. J Vasc Intervent Radiol 1993;4:347–351.

55. Lang EK, Brown CL. Colorectal metastases to the liver: selective chemoembolization. Radiology 1993;189:417–422.

56. Hatanaka Y, Yamashita Y, Takahashi M, et al. Unresectable hepatocellular carcinoma: analysis of prognostic factors in transcatheter management. Radiology 1995;195:747–752.

57. Bronowicki JP, Vetter D, Dumas F, et al. Transcatheter oily chemoembolization for hepatocellular carcinoma. A 4-year study of 127 French patients. Cancer 1994;74:16–24.

58. Matsui O, Kadoya M, Yoshikawa J, et al. Small hepatocellular carcinoma: treatment with subsegmental transcatheter arterial embolization. Radiology 1993;188:79–83.

59. Bismuth H, Morino M, Sherlock D, et al. Primary treatment of hepatocellular carcinoma by arterial chemoembolization. Am J Surg 1992;163:387–393.

60. Nakao N, Kamino K, Miura K, et al. Recurrent hepatocellular carcinoma after partial hepatectomy: value of treatment with transcatheter arterial chemoembolization. AJR Am J Roengenol 1991;156:1177–1179.

61. Yu YQ, Xu DB, Zhou XD, et al. Experience with liver resection after hepatic arterial chemoembolization for hepatocellular carcinoma. Cancer 1993;71:62–65.

62. Katsumori T, Fujita M, Takahashi T, et al. Effective segmental chemoembolization of advanced hepatocellular carcinoma with tumor thrombus in the portal vein. Cardiovasc Intervent Radiol 1995;18:217–221.

63. Groupe D'Etude et de Traitement du Carcinome Hepatocellulaire. A comparison of lipiodol chemoembolization and conservative treatment for unresectable hepatocellular carcinoma. N Engl J Med 1995;332:1256–1261.

64. Nakagawa N, Cornelius AS, Kao SCS, et al. Transcatheter oily chemoembolization for unresectable malignant liver tumors in children. J Vasc Intervent Radiol 1993;4:353–358.

65. Therasse E, Breittmayer F, Roche A, et al. Transcatheter chemoembolization of progressive carcinoid liver metastasis. Radiology 1993;189:541–547.

66. Yamashita Y, Takahashi M, Koga Y, et al. Prognostic factors in the treatment of hepatocellular carcinoma with transcatheter arterial embolization and arterial infusion. Cancer 1991;67:385–391.

67. Clouse ME, Stokes KR, Kruskal JB, et al. Chemoembolization for hepatocellular carcinoma: epinephrine followed by a doxorubicin-ethiodized oil emulsion and gelatin sponge powder. J Vasc Intervent Radiol 1993;4:717–725.

68. Perry LJ, Stuart K, Stokes KR, et al. Hepatic arterial chemoembolization for metastatic neuroendocrine tumors. Surgery 1994;116:1111–1115.

69. Ruszniewski P, Rougier P, Roche A, et al. Hepatic arterial chemoembolization in patients with liver metastases of endocrine tumors: a prospective phase II study in 24 patients. Cancer 1993;71:2624–2630.

70. Carrasco CH, Charnsangavey C, Ajani J, et al. The carcinoid syndrome: palliation by hepatic artery embolization. AJR Am T Radiol 1986;147:149–154.

71. Feun LG, Reddy KR, ?? JM, et al. A phase 1 study of chemoembolization with cisplatin and lipiodol for primary and metastatic liver cancer. Am J Clin Oneal 1994;17:405–410.

72. Martinelli DJ, Wadler S, Bakal CW, et al. Utility of embolization orchemoembolization as second-line treatment in patients with advanced or recurrent colorectal carcinoma. Cancer 1994;1706–1712.

73. Reed RA, Teitelbaum G, Daniels JR, et al. Prevalence of infection following hepatic chemoembolization with cross-linked collagen with administration of prophylaclic antibiotics. J Vasc Intervent Radiol 1994;5:367–371.

9

Organ Access Techniques
General Principles for Localization, Drainage, and Stenting

THOMAS J. DIBARTHOLOMEO AND CURTIS W. BAKAL

Percutaneous techniques for localization, drainage, and stent placement are now routine, daily procedures in the interventional radiology suite. Utilization of multiple imaging modalities allows access to almost all organs and body compartments. The goal of this chapter is to describe the general principles of localizing and accessing a target organ for draining collections and for stenting obstructive lesions.

Virtually any organ or body cavity can be accessed from a percutaneous route. It is essential to avoid traversing pleura, bowel, and major vascular structures en route to the target. On occasion, however, the stomach may be used as a pathway or ultimate drainage site for pancreatic collections. In addition to direct, percutaneous access, the liver can be biopsied via the hepatic veins. If necessary, some solid organs, for example, the liver and kidney, may be traversed during percutaneous biopsies, aspiration for diagnosis, or drainage.

■ Imaging Modalities Used for Localization

All radiographic and imaging modalities may be used for accurate localization of the target. A careful review of relevant preprocedure images should be made. This is necessary to select the optimal imaging modality for the procedure, plan the route of access, and determine material requirements for the procedure.

On plain films, some landmarks are especially helpful and will aid the subsequent fluoroscopic access. A collection may be identified by amorphous-appearing gas. Renal shadows sometimes are seen, especially in the hydronephrotic, enlarged kidney. Renal calculi aid greatly in localiza-

tion of the kidney. Contrast material may be administered intravenously to opacify the renal collecting system if renal function allows. Dilatation of the gallbladder frequently occurs with biliary tract obstruction. The gallbladder shadow occasionally is seen, assisting in localization during percutaneous cholecystostomy. Patients who are postcholecystectomy frequently have surgical clips, which localize the gallbladder bed.

Under real-time fluoroscopic guidance, the needle, catheter, or guidewire can be visualized directly, which permits immediate redirection of the catheter or guidewire when its course deviates from the desired approach. A damaged catheter or wire can be exchanged immediately.

The benefits of fluoroscopic guidance tend to result in an expedient procedure. The disadvantages include relatively poor contrast resolution. Often the target cannot be seen readily, which may necessitate additional localization punctures. Also, vital structures (e.g., blood vessels) in the anticipated course may not be readily apparent. Thus, it is often helpful to do a cross-sectional image [usually computed tomography (CT)] before a fluoroscopically guided procedure.[1] Real-time imaging requires patient cooperation (i.e., breathhold for limited motion). There is also radiation exposure to the patient and physician, although this can be minimized by proper technique.

Ultrasound (US) has increasingly become an extremely useful modality for target localization. In some practices, it has become a primary guidance modality for organ localization. US offers real-time imaging, with potentially excellent tissue contrast for both localization and needle/catheter tract identification. US is often used in combination with fluoroscopy. For example, during percutaneous nephrostomy, after localizing puncture with US, aspiration of about 5 mL of urine is performed, and the needle is injected with an equal amount of contrast to opacify the system for subsequent fluoroscopic guidance.[1] US optimally requires specialized needles, guidewires, and catheters that are sufficiently echogenic for proper visualization. It is usually cost-effective but is highly operator and patient dependent.

Computed tomography (CT) is an extremely useful modality because it provides excellent tissue contrast. CT provides clear visualization of the course of the anticipated needle tract and will demonstrate any intervening structures that might preclude placement of the desired drainage catheter.[2,3] The target lesion or anatomic structure is shown clearly on CT. The disadvantages include lack of real-time monitoring and delays to check the progress of needle placement by repeated scanning. Patient cooperation is a necessity because variations in breathing or breath-holding can result in large variability in needle placement. CT is a more expensive guidance technology than fluoroscopy or US. With the advent of fast CT scans, procedures can be done more expeditiously, although not in real time.

Magnetic resonance imaging (MRI) also provides excellent tissue contrast, imaging in any plane required for diagnosis, and visualization of the needle/catheter tract; however, specialized instruments that are nonferromagnetic are required. Conventional MRI does not offer real-time imaging and is presently the most expensive guidance modality. Its primary interventional use is in neuroradiologic procedures. Real-time MRI "fluoroscopy" is in early development.

■ Goal of Access

Percutaneous access to an organ, abscess cavity, or infected or obstructed anatomic pathway can be performed for biopsy, as described elsewhere in this book. Aspiration of a fluid collection may be performed for diagnosis (i.e., culture and sensitivity) or for therapeutic drainage. In less frequent circumstances, a cavity or pseudocyst can be sclerosed by alcohol or other agents to facilitate its closure. Urinary and biliary tract obstructions can be relieved by diverting the path of urine or bile into an external drainage bag (e.g., biliary drainage) or by crossing the site of obstruction and reestablishing the normal antegrade anatomic pathway (e.g., biliary stenting).

Obstructions are typically caused by calculi, tumor, or inflammation. Calculi are frequently the cause of urinary tract obstruction and can result in compromised function of the affected kidney and infection of the stagnant urine. Therefore, rapid relief of urinary tract obstruction is im-

portant. The therapeutic drainage procedure is termed *percutaneous nephrostomy tube placement*. Tumor is also a frequent cause of obstruction in the urinary tract and biliary tree. Primary urinary bladder or ureteral tumors (usually transitional cell) as well as primary pelvic malignancies or metastases are additional causes of urinary tract obstruction that require nephrostomy. Ureteral stent placement can be performed percutaneously, but cystoscopic retrograde stent placement usually is attempted first because it is less invasive than the percutaneous procedure. Percutaneous nephrostomy or ureteral stenting frequently is performed when the tumor causing the obstruction is inoperable or is radiosensitive. The ureter frequently responds to radiation therapy with stricture formation. Therefore, a ureteral stent can be placed prophylactically or when a stricture becomes symptomatic. Other causes of stricture include postoperative injury, ischemia, or passage of ureteral calculi. Percutaneous nephrostomy also is indicated for bladder dysfunction, colovesicular or coloureteral fistulae, or bladder leaks of any cause. Urinary diversion by nephrostomy drainage or stenting across a ureteral tear may be used to aid healing.[4]

The most common cause of biliary obstruction in the United States is carcinoma of the pancreatic head. Other causes include primary bile duct tumors, bile duct stones, and postoperative injury. Biliary obstruction that results in pruritis or sepsis requires decompression of the biliary tree. A temporary stent is used before a planned operative procedure is done or if resolution of the bile duct obstruction is expected. Typically, permanent stent placement is reserved for inoperable carcinomas. Often a diagnostic cholangiogram and stenting can be performed in one sitting. It is sometimes helpful to perform a Gram stain to determine immediately whether a cavity is infected if this is not readily clinically apparent. If positive, the original puncture then may be used immediately for placement of a drainage catheter.

■ Materials

Needles

Although a large number and type of needles are available for aspiration and biopsy, only a limited number are used for organ access and catheter placement. The prototype is the Chiba needle, a type of aspiration biopsy needle. The Chiba needle is available in multiple gauge sizes, although the 21- or 22-gauge "skinny" needles are used most frequently. If inadvertent nontarget or vascular puncture occurs or if multiple passes are needed, this small gauge is relatively atraumatic. Chiba needles range in length from 10 to 20/cm. The needle tip is beveled at 25 degrees. Originally designed to obtain cytologic or bacteriologic samples, skinny needles are used increasingly to access visceral organs for drainage and stenting. (Needles with a greater ability to cut typically are used for biopsy; these are available from a wide variety of manufacturers and are typically "gun"-type spring-loaded devices.) For organ access, skinny needles are used for atraumatic access to the target, for example, the biliary tree or intrarenal collecting system. The initial skinny needle approach is completed with contrast opacification of the target for localization and diagnosis. Vendor-specific skinny needles are also incorporated as the initial components of "one-stick" systems used for upsizing the initial puncture site to allow for drainage or stenting.

Access to the kidney and biliary trees which are deep, vascular organs, as well as to many more superficial targets, is typically done with the Seldinger technique; that is, a needle is first placed into the target and exchanged over a guidewire for the drainage catheter. Intermediate dilatation of the track is usually needed. Traditionally, 18- or 19-gauge, 15-cm long, hollow-core needles were used with exchange over a 0.035-inch to 0.038-inch stiff working wire (Rosen or Amplatz type). Many interventional radiologists now prefer "one-stick" systems that allow relatively atraumatic localization with a 21-gauge needle and 0.18-inch wire, with subsequent exchange for a triple coaxial dilator that will accommodate a 0.035-inch or 0.038-inch working wire. (After this wire is placed, the track can be dilated to accommodate a standard 8Fr to 12Fr catheter) (Fig. 9-1). An additional drainage-type catheter is the single-stick trocar. This catheter is loaded coaxially over a sharp tipped, stiffening needle/cannula and is inserted directly through a small dermatotomy into the target site. The catheter is advanced (payed off) into the target, and the sharp-tipped inner trochar is removed, leaving the drainage catheter in place (Fig. 9-2). These devices offer the advantage of limited manipulation and speed of insertions, but they must be used only when a simple, clear path to the target site from the skin is available. The trocar catheter is used only after a commitment to therapy via an indwelling drainage catheter already has been made; it is inappropriate to use this device for simple diagnostic aspiration.

Catheters

Standard directional angiographic catheters and guidewires are used for providing steerability, maneuverability, and pushability while attempting to negotiate anatomy, for example, through a stricture, or down a branch duct. Drainage catheters differ from angiographic flush pigtail catheters and are generally large-bore (8Fr to 12Fr) to expedite flow of tenacious material. They have distal configurations (i.e., pigtail), which are larger than the catheter diameter to help secure

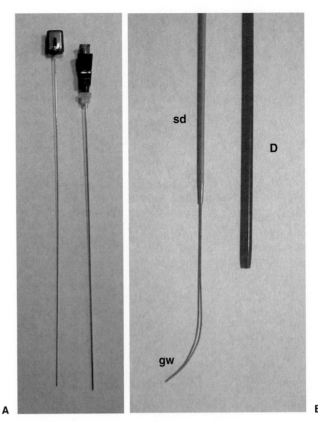

FIGURE 9-1. One-stick technique. **A:** Skinny needle (21 gauge). After entering target, the stylet (*left*) is removed to allow passage of an 0.018 inch stiff mandrel guidewire into the target. **B:** Coaxial dilator set. The 0.018-inch guidewire (gw) can support passage of a triple coaxial dilator, which is passed as a unit. The metal stiffener and inner dilator (sd) are removed; the outer dilator (D) is left in place, allowing passage of a stiff 0.035-inch or 0.038-inch guidewire, used to support passage of the final catheter or drain (Cook, Inc., Bloomington, IN, U.S.A.).

the catheter. Self-locking mechanisms have been designed to minimize dislodgement.[5] A drainage catheter has multiple large side holes placed along the distal aspect of the catheter, typically on the inside surface of the pigtail only and not extending up the catheter shaft (Fig. 9-2). This circumscribed drainage area ensures that drainage holes are placed only within the target collection, cavity, or organ. Side-hole location exclusively on the inner surface allows continued function as the target shrinks down to abut the outer surface of the pigtail. Furthermore, the circumscribed location of holes within the pigtail contains drainage to the target and decreases the likelihood of leakage back along the track. Side holes in the track would allow leakage of material into the track or subcutaneous tissues, leading to infection and wound breakdown. The drainage holes of abscess drainage catheters are large to permit the egress of thick, purulent material. The holes of nephrostomy catheters may be of only moderate size, allowing drain-

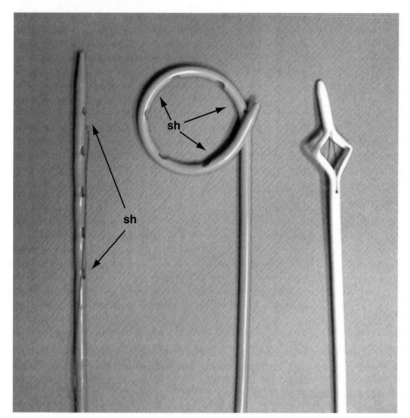

FIGURE 9-2. Drainage catheters. Drainage catheters can be placed over a guidewire via the Seldinger technique or primarily over a stiff trocar (*left*). After trocar or guidewire removal, the pigtail can reform. Note the placement of drainage side holes near the tip only, on the inside of the pigtail (*left, center:* sh). A self-retaining suture can be pulled to lock the tip. The pigtail locking loop (*center*) is compared with an Amplatz-type mushroom lock (*right*), which can be used in small targets, such as nondilated intrarenal collecting systems (CR Bard Inc., Covington GA; Boston Scientific Co., Watertown MA, U.S.A.; Cook, Inc. Bloomington, IN, U.S.A.).

age of urine while better maintaining structural integrity and rigidity of the catheter tip and pigtail. Unlike side holes of standard angiographic catheters, the side holes on a drainage catheter are larger than standard 0.038-inch guidewires, which can exit the catheter during wire advancement. Usually, this can be avoided by using straight-tipped rather than "J"-tipped guidwires or by using angled wires, which can be torqued away from the side holes during wire passage. The drainage holes are relatively widely spaced to maximize catheter body and pushing strength when inserting the catheter through tissue. The catheter typically has a slippery or low resistance coating to ease its passage through the skin tracks and deeper tissues. Typical drainage catheters are designed to be inserted over a 0.038-inch guidewire. Stiff guidewires generally should be used. Rarely, a sump catheter is utilized for drainage of purulent, thick material. The second lumen of a sump permits the catheter to be placed to suction rather than for gravity drainage only.[6]

Aspiration of fluid may be used for diagnostic purposes and may be therapeutic for small collections. The needle is removed after aspiration. Drainage catheters are left in place to conduct fluid retrograde to an external collection device, typically a bag. These are placed in a cavity or above an obstructing lesion. *Stent catheters* cross the obstruction and conduct fluid in an antegrade fashion, typi-

cally toward the anatomic recipient, such as duodenum (*biliary stent*) or urinary bladder (*ureteral stent*) (Fig. 9-3). Stents can be entirely internal (double-J pigtail plastic ureteral stent, biliary metallic stent, biliary Carey–Coons plastic stent) (Fig. 9-4). Plastic stents must be exchanged for new ones at regular intervals (usually 3 to 5 months). If entirely internal, they are best changed from below (endoscopically for biliary stents, cystoscopically for ureteral double-J stents) (Fig. 9-4). Metallic stents, which are permanent, occlude from tumor progression or debris. They usually can be salvaged by balloon dilatation or through–lumen placement of an internal–external plastic stent. Internal–external designs (e.g., nephroureteral stents, internal–external biliary stent) have an externalized portion that is easy to access for flushing and over-the-wire exchange; one typical use of such a device is during a multistage procedure during which initial catheter placement encountered infected material or periprocedural bleeding and catheter flushing are necessary for patency (Fig. 9-5).

Guidewires

Guidewires are used in three ways: The first is for access, with the guidewire typically passed through the puncture needle into the target. An angiographic catheter for directed manipulation or a drainage catheter then may be

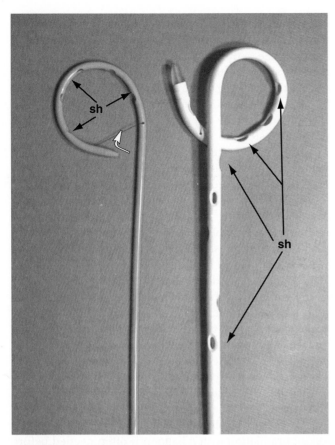

FIGURE 9-3. Placement of side holes. A partially opened 8Fr external drainage catheter (*left*) has side holes (sh) on the inner aspect of the pigtail. The 10Fr biliary drain (*right*) demonstrates side holes in the pigtail and for a distance down the shaft to allow antegrade drainage through an obstructed segment. The self-locking suture is seen in the drainage pigtail (*left, curved arrow*)

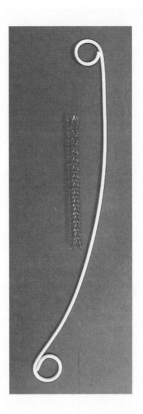

FIGURE 9-4. Internal stents. Metallic flexible stent (*left*) often used for malignant biliary obstruction. Double-J pigtail stent (*right*) used for internal uereteral drainage (Flexstent CR Bard, Inc., Covington GA, U.S.A.; ureteral double-J stent, Boston Scientific Corp., Watertown, MA, U.S.A.).

placed after exchanging out the needle over the wire. Typical access wires are 0.018 inches in diameter, allowing passage through a skinny needle or 0.035-inch to 0.038-inch stiff guidewires, such as the Rosen or Amplatz, which are used with 18- and 19-gauge needles. Second, various angiographic guidewires may be used with directional catheters for negotiation of the path to the target site. Angled and straight-tipped 0.035-inch to 0.038-inch hydrophilic and coil-spring guidewires (e.g., Bentson, Cook, Bloomington, IN, U.S.A.) typically are used for this purpose. Third, after the final site has been reached, a stiff guidewire is used to exchange the angiographic catheter for the drainage or stent catheter. The essential properties of this wire are (1) sufficient length to accommodate removal of the catheter while positioned and (2) sufficient stiffness to support the advance of the large-bore drainage catheter. Typically, 0.035-inch Amplatz-type stiffwires or 0.038-inch Rosen guidewires are used for this purpose.

■ General Procedural Principles: A Summary

Preprocedural review of any relevant imaging study is essential to planning the best potential approach. We prefer retrograde endoscopic/cystoscopic stenting to percutaneous drainage or stenting, if possible, because of the lower risk of hemorrhage.

Visualization of the target organ may be accomplished under CT, real-time US, or fluoroscopy. If fluoroscopy is used, the approach is best made using a skinny needle to enter and opacify the target organ. Residual infrarenal contrast from a CT, intravenous urogram, or previous retrograde stent attempt may be helpful. Multiple views are obtained during contrast opacification for an adequate diagnostic study, if necessary. This may be the optimal time to delineate the nature of a stricture because further manipulation (with possible bleeding or edema) or passage of a stent may subsequently obscure the lesion. Aspiration of diagnostic samples (e.g., for culture and sensitivity) may be done at this time.

The passage of a drainage catheter with dilation of the

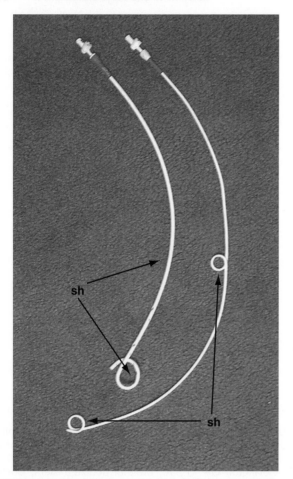

FIGURE 9-5. Internal/external stent. Biliary stent (*left*) with side holes in pigtail and on shaft (*sh*). The nephroureteral stent (*right*) has a self-locking loop pigtail for in the renal pelvis and a distal pigtail for the bladder, with a long length of side holes. For maximum bidirectional drainage, the external hubs may be kept open to a bag; closing them allows antegrade internal drainage, which, if successful, obviates the need for a collection bag. The external hubs allow exchange over a guidewire or access for flushing.

tract to 8Fr, 10Fr, or larger French sizes is best done through a vascular parenchymal tract away from the central hilus, minimizing the likelihood of major bleeding. Parenchymal tracts also help to hold catheters in place and tamponade leaks. Posterolateral approaches through Brodel's avascular area into a renal calyx or peripheral puncture of a biliary radicle are thus safest and optimal for device placement.

It is also desirable for the organ entrance site to be at some distance from the obstruction to allow for both catheter manipulation and stent placement. Good stent "purchase" well above the obstruction will allow a sufficient number of proximal side holes for drainage and will allow for continued patency if there is subsequent retrograde malignant encroachment.

If the initial puncture is well positioned, it can be used

for placement of the drainage catheter or stent. A "one-stick" system may be used to convert the skinny needle to the drainage catheter. If the initial puncture is not optimal, the skinny needle is left in place and can be used to opacify the target to optimize the second puncture under fluoroscopy. A working wire is passed into the target to allow dilation of the tract and placement of the drainage catheter or stent.

During a drainage procedure, care must be taken to minimize the risk of procedure-related septicemia.[7] Pre-procedure antibiotics are usually appropriate (e.g., before biliary drainage). Overdistention of the target with contrast should be avoided. Achieving rapid external drainage is preferable to prolonged attempts at crossing an obstruction for stenting, which increases the risk of sepsis.[8] Stenting can be done at a second session. A 24- to 72-hour period of decompression usually allows better delineation of the stricture, with easier cannulation and stent passage. Conversion of an external drain to an internal stent is often straightforward. The drainage catheter is exchanged out over a stiff guidewire for a steerable angiographic catheter. This catheter, in combination with a standard or hydrophilic guidewire, can be advanced through the obstructing lesion. The guidewire is replaced by a stiff one, and the angiographic catheter is exchanged for the stent, which is passed antegrade through the lesion; predilation with a balloon is often needed before stent passage.

In the biliary tree and urinary tract, stent placement is usually preferable to external drainage for several reasons. First, it is more physiologic; for example, biliary-enteric circulation is preserved. Second, with internal stents or internal–external stents that have long internal purchase, the problem of accidental catheter dislodgement is alleviated. Third, the presence of an external appliance and drainage bag may present a physical and psychological problem for the patient. Choice of a particular stent type depends on clinical circumstances. Wholly internal stents are generally preferred to internal–external devices; however, at initial placement, consideration must be given to future maintenance. New biocompatible co-polymers have increased plastic stent durability, but occlusion usually still occurs within 5 to 6 months, and all stents eventually occlude.[9–11] In malignant biliary tract disease with limited patient prognosis, interventional radiologists typically place a permanent metal stent because the predicted stent durability is long relative to predicted life span [e.g., Wallstent (Schneider, Inc.), Boston Scientific (Watertown, MA), Memotherm stent, (CR Bard Covington, GA, U.S.A.)]. Techniques have been devised to recanalize occluded internal stents, but these typically require repeat percutaneous puncture, especially with nonampullary lesions.[12] Plastic internal stents, such as double-J ureteral stents or Carey–Coons biliary stents, typically are exchanged endoscopically from the bladder or duodenum; however, if anatomy precludes this, it may be preferable to place an internal–external device, which is amenable to flushing and exchange over a guidewire. Covered metallic biliary prostheses may prove to enhance durability and management of selected biliary lesions, but their use is not yet widespread.[13]

If the target site is small, or if careful positioning through a narrow tract is necessary, a purposeful localizing puncture can be used. In this case, the target is punctured directly with a 21- or 22-gauge needle, and contrast is administered to distend and opacify the system gently or to elucidate a safer access point. Many interventionalists use this technique for percutaneous nephrostomy. The renal pelvis can be punctured directly from a posterior approach and opacified. A sample of urine may be aspirated for culture and sensitivity. The collecting system may be opacified with contrast, and a suitable peripheral puncture site is localized. In the kidney, this is most frequently a lower pole, posterior calyx. Puncture into a calyx provides an excellent track through renal

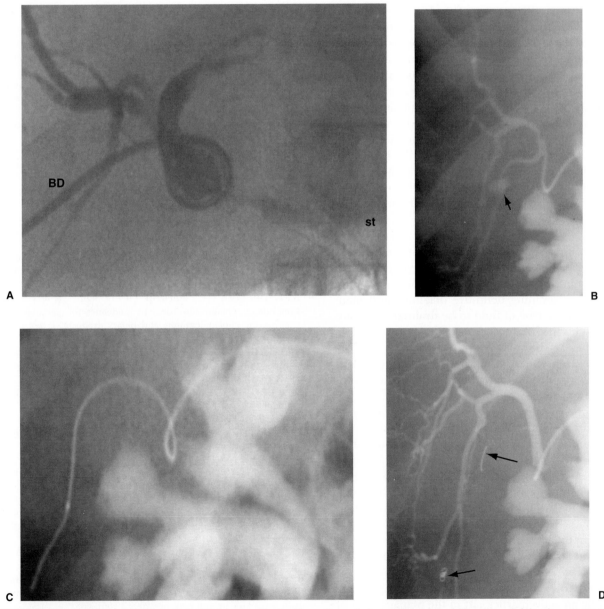

FIGURE 9-6. A: External biliary drain (BD) in a patient with malignant obstruction of the biliary tree, left in place temporarily until antegrade function of a metallic (st) stent could be confirmed. **B:** After removal of the drain, the patient developed hematochezia and hyperbilirubinemia. Arteriogram demonstrates pseudoaneurysm of a right hepatic artery branch (*arrow*). **C:** Superselective catheterization and embolization. **D:** The pseudoaneurysm is occluded by a sandwich of microcoils in the arterial branch distal and proximal to the lesion (*arrows*). Symptoms and signs resolved.

parenchyma, which is essential for catheter retention. Access by a lower pole tract ensures that the relatively large French drainage catheters or stents (8Fr or 10Fr) are kept away from the renal vascular pedicle. Although puncture of these structures is tolerated well when performed with the small, 21-gauge needle, passage of an 8Fr or 10Fr catheter through the renal vessels will result in significant hemorrhage.

The localizing puncture during percutaneous transhepatic cholangiogram and drainage likewise starts with aspiration of bile and injection of contrast to select accurately a peripheral bile duct for puncture anticipating drainage. Again, selecting a peripheral duct ensures a parenchymal tract. Placement of a drainage catheter through solid-organ parenchyma provides an anchor that helps to hold the catheter in position. A localizing puncture is almost exclusively used with fluoroscopically guided procedures, especially percutaneous transhepatic drainage of the biliary tree and percutaneous nephrostomy placement. CT guidance and US guidance often allow good visualization of the peripheral ducts or calyses, obviating a preliminary stick. Some interventional radiologists use US guidance for puncture of the bile ducts for biliary drainage; with this technology, a single puncture of a peripheral duct can suffice both to obtain a diagnostic cholangiogram and to place a drainage catheter.

After a wire is in adequate position, an external drainage catheter, internal–external stent, or internal stent is chosen for placement. As stated, the choice of catheter is based on the individual patient's needs, the stage of the procedure (i.e., awaiting definitive diagnosis and management), and the type of fluid to be drained. Typically, infected fluid is first drained externally. An unresectable pancreatic head tumor with symptomatic biliary duct obstruction may be stented primarily. Tenacious, purulent material may require placement of a sump catheter or a large 14F drainage.

Hypotension or other signs of procedure-related hemorrhage must be evaluated urgently. A CT may be obtained to confirm hematoma around the track or catheter site. Urgent selective or subselective arteriography may be needed to assess whether there is an arterial source of bleeding (extravasation, arteriovenous fistula, or pseudoaneurysm) that can be treated by percutaneous embolization.[14,15] The drainage catheter itself may obscure or tamponade such a lesion; a repeat arteriogram with the catheter pulled back over a wire then should be performed (Fig. 9-6). Other complications include sepsis and pneumothorax. The interventional radiologist is obligated to be an active participant in the management of

these appliances.[7,8] Gentle forward flushing with 5 to 10 mL of sterile saline every 8 to 24 hours will help maintain catheter patency.

■ Conclusion

Percutaneous access to organs and body cavities is a mainstay of interventional radiology practice. These techniques permit safe, minimally invasive procedures for the diagnosis and management of collections and obstructed organ systems.

REFERENCES

1. Millward SF. Percutaneous nephrostomy: a practical approach. *J Vasc Interv Radiol* 2000;1:955–964.
2. Gerzof SG, Robbins AH, Johnson WC, et al. Percutaneous catheter drainage of abdominal abscesses: a five-year experience. *N Engl J Med* 1981;305:653–657.
3. VanSonnenberg E, Ferruci JT Jr, Mueller PR, et al. Percutaneous drainage of abscesses and fluid collections: technique, results, and applications. *Radiology* 1982;142:1–10.
4. Lang EK. Antegrade ureteral stenting for dehiscence, strictures, and fistulae. *AJR Am J Roentgenol* 1984;143:795–801.
5. Cope C. Improved anchoring of nephrostomy catheters: loop technique. *AJR Am J Roentgenol* 1980;135:402–403.
6. Van Sonnenberg E, Mueller PR, Ferrucci JT Jr, et al. Sump catheter for percutaneous abscess and fluid drainage by trocar or Seldinger technique. *AJR Am J Roentgenol* 1982;139:6134.
7. SCVIR Standards of Practice Committee. Quality Improvement guidelines for adult percutaneous abscess fluid drainage. *J Vasc Interv Radiol* 1995;6:68–70.
8. Burke DR, Lewis CA, Cardella JF (SCVIR Standards of Practice Committee). Quality improvement guidelines for percutaneous transhepatic cholangiography and biliary drainage. *J Vasc Interv Radiol* 1997;8:677–681.
9. Cardella JF, Castaneda-Zuniga WR, Hunter DW, et al. Urine-compatible polymer for long-term ureteral stenting. *Radiology* 1986;161:313–318.
10. Mitty HA, Dan SJ, Train JS. Antegrade ureteral stents: technical and catheter-related problems with polyethylene and polyurethane. *Radiology* 1987;165:439–443.
11. Mitty HA, Rackson ME, Dan SJ, et al. Experience with a new ureteral stent made of a biocompatible copolymer. *Radiology* 1988;168:557–559.
12. Cwikiel W. Percutaneous management of occluded biliary duct endoprostheses. *Acta Radiol* 2000;1:338–342.
13. Petersen BD, Timmermans HA, Uchida BT, et al. Treatment of refractory benign stenoses in liver transplant patients by placement and retrieval of a temporary stent-graft: work in progress. *J Vasc Interv Radiol* 2000;1:919–929.
14. Cope C, Zeit RM. Pseudoaneurysms after nephrostomy. *AJR Am J Roentgenol* 1982;139:255–261.
15. Gardiner MF, Long WB, Haskal ZJ, et al. Upper gastrointestinal hemorrhage secondary to erosion of a biliary Wallstent in a woman with pancreatic cancer. *Endoscopy* 2000;32:661–663.

10

Percutaneous Needle Biopsy and Drainage

ALLA ROZENBLIT AND SAMUEL I. WAHL

The use of needle biopsy for nonoperative diagnosis became an acceptable diagnostic procedure in the 1930s, but it gained wide popularity in the 1970s, when computed tomography (CT) and sonography became available to guide interventional procedures.[1] The original needles were large (16- or 14-gauge) and often placed blindly for tissue diagnosis of diffuse liver disease and palpable masses. With recent innovations in imaging techniques, instruments, and cytopathology, percutaneous biopsy now plays a significant role in patient care. Today, needle biopsy is the most frequently performed interventional procedure in radiology practice.[2,3] Similarly, in the last two decades, percutaneous drainage (PD) has become a widely accepted treatment for intraabdominal abscesses.

The advantages of percutaneous procedures include lower morbidity rates, the use of local rather than general anesthesia, the elimination of surgical stress, shorter hospitalization, and decreased cost.[4] Many uncomplicated and some complicated abscesses can be completely and permanently cured by PD. Other lesions can be treated temporarily with resolved infection, but a curative surgical procedure still would be necessary to eliminate any underlying cause. PD may render palliation, achieving symptomatic relief and defervescene in patients with limited life expectancy who are not candidates for curative surgery because of underlying comorbid conditions.[5]

■ Procedure Planning

Because most biopsies and drainages are done under CT, the following discussion concentrates on CT approaches.

Many of these concepts also apply to ultrasound. Percutaneous biopsy and abscess drainage should be planned on the basis of a recent high-quality diagnostic CT performed with intravenous (IV) contrast, which helps to assess the vascularity of the lesion and to identify adjacent vascular structures. Based on the available information, diagnostic possibilities should be discussed with the referring physician to plan an appropriate procedure. If a vascular lesion, such as hemangioma, arteriovenous malformation, or aneurysm, is suspected, additional noninvasive studies may be necessary for confirmation. All other lesions can be safely biopsied using at least a fine needle.

At the time of the procedure, a needle trajectory is drawn on the chosen section, and the level is marked on the scout view. In general, the shortest distance between the skin and the lesion should be traversed. This rule, however, is not always feasible because the shortest distance to the lesion may cross anatomic structures that should be avoided. Obviously, major vascular structures should be avoided, as should large nerves. The lung should not be intentionally traversed for investigation of subdiaphragmatic abnormalities. It is advisable not to cross large muscle groups because they are vascular, and a spontaneous muscle contraction may deflect the needle.[6] Unnecessary puncture of parenchymal organs, particularly the spleen, should be avoided. Liver parenchyma, however, often is traversed with a fine needle for sampling of porta hepatic lymph nodes and adrenal, pancreatic, or biliary lesions as well as for gaining access to intrahepatic collections. We avoid penetration of the large bowel, even with fine needles, because of the possibility of infection. Although the risk of infectious complications is low in the immunocompetent population, a higher risk may exist for immunocompromised patients.[6,7] Small bowel, stomach, and duodenum can be traversed with relative impunity using a fine needle.[6,8] However, penetration of a hollow viscous with a large needle is inappropriate for tissue sampling. Small bowel and transverse and sigmoid colon often may be moved out of the path of the needle simply by repositioning the patient from a supine to a lateral decubitus position.[6]

■ Preprocedure Patient Evaluation

Referring physicians and careful chart review by the radiologist usually provide patient history and determine the presence or absence of serious concomitant conditions, such as cardiovascular, pulmonary, or neurologic disorders, as well as the ability of the patient to cooperate. We do not perform biopsies or drainages in an uncooperative patient without general anesthesia. Aspirin and other medications that potentially could alter coagulation and platelets should be discontinued one week prior to the scheduled procedure. Percutaneous procedures can be performed safely at any hematocrit level when coagulation is normal. When the hematocrit is below 32% or coagulation is abnormal, the risk of bleeding has more serious consequences. Patients with a history of abnormal bleeding and those with known clotting abnormalities also pose a higher risk. Most radiologists screen all patients for prothrombin time (PT), partial prothrombin time (PTT) and a platelet count. An acceptable PT is within 2 seconds of normal, PTT within 25%, and a platelet count above 70,000. When these parameters deviate from the acceptable levels, hematology consultation and appropriate corrective measures are mandated.

The patient is required to fast after midnight before the procedure. When the patient arrives in the radiology department, the procedure, alternatives, possible complications, and benefits are discussed, and the patient signs an informed consent form. A brief medical history is obtained, and vital signs are recorded. Prior to the procedure a peripheral IV line is placed. Anxious patients are premedicated according to the institutional conscious sedation protocol; however, this is rarely required for biopsies and actually may alter the patient's ability to cooperate. During the procedure, the patient's pulse rate and oxygenation are monitored by means of a pulse oximeter. Prior to percutaneous abscess drainage, patients should intravenously receive broad-spectrum antibiotics.

■ Percutaneous Needle Biopsy

Indications for percutaneous needle biopsy include (1) diagnosis of primary or metastatic malignancy in a newly discovered mass, (2) diagnosis of tumor recurrence in patients with known malignancy, (3) diagnosis of infection, and (4) diagnosis of benign disease. Common contraindications include (1) uncorrectable coagulopathy, (2) inability of the patient to cooperate, (3) a patient with uncontrollable cough (lung biopsy), and (4) lack of a safe needle path (with large–gauge needles).

Procedures and instruments

Percutaneous needle biopsy requires the accurate positioning of a needle into a lesion to obtain an adequate sample representative of the lesion. A sample can be obtained by either aspiration of pathologic material or by the mechanical cutting of tissues without suction. Typically, aspiration biopsy is performed with fine needles, most commonly 20- to 22-gauge, and is referred to as *fine-needle aspiration biopsy* (FNAB). A nonaspiration fine-needle technique (i.e., cutting tissue without the use of suction) may play a role in the diagnosis of extremely vascular lesions; otherwise, the aspiration technique is preferred for abdominal biopsies.[9]

FNAB is performed using needles with a variety of tip and stylet designs intended to improve diagnostic yield (Fig. 10-1). Some needles have blunt or beveled tips without cutting edges (aspiration needles) and are suitable for sampling practically any lesion.[2] End-cutting needles have sharpened tips that can be hooked, notched, spiraled, or trephined, and they often are better for recovering diagnostic material from firm hypovascular masses. Needles with a beveled tip tend to recover better samples, because the small angle of the bevel allows superior diagnostic material to be obtained.[10] Such needles, however, tend to deviate along the direction of the slant. Chiba and spinal needles appear to be a viable compromise.

The aspirated material then undergoes cytologic evaluation and occasionally is sent for histologic analysis when tissue fragments are present. Histologic material is more commonly obtained by using end-cutting rather than aspiration needles. Generally, the larger the needle, the greater the yield of diagnostic material.[6,11] Several investigators reported higher diagnostic yields, without additional complications, using 20-gauge needles rather than 22- or 23-gauge needles.[12,13] When overlying structures, such as liver, stomach, small bowel, and small vessels, are unavoidable, fine needles can be safely directed into the target lesion through these structures.[8,14] The choice of a specific needle depends on the size, location, and vascularity of the lesion; the presence of intervening structures along the needle path; the amount of tissue required to satisfy diagnostic considerations; and the experience and preference of the operator. The Franseen and Westcott needles have the best overall performance, closely followed by the spinal needle.[15]

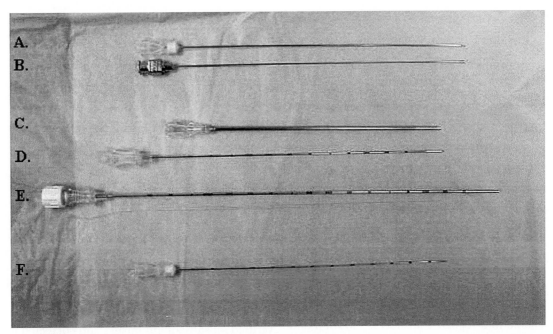

FIGURE 10-1. Various 22-gauge needles used for cytologic biopsies. (**A**) Chiba. (**B**) Spinal. (**C**) Turner. (**D**) Franseen. (**E**) Madayag. (**F**) Westcott.

Usually, FNAB is sufficient for the diagnosis of carcinoma and recurrent malignancies as well as sampling of fluid. For the diagnosis of lymphoma, unusual tumors, or benign disease, however, large-bore cutting needle biopsies (LNB) are considered more accurate.[16–18] This technique provides a sufficient histologic specimen while preserving the architecture of the lesion; however, the potential risks to the patient increase in quadratic proportion to the diameter of the needle.[19] A variety of needles ranging from 14 to 19 gauge can be used for cutting biopsy and frequently are divided into end-cutting and side-cutting types. The former requires application of suction either by a syringe or a self-aspirating device, and the latter cuts along a gap in the inner stylet while an outer needle slides over the stylet, similar to a Tru-cut needle. Both the stylet and the outer needle can be moved manually or by using automated spring-loaded biopsy gun devices. In general, a superior specimen can

be obtained by using side-cutting needles compared with end-cutting needles.

Automated biopsy devices consistently provide high-quality diagnostic tissue with minimal patient discomfort and no significant increase in the complication rate compared with FNAB.[16,17,20] There is a variety of commercially available automated biopsy devices with different loading and safety mechanisms and with different throw lengths. Some devices have an adjustable throw ranging from 1 to 2 cm that can be tailored to the lesion size. Many automated biopsy gun devices are packaged with guiding cannulas for coaxial insertion of the needle. Instructions should be studied carefully before any new device is used. Some of these devices are unacceptably bulky and cumbersome, but overall automated devices are easy to use and consistently provide good-quality histologic specimens. We prefer an 18-gauge biopsy gun, which has a strong spring mechanism and is light weight, requiring no added support, with an optional feature of coaxial insertion and suitable for lesions of variable depths (Fig. 10-2).

Imaging guidance

Percutaneous biopsy can be performed with fluoroscopic, sonographic, CT or occasionally magnetic resonance imaging (MRI) guidance.[21] The choice of imaging depends on the ability of the modality to visualize both the lesion and the needle with adequate depiction of the surrounding anatomy as well as the experience and per-

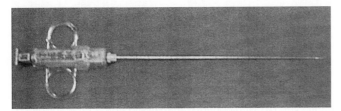

FIGURE 10-2. An example of a spring-loaded 18-gauge core biopsy needle.

sonal preference of the radiologist and the availability of the equipment.

Fluoroscopy is a simple, fast, cost-effective, real-time technique used primarily for lung lesions that are well visualized in the frontal and lateral views. For small, difficult, ill-defined, or anatomically challenging lesions near the hilum or mediastinum, CT is the method of choice. Most abdominal biopsies are best performed with ultrasound or CT because these lesions cannot be visualized by fluoroscopy.

Previously limited to the liver and superficial lesion sampling, ultrasound guidance is currently being used with considerable success to biopsy lesions throughout the abdominal cavity and certain chest lesions.[22,23] Ultrasound is less expensive and often less time-consuming than CT, and its multiplanar capability allows for needle passage in any plane in real time.

The procedure can be performed by using a freehand technique, a dedicated biopsy transducer, or biopsy guides attachable to a regular transducer.[24] Motion and high-level echoes from the needle tip indenting adjacent tissues should be observed during the needle placement. A number of technical innovations and needle designs that improve visualization of the needle have been reported.[25–27] Despite recent advances in ultrasonographic (US) guidance, the basic limitations still are related to difficulties in visualization of the needle tip, poor acoustic windows, interposed bowel gas, and large patient size.

In our experience and that of others,[6,28] CT is the most effective modality for accurate needle biopsy, allowing visualization of most lesions and surrounding anatomy, therefore providing a safe biopsy route. The entire needle is readily visible on CT, allowing precise sampling of small and difficult lesions in complex anatomic regions such as the pelvis and retroperitoneum or near major vessels in the chest and abdomen. Repeat of previously failed biopsy should be performed with CT guidance to ensure the accuracy of needle placement. The disadvantages of CT guidance include high cost, often long procedure time, inability to scan in real time, and the limitation of a single scanning plane.

Biopsy techniques

Localization

The patient is placed on the CT table in a comfortable predetermined position that is appropriate for the planned needle insertion. Several axial sections are obtained that include the lesion. The proper level is marked on the skin with the gantry laser light, and the lesion's projection on the skin is marked with a radioopaque marker (e.g., a paper clip or a commercially available, thin radioopaque grid). The position of the marker is verified on subsequent images and corrected if necessary to obtain the optimal entry point (Fig. 10-3). After sterile skin preparation, the entry site is infiltrated with 2% lidocaine to the level of the peritoneum, organ capsule, or pleura. All subsequent needle manipulations within the thoracic and abdominal cavity should be performed with suspended respiration to prevent a tearing effect of the needle tip.

A biopsy needle then is inserted into the lesion either by a single pass for superficial lesions or with incremental adjustment of depth and angulation for more difficult masses. To correct for inaccurate angulation, the needle should be withdrawn completely before any adjustment is made. After each adjustment, the position of the needle tip is radiographically verified. In-plane biopsies include

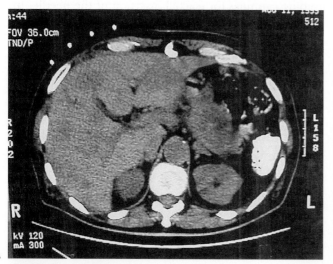
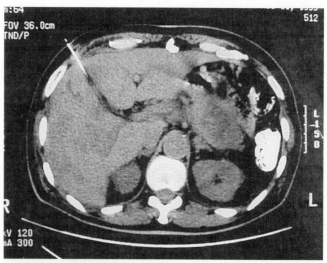

FIGURE 10-3. Single axial computed tomography image through the liver. (**A**) Radioopaque markers in preparation for percutaneous needle biopsy of a low-attenuation liver lesion. Note the mass in the pancreatic tail. (**B**) Needle tip is positioned well within the liver lesion.

lesions located at the same axial level as the skin entry plane. The procedure is simple; if any angulation is required, it is easily achieved in the same axial plane. In general, three 5- or 10-mm sections are obtained to verify the needle position.

Out-of-plane (angled) biopsies involve the sampling of lesions located above or below the skin entry point; thus, angulation in the longitudinal plane is required to reach the target. Often, additional angulation in the axial plane is also necessary. This procedure is more demanding and often lengthy because multiple adjustments of the needle are often required. Angulation of the scanning gantry may help to bring both the lesion and the needle in the same oblique plane, avoiding intervening structures.[29,30]

A longitudinal angle can be calculated using a "triangulation method"; however, it is difficult to implement precisely; therefore, this calculation is not practical.

Commercially available needle-guiding devices can be used for proper angulation. Increased accuracy and safety with these devices have been reported.[31–33] Stereotactic devices for abdominal biopsy have shown a decrease in the number of needle manipulations by 75% and procedure time by 50% compared with hand guidance,[34] but stereotactic systems are expensive and may be difficult to use.

Hand guidance, most commonly used for out of plane procedures, requires experience.[6] We simply estimate the longitudinal angle evaluating sequential images. Once the angulation in the axial plane is correct, the needle is angled longitudinally and then moved incrementally toward the lesion. To verify the needle tip position, sequential images should be obtained from the needle entry point to at least 10 mm past the lesion. Sometimes four or more sections are needed to visualize the needle in its entirety. Sonographic guidance is often a better alternative for angled procedures.

To improve the efficiency and accuracy of multiple needle placements, a coaxial technique can be used for both FNAB and LNB, including automated devices.[6,7] First, a short guiding cannula is inserted in the body wall and adjusted to achieve the proper direction. Then a biopsy needle is placed through the cannula to the desired depth.

FNAB sample

With the needle tip in satisfactory position, the stylet is removed, and a 20-mL syringe is attached to the needle; 5 to 10 mL of suction is applied while 1- to 2-cm quick, vigorous excursions are made through the lesion with some rotation of the needle. Suction can be maintained or slowly released during withdrawal of the needle. The aspirated material is expelled from the needle onto glass slides for cytologic smears and immersed in 95% alcohol for fixation prior to staining. The specimen should be examined by a cytopathologist in the biopsy suite. The aspirated syringe content is rinsed for cell-block preparation that is processed as a histologic specimen. Any tissue

fragments are immersed in a 10% buffered formalin solution for histologic processing.

Multiple passes are often necessary to obtain diagnostic material.[35,36] We limit the total number of passes to four. Regardless of the needle tip configuration, four passes with a 20-gauge needle yield diagnostic material in 95% of cases.[15]

Large-needle biopsy sample

At least one fine needle pass usually precedes LNB for obtaining cytology and as a test for lesion vascularity. Extremely vascular lesions are not sampled with large needles.

Once a large end-cutting needle is passed into the lesion, aspiration techniques are applied in a similar manner as FNAB. A side-cutting needle is placed at the margin of the lesion, and the position is checked. In some automated devices, the instrument is ready to fire at that time, and so the position of the cutting portion of the needle within the lesion cannot be verified. In other devices, the position of the inner stylet can be documented (and repositioned if necessary) after it is manually moved into the lesion. The obtained material is processed histologically.

Diagnostic yield

Image-guided percutaneous biopsy is an accurate procedure. The diagnostic accuracy varies because of differences in technique, the needles used, and the organ and lesions sampled. The range of sensitivities and specificities of CT-guided biopsies in general is 73 to 93% and 81 to 100%, respectively.[37,38]

Complications

The overall reported complication rates for abdominal needle biopsy range from 0 to 3%,[6,39] with minor bleeding the most frequent and common complication; infection, pancreatitis, and pneumothorax are less common. Fatalities and needle-tract tumor seeding have been reported only rarely. One multiinstitutional survey of 16,381 biopsies reported 33 deaths related to FNAB,[40] including 21 liver, 6 pancreatic, 2 adrenal, and 4 miscellaneous biopsies; the mean mortality rate was 0.031%. For cutting needles, serious complications are more common; however, a similar mortality rate of 0.027% was reported in more than 11,000 abdominal procedures.[41] Seeding of malignant cells via the needle tract has been reported in 0.003 to 0.009% of FNAB, more commonly with renal cell carcinoma and pancreatic and musculoskeletal masses.[40]

Specific biopsy sites

Chest

Patient cooperation is absolutely essential when obtaining a chest biopsy because the patient must suspend respiration after a midexpiration. The goal of lung biopsy is to establish the presence of malignant cells, distinguish small cell from non–small cell tumor, and diagnose benign disease. Cytologic material is usually sufficient for nonlymphomatous malignancies; however, some common mediastinal masses (e.g., lymphoma and thymoma) and benign lung lesions often require large needle samples. Peripheral lung lesions are more commonly biopsied. Central lesions can be sampled percutaneously; however, a transbronchial approach is preferred to reduce the risk of significant hemorrhage and pneumothorax. An extrapleural (either anterior parasternal or posterior paravertebral) approach using CT or fluoroscopic guidance is preferred for mediastinal biopsy.[42] This may be difficult because of the proximity of major vessels and interposed lung. Creation of an extrapleural window[43] for the safe approach to mediastinal lesions is an attractive technique, but it is time consuming and requires considerable experience. For routine lung biopsy, we use a 22- or 20-gauge Westcott needle either as a single needle method or with a coaxial technique. Large needles, including biopsy guns, can be used for suitable lung and mediastinal lesions. A safer way to approach these lesions is via preexisting areas of pleural thickening, effusion, fibrosis, or consolidation.[44,45] All necessary needle adjustments should be made superficial to the pleura to prevent pneumothorax, the most common complication of lung biopsy. Moore et al[46] showed a decreased incidence of postbiopsy pneumothorax by positioning the patient with the puncture site down after the procedure. This likely is a result of diminished mobility of the lung compressed by the patient's own body weight.

We prefer to position the lung for biopsy in a similar compressed position; therefore, the patient is placed in an ipsilateral decubitus position when a lesion can be sampled from either an anterior or a posterior approach. This maneuver seems to decrease the incidence of pneumothorax; however, no large series have been done to date to demonstrate this decrease. With CT guidance, the frequency of pneumothorax after lung biopsy ranges from 30% to as high as 50%. However, chest-tube treatment will be needed in only about 10% of patients.[42,44,47–50] Increased lesion depth, small lesion size, and preexisting lung disease have been shown to add to the development of pneumothorax.[48,51] When a pneumothorax is present, it almost always is detected on a chest film within 1 hour.[52] We thus screen for complications with an immediate postbiopsy CT and obtain a chest x-ray within 1 hour of the procedure. Patients who require chest-tube placement are admitted to the hospital for additional management; small asymptomatic pneumothoraces are followed with serial plain films. If the pneumothorax remains stable, the patient usually is sent home.

Hemoptysis reportedly occurs in 5 to 21% of patients[36,53] and is more likely to occur with the use of large needles and with more central lesions. Serious hemorrhage rarely occurs. Air embolism is an extremely rare occurrence thought to be related to coughing during the procedure. Fatalities have been reported with both endobronchial bleeding and air embolism.[6] If the patient develops a cough during biopsy, the procedure is aborted.

Liver

The liver is the abdominal organ on which biopsy is most commonly done.[54,55] Unfortunately, a significant portion of the liver projects into the chest, making lesions here difficult to biopsy because they often require a steep or straight intercostal approach. We prefer the intercostal approach for its simplicity and ultimate benefit to the patient. Even though the needle transgresses the pleura, if aerated lung is avoided (a must), this does not result in pneumothorax.[6] We routinely obtain a chest radiograph after any intercostal manipulations. Biopsies of small lesions in the dome of the liver are difficult regardless of the guidance modality used; therefore, only fine needles are used. When multiple lesions are present, the most accessible one with least necrosis should be sampled. Subcapsular lesions are approached with caution because of the possibility of subcapsular extension from potential bleeding. Such a lesion should be approached through at least some liver parenchyma, which theoretically will tamponade any possible bleeding, although some needle angulation is often required for this simple maneuver.[56] Biopsy should not be done on suspected echinococcal cysts because of the threat of potential peritoneal spillage of daughter cysts and possible anaphylactic reaction.[57]

Pancreas

The diagnostic yield of pancreatic biopsies is lower than that of the liver, particularly with pancreatic head lesions.[58–60] One possible explanation is that pancreatic masses are often difficult to separate from a peritumoral inflammatory response. A good-quality diagnostic scan, preferably helical, helps to identify relatively well-defined hypodense regions that should be biopsied. Cytologic material is often insufficient to make a diagnosis of pancreatic carcinoma,[58] often requiring larger needles or multiple samples. Complications associated with pancreatic biopsy include pancreatitis, fistula formation, peritonitis, and hemorrhage.[2,40,61] Biopsy of functioning endocrine pancreatic tumors should not be done percutaneously because it is both unnecessary and inaccurate.[6]

Biopsy of cystic pancreatic masses with the intent to differentiate benign from malignant lesions have shown to be unreliable largely as a result of sampling error.[62] Additionally, the risk of spillage of malignant cells is increased when sampling a cystic lesion.[49]

Adrenal glands

Oncologic patients who are normotensive and are found to have an adrenal mass undergo percutaneous biopsy after a non-hyperfunctioning adenoma is excluded by MRI. In a hypertensive patient, normal endocrine biochemical profile helps to exclude a pheochromocytoma or other functioning tumors unsuitable for biopsy. The role of needle biopsy of incidentally discovered adrenal masses is not well defined. Similar to other endocrine tissues, the distinction between a well-differentiated adrenal carcinoma and an adenoma may be difficult, even with large samples.[63] FNAB is usually sufficient to make a diagnosis of adrenal metastases. For unusual and benign masses, large needles can be used. Among the different approaches to adrenal lesions, a direct posterior paraspinal approach with the patient in the ipsilateral decubitus position is safe and relatively simple.[64] Alternatively, a posterior approach with cephalad angulation or a transhepatic or transrenal approach can be used to avoid the lung.[65] Gantry angulation can be helpful for adrenal biopsies when scanning patients in a prone position.[30] Reported complications include bleeding and pneumothorax. Hypertensive crisis is also a reported complication that results from inadvertent biopsy of functioning tumors. The overall complication rate is less than 5%.[2,65–67]

Kidney

The reported diagnostic accuracy for solid renal masses is quite high,[3,67] but the procedure is now uncommonly performed for diagnosis of focal renal lesions. Definitively benign lesions such as cysts and angiomyolipomas are diagnosed on the basis of imaging. Frankly malignant and indeterminate masses require surgical exploration. Patients with advanced disease and those who are poor surgical candidates undergo needle biopsy prior to the initiation of chemotherapy. Hemorrhagic complications range from 0 to 12%.[49] Tumor seeding along the needle tract also has been reported.[40]

■ Percutaneous Abscess Drainage

Because untreated abdominal abscesses are almost invariably fatal, no absolute contraindications to PD exist; however, some abscesses respond to surgical drainage (SD) rather than PD. Obviously, any abscess without a safe percutaneous pathway should be treated surgically. Additionally, collections that contain tissue debris rather than fluid (infected hematomas, fungal abscess, pancreatic necrosis and abscess, phlegmon without liquefaction, necrotic tumors) and abscesses containing foreign bodies and septated peritonitis are unlikely to respond to PD.[68,69]

Guidance choices

Like percutaneous biopsy, PD can be performed under fluoroscopic, sonographic, or CT guidance. CT is the modality of choice because of its ability to survey the entire abdomen and pelvis; visualize abnormal fluid and air collections; identify surgical staples, drains, and lines; and assess bowel wall thickness and other associated abnormalities potentially contributing to the patient's symptomatology.[6,70] CT is also most effective for guiding drainage procedures because the pathway of the catheter insertion can be more accurately planned. When a drainage procedure is attempted fluoroscopically, a recent CT scan should be available for indirect guidance. US is fast, inexpensive, and particularly attractive because of its portable capability, which allows some drainage procedures to be performed in the intensive care unit. Large and superficial collections can be readily drained with US and fluoroscopic guidance. The choice of guidance modality varies among institutions and depends on the experience and preference of radiologists and the availability of the equipment. We perform the vast majority of PDs using CT guidance. Dual guidance can be used when the regional puncture and guidewire insertion are performed under CT or US guidance. Subsequently, the procedure can be completed under fluoroscopic guidance.[6]

Drainage procedure

The procedure usually is accomplished in several stages, starting with needle aspiration and catheter insertion, followed by catheter management, follow-up, and, finally, catheter removal.

Fluid aspiration

Not all intraabdominal collections represent abscesses. Hematoma, biloma, seroma, lymphocele, and loculated ascitis all can have a similar appearance. If any clinical suspicion of infection exists, these collections should be aspirated and examined by Gram stain, culture, sensitivity, and biochemical analysis. A diagnostic sample (10 to 15 mL) is initially obtained using sterile technique and local anesthesia. For aspiration of a near-water density collection; a 20-gauge needle is sufficient. More commonly, we use a 19-gauge needle with an 18-gauge Teflon sheath, which allows aspiration of a more viscous fluid. If purulent material is obtained, the Teflon sheath can be easily exchanged over a guidewire for a larger-bore drainage catheter. Clear, thin fluid is usually sterile, and drainage is not indicated. Care must be taken to sample a deep portion of the collection because supernatant layers may be free of bacteria and debris, resulting in a false-negative Gram stain. Borderline cloudy and hemorrhagic fluid should undergo laboratory evaluation before the decision to drain these collections is made.

Fluid aspiration techniques use the same principles as needle biopsy. A needle trajectory should be precise and preferably free of any intervening structures to allow safe drainage catheter placement. Transgression of bowel should be carefully avoided, even for diagnostic aspiration, because it may give spurious results and may increase the chance of infection in the adjacent fluid collection.[6] Inadvertent enterostomy that follows such a transgression can increase morbidity, but usually it is not a disastrous complication and can be successfully managed using catheter drainage.[71] A transgastric approach can be safely used for aspiration and drainage of collections within the lesser sac. Transhepatic needle and catheter placement is acceptable in selective cases.[6] We try to avoid the diaphragm and pleura when we approach subphrenic abscesses.

Catheter insertion and management

The ideal catheter for abscess drainage possesses several important but often contradictory qualities. It should be smooth and relatively rigid for easy insertion, but it also should be soft enough to avoid pressure erosion. The inner lumen should be as large as possible for the given size, but the walls must be strong to withstand collapsing and kinking forces. A maximum number of sideholes is desired, preferably along the inner portion of the pigtail catheter, but without any weakening of the walls. We have yet to find such an ideal catheter.

Currently, two types of catheters are commercially available: single-lumen and double-lumen, or sump, type. The latter has some advantages in preventing catheter clogging by the presence of a second air lumen around the drainage lumen. These sump catheters tend to perform better with suction; however, their effective drainage lumen is smaller, and therefore evacuation of fluid is slower than in the same-size single-lumen catheter. We currently prefer the single-lumen type (Fig. 10-4). Either a Seldinger or trocar technique can be implemented for catheter insertion. The latter method is reserved for large, superficial collections; the entire assembly of a catheter, an inner stiffening cannula, and a sharp stylet is inserted into the abscess cavity in one motion. The stylet then is removed, and the catheter is advanced while the stiffener is held in a fixed position.

The more controlled and safer Seldinger technique is preferred and always is used for deep and difficult abscesses. With this technique, a soft-tipped 0.035 or 0.038 80-cm J guidewire is inserted through the aspiration needle into the abscess cavity; the needle then is removed. The position and coiling of the wire are checked by a digital scout film. The needle track then is gradually dilated to the desired catheter size by using standard angiographic dilators. Dilators are inserted to a predetermined depth to prevent bending of the guidewire and possible transgression of the backwall of the abscess cavity. A drainage catheter with an inner stiffener then is inserted over the guidewire to the same depth; while the stiffener is held in place, the catheter is "payed-off" over the wire. After removal of the stiffener, the catheter position is checked by a scout film and subsequent axial images, and all necessary adjustments are made. The wire then is removed. The content of the abscess is aspirated as fully as possible until mild resistance is met. No irrigation or contrast injection is performed at this time to avoid the possibility of bacteremia. After the fixation of a locking mechanism, the catheter is sutured to the skin or to an enterostomy ring, and the insertion site is covered with a sterile dressing. Then the catheter is attached to a drainage bag for a gravity drainage. We recommend irrigation of the lumen with 10 to 15 mL of saline every 6 to 8 hours. For abscess collections communicating with the gastrointestinal or biliary tracts, continuous low suction is not advised as an initial treatment, but it can be implemented later, when the risk of bacteremia is no longer present.[6] Lahorra et al showed that intracavitary instillation of urokinase improves drainage in abscess collections that contain extremely viscous material or septations without any associated systemic effects.[72]

Follow-up

Typically, a positive response to abscess drainage is observed within 24 to 48 hours after the procedure and is evident by overall clinical improvement, defervescence, and a drop in white cell count. Over a period of several days to weeks, a predictable change occurs in the appearance of the draining fluid, ranging from purulent to cloudy to serosanguinous and ultimately to clear. The volume of drainage material should decrease within the first few days. Continuous drainage of a large amount of fluid is suspicious for a fistulous communication.[73]

In patients with a poor clinical response to PD, a repeat CT scan is taken to identify undrained collections, possible additional abscess collections, or other unrelated abnormalities (e.g., acute cholecystitis, ischemic bowel). Depending on the nature of the problem, additional

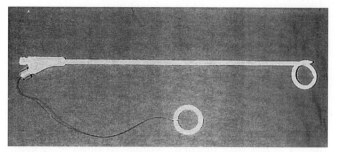

FIGURE 10-4. Example of an all-purpose pigtail-type drainage catheter and stylet, with locking pigtail loop.

percutaneous catheters may be placed or an open drainage procedure can be undertaken.

Sinogram

An initial sinogram usually is performed 48 to 72 hours after the procedure. The purpose of the study is to assess the extent of the abscess cavity, identify fistulous communications, and evaluate the position of the catheter. A suboptimally located catheter can be manipulated into a more effective position, or it can be exchanged for a larger one if the cavity is incompletely drained. An additional sinogram can be repeated 5 to 7 days later for follow-up of the cavity size.[6]

Catheter removal

In an afebrile patient who clinically demonstrates resolution of infection, cessation of drainage (< 10 mL/day) in an otherwise patent catheter, and a diminished abscess cavity by sinogram or CT, the drainage catheter can be removed. Some radiologists prefer to withdraw the catheter gradually (1 to 2 cm per day over several days).

Efficacy

Early studies of percutaneous abscess drainage have reported an overall success rate between 62.4 and 94%, with a mortality rate between 1 and 4.6%,[70,74,75] considerably lower than the reported surgical mortality rates. Many investigators have attempted to compare PD with surgical drainage (SD), suggesting that PD is as safe as SD with equal or better success.[76–80] These studies were appropriately criticized for the lack of stratification based on the severity of illness, with a larger number of critically ill patients having been treated with SD than with PD. Other investigators found a direct correlation between severity of illness and patient mortality in patients with abscess[81,82] often related to multiple organ failure.[83] The severity of illness in patients with intraabdominal infections can be assessed objectively using the Acute Physiology and Chronic Health Evaluation (APACHE II) scoring system.[84,85] Although the absolute number of survivors with APACHE II scores of 15 or higher was greater with SD, the difference was not statistically significant. The drainage technique does not affect survival of patients with abscesses, but early detection and treatment can prevent multiple organ failure (with subsequent rise in APACHE II score), contributing to decreased mortality rates.

Complications

The overall complication rate is less than 10%.[5] Sepsis following catheter insertion is the most common complication, occurring in 4 to 6% of patients. Other complications include hemorrhage, inadvertent enterostomy, spillage of infected material, pneumothorax, and empyema.

Specific sites

Subphrenic abscess

Avoiding contamination of the pleural space is an important technical consideration and can be accomplished by using an anterior or lateral subcostal transperitoneal approach with cephalad angulation. Favorable results with the more risky intercostal approach have been reported, however, with overall success rates approaching 85% and a complication rate of 4.8%.[86]

Hepatic abscess

Success rates of PD for liver abscesses are reported to range between 69 and 89%, with complication rates between 1.7 and 7.3%.[73,87] Unlike infected liver tumors or infected hematomas, primary pyogenic liver abscesses respond well to PD. PD of infected tumors have shown palliative effects in some patients.[88] Amoebic abscess usually responds to a conservative treatment and does not require drainage.[5] The diagnosis can be made by the characteristic "anchovy paste" appearance of the abscess material and by uncovering amoebae in the aspirate. Both sampling and drainage of echinococcal cysts should be avoided, as discussed.[6]

Renal and related retroperitoneal abscesses

Renal, perirenal, pararenal and psoas collections are highly amenable to treatment with PD.[89–91] Open drainage of these locations is rarely performed. The best approach is posterolateral, with a success rate between 61 and 94%. Some patients with renal and perirenal abscesses require concomitant urinary diversion. Complications are reported in 3 to 6% of cases.[5,91]

Abscesses with enteric communication

Gastrointestinal fistulas that may be either a cause or sequela of abscess formation are found in 40% of abdominal abscesses.[92] Fistulas with low output (< 200 mL per day) close spontaneously in 80% of cases, with adequate catheter drainage in the dependent portion of the abscess and with low suction.[5,92] Usually, longer drainage time is required for fistula closure compared with a simple abscess. Percutaneous treatment of high-output fistulas (> 200 mL per day) is much more difficult and includes proximal bowel diversion or nasogastric intubation with suction and hyperalimentation as well as high-level catheter suction. Surgery is often required for the definitive treatment. An overall cure rate of 77% for abscesses with enteric communication and underlying normal bowel has been reported. In patients with diseased bowel, temporization was achieved in 86%.[5]

Pancreatic collections

An uncomplicated pancreatic pseudocyst without communication to the pancreatic duct can be treated with simple aspiration, with a success rate of less than 25%.[6] A pseudocyst also can be drained externally with a catheter. There is, however, an increased risk of developing a cutaneous fistula for lesions communicating with the pancreatic duct. For large pseudocysts in the inferior recess of the lesser sac, an anterior infragastric approach is appropriate. Collections in the lateral recess are best accessed through the gastrosplenic ligament or by a transgastric route. A transhepatic approach through the left lobe of the liver is a viable alternative in some cases. Transgastric drainage of pancreatic pseudocysts is the method of choice.[93–95] A catheter is inserted through the stomach into the lesser sac, providing both internal and external drainage until the pseudocyst is resolved. After removal of the catheter, residual drainage into the stomach may continue, and cutaneous fistulae have not been reported with this method.[93] A similar transgastric drainage via percutaneous gastrostomy has been advocated.[6] Infected pseudocysts that are well defined and contain primarily liquid material usually respond well to external drainage.[96,97] Unlike pancreatic pseudocysts (with or without infection), pancreatic abscess and noninfected pancreatic necrosis containing primarily solid debris are difficult to treat percutaneously.[68,69] These collections should be managed surgically.

Splenic abscess

Experience with PD of splenic abscesses is limited; one series reported a 75% success rate and low morbidity and mortality rates.[98] Nevertheless, potential hemorrhagic complications may be disastrous, and currently PD of the spleen is at best controversial.[6] Splenectomy remains the treatment of choice for splenic abscesses.[83]

Pelvic abscess

Depending on the location of the pelvic abscess, a variety of approaches can be used. For anterior collections, an anterior transabdominal route should be used. Posterior collections, however, can be approached either by a translumbar puncture with caudal angulation or via the sciatic notch. With the transsciatic approach, the rectal wall, sciatic nerve, and hypogastric vessels should be avoided by choosing an entry point near the sacrum. Transrectal and transvaginal approaches also can be used successfully for many pelvic abscesses.[83,99]

Diverticular abscess

Surgery is the definitive treatment for diverticular abscess. It usually includes drainage with colonic diversion as a first stage and segmental colon resection with reanastomosis as a second stage. The primary goal of percutaneous drainage is temporizing with an intent to convert a potential two-stage operation into a one-stage surgical procedure. PD should be limited to large fluid-containing collections because small collections and phlegmons

may respond to antibiotic therapy. Successful temporization of diverticular abscess has been reported in 57 to 69% of cases.[5]

Appendiceal abscess

The role of PD for the treatment of appendiceal abscess is controversial, and the need for an interval appendectomy after successful drainage is uncertain. Fluid-containing abscesses can be drained for either temporization or perhaps cure, with success rates of 84 to 90%.[5]

Percutaneous drainage in the chest

Empyema

External drainage is indicated for frank empyemas and complicated parapneumonic effusions [with low pH, elevated lactate dehydrogenase (LDH), or low glucose].[100] Diagnostic thoracentesis performed using sonographic or fluoroscopic guidance defines the nature of the pleural collection. If fluid cannot be aspirated using an 18-gauge needle, surgical rather than percutaneous drainage is indicated. Cloudy, serosanguinous and hemorrhagic fluid should undergo laboratory evaluation to determine the appropriate therapeutic action. Once purulent fluid is obtained, a drainage procedure can follow. The catheter size is determined by the viscosity of fluid and usually will be between 10 and 14 Fr. Any diagnostic modality can be used for guidance. A skin puncture site is chosen at the thickest portion of the collection above the underlying rib to avoid neurovascular structures. A catheter can be placed by either the trocar or Seldinger techniques, as described previously. After manual evacuation of the contents, the catheter is attached to an underwater seal suction device such as a Pleur-evac (Deknatel, Fall River, MA, U.S.A.). For extremely viscous fluid, the use of both urokinase and streptokinase have shown improved results.[101] Overall success of image-guided pleural drainage is between 70 and 88%, compared with 66 to 83% success rates for thoracostomy tube drainage.[100] Better success rates are seen with parapneumonic than with postoperative empyema. The former condition is likely treated in the early stages before the accumulation of fibrin in the pleural space.[5]

Lung abscess

Lung abscesses refractory to medical therapy or complicated by empyema require external drainage.[100] CT usually is preferred as the guiding modality. The technique is identical to pleural drainage, with the exception of catheter placement through a zone of thickened pleura adjacent to the abscess.[102] Normal aerated lung should be avoided if at all possible. Reported complications, usually associated with traversing the lung, include pneumothorax, bronchopleural fistula, empyema and hemorrhage. VanSonnenberg et al reported an overall success rate of 84%, and the need for surgery was avoided in these patients.[102]

REFERENCES

1. Hopper KD. Percutaneous, radiographically guided biopsy: a history. *Radiology* 1995;196:329–333.
2. Gazelle GS, Haaga JR. Guided percutaneous biopsy of intraabdominal lesions. *AJR Am J Roentgenol* 1989;153:929–935.
3. Mueller PR, Van Sonnenberg E. Interventional radiology in the chest and abdomen. *JAMA* 1990;322:1364–1374.
4. Fisher HW. Cost and benefits of interventional radiologic procedures. *Radiol Clin North Am* 1979;17:371–373.
5. Lambiase RE, et al. Percutaneous drainage of 335 consecutive abscesses: results of primary drainage with 1-year follow-up. *Radiology* 1992;184:167–179.
6. Haaga J Jr. *Computed Tomography and Magnetic Resonance Imaging of the Whole Body.* St. Louis: Mosby, 3rd ed. 1994.
7. Hopper KD, Grenko RT, TenHave TR, et al. Percutaneous biopsy of the liver and kidney by using coxial technique: adequacy of the specimen obtained with three different needles in vitro. *AJR Am J Roentgenol* 1995;164:221–224.
8. Wittenberg J, Mueller PR, Ferrucci JT Jr, et al. Percutaneous core biopsy of abdominal tumors using 22 gauge needles: further observations. *AJR Am J Roentgenol* 1982;139:75–80.
9. Kinney TB, Lee MJ, Filomena CA, et al. Fine-needle biopsy: prospective comparison of aspiration versus nonaspiration techniques in the abdomen. *Radiology* 1993;186:549–552
10. Andriole JG, Haaga JR, Adams RB, et al. Biopsy needle characteristics assessed in the laboratory. *Radiology* 1983;148:659–662.
11. Haaga JR, LiPuma JP, Bryan PJ, et al. Clinical comparison of small and large caliber cutting needles for biopsy. *Radiology* 1983;146:665–667.
12. Pagani JJ. Biopsy of focal hepatic lesions. *Radiology* 1983;147:673–675.
13. Dickey JE, Haaga JR, Stellato TA, et al. Evaluation of computed tomography guided percutaneous biopsy of the pancreas. *Surg Gynecol Obstet* 1986;163:497–503.
14. Hall-Craggs MA, Lees WR. Fine-needle aspiration biopsy: pancreatic and biliary tumors. *AJR Am J Roentgenol* 1986;147:399–403.
15. Dahnert WF, Hoagland MH, Hamper UM, et al. Fine-needle aspiration biopsy of abdominal lesions: diagnostic yield for different needle tip configurations. *Radiology* 1992;185:263–268.
16. Moulton JS, Moore PT. Coaxial percutaneous biopsy technique with automated biopsy devices: value in improving accuracy and negative predictive value. *Radiology* 1993;186:515–522.
17. Bernadino ME. Automated biopsy devices: significance and safety. *Radiology* 1990;176:615–616.
18. Ha HK, Sachs PB, Haaga JR, et al. CT-guided liver biopsy: an update. *Clin Imaging* 1991;15:99–104.
19. Menghini G. One second biopsy of the liver: problems of its clinical application. *N Engl J Med* 1970;283:582–585.
20. Nyman RS, Cappelen-Smith J, Brismar J, et al. Yield and complications in ultrasound-guided biopsy of abdominal lesions: comparison of fine-needle aspiration biopsy and 1.2-mm meedle core biopsy using an automated biopsy gun. *Acta Radiol* 1995;36:485–490.
21. Mueller PR, Stark DD, Simeone JF, et al. MR-guided aspiration biopsy: needle design and clinical trials. *Radiology* 1986;161:605–609.
22. Matalon TAS, Silver B. US guidance of interventional procedures. *Radiology* 1986;161:605–609.
23. Reading CC, Charboneau JW, James EM, et al. Sonographically guided percutaneous biopsy of small (3 cm or less) masses. *AJR Am J Roentgenol* 1988;151:189–192.
24. Holm HH, Torp-Pedersen S, Juul N, et al. Instrumentation for sonographic interventional procedures. *Clin Diagn Ultrasound* 1987;21:9–40.
25. Bisceglia M, Matalon TAS, Silver B. The pump maneuver an atraumatic adjunct to enhance US needle tip localization. *Radiology* 1990;176:867–868.
26. Winsberg F, Mitty HA, Shapiro RS, et al. Use of an accoustic transponder for US visualization of biopsy needles. *Radiology* 1991;877–878.
27. Hamper UM, Savader BL, Sheth S. Improved needle-tip visualization by color Doppler sonography. *AJR Am J Roentgenol* 1991;156:401–402.
28. Welch TJ, Sheedy II PF, Stephens DH, et al. Percutaneous adrenal biopsy: review of a 10-year experience. *Radiology* 1994;193:341–344.
29. Yueh N, Halvorsen RA, Letourneau JG, et al. Gantry tilt technique for CT-guided biopsy and drainage. *J Comput Assist Tomogr* 1989;13:182–184.
30. Hussain S. Gaintry angulation in CT-guided percutaneous adrenal biopsy. *AJR Am J Roentgenol* 1996;166:537–539.
31. Palestrant AM. Comprehensive approach to CT-guided procedures. *Radiology* 1990;174:270–272.
32. Reyes GD. A guidance device for CT-guided procedures. *Radiology* 1990;176:863–864.
33. Reuther G. A device for CT-guided needle punctures: technical note. *Cardiovasc Interv Radiol* 1991;14:191–194.
34. Onik G, Cosman ER, Wells TH, et al. CT-guided aspirations for the body: comparison of hand guidance with sterotaxis. *Radiology* 1988;166:389–394.
35. Brown KT, Fulbright RK, Avitabile AM, et al. Cytologic analysis in fine-needle aspiration biopsy: smears vs. cell blocks. *AJR Am J Roentgenol* 1993;161:629–631.
36. Ferrucci JT, Wittenberg J, Mueller PR, et al. Diagnosis of abdominal malignancy by radiologic fine-needle aspiration biopsy. *AJR Am J Roentgenol* 1980;134:323–330.
37. Welch TJ, et al. CT guided biopsy: prospective analysis of 1,000 procedures. *Radiology* 1989;171:493–496.
38. Lees WR, Hall-Craggs MA, Manhire A. Five years experience with fine needle aspiration biopsy: 454 cases. *Clin Radiol* 1985;36:517–520.
39. Charboneau JW, Reading CC, Welch TJ. CT and sonographically guided needle biopsy: current techniques and new innovations. *AJR Am J Roentgenol* 1990;154:1–10.
40. Smith EH. Complications of percutaneous abdominal fine-needle biopsy. *Radiology* 1986;178:253–258.
41. Weiss H, Duntsch U, Weiss A. Risiken der Feinnadelpunktion: ergebnisse einer Umfrage in der BRD (DEGUM-umfrage). *Ultraschall Med* 1988;9:121–127.
42. Westcott JL. Percutaneous needle aspiration of hilar and mediastinal masses. *Radiology* 1981;141:323–329.
43. Moulton JS. Artificial extrapleural window for mediastinal biopsy. *J Vasc Interv Radiol* 1993;4:825.
44. Van Sonnenberg E, Lin AS, Deutsch AL, et al. Percutaneous biopsy of difficult mediastinal, hilar, and pulmonary lesions by computed tomographic guidance and a modified coaxial technique. *Radiology* 1983;148:300–302.
45. Haramati LB, Austin JHM. Complications after CT-guided needle biopsy through aerated versus nonaerated lung. *Radiology* 1991;181:778.
46. Moore EH, et al. Effect of patient positioning after needle aspiration lung biopsy. *Radiology* 181:385–387.
47. Klein JS, Salomon G, Steward EA, Transthoracic needle biopsy with a coaxially placed 20-gauge automated cutting needle: results in 122 patients. *Radiology* 1996;198:715–720.
48. Kazerooni EA, Lim FT, Mikhail A, et al. Risk of pneumothorax in

CT-guided transthoracic needle aspiration biopsy of the lung. *Radiology* 1996;198:371–375.

49. Bernardino ME. Percutaneous biopsy. *AJR Am J Roentgenol* 1984; 142:41–45.

50. Cardella J, Bakal CW, Bertino RE, et al, for the Standards of Practice Committee of the Society of Cardiovascular and Interventional Radiology. Quality improvement guidelines for image-guided percutaneous biopsy in adults: Society of Cardiovascular and Interventional Radiology Standards of Practice Committee. *J Vasc Interv Radiol* 1996;7:943–946.

51. Fish GD, Stanley JH, Miller KS, et al. Postbiopsy pneumothorax: estimating the risk by chest radiography and pulmonary function tests. *AJR Am J Roentgenol* 1988;150:71–74.

52. Perlmutt LM, Braun SD, Newman GE, et al. Timing of chest film follow-up after transthoracic needle aspiration. *Am J Roentgenol* 1986;146:1049–1050.

53. Khouri NF, Stitik FP, Erozan YS. Transthoracic needle aspiration biopsy of benign and malignant lung lesions. *Am J Roentgenol* 1985;144:281–288.

54. Martino CR, Haaga JR, Bryan PJ, et al. CT-guided liver biopsies: eight years' experience. *Radiology* 1984;152:755–757.

55. Kasugai H, Yamamoto R, Tatsuta M, et al. Value of heparinized fine-needle aspiration biopsy in liver malignancy. *Am J Roentgenol* 1985;144:243–244.

56. Alspaugh JP, Bernardino ME, Sewell CW, et al. CT directed hepatic biopsies: increased diagnostic accuracy with low patient risk. *J Comput Assist Tomogr* 1983;7:1012–1017.

57. Schiller CF. Complications of echinococcus cyst rupture. *JAMA* 1966;195:220–222.

58. Brandt KR, Charboneau JW, Stephens DH, et al. CT- and US-guided biopsy of the pancreas. *Radiology* 1993;187:99–104.

59. Yamamoto R, Tatsuta M, Noguchi S, et al. Histocytologic diagnosis of pancreatic cancer by percutaneious aspiration biopsy under ultrasonic guidance. *Am J Clin Patho* 1985:83:409–414.

60. Mitty HA, Efremidis SC, Yeh H-C. Impact of fine-needle biopsy on the management of patients with carcinoma of the pancreas. *Am J Roentgenol* 1981;137:1119–1121.

61. Mueller PR, Miketic LM, Simeone JF, et al. Severe acute pancreatitis after percutaneous biopsy of the pancres. *AJR Am J Roentgenol* 1988;151:493–494.

62. Vellet D, Leiman G, Mair S, et al. Fine needle aspiration cytology of mucinous cystadenocarcinoma of the pancreas: further observations. *Acta Cytol* 1988;32:43–48.

63. Kloos RT, Gross MD, Francis IR, et al. *Endocr Rev* 1995;16:460–480.

64. Heiberg E, Wolverson MK. Ipsilateral decubitus position for percutaneous CT-guided adrenal biopsy. *J Comput Assist Tomogr* 1985; 9:217–218.

65. Bernardino ME, McClellan WM, Phillips VM, et al. CT-guided adrenal biopsy: accuracy, safety, and indications. *AJR Am J Roentgenol* 1985;144:67–69.

66. Montali G, Solbiati L, Bossi MC, et al. Sonographically guided fine-needle aspiration biopsy of adrenal masses. *AJR Am J Roentgenol* 1984;143:1081–1084.

67. Nadel L, Baumgarner BR, Bernardino ME. Percutaneous renal biopsies: accuracy, safety, and indications. *Urol Radiol* 1986;8: 67–71.

68. Gerzof SG, Johnson WC, Robbins AH, et al. Percutaneous drainage of infected pancreatic pseudocysts. *Arch Surg* 1984;119:888.

69. Pruett TL, Rotstein OD, Crass J, et al. Percutaneous aspiration and drainage for suspected abdominal infection. *Surgery* 1984;96:731.

70. Van Sonnenberg E, Mueller PR, Ferucci JT. Percutaneous drainage of 250 abdominal abscess and fluid collections. *Radiology* 1984;151:337–341.

71. Mueller PR, Ferrucci JT Jr, Butch RJ, et al. Inadvertent percu-

taneous catheter gastroenterostomy during abscess drainage: significance and management. *Am J Roentgenol* 1985;145: 387–391.

72. Lahorra JM, Haaga JR, Stellato T, et al. Safety of intracavitary urokinase with percutaneous abscess drainage. *AJR Am J Roentgenol* 1993;160:171–174.

73. Johnson RD, et al. Percutaneous drainage of pyogenic liver abscesses. *AJR Am J Roentgenol* 1985;144:463–467.

74. Van Sonnenberg E, Ferrucci JT Jr, Mueller PR, et al. Perctaneous drainage of abscesses and fluid collection: technique, results and applications. *Radiology* 1982;142:821–826.

75. Haaga JR, Weinstein AJ. CT-guided percutaneous aspiration and drainage of abscesses. *AJR Am J Roentgenol* 1980;135:1187–1194.

76. Aeder MI, Wellman JL, Haaga Jr, et al. Role of surgical and percutaneous drainage in the treatment of abdominal abscesses. *Arch Surg* 1983;118:273.

77. Glass CA, Cohn I. Drainage of intra-abdominal abscesses: a comparison of surgical and computerized tomography guided catheter drainage. *Am J Surg* 1984;147:315.

78. Halasz NA, van Sonnenberg E. Drainage of intra-abdominal abscesses: tactics and choices. *Am J Surg* 1983;146:112.

79. Johnson WC, Gerzhof SG, Robbins AA, et al. Treatment of abdominal abscesses: comparative evaluation of operative drainage versus percutaneous catheter drainage guided by computed tomography or ultrasound. *Ann Surg* 1981:194:510.

80. Olak J, Gristou NV, Stein LA, et al. Operative vs percutaneous drainage of intra-abdominal abscesses: comparison of morbidity and mortality. *Arch Surg* 1986;121:141.

81. Dellinger EP, Wertz MJ, Meakins JL, et al. Surgical infection stratification system for intra-abdominal infection: multicenter trial. *Arch Surg* 1985;120:21.

82. Hemming A, Davis NL, Robins RE. Surgical versus percutaneous drainage of intra-abdominal abscesses. *Am J Surg* 1991;161:593.

83. Levison MA. Percutaneous versus open operative drainage of intra-abdominal abscesses. *Infect Dis Clin North Am* 1992;6:525–544.

84. Levison, Zeiger. Correlation of APACHE II. *Surg Gynecol Obstet* 1991;72:89–94.

85. Nystrom P-O, Bax R, Dellinger EP, et al. Proposed definitions for diagnosis, severity scoring, stratification, and outcome for trials on intra-abdominal infection. *World J Surg* 1990;14:148.

86. Mueller PR, Simeone JF, Butch RJ, et al. Percutaneous drainage of subphrenic abscess: a review of 62 patients. *AJR Am J Roentgenol* 1986;147:1237–1240.

87. Hochbergs P, Forsberg L, Hederstrom E, et al. Diagnosis and percutaneous treatment of pyogenic hepatic abscesses. *Acta Radiol* 1990;31:351–353.

88. Mueller PR, et al. Infected abdominal tumors: percutaneous catheter drainage. *Radiology* 1989;173:627–629.

89. Deyoe LA, Cronan JJ, Lambiase RE, et al. Percutaneous drainage in renal and perirenal abscesses: results in 30 patients. *AJR Am J Roentgenol* 1990;155:81.

90. Mueller PR, Ferrucci JT Jr, Wittenberg J, et al. Iliopsoas abscess: treatment by CT-guided percutaneous catheter drainage. *AJR Am J Roentgenol* 1984;142:359.

91. Lang EK. Renal, perirenal, and pararenal abscesses: percutaneous drainage. *Radiology* 1990;174:109–113.

92. Papanicolaou N, Mueller PR, Ferrucci JT Jr, et al. Abscess-fistula association: radiologic recognition and percutaneos management. *AJR Am J Roentgenol* 1984;143:811–815.

93. Nunez D, Yrizarry JM, Russell E, et al. Transgastric drainage of pancreatic fluid collections. *AJR Am J Roentgenol* 1985;145:815.

94. Bilbao JI, Rodriquez-Cabello J, Longo JM, et al. Pancreatic pseudocyst in a gastrectomized patient: treatment with internalized endoprosthesis. *Gastrointest Radiol* 1991;16:70–72.

95. Bernardino ME, Amerson JR. Percutaneous gastrocystostomy: a new approach to pancreatic pseudocyst drainage. *AJR Am J Roentgenol* 1984;143:1096.

96. VanSonnenberg E, Wittich GR, Casola G, et al. Percutaneous drainage of infected and noninfected pancreatic pseudocysts: experience in 101 cases. *Radiology* 1989;170:757–761.

97. VanSonnenberg E, D'Agostino HB, Casola G, et al. Percutaneous abscess drainage: current concepts. *Radiology* 1991:181:617–626.

98. Quinn SF, vanSonnenberg E, Casola G, et al. Interventional radiology in the spleen. *Radiology* 1986;161:289.

99. Gazelle GS, Haaga JR, Stellalto TA, et al. Pelvic abscesses: CT guided transrectal drainage. *Radiology* 1991;181:49.

100. Klein JS, Schultz S, Heffner JE. Interventional radiology in the chest: image-guided percutaneous drainage of pleural effusions, lung abscesses, and pneumothorax. *AJR Am J Roentgenol* 1995;164:581–588.

101. Robinson LA, Moulton AL, Fleming WH, et al. Intrapleural fibrinolytic treatment of multiloculated thoracic empyema. *Ann Thorac Surg* 1994;57:803–814.

102. VanSonnenberg E, D'Agostino HB, Casola G, et al. Lung abscess: CT-guided drainage. *Radiology* 1991;178:347–351.

11

Radiologic Gastrostomy and Gastrojejunostomy

J. MARK RYAN and STEVEN DAWSON

Provision of adequate nutritional support is a challenging problem in managing patients who are unable to take food orally. For these patients, nutrition may be provided either enterally or by means of total parenteral nutrition. Total parenteral nutritional support is a labor-intensive, expensive technique that is fraught with problems such as recurrent sepsis and maintenance of adequate central venous access. Provision of adequate trace elements and essential amino acids is more difficult with total parenteral nutrition, as a result of its nonphysiological nature, than with enteral nutrition.

For patients who have a functioning gastrointestinal tract, enteral nutrition is the method of choice. Feeding in these patients can be accomplished by placement of a nasogastric tube, which is usually adequate for short-term nutritional support; however, for long-term feeding, the method of choice is placement of a gastrostomy or gastrojejunostomy tube.

Placement of a gastrostomy tube can be done by surgical, endoscopic, or percutaneous radiological methods. Surgical gastrostomy was first performed by Vernueil in France in 1876, and it remained the sole method for gastrostomy tube placement until 1979. The complication rate of surgical gastrostomy is acceptably low but increases sharply in patients who are in poor physical condition, as many patients requiring gastrostomy tube placement tend to be. In a study of 147 patients who underwent surgical placement of a gastrostomy tube, 15.7% had complications, of which half were major complications such as hemorrhage, wound breakdown, or stoma leak.[1] Overall 30-day mortality was 6.1%, most of which was related to respiratory complications. In a recent metanalysis of the literature on gastrostomy placement, the 30-day mortality rate as well as both the major and minor complication rates for surgical placement of a gastrostomy tube were statistically significantly higher than for either endoscopic or radiologic methods of placement.[2] Gastrostomy placement was associated with a much higher cost than the endoscopic or percutaneous radiologic methods. For these reasons, there is now an increasing emphasis on nonsurgical placement of gastrostomy tubes.

Endoscopic gastrostomy was introduced by Gauderer and Ponsky in 1980 as an alternative to the surgical gastrostomy procedure.[3] Essentially, the original technique and the subsequent modifications involve introduction of an endoscope into the stomach and transillumination of the anterior abdominal wall. The abdominal wall then is pierced from the exterior over the region of transillumination, and a guidewire is passed out through the incision. The percutaneous endoscopic gastrostomy (PEG) tube is then passed over the wire into the stomach. A variety of fixation techniques have been developed. Endoscopic placement affords the potential advantages of detection of coexisting lesions in the esophagus or stomach. Wollman's study reported that additional abnormal findings were detected in 26% of patients who underwent endoscopic gastrostomy placement.[2] The endoscopic method is unsuitable for patients requiring gastric decompression for chronic bowel obstruction, in which case the fluoroscopic method offers a more facile placement of primary gastrostomy catheter.

In 1983, several radiology groups, working independently, described a percutaneous method for primary gastrostomy tube placement using a Seldinger technique.[4,5] Since the original technique was described, several technical advances and modifications have been made, and considerable clinical experience has been gained. Presently, fluoroscopic placement of gastrostomy tubes is a well-recognized, clinically important technique. In many institutions, it has become the method of choice for placement of gastrostomy feeding tubes as a result of its low complication rate and low cost compared with other available methods.

■ Indications for Gastrostomy Tube Placement

The most common indication for gastrostomy tube placement is to provide nutritional support for patients with dysphagia. For most patients, the dysphagia is a result of a debilitating neurological disorder, such as cerebrovascular accident, trauma, dysmyelinating and demyelinating disease, or postsurgical sequelae, such as a neurological deficit following resection of an intracranial neoplasm. A second important group of patients are those with swallowing disorders secondary to oropharyngeal or esophageal tumors. An infrequent but important indication is small bowel disease, such as Crohn's disease, short bowel syndrome, or radiation enteropathy. Because patients with small bowel disease cannot tolerate a normal diet, nutrition must be presented in a form that can be absorbed, which is achieved by providing an elemental diet through a gastrostomy or gastrojejunostomy tube.

Other less common indications for gastrostomy tube placement include decompression of the upper gastrointestinal tract in a patient with advanced malignant obstruction, chronic adynamic gastroparesis, or ileus, and anorexia with underlying psychiatric or malignant illness. Percutaneous gastrostomy also has been used for the removal of intragastric foreign bodies, such as displaced esophageal stents, and for transgastric drainage of pancreatic pseudocyst fluid collections.

■ Contraindications to Percutaneous Gastrostomy

Relative contraindications for radiologic gastrostomy tube placement include portal hypertension with gastric varices, severe gastritis, and massive ascites, which can increase the tendency for leakage of gastric contents from the stomach after tube placement. Many radiologists consider large ascites to be an absolute contraindication; however, this is not the case in our practice. We perform decompression gastrostomy in patients with chronic bowel obstruction and ascites, most commonly secondary to intraperitoneal metastatic spread of ovarian carcinoma. For these patients, we perform preprocedural paracentesis, and we routinely use the radiologic T-fas-

tener gastropexy to reduce the incidence of intraperitoneal leakage of gastric contents. We also perform serial paracentesis after gastrostomy tube placement to prevent massive ascites buildup, which can cause necrosis of the gastropexy.

Percutaneous placement of a gastrostomy tube requires a safe percutaneous access to the stomach. Occasionally, a patient's stomach is overlaid by transverse colon or the left lobe of the liver. The stomach may have a high subcostal position in some patients as an anatomic variant or in patients who have had a previous partial gastrectomy. These problems are usually surmountable by performing the initial gastric puncture under computed tomography (CT) guidance, after which the patient is transferred to the interventional fluoroscopy suite for track dilation and tube placement.

Encasement of the stomach by tumor is also a relative contraindication for several reasons. One reason is that healing does not occur normally, and a fistulous track therefore does not readily form between the stomach and the skin. A second reason is that tumor tissue is abnormally vascularized by neovessels that have an increased propensity to bleed if they are transgressed. Lack of distensibility of a tumor-encased stomach also may make tube placement extremely difficult. The symptoms of anorexia and nausea that patients with tumor encasement of the stomach experience often remain unrelieved by gastrostomy tube placement because the symptoms are due largely to effects of the tumor on the autonomic nervous system.

Gastrostomy tube placement is relatively contraindicated in patients who are taking long-term corticosteriod treatment because they may have a higher complication rate of gastric perforation as a result of stomach wall atrophy and poor healing, leading to increased risk for gastric perforation and leakage of gastric contents. Patients with active or chronic duodenal ulcers should have a gastrostomy tube placed rather than undergo a transgastric jejunostomy or gastrojejunostomy tube because the mechanical irritation from a tube passing through the duodenal bulb may cause serious bleeding.

In some patients, the presence of a tube through the pylorus can cause a partial or complete gastric outlet obstruction syndrome, which may be overcome by placement of either a single gastrojejunostomy tube, which incorporates both a draining gastrostomy port and a feeding jejunal port, or by a two-tube technique, in which both a gastrostomy and a transgastric jejunostomy are placed through separate tracks. Our experience leads us to favor the two-tube approach because better gastric drainage may be achieved by using this approach. To achieve optimum gastric drainage, the drainage tube should be situated at the most dependent portion of the stomach, which in most patients requiring gastrostomy is the fundus because of the patient's supine position.

The two-tube approach allows a tube to be placed directly in the fundus, whereas the use of a single gastrojejunostomy catheter allows only for the gastrostomy drainage port to be placed in the antrum, resulting in suboptimal drainage. The two-tube approach also allows a large 14 Fr catheter to be used for drainage and a separate 14 Fr tube to be used for jejunal feeding. We routinely use gastrostomy tubes that are 30 cm working length and transgastric jejunostomy tubes that are 53 cm working length.

■ Preprocedural Assessment and Preparation

Informed written consent is necessary before the procedure is performed. Because many patients who require a gastrostomy tube cannot give consent themselves, consent should be obtained in advance from the next of kin. Preprocedural blood workup, such as prothrombin time, partial thromboplastin time, and platelet count, although not routinely performed on every patient, should be requested for patients in whom a coagulopathy may preexist, such as patients who have been treated with anticoagulants or who are malnourished. The patient's medical records are reviewed with particular attention to previous gastric surgery or medical conditions that preclude the use of hypotonic agents, sedation, or narcotics. Patients with a coagulopathy should receive treatment to correct clotting parameters before the procedure is done.

In our institution the patient is given a cupful of barium by mouth or through nasogastric tube the evening before the procedure. By the time the procedure commences, the barium will opacify the transverse colon, thus preventing inadvertent colonic puncture. If the patient is unable to take barium orally, a limited barium enema may be performed immediately before the procedure in the general fluoroscopy suite to opacify the transverse colon. An alternative approach, which we favor, is to perform the initial stomach puncture under CT guidance with subsequent transfer of the patient to the interventional fluoroscopy suite for completion of the procedure.

The patient's fast begins at midnight the night preceding the procedure. When the patient arrives in the fluoroscopy suite, a nasogastric tube and intravenous access should be in position to expedite the procedure. If problems are encountered in inserting the nasogastric tube, placement can be done under fluoroscopic guidance before the procedure. An enteroclysis catheter or an angled angiographic catheter usually can be inserted successfully under fluoroscopic guidance, even in the presence of high-grade esophageal obstruction.

Intravenous sedation is administered to patients who are anxious or restless. A combination of midazolam (Versed, Roche) and fentanyl (Sublimaze, Janssen) is used in our institution. A nurse experienced in the administration of sedation monitors the patient's vital signs throughout the procedure using an automatic blood pressure cuff, continuous electrocardiographic (ECG) monitoring, and continuous transcutaneous pulse oximetry. Supplemental oxygen is administered through nasal prongs during the procedure. It is important to have a suction apparatus available so that any spontaneous reflux into the esophagus can be removed before aspiration occurs. We do not routinely administer antibiotics to the patient before the gastrostomy procedure, although some institutions prefer to do so.

■ Technique and Modifications

Traditional method of tube placement

The gastropexy technique, which is the traditional method of tube placement, is illustrated in Figure 11-1.

Initial access to the stomach

The patient is positioned supine on the fluoroscopic table for a left-sided approach to the abdomen. The margin of the left lobe of the liver is noted, as is the position of the transverse colon, which is opacified by the barium administered the preceding evening. Air is insufflated through the nasogastric tube to distend the stomach. Some authors have described the use of ultrasound as an additional guidance modality.[6,7] The stomach is filled with water instead of air. No complications occurred in 27 patients for whom this method was used.[6] Hypotonia (intravenous glucagon, 0.5–1 mg) is used to maintain gastric distention, and fluoroscopy is performed to select a site of entry. The preferred entry site is just distal to the incisura in a plane equidistant from the greater and lesser curves of the stomach, thus avoiding both gastric and gastroepiploic vessels. The puncture site is also ideally located lateral to the rectus muscle to avoid damage to the superior epigastric artery.

The skin is infiltrated using 20 mL of 1% lidocaine, and a small skin incision is made with a no. 11 scalpel blade. Using an 18-gauge sheathed needle angled toward the pylorus, a quick thrust is made to introduce the needle into the stomach. Aspiration of air into a syringe containing 4 mL of saline is usually sufficient evidence of gastric puncture; however, iodinated contrast medium or a guidewire may be introduced if further confirmation of position is required. The Teflon sheath then is advanced over the needle while ensuring that the sheath is in optimal position in the stomach. In patients undergoing gastrostomy placement for gastric decompression, the sheath is directed toward the fundus of the stomach. The needle then is withdrawn, and a straight tip 0.038-inch guidewire is

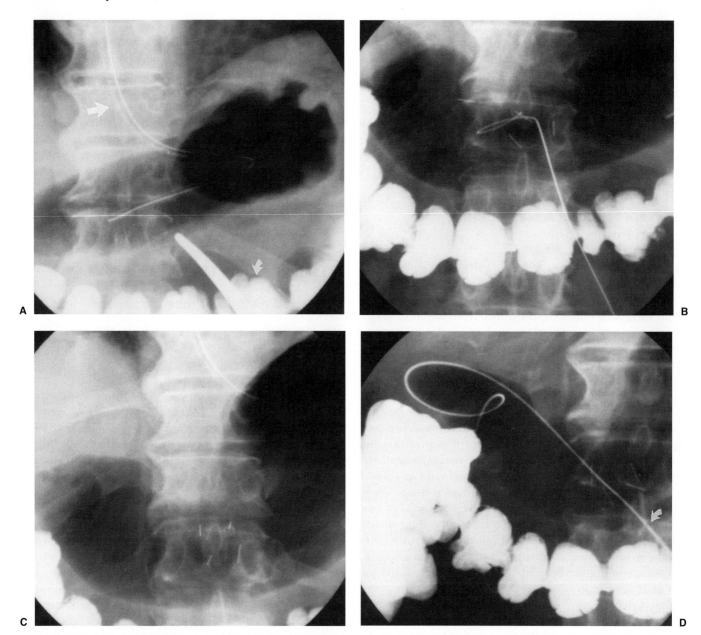

FIGURE 11-1. Gastrojejunostomy insertion (using the gastropexy technique). **A:** The stomach is distended with air insufflated through the nasogastric tube (*white arrow*). Note the presence of barium in the transverse colon (*curved arrow*). **B:** T-fastener insertion. A guidewire is passed through the insertion needle in order to release the T-fastener. **C:** The four T-fasteners in position in the midantrum. **D:** Eighteen-gauge sheathed needle (*arrow*) is inserted through the center of the square bordered by the four T-fasteners and is angled toward the pylorus. A 0.38-inch guidewire has been inserted through the sheathed needle into the prepyloric region.

introduced through the sheath into the stomach. The sheath then is withdrawn and serial dilatation is performed.

Cannulation of pylorus and duodenum

Cannulation of the pyloric canal is required for transgastric jejunal feeding and for gastrojejunostomy tube placement, because positioning of the tube in the jejunum greatly reduces the risk of esophageal reflux with

aspiration following feeding (Fig. 11-2). Aspiration pneumonia has caused several deaths in patients after gastrostomy tube placement.[8] After the initial needle puncture, the needle is angled toward the antrum so that the guidewire advances in the direction of the pylorus. Occasionally, pyloric cannulation can be achieved at this stage simply by advancing the wire along the greater curve of the stomach. If the guidewire does not enter the pylorus, a dilator or a torquable catheter can be used to assist

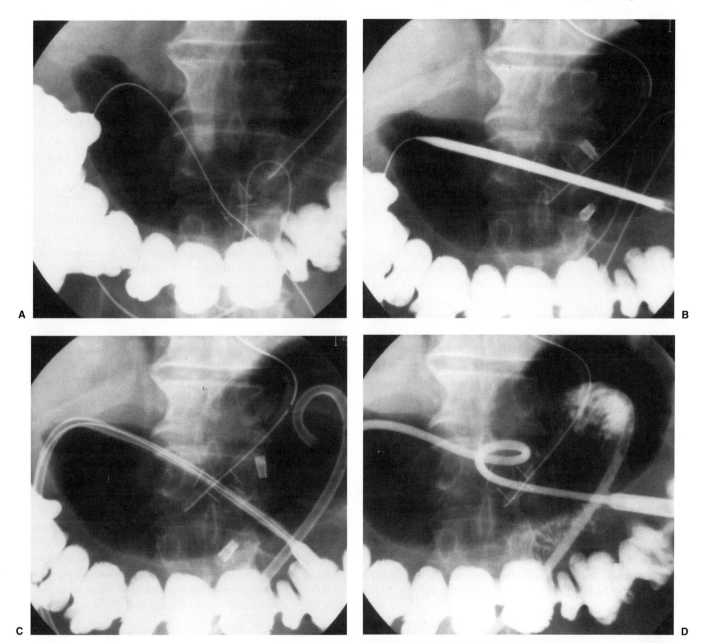

FIGURE 11-2. Gastrojejunostomy insertion. **A:** The guidewire has been manipulated beyond the ligament of Treitz using an angiographic catheter. **B:** Track is serially dilated using 6, 10, and 12 Fr dilators. **C:** Gastrojejunostomy catheter is inserted over the guidewire so that its tip position is beyond the ligament of Treitz. **D:** Catheter is locked in position. Contrast has been injected to demonstrate mucosal folds in the proximal jejunum.

cannulation. Most often, an angled angiographic catheter is required to pass through the pylorus; once this step is achieved, the wire tip is advanced to the ligament of Treitz. During cannulation of the pylorus, care must be taken to avoid looping the guidewire in the fundus of the stomach, which can occur when the catheter or guidewire is advanced against resistance and will prevent correct tube position from being achieved.

Dilatation of the track

With the tip of the guidewire at the ligament of Treitz, the transgastric jejunostomy (or gastrojejunostomy) track is serially dilated to 9 and 12 Fr. The dilator must be inserted with controlled force because the stomach wall is thick and will indent easily. A rotational action aids the dilatation. The dilator should advance smoothly along the course of the guidewire to avoid kinking or buckling of the guidewire into the peritoneal cavity. Overdilatation of the track is to be avoided. A snug fit between the tube and the stomach wall usually is achieved by using the percutaneous fluoroscopic technique, thus reducing the potential of intraperitoneal leakage and peritonitis.

After dilatation has been achieved and a sheath placed, the transgastric jejunal feeding (or gastrojejunostomy) catheter is introduced over the guidewire and advanced with its inner stiffener in position to the level of the pylorus. After the stiffener has been advanced distal to the pylorus, the catheter is advanced off the stiffener into the duodenum and out to the ligament of Treitz, where it is locked in position (Fig. 11-3). This maneuver avoids buckling of the catheter into either the peritoneum or the fundus of the stomach.

Technical modifications

Nylon T-fasteners

Unlike endoscopic or surgical gastrostomies, the percutaneous technique described herein does not appose the anterior gastric wall to the anterior abdominal wall, which may lead to an increased incidence of intraperitoneal leakage of gastric contents with resultant peritonitis. Brown and colleagues at Massachusetts General Hospital

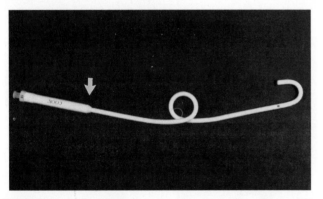

FIGURE 11-3. Gastrostomy catheter with locking device. The collar of the tube is retracted to activate the locking device (*arrow*).

described a percutaneous method to simulate surgical gastropexy by means of nylon T-fasteners (Fig. 11-4),[9] and Coleman et al. also described a percutaneous radiologic gastropexy technique.[10] The necessity for the use of gastropexy with radiologic gastrostomy remains controversial.

The T-fastener technique closely simulates the Stamm surgical gastropexy and is the method we use routinely in our institution. We have reported a study of 316 patients in whom radiologic gastrostomy with T-fastener gastropexy was performed, which supported the opinion that a low rate of pericatheteral leakage, low catheter displacement rates, and the ability to perform gastrostomy on small postsurgical gastric remnants and in patients with ascites were the principal benefits of the gastropexy technique.[11,12] In that study, successful catheter placement was achieved in 99.4% of patients, with a major complication rate of 1.9% and a minor complication of 3.2%. These results compare favorably with those in the literature, despite a large number of patients ($n = 43$) in the study who had ascites and tumor encasement of the stomach.[13–16]

The technique for performing a radiologic gastropexy is easily learned and adds only a short additional duration to a procedure. A specially designed 18-gauge needle with a 5-mm longitudinal side-slot cut from the heel of the bevel to load the fastener (Brown-Mueller T-fastener kit, Medi-tech, Natick, MA) is used to introduce the T-fastener into the stomach. Four fasteners are introduced, one at each corner of a 2.5 cm square, the central point of which has been selected for the entry of the gastrostomy catheter. The needle with a syringe containing 4 mL of saline is inserted through the abdominal and gastric walls in a single motion. Aspiration of air into the syringe confirms intragastric position. The T-fastener is dislodged from the shaft of the needle by inserting a guidewire through the needle. This step is repeated for each of the four fasteners. The fasteners then are pulled taut, and the metallic lock-

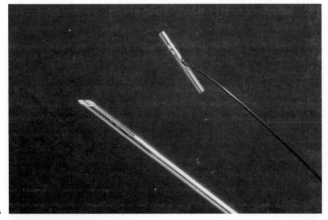
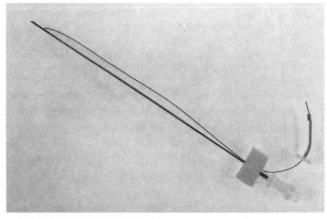

FIGURE 11-4. A: T-fastener and specially adapted needle with a groove cut for T-fastener insertion. **B:** Insertion needle with T-fastener in situ.

ing device on each fastener is cinched with a metal forceps. The anterior gastric wall and the abdominal wall are now apposed, simulating a surgical gastropexy. Overtightening of the T-fasteners is to be avoided because this can potentially cause necrosis around the gastropexy site. The gastrostomy catheter then can be introduced by either the Seldinger or the trocar technique.

Intragastric balloon support

Direct puncture of the stomach with a large trocar catheter (12 Fr) is possible with the stomach supported from within by a fluid-filled balloon. A commercially available balloon, sutured into a 12 Fr feeding tube to cover the most proximal side hole and the tube, is passed into the stomach. The balloon then is distended with air or dilute contrast medium to aid in gastric wall puncture. The passage of such a balloon can be difficult and sometimes impossible in patients with obstructing esophageal lesions, and it may not be well tolerated by these patients. This technique is not used commonly.

Transgastric jejunostomy feeding tubes

Placement of a transgastric jejunostomy tube may be preferred to a simple gastrostomy in patients with esophageal reflux because positioning of the catheter in the jejunum provides protection against regurgitation and aspiration. Patients with poor gastric emptying also benefit from the delivery of feeding materials into the jejunum. Patients with feeding gastrostomy tubes may require later conversion to a transgastric jejunostomy feeding tube as a result of problems with esophageal reflux or delayed gastric emptying with a resultant risk of aspiration pneumonia.

The gastric puncture site and the method used for transgastric jejunostomy feeding tube placement are similar to those for a simple gastrostomy tube, except that cannulation of the pylorus is required for the former technique. An angled gastric puncture with the needle tip pointing toward the pylorus is useful when performing transgastric jejunostomy or gastrojejunostomy, because this facilitates maneuvers required to pass the guidewire and catheter from stomach into jejunum.

■ Complications

Complications encountered in patients undergoing surgical gastrostomy have been categorized by Shellito and Malt.[1] This classification is used for assessment of complications for all methods of gastrostomy placement, with some modifications, because it allows valid comparisons to be made between the different methods of gastrostomy tube placement.

Major complications, according to this classification, include severe wound infection, tube displacement requiring a repeat of the procedure, significant leakage of gastric contents requiring intervention, gastric hemorrhage requiring transfusion or surgery,[17] aspiration pneumonia associated with feeding, profound procedure-related gastroparesis, persistent gastrocutaneous fistula after tube removal, and deep venous thrombosis. Saini et al. added emergency exploratory laparotomy and the formation of a gastrocolic fistula to the original classification to account for complications specific to the radiologic percutaneous gastrostomy technique.[12]

Shellito and Malt classified minor complications as tube migration that produces bowel obstruction, functional failure of the tube due to kinking or blockage, inadvertent premature removal of the tube, abscess formation, and self-limiting peritonitis not necessitating laparotomy.

Catheter displacement and blockage have been reported with varying frequencies in different studies. If a gastrostomy tube without a gastropexy becomes dislodged within a week of insertion, the stomach must be decompressed rapidly using a nasogastric tube to prevent gastric leakage from the immature gastrostomy into the peritoneal cavity. This procedure is not necessary for patients who have a gastropexy because gastric leakage is prevented by the apposed stomach and anterior abdominal wall. It also may be possible to replace the tube immediately in patients with gastropexy by probing the track with a feeding tube and a guidewire.

If the catheter has been present for more than several weeks, a mature gastrocutaneous fistula will have formed, and if the catheter becomes displaced, it usually can be replaced easily if done within 24 to 48 hours. To do so, the gastrostomy is probed with a straight guidewire or infant feeding tube to enter the stomach. Once the stomach is entered, a catheter is passed over the guidewire and the stomach is reinsufflated with air. If a mature gastrocutaneous fistula has not formed or if the gastrostomy has closed completely, a new primary procedure is necessary.

Long-term complications of gastrostomy tube placement can include gastric outlet obstruction or migration of the tube into the esophagus or peritoneal cavity. Catheter blockage is often the result of the administration of incompletely crushed pills via the gastrostomy tube. The catheter should be flushed well after each feed or administration of tablets. The morbidity and mortality rates of the percutaneous method compare favorably with those of both endoscopic and surgical gastrostomy.[2]

■ Immediate and Long-Term Management of Percutaneous Feeding Tubes

Immediate management of a patient involves monitoring the patient's postprocedural recovery from the sedation and the detection of early complications such as hemorrhage. Nasogastric suction is continued for 24 hours and then is discontinued if the patient is free of pain or signs of peritoneal irritation. Enteral feeding may be commenced as soon as the patient's bowel sounds return. The patient should be monitored carefully during the initial feedings for evidence of aspiration or obstruction.

The long-term care of percutaneous feeding tubes should be the responsibility of the radiologist who placed the tube. Therefore, the patient should have direct access to the interventional radiologist to report problems that may arise. The skin around the tube should be cleaned and dried daily, and protective hydrophobic creams should be applied for any skin irritation. Granulation tissue around the skin entry site can be treated with topical silver nitrate sticks. Bacterial, candidal, or fungal skin infections around the tube are treated with topical antibiotics, although more severe infections require oral antibiotic medication. Reflux of gastric contents onto the skin may cause cutaneous erosion which must be treated promptly with wet skin dressings soaked in antacids that will neutralize the acid pH of the gastric fluid. H_2-blocker therapy also may be required.

For patients who have undergone a gastropexy, the T-fasteners are cut after 3 weeks. The gastrostomy tube is changed routinely after 6 months for all patients.

■ Summary

In summary, percutaneous radiologic gastrostomy is a safe and inexpensive technique for providing enteral feeding.[18] Recent studies have shown it to be a safer and more cost-effective technique than either the endoscopic or surgical methods of gastrostomy tube placement. The addition of a gastropexy appears to decrease the incidence of leakage of gastric contents and also makes tube displacement less of a problem should it occur. For these reasons, in many institutions radiologic gastrostomy has become the method of choice for gastrostomy placement.

REFERENCES

1. Shellito PC, Malt RA. Tube gastrostomy: techniques and complications. *Ann Surg* 1985;201:180–185.
2. Wollman B, D'Agostino HB, Walus-Wigle JR, et al. Radiologic, endoscopic, and surgical gastrostomy: an institutional evaluation and metanalysis of the literature. *Radiology* 1995;197: 699–704.
3. Gauderer MWL, Ponsky JL, Izant RJ. Gastrostomy without laparotomy: a percutaneous endoscopic technique. *J Pediatr Surg* 1980; 15:872–875.
4. Ho CS. Percutaneous gastrostomy for jejunal feeding. *Radiology* 1983;149:595–596.
5. Tao HH, Gillies RR. Percutaneous feeding gastrostomy. *AJR Am J Roentgenol* 1983;141:793–794.
6. Lorentzen T, Skjoldbye S, Nolsoe C, et al. Percutaneous gastrostomy guided by ultrasound and fluoroscopy. *Acta Radiol* 1995;369:159–162.
7. Pugash RA, Brady AP, Isaacson S. Ultrasound guidance in percutaneous gastrostomy and gastrojejunostomy. *Can Assoc Radiol J* 1995;46:196–198.
8. Laing B, Smithers M, Harper J. Percutaneous fluoroscopic gastrostomy: a safe option? *Med J Aust* 1994;161:308–310.
9. Brown AS, Mueller PR, Ferrucci JT. Controlled percutaneous gastrostomy: nylon T-fastener for fixation of the anterior wall. *Radiology* 1986;158:543–545.
10. Coleman CC, Coons HG, Cope C, et al. Percutaneous enterostomy with the Cope suture anchor. *Radiology* 1990;174:889–891.
11. Ryan JM, Hahn PF, Boland GW, et al. Percutaneous gastrostomy with T-fastener gastropexy: results in 316 consecutive patients. *Radiology* 1997;203:496–500.
12. Saini S, Mueller PR, Gaa J, et al. Percutaneous gastrostomy with gastropexy: experience in 125 patients. *AJR Am J Roentgenol* 1990;154: 1003–1006.
13. Halkier B, McGloughlin MJ, Ho CS. Percutaneous gastrostomy and cystogastrostomy. *Semin Intervent Radiol* 1988;3:223–229.
14. Wasiljew BK, Ujiki GT, Beal JM. Feeding gastrostomy: complications and mortality. *Am J Surg* 1982;143:194–195.
15. Larson DE, Burton DD, Schroeder KW, et al. Percutaneous endoscopic gastrostomy: indications, success, complications, and mortality in 314 consecutive patients. *Gastroenterology* 1987;93: 48–52.
16. Bell SD, Carmody EA, Yeung EY, et al. Percutaneous gastrostomy and gastrojejunostomy: additional experience in 519 procedures. *Radiology* 1995;194:817–820.
17. Rose DB, Wolman SL, Ho CS. Gastric hemorrhage complicating percutaneous transgastric jejunostomy. *Radiology* 1986;161:835–836.
18. Bodley R, Banerjee S. Radiological percutaneous gastrostomy placement for enteral feeding. *Paraplegia* 1995;33:153–155.

12

Radiation Protection

ALAN H. SCHOENFELD

Persons who work in the interventional radiology suite have the potential for receiving a relatively high radiation dose as a result of diagnostic and interventional procedures that may require relatively long fluoroscopy exposure times. This section reviews the principles of radiation protection specific to the angiosuite that will minimize the exposure to the patient and the radiologist. With careful attention to technology and the use of proper fluoroscopy and personal protective equipment, radiation exposure can be kept to well within accepted limits.

■ Radiation Units and Dose Limits

The measurement of radiation is based on its ability to ionize air. The units used to measure radiation are numerous and usually are expressed in both the older, more familiar "conventional" system and the newer International System of Units (SI). For diagnostic x-rays, the units used most often are the roentgen (R), radiation absorbed dose (rad), Gray (Gy), and Sievert (Sv). For absorption of x-rays in soft tissue, a rule of thumb is

$$1 \text{ R} \approx 1 \text{ rad} = 10 \text{ mGy} = 10 \text{ mSv}$$

The National Council on Radiation Protection and Measurements (NCRP),[1] a nonprofit corporation chartered by the U.S. Congress in 1964 to provide expertise and guidance with regard to radiation, currently recommends an annual dose limit for occupational exposure of 50 mSv (5 rem) and a cumulative dose limit, in mSv, of 10 × the person's age (in years) (Table 12-1).

The annual dose limit recommended by the NCRP as-

sumes a uniform irradiation of the individual person's body. In situations where this is not the case, the concept of the effective dose (E) is introduced, which has associated with it the same probability of the occurrence of cancer and genetic effects whether received by the whole body by uniform irradiation or by partial body or individual organ irradiation. In the case of partial body irradiation, if the dose received by different organs is known, the effective dose can be calculated by multiplying each organ dose by the appropriate weighting factor and then summing these values:

$$E = \Sigma_\text{I}(\text{organ dose})_\text{I} \times (\text{weighting factor})_\text{I},$$

with I, irradiation (Table 12-2). Note that there is no longer a separate dose limit for the thyroid because it is incorporated into the effective dose.

Occupational doses are measured by personnel monitors such as film badges or thermoluminescent detectors. At a minimum, a single monitor should be worn outside the lead apron at collar level to monitor the thyroid and eye lens doses. The use of a second monitor, worn under the apron at waist level, is recommended for a more accurate determination of the effective dose and should be mandatory for pregnant personnel. A finger dosimeter should be worn if the individual's hands will be exposed to the primary x-ray beam.

It should be noted that a relatively high reading of the dosimeter worn outside the apron at the neck does not represent the effective dose. The NCRP recommends that the effective dose E can be estimated by the formulas, $E = 0.5 \, H_\text{W} + 0.025 \, H_\text{N}$ when two monitors are worn and by $E = (H_\text{N}/21)$ for a single monitor,[2] where H_W and

TABLE 12-1. *Recommended dose limits (1)*

Exposures	mSv	Dose Limit (rem)
Occupational		
Effective dose limits		
Annual	50	(5)
Cumulative	10 × Age (yrs)	[1 × Age (yrs)]
Equivalent dose annual limits for tissues and organs		
Lens of eye	150	(15)
Skin, hands, and feet	500	(50)
Members of the Public (annual)		
1. Effective dose limit, continuous or frequent exposure	1.0	(0.1)
2. Effective dose limit, infrequent exposure	5.0	(0.5)
3. Equivalent dose limits for tissues and organs		
Lens of eye	15	(1.5)
Skin, hands, and feet	50	(5)
Embryo-fetus (monthly)		
Equivalent dose limit	0.5	(0.05)

H_N are the recorded values of the monitors under the apron and outside the apron at the neck, respectively.

One study, which involved 28 interventional radiologists from 17 institutions who performed an average of 972 interventional procedures per year, calculated the effective dose from the personnel dosimetry readings of these persons using tables of weighting factors, organ doses, and depth dose charts.[3] The average yearly estimate of the collar and under apron badges for this group was 48.0 mSv (4.80 rem) and 0.88 mSv (88 mrem), respectively. Conversion of these badge readings to mean annual effective dose resulted in a value of 3.16 mSv (316 mrem), substantially less than the annual limit of 50 mSv. The authors also found that Webster's formula for effective dose from two personnel monitors, $H_E = 1.5 H_W + 0.04 H_N$, overestimates the effective dose by 70% for those who wear a thyroid shield but underestimates the value by 21% for those who do not wear a shield.

Personnel dosimeters always should be kept in a radiation-free area when not in use. If film badges are left on a lead apron hanging inside the room, they may be exposed to scatter during interventional cases, or they may accidentally be worn by another staff member.

TABLE 12-2. *Weighting factors used in calculation of effective dose during partial body irradiation[a]*

Tissue or Organ	Weighting Factor
Bone surface, skin	0.01
Bladder, breast, liver, esophagus, thyroid, remainder [a]	0.05
Bone marrow, colon, lung, stomach	0.12
Gonads	0.20

[a] The remainder includes adrenals, brain, small intestine, large intestine, kidney, muscle, pancreas, spleen, thymus, and uterus.

■ Basic Principles of Radiation Protection

The often quoted basic principles of radiation protection used techniques associated with time, distance, and shielding. All fluoroscopic examinations clearly should be performed with the lowest exposure time possible. Fluoroscopic units are designed to meet the U.S. Food and Drug Administration (FDA) limits for entrance exposure rate to the patient, which for units with automatic exposure control are 5 R/min for the average patient, with a maximum limit of 10 R/min. Some units have a "high-level control," which allows entrance exposure rates in excess of 10 R/min as long as an audible signal is present to indicate that the high-level mode is activated. Under high-level control, the entrance exposure rate may reach levels as high as 20 to 40 R/min although a recent FDA performance standard limits the value to 20 R/min. The amount of scatter radiation that exposes the radiologist is directly proportional to the patient exposure. A rule of thumb is that the radiation exposure rate at a 90-degree angle measured at 1 m (≈ 40 inches) from the central ray is approximately 0.1% of the entrance exposure to the patient; thus, limiting the total exposure time will reduce both the patient and the radiologist dose.

The distance factor in radiation protection refers to the inverse square law. The radiation intensity of the x-ray beam decreases with distance from the x-ray tube and is inversely proportional to the square of the distance. The same relationship is approximately true regarding the intensity of the scattered radiation beam and the distance between the radiologist and the scattering medium (i.e., the patient). Thus, whenever possible, persons in the radiology suite should remain as far away as possible from the patient.

Because the interventional radiologist is usually standing close to the patient and cannot take advantage of the inverse square law, shielding materials must be used to intercept the scattered beam. These shielding materials include aprons made of lead rubber (Z = 82) or composites consisting of lead and other high-atomic-number elements, thyroid shields, and leaded eyeglasses. Lead aprons come in thickness of 0.25, 0.50, and 1.00 mm. The NCRP[4] recommends protective aprons of at least 0.5 mm lead equivalent for every person (except the patient) in the fluoroscopy room, which provides an attenuation factor of approximately 95% at 70 kVp. Persons who must move around the room during the procedure should wear a wraparound protective garment, which usually has 0.5 mm of lead in the front panels and 0.25 mm in the back section.

The NCRP also recommends lead gloves of at least 0.25 mm lead equivalent for the fluoroscopist if the hand is placed in the useful beam (after attenuation by the patient). Conventional lead gloves are too thick and heavy to be used by interventionalists, but several manufacturers produce flexible surgical gloves that have some degree of radiation attenuation. A recent study of these gloves found that the protection they provide varied widely among manufacturers, ranging from 2 to 35% reduction at 90 kVp,[5] and their cost effectiveness may not be adequate. The authors suggested that the most effective way to reduce exposure of the hands is to keep them out of the primary beam.

Protection for the lens of the eye can be accomplished by using ceiling-mounted lead glass panels, leaded eyeglasses, and even regular prescription glass lenses. Ceiling-mounted lead glass shields secured to a concentric ball-and-socket joint with spring loaded extension arms can be rotated and tilted in all directions for flexibility of positioning. Leaded eyeglasses are available with wraparound side shields with 0.5-mm lead equivalence. At the least, for 84-kVp x-rays conventional white crown glass lenses provide 44% attenuation; photochromic lenses that turn dark in sunlight result in 70% attenuation.[6] Plastic lenses, however, offer little protection.

Other protective highly recommended devices include thyroid shields and lead rubber drapes that can hang along the side of the table, shielding the lower body of the operator from leakage and scatter.

■ Factors That Affect Patient Dose

The major factors that affect patient dose rate (roentgen per minute) during fluoroscopy are the automatic brightness-control system, filtration in the beam, geometry of the x-ray tube and image intensifier, diameter of the x-ray beam (image intensifier magnification mode), and patient size. Keeping the patient dose low ultimately reduces the dose to the operator.

Fluoroscopy is almost always conducted under auto-

matic brightness control, during which the kVp and tube current (mA) are established automatically by the generator, depending on the patient's size and the entrance exposure requirements of the image intensifier. In some units, however, the minimum fluoroscopic kVp can be set by the radiologist. The use of a higher kVp results in a more penetrating x-ray beam and lower patient dose, but the image contrast will be reduced.

Some systems also provide a low-dose and a high-dose selection. When the low-dose mode is selected, the television gain is increased with a subsequent reduction of the tube current or kVp, resulting in a lower patient dose. The resulting image, however, will have increased noise. When a heavy patient is examined, the high-dose mode will increase the technique factors and patient dose to improve the image.

Pulsed fluoroscopy also may be available; this procedure allows the radiologist to produce the fluoroscopic image at rates of 7.5, 15, or 30 pulses per second instead of the continuous mode. This option, along with the last-image hold feature, can result in reductions in entrance exposure rates to the patient and scatter to the physician by as much as 75%.[7]

The NCRP (4) recommends a minimum total filtration of 2.5 mm of aluminum for x-ray tubes operating above 70 kVp. Some fluoroscopic units, however, allow the radiologist to vary the amount of filtration, usually specified in millimeters of aluminum or copper, in the x-ray beam. As in the case of kVp, an increase in added filtration will result in a lower dose and reduced contrast. One study applied a supplemental filter of 0.5 mm aluminum and 0.076 mm copper for use in neurointerventional procedures, resulting in a dose reduction of 36%.[8] In addition, when the positions of the x-ray tube and image intensifier were rotated every 5 min and the techniques were monitored carefully, the maximum skin dose was reduced by 63%.

The distance of the patient from the x-ray tube usually is set at a minimum of 15 inches in a conventional fluoroscopic unit with an undertable x-ray tube. With a c-arm type of unit, which is used in the special procedures suite, the distance can be varied as the table and image intensifier are repositioned. The minimum distance that the table can be placed above the x-ray tube is usually 12 to 15 inches. Under automatic brightness control, the exposure rate will increase if the image intensifier is moved away from the patient, which also will increase the magnification factor and decrease the field of view. For these reasons, the image intensifier should be placed as close to the patient as possible.

Most special procedure units contain image intensifiers whose diameters are 14 to 16 inches with three to five magnification modes of operation. If one of the magnification modes is chosen, the minification gain is reduced and the system compensates by increasing the exposure rate. The smaller diameter chosen with the magnification mode results in a smaller volume of tissue irradiated and a lower intensity of scattered radiation. The x-ray beam always should be collimated to the smallest size needed for viewing to minimize scatter to the operator and improve visualization.

The size of the patient as a determining factor in patient dose cannot be controlled. It is obvious that a larger patient attenuates a greater fraction of the incident x-ray beam; thus, the kVp and exposure rate must increase to maintain the proper image brightness.

The use of cut film and digital subtraction angiographic (DSA) techniques during interventional procedures also contributes to the total effective dose equivalent the patient will receive. One study of ten patients undergoing cerebral angiography revealed that, on average, 67% of the effective dose equivalent to the patient was due to fluoroscopy with 26% contributed by cut film and 7% by DSA.[9]

■ Factors Affecting the Dose to the Radiologist

Exposure to the radiologist in the interventional suite is due to scattered radiation resulting mainly from the Compton interaction and also from leakage radiation. All x-ray units are required to have a protective tube housing that limits the leakage radiation to 100 mR/hr at 1 m when the unit is operating at the maximum technique factors for continous radiation production.

The intensity of the scatter radiation levels in the room depends on the exposure rate incident on the patient and the volume of tissue in the beam. As mentioned, the amount of scattered radiation at a distance of 1 m from the patient is approximately 0.1% of the incident beam intensity.

If the area of the x-ray beam entering the patient is increased, the fraction of the beam that is scattered increases approximately in direct proportion. Thus, it is clearly advantageous to collimate the beam as closely as possible to minimize the scatter component, which will decrease the exposure to the operator and improve image quality.

The patient's size affects operator exposure because increases in attenuation of the x-ray beam as a result of greater patient diameter will result in higher mA and kVp values with more scattered photons and a greater degree of stray radiation to the radiologist.

The location of the x-ray tube also can affect the stray radiation dose levels received by the radiologist and other personnel in the room. In general, it is preferable to position the x-ray tube underneath the table rather than above it, as most of the scatter is produced near the side of the patient first intercepted by the beam. If the tube is placed in the lateral position, the radiologist will be ex-

TABLE 12-3. *Summary of techniques to minimize radiation exposure to patient and operator*

Minimize total fluoroscopy time.
Keep image intensifier as close as possible to patient.
Do not use high level mode, if available, unless absolutely necessary.
Keep x-ray tube underneath patient whenever possible.
Try to maintain distance from x-ray tube and patient.
Always wear lead apron and film badge(s).
Try to limit use of magnification mode.
Collimate x-ray beam to area of interest.
Keep hands out of primary beam as much as possible.
If kV is manually adjusted, use higher kV ($\geq$75) and lower mA techniques.
Use the last image hold and pulsed fluoroscopy if available.

posed to lower radiation levels near the image intensifier rather than near the x-ray tube.

■ Potential for Skin Injuries to the Patient

Although fluoroscopically guided interventional procedures are often the treatment of choice for critically ill patients, there is some potential for radiation induced injury.[10] Certain interventional procedures may require long fluoroscopic exposure times along with recording of images, which may lead to entrance skin doses of 2 Gy (200 rad) or more with subsequent skin injuries. During an interval of approximately 4 years, the FDA received reports of skin injuries to 26 patients, including erythema, moist desquamation, and skin necrosis.[11] The procedures resulting in skin injuries included radiofrequency cardiac catheter ablation, catheter placement for chemotherapy, transjugular interhepatic portosystemic shunt placement, coronary angioplasty, renal angioplasty, multiple hepatic or biliary procedures, and percutaneous cholangiography followed by multiple embolization procedures.

The FDA[12] recommends that information be recorded for patients that might receive a threshold dose to the skin of 1 Gy (100 rad) or more, including identification of those areas of the patient's skin that may receive the dose threshold and an estimate of the dose received or information that would allow estimation of the dose to those areas. The dose to the skin may be estimated by direct measurement with placement of dosimeters on the skin during the procedure. Alternatively, the radiation exposure rates may be measured for the particular x-ray system and the skin dose may be calculated if the system geometry and the technique factors are recorded, such as kVp, mA, total exposure time during fluoroscopy and kVp, mAs per image, and the total number of images during digital or conventional image acquisition. Although the FDA recommends recording information for dose estimation in cases that may approach the threshold of 1 Gy, it is prudent to record this information for all interventional cases.

■ Summary

A summary of techniques to minimize radiation exposure to the patient and the operator is given in Table 12-3.

REFERENCES

1. Limitation of exposure to ionizing radiation. NCRP Report no. 116. Bethesda, MD: National Council on Radiation Protection and Measurements, 1993.
2. Use of personal monitors to estimate effective dose equivalent and effective dose to workers for external exposure to low-LET radiation. NCRP Report no. 122. Bethesda, MD: National Council on Radiation Protection and Measurements, 1995.
3. Niklason LT, Marx MV, Chan H-P. Interventional radiologists: occupational radiation doses and risks. *Radiology* 1993;187:729–733.
4. Medical x-ray, electron beam and gamma-ray protection for energies up to 50 MeV (equipment design, performance and use). NCRP Report no. 102. Bethesda, MD: National Council on Radiation Protection and Measurements, 1989.
5. Wagner LK, Mulhern BS. Radiation-attenuating surgical gloves: effects of scatter and secondary electron production. *Radiology* 1996;200:45–48.
6. Agarwal SK, Friesen EJ, Huddleston AL, et al. The effectiveness of glass lenses in reducing exposure to the eyes. *Radiology* 1978; 129:810–811.
7. Tidwell A, Brahmavar S, Breton R, et al. Radiation exposures in pulsed fluoroscopy systems: patient and physician. *Med Phys* 1994;21:943. (abst.)
8. Norbash AM, Busick D, Marks MP. Techniques for reducing interventional neuroradiologic skin dose: tube position rotation and supplemental beam filtration. *AJNR Am J Neuroradiol* 1996;17: 41–49.
9. Feygelman VM, Huda W, Peters KR. Effective dose equivalent to patients udergoing cerebral angiography. *AJNR Am J Neuroradiol* 1992;13:845–849.
10. Wagner LK, Eifel PJ, Geise RA. Potential biological effects following high x-ray dose interventional procedures. *J Vasc Intervent Radiol* 1994;5:71–84.
11. Shope TB. Radiation-induced skin injuries from fluoroscopy. *Radiographics* 1996;16:1195–1199.
12. Recording information in the patient's medical record that identifies the potential for serious x-ray induced skin injuries following fluoroscopically guided procedures. Rockville, MD: Food and Drug Administration (FDA), Department of Health and Human Services, September 15, 1995.

13

Physician Health and Safety in the Angiography Suite

MARGARET E. HANSEN

■ Infectious Risks

Non-bloodborne pathogens

Although blood-borne pathogens may stimulate more concern among health care workers (HCWs) and patients, certain non-bloodborne agents are also important, particularly in hospital settings. Many pathogens are transmitted by droplet infection or by direct contact. Influenza and childhood diseases such as measles and rubella can be transmitted between HCWs and patients. Patients can be infected by asymptomatic HCWs harboring these viruses, hence the recommendation that all HCWs be vaccinated against these three diseases. The elderly, the immunocompromised, and those with chronic diseases are at greatest risk for influenza. Immunity to rubella is important for women of childbearing age because severe fetal damage may result from congenital infection.

The incidence of tuberculosis (TB) is increasing across the United States, especially in large cities.[1,2] Most worrisome is the emergence of multidrug resistant (MDR) strains, which can cause fulminant, rapidly fatal infection, particularly (but not only) in human immunodeficiency virus (HIV) -positive persons. HCWs in several cities have been infected on the job, and several have died as a result.[3] Patients with known or suspected active TB infection should wear masks or particulate respirators, if possible, while undergoing procedures outside approved isolation rooms. Standard face masks do not filter particles in the droplet size range (1–5 µm) and are not adequate to prevent the spread of TB; for this reason, particulate respirators are preferred.[4] All radiology personnel involved in procedures on patients with active TB should wear respirators if possible.

Methicillin-resistant *Staphylococcus aureus* (MRSA), a serious problem in many hospitals, may be found in the nares or on the skin of HCWs and is spread primarily by the hands (5). Handwashing is critical in preventing transmission of MRSA; gloves, gowns, and masks should be used when caring for patients with this infection.[5]

Bloodborne pathogens

The most important agents in this category are HIV and the hepatitis viruses. Concern about nosocomial transmission of these agents has increased dramatically in the past few years.

Scope of the problem

Although a great deal of publicity and concern has centered on HIV, hepatitis B and C should be regarded as equally serious because these viruses are both more prevalent and more infectious than HIV.[6] More than 20 outbreaks of HCW to patient transmission of hepatitis B virus (HBV) have been reported, and the Centers for Disease Control and Prevention (CDC) estimates that 8,000 to 12,000 HCWs are infected with HBV on the job each year. Of these, 10% will become chronic viral carriers; about 200 deaths of HCWs are attributed to HBV-related disease each year.[7] Between 3 and 14% of the general population have serologic evidence of HBV exposure (>50% for foreign-born Asians), and 0.2 to 13% are chronic carriers. Among hospitalized patients, at least 1% are HBV carriers, most asymptomatic and unaware of their carrier status.[7] Hepatitis C virus (HCV) is also prevalent in certain groups: studies indicate exposure in 1 to 4% of HCWs, 12% of dialysis patients, and 50 to 80% of injecting drug users and hemophiliacs.[8,9]

The prevalence of HIV infection in the United States is estimated to be about 1% in the general population,[10] although it is higher in certain groups, such as emergency department patients (6%)[11] and young urban adults treated for penetrating trauma (19% in one study).[12] The prevalence of HIV infection among patients in acute care hospitals ranges from 0.2% to 14.2%.[13]

Means and risk of transmission

Transmission of HIV, HBV, and HCV occurs through blood contact and sexual contact. In the health care setting, this generally involves needlestick injuries, but contact with mucous membranes or nonintact skin also has resulted in HIV infection.[14] Transmission after contact with intact skin has not been reported. In addition to blood, other body fluids may be infectious. HIV has been detected in saliva, semen, vaginal secretions, breast milk, amniotic fluid, synovial fluid, cerebrospinal fluid, and serous exudates from infected persons.[7] HBV can be present in most of these fluids, too, as well as in urine and feces.[7] HCV has not been recovered from vaginal fluid, semen, or saliva of chronically infected persons even when viremia is present, but otherwise has a distribution similar to that of HBV.[7]

HBV is a fairly hardy virus, able to survive on environmental surfaces for up to 7 days at room temperature, but it is killed by bleach and other high-level disinfectants.[7] HIV is also readily inactivated by household bleach and other high-level disinfectants, but it is less robust and survives only briefly on surfaces at room temperature.[7]

The risk of infection after a single parenteral exposure depends on the infectivity of the source, the amount of blood or other fluid transferred, and other factors. Infectivity depends on the viral titers of the source. For HBV, the most infectious of the three viruses, the type of viral particle present in the blood is also important; hepatitis B e antigen (HBeAg) is the most infectious. Infection risk after one parenteral contact with HBV ranges from 7 to 30%;[7] with HCV from 2 to 4%,[7] and with HIV is about 0.4%.[15,16] For a given procedure, the risk of infection depends on the likelihood of parenteral contact during the procedure and the source's likelihood of infection in addition to the above factors.

The risk of HCW-to-patient transmission is unknown but probably is much lower than the risk in the opposite direction. For such transmission to occur, the HCW must be infected with a blood-borne agent and sustain an injury that causes bleeding (or have open, exudative skin lesions, in which case the HCW should avoid patient contact), and then his or her blood must come into parenteral contact with the patient. Perhaps the most common scenario in which this might occur in the angiography suite is if a needle is reused on the patient after being contaminated with the blood of an HCW after a needlestick injury. If such contact occurs and the HCW is HIV positive, the risk of infecting the patient probably would be about 0.4% (the same as for infection of an HCW after a single needlestick exposure).[15,16] Computer modeling done by the CDC to estimate the risk of an HIV positive surgeon infecting a patient during a procedure yielded a range of 1/42,000 to 1/420,000 procedures.[17] Modeling specific to vascular and interventional radiology has produced similar results, estimating the risk of infecting a patient to be 0.03 per million procedures if the radiologist's HIV status is unknown and 7.5 per million procedures if the physician is HIV positive.[18] The estimated risk of patient-to-physician transmission of HIV for a single procedure ranges from 0.03 to 7.5 per million.[18]

Blood contacts and injuries in vascular/interventional radiology

Needlestick injuries occur less often in interventional radiology than in surgery. A recent prospective study noted needlestick injuries in 0.6% of interventional radiologic procedures,[19] compared with previously reported rates of 1.7 to 15.4% for surgical procedures.[20–24] A national survey of interventional radiologists found an annual median injury rate of 0.3,[25] compared with an annual median of 2 in a survey of surgeons.[26] Improper handling of sharps, such as leaving exposed sharps in the folds of a drape or under a towel, or recapping needles was a common source of injury to radiologists.[19,25] Procedure duration, operator experience level, and elective versus emergency procedure status had no effect on the risk of injury, but the risk for nonvascular interventional procedures was slightly higher than for other types of cases.[19] Cutaneous or mucous membrane exposures, including splashes to the face, eyes, or other areas, occured in 3% of cases.[19] More than 70% of these blood contacts could have been avoided by using appropriate protective gear, such as gowns and goggles. Longer procedure duration was strongly associated with higher risk of such exposures,[19] although not with higher risk of injury.

Glove perforations are another potentially important means of blood contact. Overall, occult perforations occur in 10% of gloves used for angiographic or interventional procedures, but the relationship between the length of time gloves are worn and the perforation rate is strong, with 2 hours being the dividing point between low and high risk.[27] For this reason, it is prudent to change gloves during lengthy procedures at or before 2 hours of wear. Most of the holes are probably attributable to mechanical stresses, such as forceful hand injection or catching glove material in a stopcock, rather than actual sharp injuries.

■ Risk-reduction Strategies

Universal precautions

The use of universal precautions (UP) has been recommended by the CDC since 1987 (Table 13-1.[28] The basic tenet of UP is the assumption that blood and body fluids from all patients should be considered potentially infectious. Rather than targeting the use of blood and body fluid precautions to "high-risk" cases only, UP mandates their routine use. Adherence to CDC infection control recommendations, including use of UP, was voluntary until 1992, when federal law made it mandatory.[7]

Safety devices and personal protective gear

Many devices have been produced in attempts to reduce the risk of injury and blood contacts during procedures. "Needleless" intravenous systems (Fig. 13-1), self-sheathing needles, and needle-capping devices are among those in current use; improved containers for the disposal of sharps are now standard in most health care settings as well.

Several products have been designed specifically for interventional radiology, such as sharps holders for procedure trays, closed flush systems, closed-system drainage kits, and "bloodless" arterial puncture systems.[29–33] Most of these products are slightly more expensive than standard versions (some of the needles may be significantly more expensive) and do not interfere with procedure performance. Tactile feel during guidewire introduction may be altered with the bloodless puncture devices, how-

ever, which should be kept in mind when these devices are used.[34]

Personal protective equipment has been available for a long time, but some improvements have been made recently. Fluid-impermeable gowns are now widely used, some of which offer added protection in areas where strike-through is most likely, such as the chest and sleeves. Clear plastic face shields and shield-mask combinations can be used by most people, including those who wear corrective eyeglasses. Most brands of goggles and shields provide side shielding as well, which is required by current safety standards.

Unfortunately, protective gear is not widely used in interventional radiology despite being affordable and readily available. Anecdotal evidence suggests that many radiologists often do not wear caps, masks, goggles, and shoe covers (or even gowns) while performing procedures. This evidence is supported by the survey of interventional radiologists mentioned earlier,[25] which found that only 20% of radiologists who do not wear corrective eyeglasses for procedures routinely used eye protection, and only 32% routinely wear a face mask or shield. Inconvenience and fogging of eyeglasses are commonly cited reasons for failure to use these items; given the many styles of masks or shields now available, one should be workable for almost everyone, and persons who have such concerns should try different brands.

Safe sharp handling

Proper handling of sharp instruments includes not recapping them by hand and prompt disposal of used sharps in an appropriate container. Preferably, sharps should not be recapped at all, but if this must be done, a mechanical device such as a sheath guard or a hemostat should be used. The one-handed method in which the cap is scooped up with the needle, fingers well away from its tip, is also acceptable but slightly more risky. Communication between team members during procedures is perhaps the most important element of safe handling of sharps so that all persons involved in a case are aware of the location and status of all sharp instruments in use. It never should be assumed by one team member that another person has seen where a sharp has been placed; verbal communication is essential. Removing sharps from the field immediately after use is also important in avoiding inadvertent injury. Leaving exposed sharps in the folds of a drape is a common cause of injury.[25] Prompt disposal of used sharps in a puncture- and spill-proof container is the final element in safe handling.

Vaccinations

Vaccination against HBV is recommended for all HCWs at risk for occupational exposure to blood or other poten-

TABLE 13-1. *Strategies for risk reduction in interventional radiology*

Adherence to universal precautions
  Blood and body fluids from *all* patients are potentially infectious

Use of safety devices and personal protective gear
  Needleless intravenous systems
  Self-sheathing needles and needle-capping devices
  Sharps holders
  Closed flush systems
  Fluid-impermeable gowns
  Face shields, masks and goggles
  Caps, shoe covers, gloves

Safe handling of sharp instruments
  Do not recap by hand unless one-handed method is used
  Maintain awareness regarding location and status of sharps during procedure
  Remove sharps from field immediately after use
  Dispose of sharps promptly in appropriate container

Vaccinations
  Hepatitis B
  Influenza, rubella, measles
  Tetanus
  Future vaccines: hepatitis C, human immunodeficiency virus?

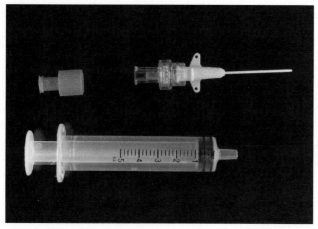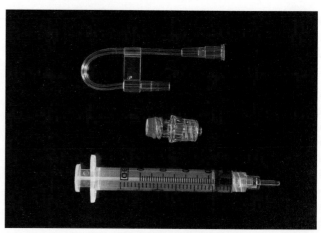

Figure 13-1. A: Saf-Site (Burron Medical Inc., Bethlehem, PA), a "needleless" intravenous access system features a one-way valve that is opened by inserting the syringe tip into the hub of the device; caps are also available. **B:** The InterLink device (Becton Dickinson, Franklin Lakes, NJ) is similar, with a hep-lock style hub that is penetrated by the special syringe tip.

tially infectious materials and now must be offered free of charge to such employees.[7] Because it is produced by recombinant DNA technology, the current vaccine carries no risk of pathogen transmission.[35] Booster doses may be needed in some cases. Currently, no vaccines are available for HCV or HIV, although intensive research effort is under way.

Vaccination against rubella, tetanus, influenza, and measles is recommended for all HCWs. Rubella vaccine is contraindicated during pregnancy, which should be avoided for 3 months after vaccination.[36] Measles vaccine also is contraindicated during pregnancy.[37] Influenza vaccines are formulated each year against strains thought to be common in the coming flu season, and revaccination is needed annually.[38]

■ What to Do If Exposure Occurs

Blood testing

After a parenteral exposure to blood or body fluid, the risk of the source individual's being infected with a blood-borne pathogen should be assessed and appropriate serologic testing performed as soon as possible (Table 13-2).[39] Both the source and the exposed person should be tested for evidence of HIV, HBV, and HCV infection initially.

If the source is HIV positive, the exposed person should be retested for HIV 3 and 6 months after exposure if the initial test has a negative result. Safe sexual practices should be followed during this period, and sharing of toothbrushes, needles, or razors should be avoided. Donation of blood, organs, and sperm should be avoided as well, and preventing pregnancy for 6 months is recommended.[39]

Repeated serologic testing is recommended to be

done 6 and 9 months after exposure to HCV. If infection is diagnosed, liver-function testing should be done to determine whether any treatment or further follow-up is needed.[39]

HIV and hepatitis prophylaxis

If the source is HIV positive, the exposed person should be counseled about antiviral prophylaxis using zidovudine (ZDV), an agent that is active against human retroviruses such as HIV, possibly in combination with other antiretroviral drugs. ZDV prophylaxis is widely used, al-

TABLE 13-2. *What to do if exposure occurs*

Determine which pathogens might be involved by initial blood testing
  Source: HIV, HBV, HCV if status unknown
  Exposed person: HIV, HBV, HCV if status unknown

HBV exposure of nonimmune person
  Start HBV vaccine series within 7 days of exposure
  Give HBV immunoglobulin within 24 hr of exposure

Repeat blood testing of exposed person based on results
of initial tests
  HIV-positive source: test at 3 and 6 mo if initial test negative
  HCV-positive source: test at 6 and 9 mo if initial test negative
  HBV-positive source: test at 4 and 6 mo after immunoglobulin
    given

Chemoprophylaxis against HIV
  Recommendations vary based on the degree of risk from exposure
  For high-risk exposure, combination of three antiretroviral drugs
    used
  For lower-risk cases, one or two drugs recommended
  Recommendations may change in the future

Counseling and follow-up
  If exposed to HIV, practice safe sex, refrain from blood and organ
    donation, and prevent pregnancy for 6 mo
  If HCV infection develops, check liver function tests as needed
  In all cases, counseling by an experienced professional is vital

,HIV, human immunodeficiency virus; HBV, hepatitis B virus, hepatitis C virus.

though side effects are common.[40–42] If prophylaxis is elected, it should be started as soon as possible after exposure, ideally within an hour, as HIV infection may be established within a few hours. Several dosage regimens have been used.[39,41–43] The most recent recommendations issued by the U.S. Public Health Service in mid-1996 vary with the level of risk (based on the route of exposure and type of material involved, i.e., blood versus other fluids) and include the use of ZDV and one or more of the newer antiretroviral agents, such as indinavir or saquinavir. Because these recommendations may change with experience, and as newer drugs become available, the best course is to report all injuries immediately and to seek appropriate counseling regarding current recommendations.

If the source has evidence of HBV infectivity (HBsAg or HBeAg in the blood) and the exposed person has not been vaccinated against HBV or had a previous infection, the HBV vaccine series should be started within 7 days of exposure.[39] Hepatitis B immunoglobulin also should be given within 24 hours of exposure, but the two injections must not be given in the same site because they might inactivate each other. Follow-up testing for development of infection or establishment of immunity should be done 4 to 6 months after immunoglobulin administration. Exposed persons who follow the recommended prophylaxis regimen pose little risk to patients and other contacts, and patient-care activities need not be restricted during the interval between tests.[39]

No effective prophylaxis against HCV infection is currently available. Immunoglobulin has not been shown to prevent HCV infection, and its use for this purpose is not recommended. Interferon alfa, although used with some success in the treatment of chronic HCV infection, has no role in preventing infection.[39]

Counseling is as important after exposure to a bloodborne pathogen as are the serologic testing and prophylactic measures described previously. Counseling should be done by a health care professional who is experienced in this area.

■ Infection Control Regulations

1992 OSHA Bloodborne pathogen standard

In 1992, the Bloodborne Pathogen Standard of the Occupational Safety and Health Administration (OSHA) became federal law.[7] This statute has several major provisions that affect all radiologists, interventional radiologists in particular (Table 13-3). The standard applies to all employees with potential occupational exposure to blood or other infectious materials, except those in certain state, county, or city facilities. Volunteers and students are not covered unless they are also employees. Exposure need

TABLE 13-3. *Infection control regulations: 1992 OSHA Bloodborne Pathogen Standard*

Employers must develop an exposure control plan
Employers must provide personal protective equipment and mandate its use
Employers must provide HBV vaccination and postexposure evaluation and treatment for HIV and hepatitis; vaccination must be free of charge
All employees must have annual training in infection control
Employers must keep records of training sessions
Employers must keep medical records for at-risk employees, including HBV vaccination, exposure, and treatment
Employers must provide facilities for handwashing and sharps disposal
Use and storage of food, drink, and cosmetics prohibited in at-risk areas
Recapping of sharps by hand prohibited
Sharps disposal containers must be leak- and puncture-proof
Contaminated laundry must be placed in labeled or color-coded bags
Specimens must be placed in labeled or color-coded bags

HBV, hepatitis B virus; HIV, human immunodeficiency virus; OSHA, Occupational Safety and Health Administration.

not occur frequently for the standard to apply, and if any part of a person's job poses an exposure risk, he or she is covered by all provisions of the standard.

Employers must develop an exposure control plan that identifies employees at risk, details how the standard will be implemented, specifies how exposures will be dealt with, is reviewed and updated at least annually, and is accessible to employees and to OSHA.

They also must provide personal protective equipment, including gloves, gowns, masks, goggles, caps, shoe covers, and other items as needed. The use of such equipment is mandatory whenever exposure to blood or body fluid may be "reasonably anticipated" (no specific procedures or situations are cited in the standard), and the equipment provided must be clean, readily available in appropriate sizes, in good repair, and free of charge to employees. Hypoallergenic gloves or glove liners must be provided if needed.

In addition, HBV vaccination and postexposure evaluation and treatment for HIV and HBV must be provided. Vaccination must be offered free of charge to all employees who are at risk an average of one or more times per month; those declining must sign a waiver. Free booster doses also must be provided.

All employees at risk must be trained in infection control, with sessions repeated at least once a year. Medical records for employees at risk must include documentation of HBV vaccination, exposures, and postexposure treatment and must be kept for the duration of employment plus 30 years.

Readily available handwashing facilities and containers for sharps disposal must be provided. Work-practice controls must be established, such as prohibiting the use or storage of food, drink, or cosmetics in at-risk areas; handwashing immediately after removal of gloves or other protective gear; prohibiting recapping of sharps; and immediate washing of skin and flushing of mucous membranes after contact with potentially infectious material.

Containers for the disposal of sharps are required to be leakproof, spillproof, closable, and located as close as possible to the point(s) of sharps use. Contaminated laundry must be placed in appropriately labeled or color-coded bags, as must specimens. Biohazard labels or red bags/containers must be used for all potentially infectious materials.

Recently, guidelines regarding bloodborne pathogens were developed and published by the Society of Cardiovascular and Interventional Radiology.[44] These guidelines incorporate many elements of the OSHA standard as well as some from other sources and are specific to interventional radiology practice.

Resources for education and training

Many resources are available for education and training in infection control and to assist physicians in complying with the OSHA standard. Many commercial products, such as videos, workbooks, and seminars, are available. Local infectious disease specialists or infection-control practitioners are a valuable resource; state or local medical or radiologic societies also may be able to provide information on these topics.

REFERENCES

1. Goldsmith MF. Medical exorcism required as revitalized revenant of tuberculosis haunts and harries the land. JAMA 1992;268:174–175.
2. Menzies D, Fanning A, Yuan L, et al. Tuberculosis among health care workers. N Engl J Med 1995;332:92–98.
3. Centers for Disease Control. Nosocomial transmission of multidrug resistant tuberculosis among HIV-infected persons—Florida and New York, 1988–1991. MMWR 1991;40:585–591.
4. Centers for Disease Control. Guidelines for preventing the transmission of tuberculosis in health-care settings, with special focus on HIV-related issues. MMWR 1990;39(RR-17):1–29.
5. Wenzel RP, Nettleman MD, Jones RN, et al. Methicillin-resistant Staphylococcus aureus: implications for the 1990s and effective control measures. Am J Med 1991;91(Suppl 3B):221S–227S.
6. Lettau LA. The A, B, C, D, and E of viral hepatitis: spelling out the risks for healthcare workers. Infect Control Hosp Epidemiol 1992;13:77–81.
7. OSHA. Occupational exposure to bloodborne pathogens: final rule (29 CFR 1910.1030). Federal Register 1991;56:64003–64182.
8. Polywka S, Laufs R. Hepatitis C virus antibodies among different groups at risk and patients with suspected non-A, non-B hepatitis. Infection 1991;19:81–84.
9. Alter MJ. Hepatitis C: a sleeping giant? Am J Med 1991;91(Suppl 3B):112S–115S.
10. Centers for Disease Control. HIV prevalence estimates and AIDS case projections for the US: report based upon a workshop. MMWR 1990;39 (RR-16):1–31.
11. Kelen GD, DiGiovanna T, Bisson L, et al. Human immunodeficiency virus infection in emergency department patients: epidemiology, clinical presentations, and risk to healthcare workers—the Johns Hopkins experience. JAMA 1989; 262:516–522.
12. Baker JL, Kelen GD, Sivertson KT, et al. Unsuspected human immunodeficiency virus in critically ill emergency patients. JAMA 1987;257:2609–2611.
13. Janssen RS, St Louis ME, Satten GA, et al. HIV infection among patients in US acute care hospitals: strategies for counseling and testing of hospital patients. N Engl J Med 1992;327:445–452.
14. Centers for Disease Control. Update: human immunodeficiency virus infections in health-care workers exposed to blood of infected patients. MMWR 1987;36:285–289.
15. Marcus R and the CDC Cooperative Needlestick Surveillance Group. Surveillance of healthcare workers exposed to blood from patients infected with the human immunodeficiency virus. N Engl J Med 1988;319:1118–1123.
16. Henderson DK, Fahey BJ, Willy M, et al. Risk for occupational transmission of human immunodeficiency virus type 1 (HIV-1) associated with clinical exposures: a prospective evaluation. Ann Intern Med 1990;113:740–746.
17. Chamberland ME, Bell DM. HIV transmission from health care worker to patient: what is the risk? Ann Intern Med 1992;116:871–872.
18. Hansen ME, McIntire DD. HIV transmission during invasive radiologic procedures: estimate based on computer modeling. AJR Am J Roentgenol 1996;166:263–267.
19. Hansen ME, Miller GL III, Redman HC, et al. Needlestick injuries and blood contacts during invasive radiologic procedures. AJR Am J Roentgenol 1993;160:1119–1122.
20. Gerberding JL, Littell C, Tarkington A, et al. Risk of exposure of surgical personnel to patients' blood during surgery at San Francisco General Hospital. N Engl J Med 1990;322:1788–1793.
21. Popejoy SL, Fry DE. Blood contact and exposure in the operating room. Surg Gynecol Obstet 1991;172:480–483.
22. Hussain SA, Latif ABA, Choudhary AAAA. Risk to surgeons: a survey of accidental injuries during operations. Br J Surg 1988;75:314–316.
23. Tokars JI, Bell DM, Culver DH, et al. Percutaneous injuries during surgical procedures. JAMA 1992;267:2899–2904.
24. Quebbeman EJ, Telford GL, Hubbard S, et al. Risk of blood contamination and injury to operating room personnel. Ann Surg 1991;214:614–620.
25. Hansen ME, Miller GL III, Redman HC, et al. HIV and interventional radiology: a national survey of physician attitudes and behaviors. J Vasc Intervent Radiol 1993;4:229–236.
26. Lowenfels AB, Wormser GP, Jain R. Frequency of puncture injuries in surgeons and estimated risk of HIV infection. Arch Surg 1989;124:1284–1286.
27. Hansen ME, McIntire DD, Miller GL III. Occult glove perforations: frequency during interventional radiologic procedures. AJR Am J Roentgenol 1992;159:131–135.
28. Centers for Disease Control. Recommendations for prevention of HIV transmission in health-care settings. MMWR 1987;36(Suppl 2S).
29. Wall SD, Olcott EW, Gerberding JL. AIDS risk and risk reduction in the radiology department. AJR Am J Roentgenol 1991;157:911–917.
30. Mueller PR, Silverman SG, Tung G, et al. New universal precautions aspiration tray. Radiology 1989;173:278–279.
31. vanSonnenberg E, Casola G, Maysey M. Simple apparatus to avoid inadvertent needle puncture. Radiology 1988;166:550.
32. Olsen WL, Jeffrey RB Jr, Tolentino CS. Closed system for arterial puncture in patients at risk for AIDS. Radiology 1988;166:551–552.
33. Palestrant AM, Esplin CA, Shaw GT. A closed irrigation and drainage system for use with percutaneous abcess drainage: technical note. Cardiovasc Intervent Radiol 1990;13:119–121.
34. Williams DM, Marx MV, Korobkin M. AIDS risk and risk reduction in the radiology department [commentary]. AJR Am J Roentgenol 1991;157:919–921.

35. Hepatitis B virus vaccine inactivated. In: McEvoy GK, ed. *AHFS Drug Information*. Bethesda, MD: American Society of Hospital Pharmacists, 1992:2026–2034.

36. Rubella virus vaccine live. In: McEvoy GK, ed. *AHFS Drug Information*. Bethesda, MD: American Society of Hospital Pharmacists, 1992: 2061–2065.

37. Measles virus vaccine live. In: McEvoy GK, ed. *AHFS Drug Information*. Bethesda, MD: American Society of Hospital Pharmacists, 1992: 2038–2043.

38. Influenza virus vaccine. In: McEvoy GK, ed. *AHFS Drug Information*. Bethesda, MD: American Society of Hospital Pharmacists, 1992: 2034–2038.

39. Gerberding JL. Management of occupational exposures to bloodborne viruses. *N Engl J Med* 1995;332:444–451.

40. Zidovudine. In: McEvoy GK, ed. *AHFS Drug Information*. Bethesda, MD: American Society of Hospital Pharmacists, 1992:392–401.1.

41. Centers for Disease Control. Public Health Service statement on management of occupational exposure to human immunodeficiency virus, including considerations regarding zidovudine postexposure use. *MMWR* 1990;39(RR-1):1–14.

42. Henderson DK. Postexposure chemoprophylaxis for occupational exposure to Human Immunodeficiency Virus type 1: current status and prospects for the future. *Am J Med* 1991;91(suppl 3B):312S–319S.

43. Centers for Disease Control. Update: provisional Public Health Service recommendations for chemoprophylaxis after occupational exposure to HIV. *MMWR* 1996;45:468–472.

44. Hansen ME, Bakal CW, Dixon GD, et al. Guidelines regarding HIV and other bloodborne pathogens in vascular/interventional radiology. *J Vasc Intervent Radiol* 1997;8:667–676.

■ PART II ■

A Systems Approach to Diagnosis and Management

14

Vascular Anatomy above the Diaphragm

JACOB CYNAMON

■ Arteries

The right and left coronary arteries arise off the right and left aortic sinuses. The brachiocephalic artery is the first branch off the arch, which bifurcates into the right subclavian and right carotid arteries. Next, the left carotid artery and, last, the left subclavian artery arise directly off the arch. (See Table 14-1 for variants of normal arch anatomy and Table 14-2 for genetic abnormalities of the thoracic arch.)

The thoracic aorta is divided into four segments[1] (Fig. 14-1): the ascending aorta, the aortic arch, the isthmus (between last great vessel and the attachment of the ductus arteriosus), and the descending aorta. Occasionally, there is a fusiform dilatation of the proximal descending aorta, a ductus diverticulum, which should not be confused with a traumatic injury. Usually, there are nine pairs of intercostal arteries, from the third through the 11th intercostal spaces. There are many variations to the intercostal anatomy. Most commonly, there are between two and four bronchial arteries; multiple bronchial arteries are more common on the left. Bronchial arteries may arise directly off the aorta or have a common origin with an intercostal artery, thus forming an intercostal bronchial trunk.[2]

The right subclavian artery originates off the brachiocephalic artery and the left subclavian artery arises directly off the aortic arch. The subclavian artery becomes the axillary artery after it crosses the lateral margin of the first rib. The subclavian artery gives rise to the following: the vertebral artery, the thyrocervical trunk, the internal mammary artery, and the costocervical trunk. There are variants to this anatomy, such as independent origins of branches of the thyrocervical trunk or the costocervical trunk.

The axillary artery gives rise to several small branches around the shoulder (Fig. 14-2A), including the superior thoracic, thoracoacromial, lateral thoracic, subscapular, and circumflex humoral arteries. There are many variants to this typical anatomy, including absent vessels and independent origins to vessels that may be normally common trunks. Occasionally (2%), the radial artery may originate from the distal axillary artery, and even more rarely (1%), the ulnar artery may originate from the distal axillary artery.

The axillary artery becomes the brachial artery at the lateral margin of the terres major muscle (Fig. 14-2A). It divides into the radial and ulnar arteries at the antecubital fossa. Its major branches include the deep brachial artery, which is a large vessel arising in the proximal upper arm and coursing posterolaterally. The deep brachial artery bifurcates into the radial collateral artery and the medial collateral artery. Variant anatomy includes a radial artery that originates off the proximal brachial artery (12%) and an ulnar artery that originates off the proximal brachial artery (1 to 2%).

The brachial artery bifurcates a few centimeters below the elbow joint into the radial and ulnar arteries. The axial remaining artery is known as the interosseous artery. The ulnar artery undergoes anastomosis with the median artery and forms a superficial palmer arch. The radial artery forms a deep palmer arch.

TABLE 14-1. Prevalence of Normal Arch Anatomy and Its Variants

Anatomy	Percent
Normal arch	70
Common origin of the brachiocephalic and left common carotid artery	22
Left vertebral artery directly off the aorta	4–6
Right and left common carotid artery have common origin	<1
Two brachiocephalic arteries	<1
All four great vessels have separate origins	0.1

TABLE 14-2. Congenital Variants for the Aortic Arch

Variant	Percent
Left aortic arch with aberrant right subclavian artery[a]	1
Right aortic arch	1–2
60% mirror image branching[b]	
35% with aberrant right subclavian and left ductus or ligamentum arteriosus[c]	
Cervical aortic arch is rare, not associated with intracardiac anomalies	
Coarctation, localized narrowing of the aorta	
50% isolated	
50% associated with congenital cardiac lesions such as bicuspid aortic valves, patent ductus arteriosus, ventricular septal defects, aneurysms of circle of Willis	

[a] Associated with congenital heart disease, 10 to 15%.
[b] Associated with cyanotic heart disease, 98%.
[c] Associated with congenital heart disease, 12%.

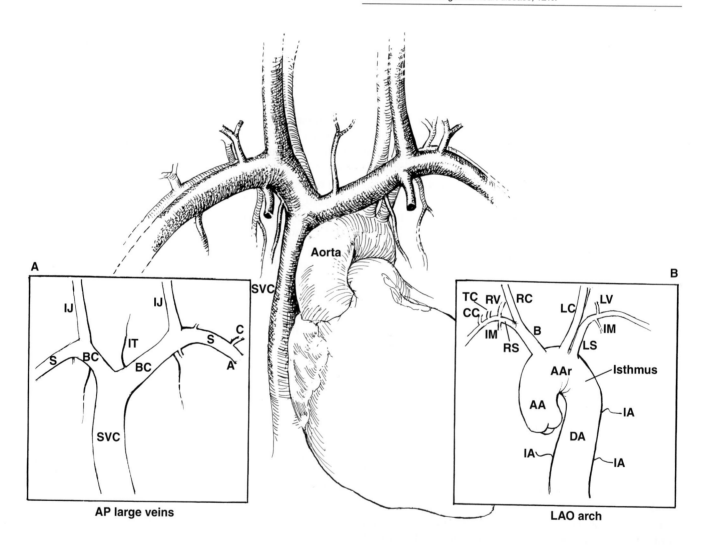

FIGURE 14-1. Superimposed arteries and veins of the thorax. **(A)** AP large veins. A, axillary; C, cephalic; BC, brachiocephalic; IJ, internal jugular; IT, inferior thyroid; S, subclavian; SVC, superior vena cava. **(B)** LAO arch. AA, ascending aorta; AAr, aortic arch; B, brachiocephalic artery; CC, costocervical; DA, descending artery; IA, intercostal arteries; IM, internal mammary artery; LC, left common carotid artery, LS, left subclavian artery; LV, left vertebral artery; RC, right common carotid artery; RS, right subclavian artery; RV, right vertebral artery; TC, thyrocervical.

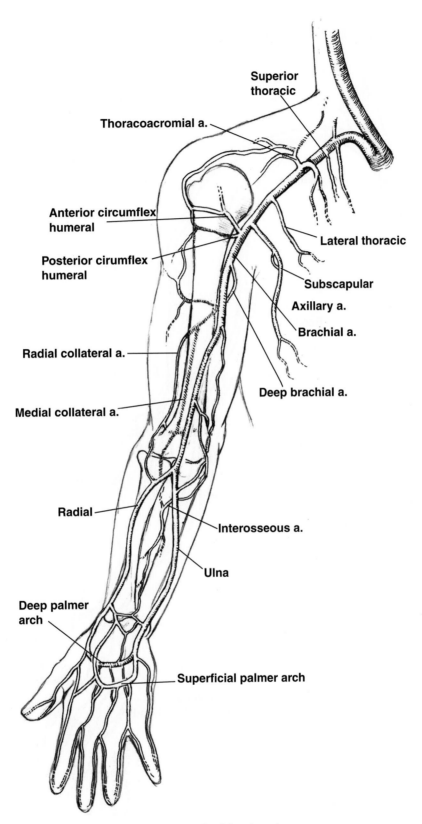

FIGURE 14-2. (A) Arteries of the upper extremity. (*Continued*)

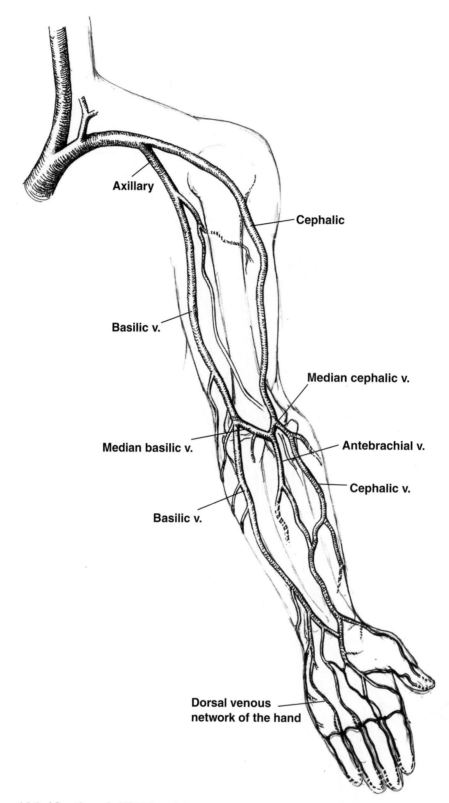

Figure 14-2. (*Continued*) (B) Veins of the upper extremity.

■ Veins

The veins of the upper extremity are composed predominantly of the superficial venous system (Fig. 14-2). The veins in the forearm are composed of the dorsal venous network of the hand, the superficial veins of the palm, the basilic vein, the cephalic vein, the antebrachial veins, and the median cephalic and basilic veins. There is a great deal of variation in the venous anatomy of the upper extremity. The cephalic vein originates dorsally and laterally. It crosses the elbow joint and enters the superior aspect of the axillary vein just below the clavicle. An accessory to the cephalic vein is frequently present. The basilic vein originates on the ulnar side of the arm and continues medial to the brachial artery. It joins the brachial vein to become the axillary vein at the border of the teri major muscle. The median cubital veins are the veins that connect the basilic and cephalic veins in the antecubital fossa. These veins are inconsistent.

The deep veins on the upper arm usually are paired and follow their respective arteries (Fig. 14-1B). The subclavian vein is a continuation of the axillary vein. As it crosses the sternum, it joins with the internal jugular vein to form the brachiocephalic vein. The left brachiocephalic vein (BCV) is longer than the right. The right and left BCVs join behind the first anterior rib to form the superior vena cava (SVC). The azygos vein forms at the L1–2 level. It travels in the anterior aspect of the posterior mediastinum slightly to the right of midline. It arches anteriorly to join the superior vena cava just above the SVC's entry into the pericardium.

Anterior and also originating at the L1–2 level slightly to the left of midline, the hemiazygos ascends and joins the azygos at the T8 level. The accessory hemiazygos is the most variable of the azygos hemiazygos system. It usually lies on the left side of the upper thorax.

REFERENCES

1. Shuford WH, Sybers RG. The aortic arch and its malformations. Springfield, IL: Charles C. Thomas; 1974.
2. Khan S, Haust MD. Variations in the aortic origin of intercostal arteries in man. *Anat Rec* 1979;195:545–552.

15

Pulmonary and Bronchial Arteries

JAMES E. SILBERZWEIG

■ PULMONARY ARTERIOGRAPHY

Pulmonary embolism

The most common indication for pulmonary arteriography is for the diagnosis of pulmonary embolism. Other indications for pulmonary arteriography include the diagnosis and treatment of arteriovenous malformations (AVMs), aneurysms, developmental abnormalities, vasculitis or inflammatory disease, neoplasms, and evaluation of pulmonary hypertension.

Pulmonary embolism is a common and potentially lethal disorder. Effective treatment of pulmonary embolism requires rapid and accurate diagnosis. Because the clinical signs and symptoms of pulmonary embolism are nonspecific, imaging procedures are used to make the diagnosis. Chest radiograph findings that may suggest the presence of pulmonary embolism include wedge-shaped, pleural-based densities (*Hampton's hump*), regional oligemia (*Westermark's sign*), and central pulmonary artery enlargement.[1] These findings are not, however, reliable indicators of pulmonary embolism. Most patients have vague parenchymal opacification, atelectasis, pleural effusion, or no abnormality. The utility of the chest radiograph in patients with suspected pulmonary embolism is to identify a nonembolic etiology for the patient's symptoms and aid in interpretation of lung ventilation-perfusion (V/Q) scintigraphy.

V/Q scintigraphy is the most commonly performed initial study for the diagnosis of pulmonary embolism; however, the results of V/Q scintigraphy are indeterminate in most patients. In these patients, the next diagnostic test performed is usually pulmonary arteriography, which serves as the "gold standard" study for making the diagnosis of acute pulmonary embolism. A negative high-quality pulmonary arteriogram excludes clinically significant pulmonary embolism.

Noninvasive imaging techniques such as magnetic resonance imaging and helical computed tomography (CT) have been used for evaluation of pulmonary embolism but are undergoing further investigation.[2–5] Some investigators have concluded that helical CT may be more useful than V/Q scintigraphy[2] for initial evaluation for pulmonary embolism; however, investigators have indicated that at this time CT cannot replace pulmonary arteriography for the diagnosis of pulmonary embolism because of its limited ability to identify emboli within subsegmental branches.[3,4]

Up to 90% of pulmonary emboli arise from the deep veins of the lower extremities.[6] Risk factors for venous thrombosis and pulmonary emboli include immobilization, prior history of thromboembolic disease, recent surgery or trauma, pregnancy, use of oral contraceptives, advanced age, cancer, and the presence of a hypercoagulable state. The initial clinical findings of pulmonary embolism are often nonspecific and include dyspnea, cough, fever, chest pain, and hemoptysis. Massive pulmonary embolism may result in cardiogenic shock. It is difficult to diagnose pulmonary embolism clinically because the symptoms may mimic other conditions, such as myocardial infarction, congestive heart failure, and pneumonia.

Pulmonary arteriography has high sensitivity and specificity in the diagnosis of pulmonary embolism in addition to being a safe procedure. The incidence of minor complications ranges from 1 to 5%. Complications include contrast reaction, transient renal dysfunction, access site hematoma, arrhythmia, and respiratory distress. Cardiac perforation is rare when pigtail catheters are used. The incidence of major complications has been reported to be less than 1%.[7,8]

The most common indication for pulmonary arteriography is for a patient with an indeterminate V/Q study. Pulmonary arteriography is often performed in patients with a low-probability V/Q study with a strong clinical suspicion of pulmonary embolism. A pulmonary arteriogram may be performed in patients with a high-probability V/Q study to confirm the diagnosis before starting anticoagulation, thrombolytic therapy, insertion of an inferior vena cava filter, or if the clinical suspicion for pulmonary embolism does not correlate with the result of the V/Q study.

Pulmonary embolization occurs to the lower lobes in more than 50% of patients and is bilateral in 25% of patients.[9] Pulmonary emboli may lyse spontaneously, organize and incorporate into the arterial wall as a plaque, or recanalize. Partial lysis of pulmonary emboli can occur within 24 hours, and complete lysis can occur within 1 to 3 weeks.[10]

The primary angiographic signs of pulmonary embolism include an intravascular filling defect (Fig. 15-1) and an abrupt vessel cutoff (Fig. 15-2). Overlying vessels must not be confused to be filling defects. Occasionally, a small branch is occluded flush with the origin of the vessel, which makes detection difficult. Secondary angiographic findings of pulmonary embolism include parenchymal staining, decreased perfusion, crowded vessels, delayed venous return from the affected area, pruning of vessels, slow flow, and shunting away from the involved lung.

Pulmonary artery catheterization most commonly is performed by the transfemoral route, but it can be performed from an upper-extremity vein or internal jugular vein approach. When using the common femoral vein approach, an iliac and inferior venacavogram is performed to exclude the presence of thrombus before the catheter is advanced into the right atrium.

Catheters used for pulmonary arteriography typically have a pigtail tip to resist catheter recoil and multiple side holes to allow for rapid contrast injection. End-hole catheters have been known to cause myocardial injury and pericardial extravasation through recoil and jet effect. The Grollman-type pigtail catheter has good torque control and is angled at the distal shaft that facilitates catheter passage through the tricuspid valve and right ventricular outflow tract (Fig. 15-3). After the right ventricle is entered, the catheter is rotated to direct the tip toward the pulmonic valve. The catheter then is advanced into the pulmonary artery. An alternative method uses a standard pigtail catheter and a tip-deflecting guidewire to angle the distal shaft of the catheter.

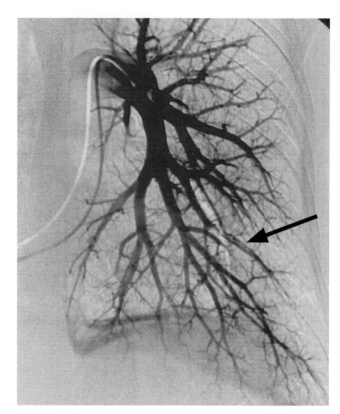

FIGURE 15-1. Pulmonary embolism. Intraluminal filling defect is present within a left lower lobe pulmonary artery branch (*arrow*).

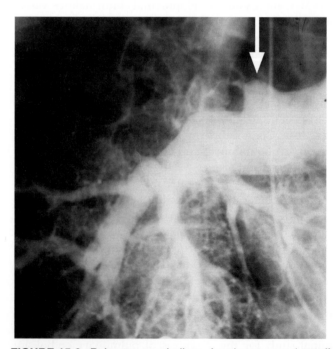

FIGURE 15-2. Pulmonary embolism. An abrupt vessel cutoff is present at the right upper lobe pulmonary artery branch (*arrow*).

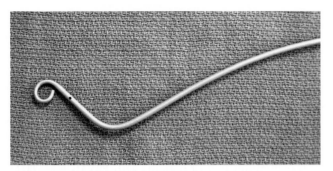

FIGURE 15-3. Grollman pigtail catheter.

The patient's electrocardiogram must be monitored continuously for the occurrence of induced ventricular ectopic beats during catheter manipulations within the cardiac chambers. Catheter-induced ventricular tachycardia usually can be reversed by immediately withdrawing the catheter. Rarely, intravenous administration of lidocaine or electroversion may be required. If left bundle-branch conduction block is present, there is a risk of inducing total heart block during catheterization, and a temporary cardiac pacemaker should be placed before

the catheter is introduced into the pulmonary artery. Pulmonary artery pressure can be measured using the diagnostic catheter. Some interventionalists recommend decreasing the contrast injection rate and volume in patients with a pulmonary artery systolic pressure greater than 40 mm Hg; however, no relationship between administered contrast dose and complications in patients with pulmonary hypertension has been demonstrated.[11]

A technically adequate pulmonary arteriogram to exclude the presence of pulmonary embolus requires selective catheterization of the right and left pulmonary arteries, with imaging in at least the frontal and one oblique projection. The ipsilateral posterior oblique view tends to produce the least amount of vascular overlap, especially of the lower lobes (Fig. 15-4). If any injection demonstrates embolus, the examination usually can be stopped.

Massive pulmonary emboli or emboli that do not respond to anticoagulation may require aggressive therapy. Catheter-directed thrombolytic therapy, thromboaspiration, mechanical clot fragmentation, and stent placement have been used to treat massive pulmonary embolism.[12–15] The role of local transcatheter therapy for acute pulmonary embolism has yet to be defined. Surgical pulmonary embolectomy is performed as a last resort in

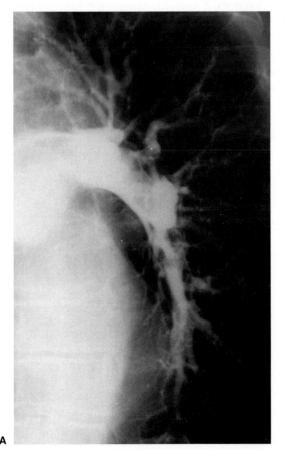

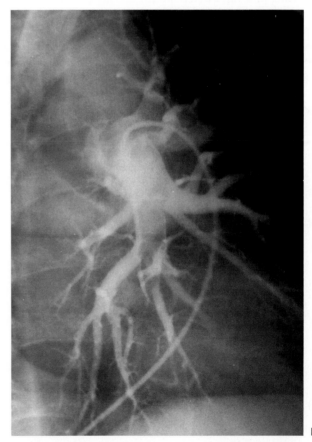

A   **B**

FIGURE 15-4. Pulmonary embolism. Selective left pulmonary arteriogram in the right posterior oblique projection **A:** shows overlap of the lower lobe branches. The left posterior oblique view **B:** clearly demonstrates a large left lower lobe embolus.

patients with cardiopulmonary collapse who do not respond to transcatheter techniques.

Chronic pulmonary embolism

Repeated episodes of pulmonary embolism with failure of the pulmonary emboli to lyse or recanalize may result in pulmonary hypertension and right ventricular dysfunction. Computed tomography (CT) and magnetic resonance imaging are useful in differentiating this disorder from other causes of chronic pulmonary artery hypertension. Angiography is the definitive diagnostic procedure performed for diagnostic confirmation and preoperative planning for open thromboendarterectomy. Chronic thromboembolic disease produces webs, luminal irregularities, segments of abrupt vessel narrowing, and obstruction (Fig. 15-5).[16] The main pulmonary arteries are usually dilated. The disease is usually bilateral.

Pulmonary arteriovenous malformations

Pulmonary arteriovenous malformations (PAVMs) are abnormal connections that develop between pulmonary artery and pulmonary vein branches originating from abnormal development of pulmonary capillaries. The PAVM results in a right-to-left shunt. PAVMs are divided into *simple* and *complex* malformations. *Simple malformations* have a single segmental artery and draining vein. *Complex malformations* have two or more arteries that supply the PAVM with one or two draining veins (Fig. 15-6). About 80 to 90% of all PAVMs are simple, and 10 to 20%

are complex. PAVMs are found most commonly in the lower lobes and are multiple in 33 to 50% of patients and bilateral in 8 to 20%.[17,18]

PAVMs may occur sporadically, but most are seen in patients with Osler–Weber–Rendu syndrome, also known as *hereditary hemorrhagic telangiectasia* (HHT), an autosomal dominant disease characterized by telangiectasias or AVMs of the respiratory tract, gastrointestinal tract, and brain. Ninety percent of patients with HHT have epistaxis.[17–19] About half of patients with PAVMs have HHT. The likelihood of having HHT is greater if the patient has multiple PAVMs rather than a single lesion. Family members should be evaluated because up to one third of them also have PAVMs.

Patients with PAVMs commonly have initial symptoms related to pulmonary-to-systemic shunting, such as low arterial blood oxygen leading to dyspnea and fatigue, or they may have systemic arterial embolization resulting in stroke or brain abscess. Rupture of a PAVM may result in hemoptysis or hemothorax.

The goal of PAVM treatment is occlusion of the shunt to prevent complications resulting from paradoxical embolization and to enhance arterial oxygen saturation. Embolotherapy is recommended when the feeding artery of a PAVM exceeds 3 mm in diameter.[18] Embolotherapy with coils or detachable balloons has become the treatment of choice.[19] The use of liquid or small-particle embolic agents for therapeutic embolization is ineffective and may result in inadvertent systemic embolization. Therapeutic embolization is performed at the pulmo-

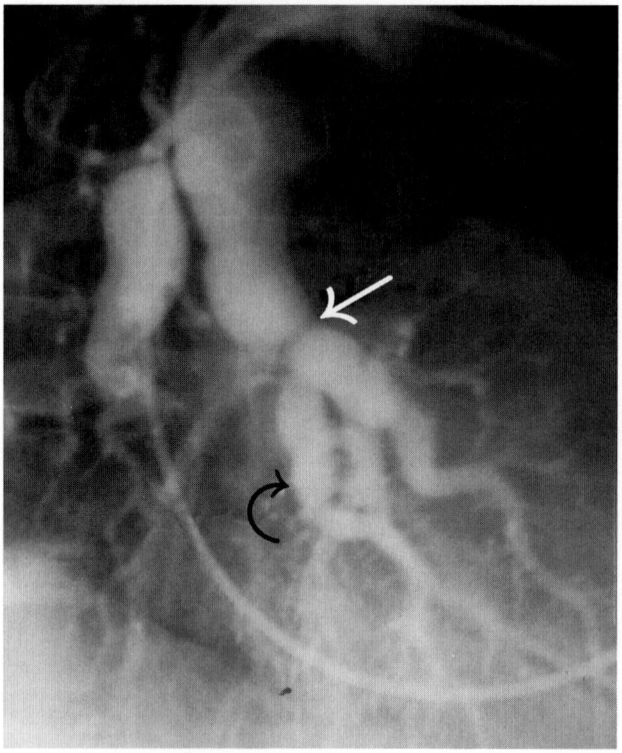

FIGURE 15-5. Chronic pulmonary thromboembolism. Webs (*arrow*) and mural irregularities (*curved arrow*) are present.

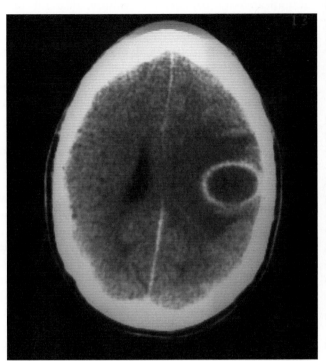

A

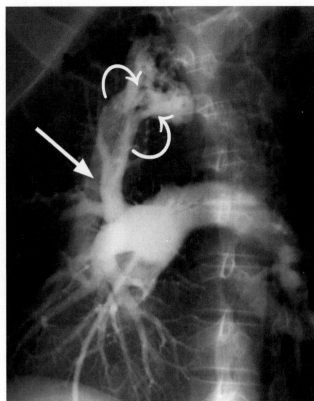

B

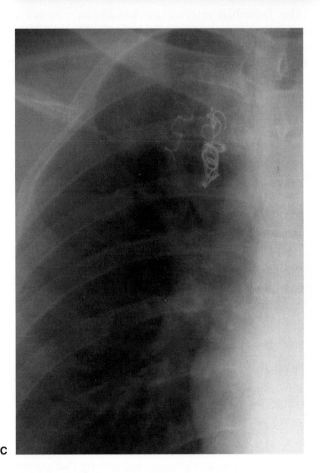

C

FIGURE 15-6. Pulmonary arteriovenous malformation (PAVM). **A:** This patient presented with a brain abscess resulting from **B:** a large complex right upper lobe AVM. There are two feeding arterial branches (*curved arrows*) and a large draining vein (*arrow*). **C:** The AVM was occluded by placement of embolization coils.

nary artery branch immediately proximal to the malformation. Embolotherapy is preferred over surgical resection in patients with multiple PAVMs because embolization spares normal lung and allows for future embolization of enlarging PAVMs.

■ Bronchial Arteriography

Management of hemoptysis is frequently a challenging clinical problem. Most patients with mild intermittent bleeding respond to supportive therapy and to medications that treat the underlying cause; however, the mortality rate in patients with acute massive hemoptysis is high in those who are inadequately treated, with death resulting from asphyxiation rather than from exsanguination. The definition of massive hemoptysis varies in the medical literature from less than 100 mL to greater than 600 mL in 24 hours.[20] Criteria for bronchial artery embolization are variable, and the amount of hemoptysis may be difficult to measure; however, a patient with any amount of hemoptysis that is life threatening may benefit from bronchial artery embolotherapy.

The most common causes of massive or repeated hemoptysis include tuberculosis, bronchiectasis, pneumoconiosis, aspergilloma, cancer, amyloidosis, sarcoidosis, and cystic fibrosis. These destructive lung processes cause massive hemoptysis by erosion of blood vessels in its vicinity. Hemorrhage usually arises from the bronchial arteries. The pulmonary artery is rarely a source of hemoptysis. Conditions that may result in hemorrhage arising from the pulmonary artery include a *Rasmussen aneurysm* (erosion of a tuberculosis cavity into a pulmonary artery branch), *traumatic pseudoaneurysm* (e.g., overinflation of a Swan–Ganz catheter balloon, penetrating thoracic trauma) (Fig. 15-7), and PAVMs.

Surgery can be a definitive treatment for massive hemoptysis but is a viable option only for patients who present with localized unilateral disease. Surgery is contraindicated for patients with diffuse, bilateral, or advanced pulmonary disease. Other contraindications to surgery include inability to localize the site of bleeding, bleeding from both lungs, and nonresectable malignancy. Bronchial artery embolization is an effective primary method to control massive or recurrent hemoptysis, especially in patients who are not suitable candidates for surgical resection. Bronchial arteriography and embolization can be performed in combination with surgery or medical therapy of the underlying condition. Angiographic localization and embolization of the bleeding vessels can be used to stabilize a patient prior to surgery.

Localization of the bleeding site is often useful before arteriography because abnormal but nonbleeding vessels may be encountered in patients with diffuse or bilateral disease. Bronchoscopy can be used to identify the side and sometimes site of bleeding; however, it may be technically challenging in patients with acute massive hemoptysis. Chest radiography and CT might indicate the source of hemorrhage, but these tests are often unreliable. If the site of hemorrhage cannot be accurately localized or if diffuse disease is present, all identifiable bronchial artery branches are embolized.

The bronchial arteries are variable in number and distribution, but most arise from the descending thoracic aorta at the level of the T5–T6 vertebral bodies and the carina. The most common bronchial artery origin variations include single arteries bilaterally (30%), two bronchial arteries on one side and a single bronchial artery on the contralateral side (45%), and four bronchial arteries with two on each side (20%) or three left and one right (4%).[21] The most common arteriographic findings in patients with bronchial artery bleeding include enlargement of the bronchial artery (diameter >3 mm), hypervascularity, aneurysmal dilatation, prominent parenchy-

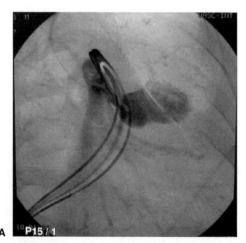
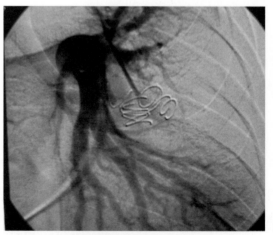

FIGURE 15-7. Traumatic pulmonary artery pseudoaneurysm. **A:** A pseudoaneurysm of the lingular branch of the left pulmonary artery resulting from a gunshot wound. **B:** Treatment was with coil embolization.

mal stain, and bronchial-to-pulmonary artery shunting (Figs. 15-8 and 15-9). In patients with neoplasms, the vascular supply is usually from bronchial arteries or parasitized intercostal arteries, and multiple feeding arteries are often present. Embolization is performed, even though no contrast extravasation is identified, because contrast extravasation into a bronchus is a rare arteriographic finding. If a potential bleeding source cannot be identified, a descending thoracic aortogram with the pigtail catheter placed near the left subclavian artery may be helpful.

Nonbronchial systemic collateral arteries are a significant bleeding source in many cases.[22] Common nonbronchial systemic collaterals include the internal mammary artery, thyrocervical trunk, branches of the subclavian or axillary artery, intercostal arteries, and inferior phrenic artery.

Occasionally, a spinal artery branch may arise from a bronchial artery. Careful consideration must be given to the arterial supply to the spinal cord when performing bronchial arteriography and embolization. The anterior spinal artery supplies the anterior portion of the cord and can be identified by its characteristic cephalic course with a hairpin bend in the midline within the ventral median sulcus. Many interventional radiologists consider the presence of spinal artery branches originating from the bronchial artery a contraindication to embolization (Fig. 15-10).[23] Some researchers, however, have described

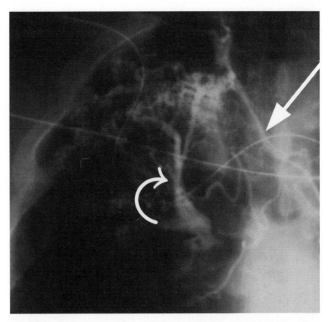

FIGURE 15-9. Bronchial artery to pulmonary artery shunting. Right bronchial arteriogram in a patient with massive hemoptysis from tuberculosis. Findings include bronchial artery (*arrow*) to pulmonary artery (*curved arrow*) shunting and hypervascularity.

successful bronchial artery embolization with no resultant neurologic complications in the presence of spinal artery branches. These procedures were performed with nonionic contrast and large embolization particles to prevent unintentional embolization of spinal feeders.[24,25] Because of the remote possibility of spinal cord injury from bronchial artery embolization, a neurologic examination should be performed before bronchial arteriography is done.

The most commonly used agents are polyvinyl alcohol (PVA) particles and Gelfoam pledgets. PVA particle sizes between 250 and 700 μ are used. Smaller particles could pass through small spinal artery branches or bronchial–pulmonary artery shunts. It is essential that the catheter be well seated and that there is no obvious risk of spinal artery embolization. If the spinal arteries are seen and the catheter can be advanced distal to their origin, embolic material can be placed from that location.

Visceral selective catheters, such as the Cobra, Simmons, or Mikaelsson, typically are used for bronchial artery catheterization. A coaxial microcatheter is often used for catheterization of bronchial artery branches.[26] Use of a conventional 5Fr catheter placed within the origin of the bronchial artery may not allow passage of embolic materials into peripheral branches because the catheter may be occlusive and prevent flow beyond the catheter tip. Use of a microcatheter permits superselective bronchial artery catheterization and embolization

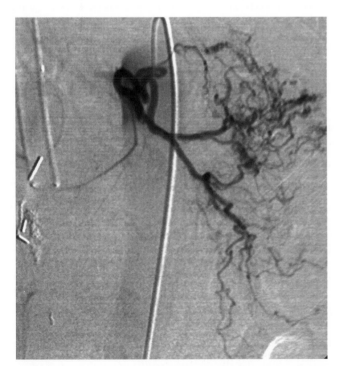

FIGURE 15-8. Bronchial arteriogram. Left bronchial arteriogram in a patient with massive hemoptysis from sarcoidosis. Findings include bronchial artery enlargement and hypervascularity.

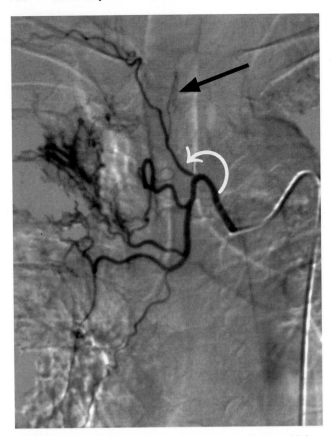

FIGURE 15-10. Spinal artery branch. The right bronchial artery and superior intercostal artery arise from a common bronchial intercostal trunk. An anterior spinal artery branch (*arrow*) arises from the superior intercostal artery (*curved arrow*). Embolization of the right bronchial artery was performed after placing a microcatheter distal to the origin of the intercostal artery and spinal artery branch.

tery embolization is ischemic injury to the spinal cord from contrast- or embolization-related injury, because radicular spinal arteries may arise from bronchial arteries or from intercostobronchial trunks. The reported frequency of this complication is less than 1%.

without occluding flow into the bronchial artery and occluding branches such as the spinal artery.

Bronchial artery embolization can be expected to provide initial control of hemorrhage in 75 to 90% of patients. Technical failure results from an inability to identify and catheterize the bronchial arteries. Failure to catheterize a bronchial artery occurs in up to 10% of patients.[23,27] The most common causes of recurrent bleeding include incomplete initial embolization or failure to identify all bleeding vessels, recruitment of collateral vessels, recanalization of embolized vessels, and progression of disease.[23,27] Late rebleeding (i.e., after 6 months) may occur in up to 20% of patients initially controlled by bronchial artery embolization. This problem is not unexpected, however, because embolization is a palliative procedure and does not directly treat the underlying disease.

Complications from embolotherapy occur in about 2 to 5% of cases and include nontarget embolization, bronchial or esophageal necrosis, and subintimal aortic injections.[26,27] The most severe complication of bronchial ar-

REFERENCES

1. Stein PD, Terrin ML, Hales CA, et al. Clinical, laboratory, roentgenographic, and electrographic findings in patients with acute pulmonary embolism and no pre-existing cardiac or pulmonary disease. *Chest* 1991;100:598–603.
2. Garg K, Welsh CH, Feyerbend AJ, et al. Pulmonary embolism: diagnosis with spiral CT and ventilation-perfusion scanning-correlation with pulmonary angiographic results or clinical outcome. *Radiology* 1998;208:201–208.
3. Drucker EA, Rivitz SM, Shephard JA, et al. Acute pulmonary embolism: assessment of helical CT for diagnosis. *Radiology* 1998;209:235–241.
4. Goodman LR, Curtin JJ, Mewissen MW, et al. Detection of pulmonary embolism in patients with unresolved clinical and scintigraphic diagnosis: helical CT versus angiography. *AJR Am J Roentgenol* 1995;164:1369–1374.
5. Erdman WA, Peshock RM, Redman HC, et al. Pulmonary embolism: comparison of MR images with radionuclide and angiographic studies. *Radiology* 1994;190:499–508.
6. Browse NL, Thomas ML. Source of non-lethal pulmonary emboli. *Lancet* 1974;1:258–259.
7. Goodman LR, Lipchik RJ. Diagnosis of acute pulmonary embolism: time for a new approach. *Radiology* 1996;199:25–27.
8. Zuckerman DA, Sterling KM, Oser RF. Safety of pulmonary angiography in the 1990s. *J Vasc Interv Radiol* 1996;7:199–205.
9. Oser RF, Zuckerman DA, Gutierrez FR, Brink JA. Anatomic distribution of pulmonary emboli at pulmonary angiography: implications for cross-section imaging. *Radiology* 1996;199:31–35.
10. Fred HL, Axelrad MA, Lewis JM, et al. Rapid resolution of pulmonary thromboemboli in man: an angiographic study. *JAMA* 1966;196:1137–1139.
11. Stein PD, Athanasoulis C, Alavi A, et al. Complications and validity of pulmonary angiography in acute pulmonary embolism. *Circulation* 1992;85:462–468.
12. Haskal ZJ, Soulen MC, Huettl EA, et al. Life-threatening pulmonary emboli and cor pulmonale: treatment with percutaneous pulmonary artery stent placement. *Radiology* 1994;191:473–475.
13. Greenfield LJ, Proctor MC, Williams DM, Wakefield TW. Long-term experience with transvenous catheter pulmonary embolectomy. *J Vasc Surg* 1993;18:450–457.
14. Uflacker R, Strange C, Vujic I. Massive pulmonary embolism: preliminary results of treatment with the Amplatz thrombectomy device. *J Vasc Interv Radiol* 1996;7:519–528.
15. Lang EV, Barnhart WH, Walton DL, Raab SS. Percutaneous pulmonary thrombectomy. *J Vasc Interv Radiol* 1997;8:261–266.
16. Auger WR, Fedullo PF, Moser KM, et al. Chronic major-vessel thromboembolic pulmonary artery obstruction: appearance at angiography. *Radiology* 1992;182:393–398.
17. Guttmacher AE, Marchuk DA, White RI Jr. Hereditary hemorrhagic telangiectasia. *N Engl J Med* 1995;333:918–924.
18. Coley SC, Jackson JE. Pulmonary arteriovenous malformations. *Clin Radiol* 1998;53:396–404.
19. White RI Jr, Pollak JS, Wirth JA. Pulmonary arteriovenous malformations: diagnosis and transcatheter embolotherapy. *J Vasc Interv Radiol* 1996;7:787–804.
20. Fernando HC, Stein M, Benfield JR, Link DP. Role of bronchial

artery embolization in the management of hemoptysis. *Arch Surg* 1998;133:862–865.

21. Kadir S. Regional anatomy of the thoracic aorta. In: *Atlas of Normal and Variant Angiographic Anatomy.* Philadelphia: WB Saunders; 1991:49.

22. Keller FS, Rosch J, Loflin TG, et al. Nonbronchial systemic collateral arteries: significance in percutaneous embolotherapy for hemoptysis. *Radiology* 1987;164:687–692.

23. Mal H, Rullon I, Mellot F, et al. Immediate and long-term results of bronchial artery embolization for life-threatening hemoptysis. *Chest* 1999;115:996–1001.

24. Mauro MA, Jaques PF, Morris S. Bronchial artery embolization for control of hemoptysis. *Semin Interv Radiol* 1992;9:45–51.

25. Uflacker R, Kaemmerer A, Picon PD, et al. Bronchial artery embolization in the management of hemoptysis: technical aspects and long-term results. *Radiology* 1985;157:637–644.

26. Tanaka N, Yamakado K, Murashima S, et al. Superselective bronchial artery embolization for hemoptysis with a coaxial microcatheter system. *J Vasc Interv Radiol* 1997;8:65–70.

27. Remy-Jardin M, Wattinne L, Remy J. Transcatheter occlusion of pulmonary arterial circulation and collateral supply: failures, incidents, and complications. *Radiology* 1991;180:699–705.

16

Diseases of the Thoracic Aorta

*HUGO SPINDOLA-FRANCO, SCOTT SEGAL, BERNARD G. FISH,
and MARK A. GREENBERG*

Medical and surgical treatment as well as recently developed interventional catheter procedures for the treatment of aortic diseases requires precise delineation of the pathological disorders. Concurrent with the development of these new techniques, the emergence of new imaging modalities such as magnetic resonance imaging (MRI), spiral computed tomography (CT), and transesophageal echocardiography (TEE) have revolutionized our ability to diagnose these complex conditions. Once considered the gold standard, angiography remains important only when other techniques are inconclusive.

Acquired diseases of the aorta such as ectasia, aneurysm, dissection, and its variants occur as a result of degenerative processes in older persons. These processes are accelerated in persons who have underlying connective tissue disorders such as Marfan syndrome and in those with hypertension and atherosclerosis. Of these entities, acute aortic dissection or rupture may represent a surgical emergency. Aortic trauma also results in an acute emergency requiring the most expeditious diagnosis and surgical management. Aortic arteritis syndromes are caused by inflammatory diseases such as giant cell arteritis and Takayasu arteritis, which may lead to aortic insufficiency or obstructive lesions. Aortitis also occurs during late stages of syphilis. Complications of catheter and surgical procedures also may require surgical intervention. Recognition of these complications has become more important as more procedures are performed. Secondary involvement of the aorta by neoplasms, abscesses, and hematomas are a challenge to the clinician. Modern imaging techniques have become essential in the diagnosis and management of these entities.

Congenital diseases of the aorta constitute a smaller segment of the population with aortic disease.[1,2] The most common entities are preoperative and postoperative coarctation of the aorta and patent ductus arteriosus. Other uncommon disorders occasionally are encountered, including vascular rings, cervical aortic arch, interruption of the aortic arch, and anomalous origin of a pulmonary artery. Pulmonary artery sling and ductus arteriosus sling are rarely encountered. Bronchial arteries are dilated in cyanotic congenital heart disease with pulmonary atresia and may be hemodynamically significant as a source of pulmonary blood flow. Coil embolization may be necessary before surgical correction of these entities. Pulmonary sequestrations are supplied by vessels arising from the aorta and may be treated by coil embolization.

■ Aortic Dissection

Aortic dissection consists of an intimal tear in the wall of the aorta that causes separation of the intramural layers, usually between the middle and outer thirds of the media, creating a false lumen (Fig. 16-1). Blood in the false lumen may reenter the true lumen via a second intimal tear, or it may rupture through the adventitia into the periaortic tissues. Most commonly, dissections are believed to be caused by cystic medial necrosis. Proximal dissections tend to occur in younger persons who often are found to have Marfan syndrome (Figs. 16-2 and 16-3). Less commonly, inherited connective tissue disorders such as osteogenesis imperfecta, Turner syndrome, and Ehlers-Danlos syndrome may be associated with proximal dissections. Distal dissections occur more commonly in older patients with hypertension. Other less common causes include

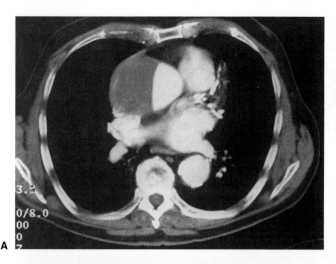

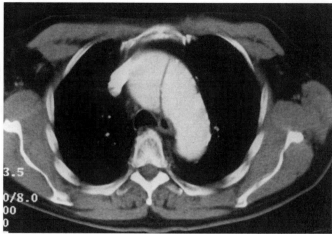

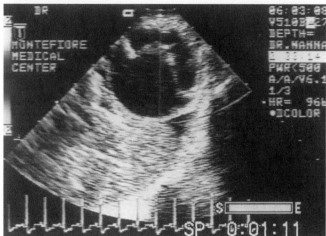

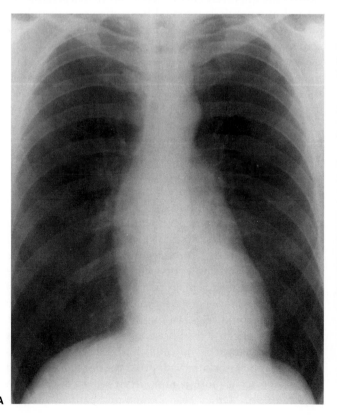

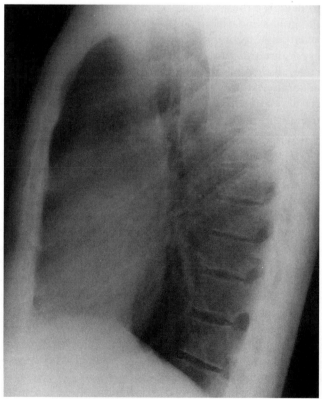

FIGURE 16-1. Type I dissection of the aorta in a 74-year-old man. The dynamic spiral computed tomography (CT) shows the characteristic flap in a type I dissection involving the ascending aorta **(A)** and the proximal aortic arch **(B).** The brachiocephalic vessels were not involved. Calcification of the wall of the aorta is noted. Transesophageal echocardiogram in a different patient with a type I dissection showing the flap in the descending aorta **(C)**. On the real-time image, the flap oscillates in the lumen of aorta. The true lumen is closest to the transducer and the false lumen is farther away. The echogenicity beyond the aorta represents extravasated blood in the mediastinum.

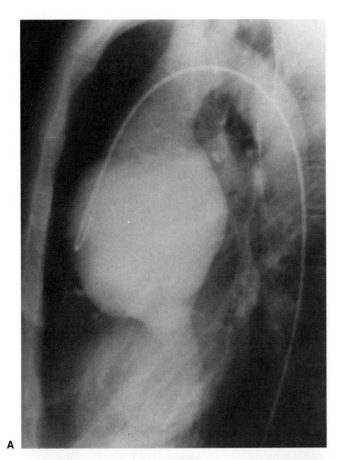

A

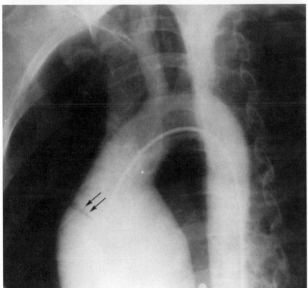

B

atherosclerosis, trauma, syphilis, idiopathic kyphoscoliosis, and congenital heart defects, such as coarctation and pseudocoarctation of the aorta. Approximately 2,000 new cases of aortic dissection are diagnosed each year in the United States.[3,4] The male-to-female ratio is approximately 2:1, with a peak incidence in the sixth and seventh decades of life.

Two major classifications of aortic dissection are widely used. The older classification, introduced by DeBakey et al., divides aortic dissections into type I, which includes those involving the ascending and descending aorta (Fig. 16-1); type II, which involves the ascending aorta only; and type III, which involves the descending aorta (Fig. 16-4).[5] A mnemonic for this classification is "BAD": type I = both aortas, type II = ascending aorta and type III = descending aorta. Another classification, introduced by Dailey et al., and often called the *Stanford classification*, divides aortic dissection into two groups. Dailey's type A includes proximal dissections as well as those distal dissections that extend retrograde to involve the arch and ascending aorta. Type B includes dissections of the distal aorta without proximal extension.[6]

Important variants of aortic dissection are caused by penetrating ulcers and by intramural hemorrhage (IMH) (Fig. 16-5).[7] Penetrating ulcers result from erosion of atherosclerotic plaque with eventual violation of the internal elastic lamina.[8] Penetrating ulcers occur most often in persons who have extensive atherosclerotic disease, but not in persons with Marfan syndrome or other diseases of connective tissue. Ulcers affect the mid-portion to distal portion of the descending thoracic aorta almost exclusively and do not result in valvular, pericardial, or neurovascular complications that occur with aortic dissection. The ulcer has a nipple-like configuration extending

←

FIGURE 16-3. Aortic insufficiency in an asymptomatic patient with Marfan syndrome. The aortogram. **A:** Lateral view. **B:** Shallow left anterior oblique (LAO) view shows that the root of the aorta is dilated symmetrically and bulbous, with effacement of the semilunar sinuses. Aortic insufficiency is present. In (**B**) a tear is demonstrated in the anterolateral wall (*arrows*). The tear was not detected on the lateral film, which emphasizes the requirement to look carefully for tears, using multiple views as necessary. This example is a "silent aortic dissection" (same patient as in Fig. 16-2). (Courtesy of Spindola-Franco H, Fish BG, eds. Radiology of the heart: cardiac imaging in infants, children, and adults. New York: Springer-Verlag, 1985:204.)

←

FIGURE 16-2. Findings on chest roentgenography in a man with Marfan syndrome. **A:** Frontal view. **B:** Lateral view. Marked dilatation of the root of the aorta produces a double density within the cardiac silhouette (pseudo left atrial enlargement). The normal angle formed between the ascending aorta and the base of the heart is effaced by the dilated ascending aorta. The aorta also displaces the main pulmonary artery superiorly and laterally, producing a bulge in the pulmonary artery segment simulating pulmonary artery dilatation. In the lateral film, the dilated aortic root obliterates the retrosternal clear space. Thus, the lateral film shows that the double density noted on the frontal view is due to the dilatation of the aortic root rather than enlargement of the left atrium. Note that the dilatation of the root of the aorta does not extend into the aortic arch. Mild left ventricular enlargement is present (same patient as in Fig. 16-3). (Courtesy of Spindola-Franco H, Fish BG, eds. Radiology of the heart: cardiac imaging in infants, children, and adults. New York: Springer-Verlag, 1985:203.)

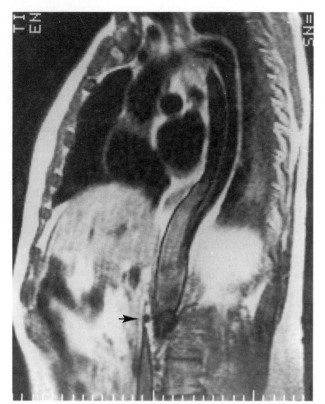

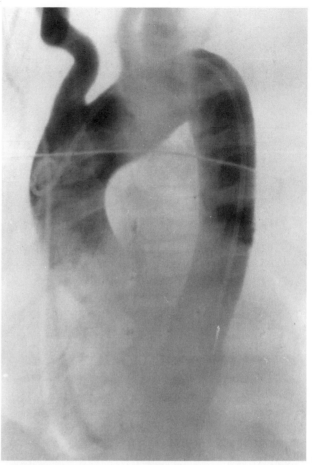

A

FIGURE 16-4. Complications of DeBakey type III aortic dissection in a patient who presented with acute abdominal pain. The left anterior oblique (LAO) plane of a T1-weighted spin-echo image shows two flaps distal to the left subclavian artery. One false lumen is confined to the distal aortic arch and proximal descending aorta. The other extends into the abdomen, compromising the superior mesenteric artery (*arrow*). Ischemia of the gut caused acute abdominal pain in this patient. Angiography was not successful because the catheter could not be advanced into the lumen of the aorta.

beyond the intima and is surrounded by hematoma. The process may be contained spontaneously or may progress to false aneurysm formation or aortic rupture (Fig. 16-6).

IMH may result from rupture of aortic vasa vasorum.[9] IMH differs from classic dissection in that hematoma forms within the aortic wall, but an intimal tear is not present.[10,11] Intramural hemorrhage may be the first stage in the development of aortic dissection, the second

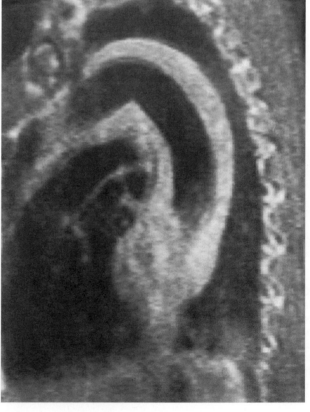

B

FIGURE 16-5. Angiogram and magnetic resonance imaging (MRI) in a patient with intramural hemorrhage (IMH). **A:** Subtraction film from the left anterior oblique (LAO) view of an aortogram. **B:** T1-weighted spin-echo pulse sequence MRI in the sagittal plane. In (**A**) the aortic lumen is normal with no intimal flap or leakage, whereas in (**B**) the high signal intensity and increased thickness of the aortic wall indicate intramural hemorrhage. The increased signal intensity indicates a subacute process. Acute hemorrhage would be isointense and may not be separated from the wall of the aorta. Blood is also present in the mediastinum, considered a typical feature of IMH.

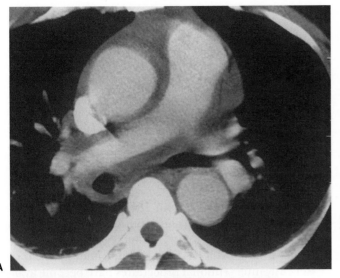

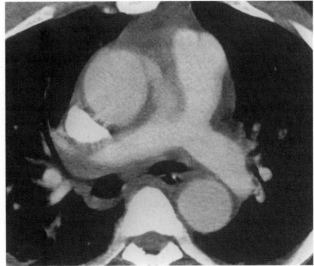

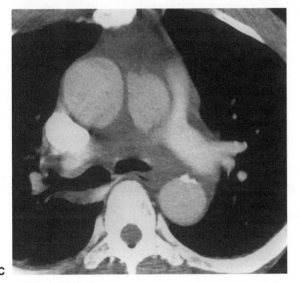

FIGURE 16-6. Acute perforation of an atherosclerotic ulcer in a 54-year-old man with sudden onset of severe chest pain. Frames from a dynamic spiral CT scan. **A:** The lowest slice, the ascending aorta is dilated, but no dissection is noted. **B:** 1 cm higher, a jet of contrast exits the aortic lumen into the mediastinum. **C:** 1 cm above (**B**), a collection of contrast is noted just under the aortic arch. The surrounding fat is dense ("dirty fat sign"), indicating infiltration with blood. These findings are consistent with rupture of an atherosclerotic plaque. Soon after the scan, the patient became more unstable and was taken to the operating room. At surgery, an aortic dissection and a hemopericardium were found, indicating that propagation of the pathologic process had occurred, accounting for the sudden deterioration after the scan.

stage being an intimal tear that allows blood to flow into the false lumen, extending the plane of dissection.[12] Complications of IMH are the same as with aortic dissection, but they are significantly less common with IMH than with aortic dissection.

Clinical features

Aortic dissection often presents with severe chest pain (anterior or posterior) with a tearing character. Pain is maximal at onset and changes in location as the dissection propagates. Painless ("silent") dissection is rare (Fig. 16-3). Acute complications include aortic insufficiency and congestive heart failure. Aortic insufficiency occurs in up to 50% of patients who undergo type A dissection secondary to either widening or distortion of the aortic annulus, causing failure of coaptation of the valve leaflets, or torn leaflets. Congestive heart failure may result from sudden onset of severe aortic insufficiency. Syncope as a present-

ing symptom may be associated with rupture into the pericardial cavity and cardiac tamponade. Physical findings with aortic dissection include shock with normal to elevated blood pressure and pseudohypotension or pulse deficits secondary to dissection of the brachiocephalic vessels. Myocardial infarction occurs in a small percentage of patients with proximal dissection, secondary to involvement of the coronary arteries. Neurological findings and renal and mesenteric infarctions occur as a result of occlusion of related vessels. Left ventricular hypertrophy is commonly noted on electrocardiography. Aortic dissection should be suspected in patients with chest pain and no electrocardiographic signs of myocardial ischemia.

Imaging modalities

On chest roentgenography, the characteristic findings of aortic dissection are a widened aortic contour and a "calcium sign" consisting of a greater than 5 mm separation of the calcification of the aortic arch from its outer contour. A left pleural effusion may be present, indicating leakage into the pleural space. The trachea may be deviated. Importantly, the chest roentgenogram may be normal in aortic dissection.

TEE (Fig. 16-1) and MRI are both very sensitive in the diagnosis of aortic dissection.[13,14] Advantages of TEE include the availability of this modality at the bedside, enabling diagnosis in acutely unstable patients. TEE is useful in proximal and distal dissections. A disadvantage is its inability to delineate the branches of the aortic arch accurately. In addition, TEE is an invasive procedure.

If available, MRI is the procedure of choice in persons with aortic dissection who are relatively stable and can tolerate a longer procedure (Fig. 16-4). The advantages of MRI include its ability to determine the exact extent and site of origin of the dissection and its anatomic relationships with neighboring organs. MRI also allows the diagnosis of associated aortic insufficiency and leakage. By using MRI, thrombus or flow in the false lumen can be detected. Cine MRI allows visualization of the oscillations of the flap separating the false lumen from the true lumen, which is a hallmark of aortic dissection.

Spiral and ultrafast CT are extremely useful in the acute assessment of aortic dissection when MRI is not available or when the patient cannot tolerate the time required by the MRI examination (Fig. 16-1). Ultrafast CT is available in only a few centers, whereas spiral CT has replaced standard CT in many centers and often is staffed through the night. The shorter time taken to perform a CT study compared with the time taken by MRI should be weighed against the radiation exposure involved and the requirement to administer angiographic contrast medium. One limitation of CT relates to difficulty in timing the injection to enhance the false lumen.

MRI, spiral CT, TEE, and angiography are all complementary, and each has an ability to identify aortic dissection; however, angiography cannot detect IMH (Fig. 16-5).[15] Atherosclerotic ulcers are detected by angiography, but the hematoma surrounding a penetrating ulcer may be missed. For this reason, angiography is not the primary diagnostic modality for these entities but should be used when the others are not definitive.

Treatment

Without treatment, aortic dissection is a lethal disease. Death occurs as a result of progression of the dissection, which causes damage to vital structures. Ninety percent of untreated patients die within one year, with the highest mortality occurring during the first week after the onset.[16] Initial treatment for all patients includes beta-blockers and aggressive control of hypertension to prevent progression. Proximal dissections are surgically repaired

early or even emergently because of the risk of catastrophic consequences such as acute aortic insufficiency, cardiac tamponade, and neurologic complications with even minimal progression. On the other hand, distal dissections may be treated medically unless they show signs of rupture, impending rupture, or renal or mesenteric compromise. Chronic dissections, which present 2 weeks or longer after onset, also may be treated medically because they already have passed the most dangerous period, suggesting a nonlethal outcome. Surgery of proximal dissections commonly consists of placement of a composite graft containing a prosthetic valve. The native ascending aorta is wrapped around the graft. The coronary arteries are reimplanted using a button of native aorta to facilitate the anastomosis. Conduit grafts also may be used to replace the aortic arch and descending aorta.

Recently interventional procedures have become available as alternatives to surgery for dissections in the descending aorta.[17-19] Placement of a self-expandable covered stent (Gianturco stent) to cover the proximal entry site reestablishes the true lumen by compressing the false lumen so that thrombosis of the residual false lumen is promoted. The catheter is inserted by way of the femoral artery into the true lumen, and the intraluminal prosthesis is deployed slightly proximal to the entry site of the dissection. The diameter of the device should be slightly larger than the aortic diameter to prevent migration. Another treatment option currently being explored is the percutaneous creation of a reentry tear in an aortic dissection, which decompresses the false lumen of a dissection, thereby limiting its progression.[20]

Long-term follow-up is necessary for patients treated medically and surgically. Blood pressure must be controlled at the lowest level tolerated. Follow-up chest roentgenograms are essential to detect changes that suggest late complications such as false aneurysms and leakage into the pleural space. Serial imaging studies are also essential to detect complications or progression. Currently, MRI is considered the procedure of choice.[21]

■ Thoracic Aortic Aneurysms

Aneurysms of the thoracic aorta are localized, sac-like dilatations of the aortic wall. All layers of the aortic wall are involved. They may be saccular, in which only part of the circumference is involved, or fusiform, if all or almost all of the circumference is involved. Fusiform aneurysms are four times more common than saccular aneurysms, which are found chiefly in the ascending aorta.

Aneurysms may be congenital or acquired. Congenital aneurysms are rare and mostly affect the sinuses of Valsalva. Causes of acquired thoracic aortic aneurysms include atherosclerosis, syphilis, trauma, cystic medial necrosis, arteritis, and infection (mycotic). Atherosclerotic aneurysms are the most common, and their incidence is increasing as a consequence of increasing longevity of the population. They are more common beyond the aortic arch. Syphilitic (luetic) aneurysms are most common in the ascending aorta. Posttraumatic aneurysms occur in a small number of persons who survive chest trauma. These are found mainly in the most proximal portion of the descending aorta, resulting from a small tear. Mycotic aneurysms, also called *infected aneurysms,* are rare and are caused by sepsis in the wall of the aorta or any vessel. Infection can cause fusiform, saccular, or even false aneurysms. They can perforate into adjacent venous structures, resulting in arteriovenous fistulae.

Annuloaortic ectasia is a specific subgroup of aortic aneurysm affecting the root of the aorta and the aortic annulus (Figs. 16-2 and 16-3). This entity is typical of Marfan syndrome and other conditions associated with cystic medial necrosis. Persons with annuloaortic ectasia should be investigated for other stigmata of Marfan syndrome. The ectasia is often progressive, leading to aortic insufficiency, congestive heart failure, dissection and rupture of the ascending aorta, sometimes resulting in sudden death. A diameter greater than 7 cm is associated with a high incidence of aortic dissection, and usually this measurement in itself constitutes sufficient grounds for replacement of the aortic root and the aortic valve with a valved conduit. The coronary arteries are reimplanted into the conduit. Cystic medial necrosis with dilatation of the aortic root also occurs in Ehlers-Danlos syndrome, osteogenesis imperfecta, homocysteinuria, Larsen syndrome, and Cogan syndrome.

Clinical features

Presenting features relate to the size and location of the aneurysm. Small aneurysms may be asymptomatic whereas large aneurysms produce symptoms by directly compressing adjacent structures. Wheezing, cough, dyspnea, stridor, hemoptysis, recurrent pneumonitis, intrapulmonary hemorrhage, and superior vena cava syndrome all may result from large thoracic aneurysms. As with aortic dissection, acute aortic insufficiency may result in acute congestive heart failure. Collapse and sudden death may be caused by rupture of an aortic aneurysm. Most patients, however, die of associated disease unrelated to the aneurysms (e.g., coronary artery disease). Patients with mycotic aneurysms have other signs of infection, such as high fever. Other features that differentiate mycotic aneurysms from uninfected aneurysms include tenderness, lack of calcification, and early vertebral erosion.

Imaging modalities

Most aneurysms are easily detectable on chest roentgenography, appearing as a dilated aorta or as a localized bulge (Fig. 16-7). The differential diagnosis includes an uncoiled aorta (*atherosclerotic elongated aorta*), kinking or buckling of the aorta (*pseudocoarctation*), and poststenotic dilatation (*aortic stenosis*). A localized aneurysm may be confused with a mediastinal mass. Calcification occurs much less commonly in thoracic aneurysms than in aneurysms involving the abdominal aorta.

Axial or spiral CT, MRI, TEE, and angiography are all definitive in the diagnosis of aneurysms of the thoracic aorta. If available and not contraindicated (e.g., pacemaker, hemodynamic instability), MRI is the procedure of choice. No radiation is involved, and no intravenous contrast needs to be administered.

Treatment

Survival is related to the size of the aneurysm. Aneurysms larger than 6 to 7 cm in diameter and those causing symptoms by compression are more likely to rupture than smaller ones. Surgical excision is indicated in aneurysms greater than 7 cm in the ascending or descending aorta and in smaller aneurysms if they produce symptoms.

■ Aortic Trauma

Injuries to the thoracic aorta may be blunt or penetrating. Blunt trauma may be associated with a sudden high-speed deceleration on impact, such as a motor vehicle accident or severe fall or explosion. Abrupt deceleration creates shearing forces at a point where a highly mobile portion of the aorta joins a relatively fixed segment. The most common site is the aortic isthmus (the portion of the aorta between the left subclavian artery and the ligamentum arteriosum), which is attached to the relatively fixed segment at the site of insertion of the ligamentum arteriosum. The second most frequent site is the ascending aorta, just above the aortic valve. Tears of the ascending aorta are associated with significantly higher mortality than those in the isthmic region. Recently, an "osseous pinch mechanism" was described in which the spine and manubrium/clavicle/first rib may play a role during acute deceleration injury.[22] Aortic trauma also may result from interventions such as cardiac catheterization or balloon dilatation of coarctation of the aorta. The tear of the aorta may be small, resulting in a localized aneurysm or false aneurysm, or it may be circumferential, resulting in transection of the aorta.

Clinical features

A high index of suspicion is needed because severe injuries of the central nervous system, visceral injury, and multiple fractures may overshadow the diagnosis. The

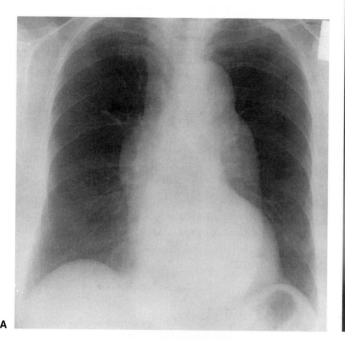

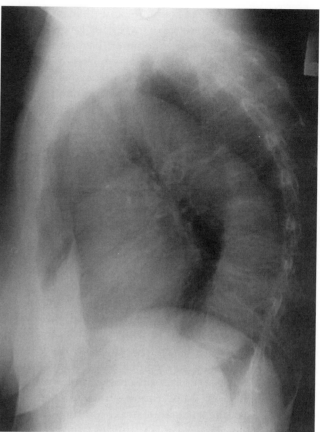

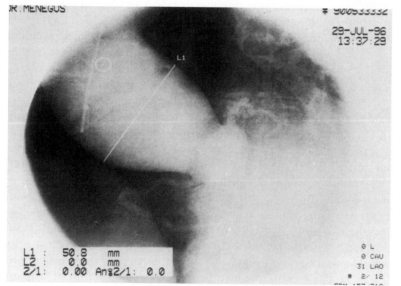

FIGURE 16-7. Aneurysmal dilatation of the aorta in a 67-year-old man noted on chest roentgenogram. **A:** Frontal. **B:** Lateral. The magnetic resonance imaging (MRI) and computed tomography (CT) scan showed no dissection. **C:** The aortogram in the left anterior oblique (LAO) view was performed at the time of coronary angiography. The ascending aorta measures 5 cm above the sinotubular junction. The coronary ostia are unobstructed. Mild aortic insufficiency was noted. The aortic arch and descending aorta also were aneurysmally dilated (not shown). The patient was monitored medically.

syndrome of "acute coarctation" (upper-extremity hypertension, low pressure in the lower extremities, systolic murmur over the precordium or in the interscapular region, and a palpable radial-femoral pulse lag) is diagnostic. Other signs of aortic trauma include hoarseness, cough, or dysphagia from compression of the adjacent recurrent laryngeal nerve, trachea, or esophagus. Additionally, swelling of the lower neck and paraplegia may be noted. An aortic insufficiency murmur is heard with significant tears of the ascending aorta.

Imaging modalities

The roentgenogram of the chest is essential in the diagnosis of trauma even in the absence of classic clinical features. Signs include a widened mediastinum, obliteration of the aortic arch (knob), a rightward tracheal shift, depression of the left mainstem bronchus, displacement of the nasogastric tube to the right, displacement of the right or left paraspinal line, and opacification of the space between the descending aorta and the pulmonary artery.[23] A pleural effusion, especially one that obliterates the left thoracic apex (apical cap sign) is an important sign.[24] An aortic transection also can occur in the absence of these signs. The portable technique and other factors occuring during the course of acute trauma may obscure the findings. Bone fractures, pulmonary contusion, pneumothorax, and pneumoperitoneum indicate severe thoracic trauma, and should result in a suspicion of aortic trauma.

Despite the advent of sophisticated noninvasive imaging modalities such as spiral CT and MRI, angiography remains the diagnostic procedure of choice when aortic transection is suspected. MRI can provide a complete diagnosis in patients with aortic trauma, but it requires a lengthy procedure and may not be practical for critically ill patients who are instrumented with multiple invasive monitoring and life support devices. High-speed CT may be a useful primary imaging modality. Abdominal CT can be performed concurrently. Associated hemorrhage and hematoma, which might be missed by both chest roentgenography and angiography, may be detected by CT scanning or MRI. It is important to note that traumatic rupture of the aorta can be missed on CT scanning unless a linear lucency inside the aortic lumen caused by the torn edge of the aortic wall is noted or a dissection is present. Irregularity of the intima of the opacified aortic lumen and periaortic or intraluminal hematoma are other confirmatory findings on CT scanning, but these may not be diagnostic. Mediastinal hematoma usually is caused by tearing of small vessels, which requires no treatment. Immediate angiography with digital subtraction should follow if the CT scan is not definitive and the patient is stable. If a patient cannot be moved, TEE may be performed at the bedside to exclude transection of the aorta. In the future, intravascular ultrasound may play an important role.[25,26]

Treatment

Surgery should be performed as soon as possible once aortic transection is diagnosed. The repair consists of resection of the torn edges and interposition of a graft. The distal circulation may be supported by a pump oxygenerator or by a conduit bypass. Late sequelae include aneurysms that may require secondary surgical excision to prevent dissection and rupture. Early animal trials that may lead to the replacement of surgical treatment using covered endovascular stents in selected subjects are ongoing.[27]

■ Penetrating trauma

Penetrating trauma to the aorta and its branches is caused by puncture or laceration, most commonly a result of a bullet or stab wound. These are likely to cause acute exsanguination and require immediate surgical exploration with or without the findings on chest roentgenography of a widened mediastinum, pleural effusions, and cardiomegaly (hemopericardium). Although signs of acute penetrating trauma may be obtained by angiography or by CT scanning, these patients are usually too unstable to allow these studies.

■ Aortic Arteritis Syndromes

Aortitis is caused by an infectious or immunologic process that affects any layer of the wall of the aorta. Aortitis may manifest as aneurysmal dilatation (*ectasia*) or as segmental narrowing. The aneurysmal form is more common, and fusiform aneurysms are more common than saccular ones. Conditions that result in ectasia of the ascending aorta frequently cause aortic insufficiency. These conditions include Takayasu's arteritis, giant cell arteritis, syphilis, rheumatoid arthritis, ankylosing spondylitis, psoriatic arthritis, ulcerative colitis, relapsing polychondritis, and Reiter syndrome. Stenosing aortitis occurs in a few conditions, including Takayasu's arteritis and radiation aortitis. In most inflammatory diseases of the aorta, the media is primarily involved, with occasional damage to the adventitia. Thickening of the intima is a reactive phenomenon. Rheumatic fever and rheumatoid arthritis cause an inflammatory reaction and fibrinoid necrosis of all three layers of the aorta, resulting in a true panaortitis.[28]

Takayasu's arteritis is a syndrome caused by a panarteritis and leads to narrowing and occlusion of the aorta and its branches. Less commonly, the coronary ostia may be involved. Localized areas of dilatation also may occur (Fig. 16-8). This syndrome usually occurs in young women, occasionally in children, and rarely in infants and middle-aged individuals. The female-to-male ratio is 8.5:1, peaking in the teenage years.

The syndrome has been classified into four subtypes according to the site of involvement. Type I (8%) involves the aortic arch and brachiocephalic vessels. Type II (11%) affects the thoracoabdominal aorta, especially the renal arteries. Type III (65%) combines the features of both types I and II. Type IV (45%) includes characteristics of the first three types along with involvement of the pulmonary arteries.[29]

Clinically, there are two recognized phases of the syndrome. The early, or systemic phase, is characterized by the signs and symptoms of a generalized inflammatory process, such as fever, anorexia, malaise, weight loss, night

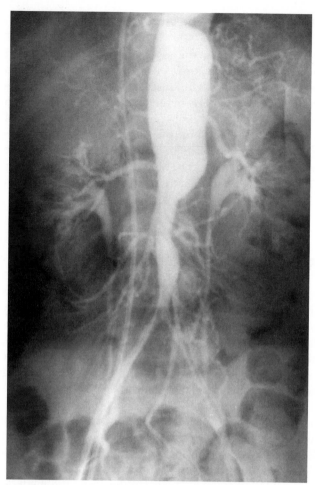

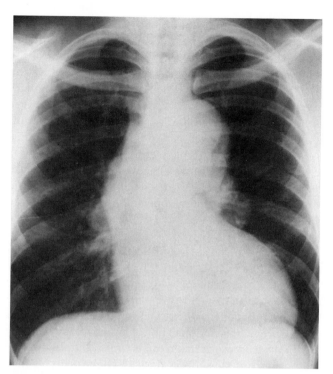

FIGURE 16-9. Aneurysmal dilatation of the aorta and severe aortic insufficiency in a 31-year-old patient with giant cell arteritis. The frontal chest roentgenogram shows cardiomegaly with moderate left ventricular dilatation. The left heart border is elongated, and the cardiac apex projects below the left hemidiaphragm. The ascending aorta and the aortic arch are markedly dilated. Mild pulmonary venous hypertension is indicated by equalization of the caliber of the upper and lower pulmonary vessels. Microscopic examination of surgical specimens of the aortic wall showed giant cell aortitis (same patient as in Fig. 16-10). (Courtesy of Spindola-Franco H, Fish BG, eds. Radiology of the heart: cardiac imaging in infants, children, and adults. New York: Springer-Verlag, 1985:200.)

FIGURE 16-8. Abdominal aortogram in a 6-year-old girl with Takayasu arteritis and severe systemic hypertension. Marked aneurysmal dilatation of the abdominal aorta is noted with minimal narrowing of the right and severe narrowing of the left common iliac artery. Similar changes were found in the thoracic aorta on magnetic resonance imaging (MRI).

sweats, arthralgias, pleuritic pain, and fatigue. This phase generally lasts from weeks to months and is followed by the occlusive features of the late phase, which include diminished or absent pulses (96%), bruits (94%), hypertension (74%), and congestive heart failure (28%). Angina or myocardial infarction may occur if coronary arteries are involved.[30]

The etiology of Takayasu's arteritis is probably autoimmune, although no specific cause has been identified. Laboratory studies in the early phase are consistent with an autoimmune etiology but are nonspecific and include elevated erythrocyte sedimentation rate, low-grade leukocytosis, and mild anemia.

Imaging modalities

In the early phase, the chest roentgenogram is frequently normal. In the late phase, nonspecific findings such as cardiomegaly and congestive heart failure may be pre-

sent. The authors observed abnormal dilatation of the descending aorta. In addition, rib notching resulting from acquired coarctation has been observed in severe cases. Angiography, spiral CT, and MRI demonstrate characteristic findings such as stenosis of the aorta and its branches and poststenotic dilatation, saccular aneurysms, and even occlusions. The aorta may present the typical "rat-tail narrowing." Echocardiography is helpful in assessing left ventricular function and in identifying the presence of thrombus in the left ventricle.

Treatment

Treatment is directed at control of the initial inflammatory process using steroids. Congestive heart failure and hypertension are treated with medical therapy. Surgical intervention occasionally is required in severe cases. Endarterectomy or bypass surgery is used for obstructive lesions. Excision of aneurysms, and rarely aortic valve replacement, may be necessary. Balloon angioplasty has been used in selected cases. Endovascular covered stents for treatment of aneurysms, or a combination of stenting and balloon dilatation for selected stenotic lesions, may be useful.

■ Giant Cell Arteritis

Giant cell arteritis, also known as *temporal arteritis,* is a granulomatous arteritis that involves medium-sized arteries in patients aged 50 years and older. The mean age of onset is 69 years, and 64% of cases occur in women. The aorta and its branches are involved in 15% of cases. The etiology is unknown, but it may be infectious or autoimmune. The disease may manifest rapidly or it may have an insidious course. The triad of severe headache, malaise, and fever, along with aching and myalgias of the shoulder and pelvic girdle musculature, neck, and proximal extremities, has been called *polymyalgia rheumatica.* The symptoms of claudication, headache, visual changes, and scalp tenderness are the result of arteritis. Claudication can occur in muscle groups in which the vascular supply is involved. Most commonly, muscles of mastication, deglutition, and the extremities are involved. Visual symptoms include diplopia, ptosis, and blindness, either partial or complete. Rarely, the aorta may be the first target,

mimicking Takayasu's arteritis. Even more rarely, aortic aneurysms, aortic insufficiency, and aortic dissection may occur. Death can occur from heart failure, aortic rupture, or dissection. Laboratory findings, such as an elevated erythrocyte sedimentation rate, are nonspecific, reflecting an inflammatory process. A definitive pathologic diagnosis usually is established by examining multiple biopsies of the temporal arteries.[28]

Imaging modalities

In patients with aortic involvement, chest roentgenography shows a widened mediastinum (Fig. 16-9). The left ventricle may be enlarged if significant aortic insufficiency is present. MRI is the procedure of choice to assess the degree of aortic involvement and the presence of aortic insufficiency. TEE may help to distinguish giant cell arteries from arteriosclerotic disease because irregularities of the wall and pedunculated plaques noted with arteriosclerosis are not present in giant cell arteritis. CT is indicated when signs of dissection are evident, and immediate diagnosis is necessary. Cardiac catheterization may be required before surgery to assess the extent of aortic insufficiency relative to the need for replacement of the aortic valve (Fig. 16-10).

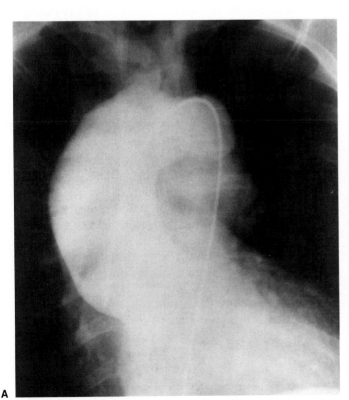

A

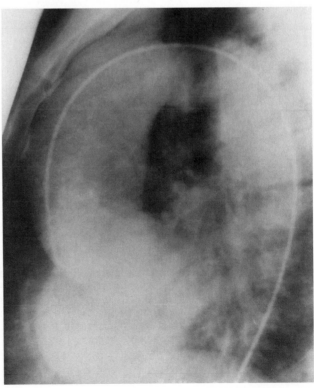

B

FIGURE 16-10. Aortogram in a 31-year-old man with giant cell arteritis and aortic insufficiency. **A:** Anteroposterior view. **B:** Lateral view. The ascending and descending aorta are dilated. The arch is also dilated but to a lesser extent. The root of the aorta and the semilunar sinuses also are dilated. The left ventricle opacifies densely because of severe aortic insufficiency. The coronary arteries usually are dilated in patients with severe aortic insufficiency (same patient as in Fig. 16-9). (Courtesy of Spindola-Franco H, Fish BG, eds. Radiology of the heart: cardiac imaging in infants, children, and adults. New York: Springer-Verlag, 1985:205.)

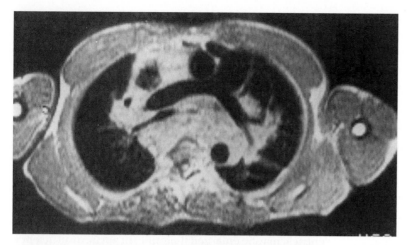

FIGURE 16-11. Periaortic neoplasm in a 19-year-old man with neurofibromatosis. The T1-weighted spin-echo magnetic resonance imaging (MRI) in an axial plane shows the neoplasm encasing all of the mediastinal structures. The superior vena and the aorta are widely separated by tumor interposition. No cleavage plane is identified between the mass and the vascular structures to permit surgical debulking.

ment must be initiated once the diagnosis is suspected in order to prevent blindness. The histopathologic findings will not be masked if the biopsy is performed within 1 week. Rarely, surgical excision of an expanding aneurysm or replacement of the aortic valve with a composite graft may be necessary.

■ Periaortic Pathology

The aorta may be secondarily involved by extrinsic pathology. Neoplasms, abscesses, and hematomas can be suspected by chest roentgenogram. MRI and CT permit precise preoperative evaluation (Fig. 16-11).

■ Congenital Diseases of the Aorta and Its Branches

Of the congenital thoracic diseases, coarctation of the aorta and pseudocoarctation of the aorta (buckled aorta) are the most common. Coarctation of the aorta is diagnosed in infants as well as in children and adults. In infants, it can cause acute congestive heart failure and often is associated with other cardiac defects such as bicuspid aortic valve, mitral valve pathology, ventricular septal defect, patent ductus arteriosus, endocardial fibroelastosis, and complex intracardiac disorders. In older children and adults, it is found in some patients during evaluation for hypertension and stroke.

Imaging

The roentgenogram of the chest may show a classic "three sign," whereas a barium esophagogram may show a "reverse three sign," or "E sign." Subtle signs include an inconspicuous aortic arch with a prominent descending aorta and a prominent left subclavian artery. Rib notch-

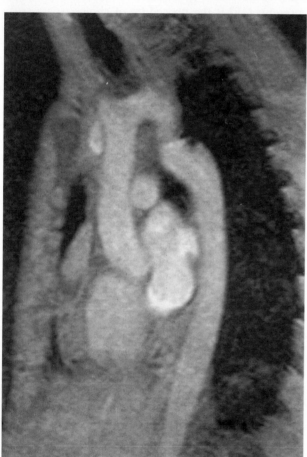

FIGURE 16-12. Magnetic resonance imaging (MRI) studies in a 16-year-old boy who had balloon angioplasty (BAP) for correction of a juxtaductal coarctation of the aorta. The fast field echo (cine gradient) MRI was performed to exclude aneurysm formation, dissection, or recoarctation at the site of the BAP. None of these sequelae was present.

Treatment

High-dose steroids will control inflammation and prevent progression of all manifestations of the disease. Treat-

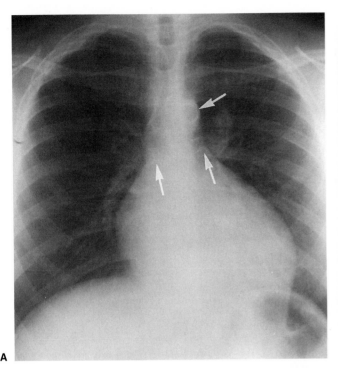

A

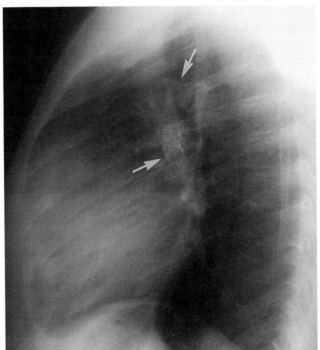

B

FIGURE 16-13. Congenital coarctation of the aorta and severe valvular and peripheral pulmonic stenosis in a 12-year-old boy treated by stenting procedures. The PA and lateral chest roentgenograms **(A,B)** show a stent in the aortic arch and in the thoracic aorta, and also one in each pulmonary artery. Coronal T1 magnetic resonance imaging (MRI) before the stenting procedure **(C)** demonstrates severe stenosis of the pulmonary valve (arrow) and marked hypoplasia of the left and right pulmonary artery. Severe biventricular hypertrophy is also evident. Fast field echo *(gradient echo)* in the left anterior oblique plane **(D)** demonstrates severe coarctation of the aorta with turbulence *(signal void)* just distal to the narrowing.

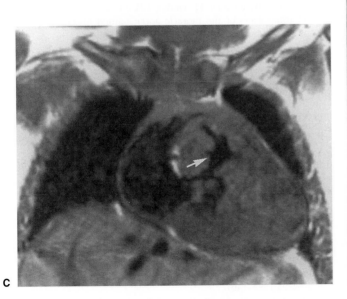

C

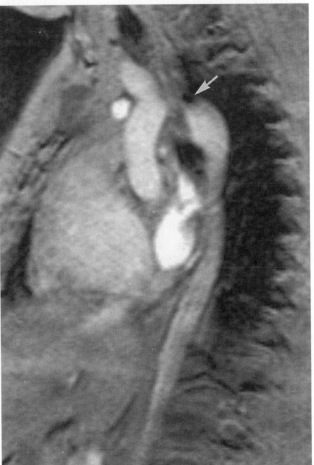

D

ing, formerly one of the classic signs of coarctation of the aorta, is now rarely noted because diagnosis and treatment occur earlier.

Pseudocoarctation is an important finding on plain chest roentgenograms caused by a buckled aorta. An acute bend in the aorta is noted at the site of the ligamentum arteriosum. A bicuspid aortic valve may be associated but this occurs less frequently than with coarctation of the aorta. Depending on the severity of the kink, no pressure gradient may be noted or a small pressure gradient may be found. Although a barium esophagogram may show two indentations in the esophagus similar to the reverse three sign or E sign noted with coarctation of the aorta, an MRI is definitive and is indicated if a pseudocoarctation cannot be differentiated from a mediastinal mass on plain films of the chest.

Treatment

Treatment in infants requires stabilization with prostaglandin E_1 (PGE_1) and cardiac inotropes, followed by surgery to correct the defect. The left subclavian artery often is used as a roof patch (also called a *subclavian flap*) to use native tissue in the repair rather than exogenous material. The left subclavian artery is ligated and divided distally. Its proximal portion is incised longitudinally to match a longitudinal split along the coarcted segment. The subclavian artery then is opened, turned down, and sutured to the two sides of the split aortic isthmus and coarcted segment forming a roof, thus enlarging the lumen of the aorta. Excision and end-to-end anastomosis or a prosthetic patch may be necessary in other persons. In infants, balloon angioplasty generally is not performed in native coarctation because of the risk of aortic rupture at the site of the ductus arteriosus. If restenosis occurs, balloon angioplasty can be used safely as a secondary repair.[31] Coarctation of the aorta in children and adults is often an isolated defect but may be associated with aortic and mitral pathology. It also may be associated with aneurysmal dilatation of the aortic root. Complications include Berry aneurysm and subarachnoid hemorrhage, aortic dissection, and infective endocarditis with mycotic aneurysm. Coarctation of the aorta also may present with congestive heart failure. In children and adults, some physicians prefer balloon angioplasty for treatment (Fig. 16-12), whereas some centers treat native coarctation in persons of any age by surgical means. In the unusual cases in which balloon angioplasty fails to dilate a coarcted segment, a stent[32] may be deployed to maintain patency of the vessel (Fig. 16-13). Persons who have severe dilatation of the aortic root will require replacement of the aortic root and aortic valve at the time of the coarctation repair. A prosthetic conduit between the ascending and the descending aorta, or between the left subclavian artery and the descending aorta, also may be used.

■ Postoperative Complications

Common thoracic procedures include aortic valve replacement, coronary artery bypass grafting, placement of a valved conduit for aortic dissection, placement of intravascular stents, surgical repair, and balloon angioplasty of coarctation of the aorta. The most common complications following these procedures include mediastinal or paravalvular leakage, infection, dissection, and true and false aneurysms. Complications should be suspected in the presence of a wide superior mediastinum, retrosternal obliteration of the clear space, pleural effusions, or an unusual cardiac silhouette.

REFERENCES

1. Spindola-Franco H, Fish BG. Abnormalities of the aortic arch and pulmonary arteries—vascular rings and slings. In: Elliot LP, ed. *Cardiac imaging in infants, children, and adults.* Philadelphia: JB Lippincott, 1991:344–368.
2. Spindola-Franco H, Fish BG. Left heart obstruction. In: Spindola-Franco H, Fish BG, eds. *Radiology of the heart: cardiac imaging in infants, children, and adults.* New York: Springer-Verlag, 1985: 540–583.
3. Wolfe WG, Moran JF. The evolution of medical and surgical management of acute aortic dissections. *Circulation* 1977;56:503–505.
4. Lindsay J Jr. Aortic dissection. In: Lindsey and Hurst, eds. *The Aorta.* New York: Grune and Stratton, 1979:239.
5. DeBakey ME, Henly WS, Cooley DA, Morris GC Jr, Crawford ES, Beall AC. Surgical management of dissecting aneurysms of the aorta. *J Thorac Cardiovasc Surg* 1965;49:130.
6. Dailey PO, Trueblood HW, Stinson EB, Wuerflein RD, Shumway NE. Management of acute aortic dissections. *Ann Thorac Surg* 1970;10:237–247.
7. O'Gara PT, DeSanctis RW. Acute aortic dissection and its variants: toward a common diagnostic and therapeutic approach. *Circulation* 1995;92:1376–1378.
8. Stanson AW, Kazmier FJ, Hollier LH, et al. Penetrating atherosclerotic ulcers of the thoracic aorta: natural history and clinic pathologic correlation. *Ann Vasc Surg* 1986;1:15–23.
9. Gore I. Pathogenesis of dissection aneurysm of the aorta. *Arch Pathol* 1952;53:142–153.
10. Nienaber CA, von Kodolitsch Y, Petersen B, et al. Intramural hemorrhage of the thoracic aorta: diagnostic and theraputic implications. *Circulation* 1995;92:1465–1472.
11. Yamada T, Tada S, Harada J. Aortic dissection without intimal tear: diagnosis with MR imaging and CT. *Radiology* 1988;168:347–352.
12. Wilson SK, Hutchins GM. Aortic dissecting aneurysms: causative factors in 204 subjects. *Arch Pathol Lab Med* 1982;106:175–180.
13. Laissy JP, Blanc F, Soyer P, et al. Thoracic aortic dissection: diagnosis with transesophageal echocardiography versus MR imaging. *Radiology* 1995;194:331–336.
14. Nienaber CA, von Kodolitsch Y, Nicolas V, et al. The diagnosis of thoracic aortic dissection by noninvasive imaging procedures. *N Engl J Med* 1993;328:1–9.
15. Bansal RC, Chandrasekaran K, Ayala K, Smith DC. Frequency and explanation of false negative diagnosis of aortic dissection by aortography and transesophageal echocardiography. *J Am Coll Cardiol* 1995;25:1393–1401.
16. Anagnostopoulos CE, Prabhakar MJS, Kittle CF. Aortic dissections and dissecting aneurysms. *Am J Cardiol* 1972;30:263–273.
17. Kato N, Hirano T, Takeda K, Nakagawa T, Mizumoto T, Yuasa H.

Treatment of acute aortic dissections with expandable metallic stents: experimental study. *J Vasc Intervent Radiol* 1994;5:417–423.

18. Marty-Ane CH, SerreCousine O, Laborde JC, Costes V, Mary H, Senac JP. Use of a balloon-expandable intravascular graft in the management of type B aortic in an animal model. *J Vasc Intervent Radiol* 1995;6:97–103.

19. Marty-Ane C, Serres-Cousine O, Laborde JC, Costes V, Alauzen M, Mary H. Use of endovascular stents for acute aortic dissection: an experimental study. *Ann Vasc Surg* 1994;8:434–442.

20. Williams DM, Andrews JC, Marx MV, Abrams GD. Creation of reentry tears in aortic dissection by means of percutaneous balloon fenestration: gross anatomic and histologic considerations. *J Vasc Intervent Radiol* 1993;4:75–83.

21. Gaubert JY, Moulin G, Mesana T, et al. Type A dissection of the thoracic aorta: use of MR imaging for long-term follow-up. *Radiology* 1995;196:363–369.

22. Cohen AM, Crass JR, Thomas HA, Fisher RG, Jacobs DG. CT evidence for the "osseous pinch" mechanism of traumatic aortic injury. *AJR Am J Roentgenol* 1992;159:271–274.

23. Marsh DG, Strum JT. Traumatic aortic rupture: roentgenographic indications for angiography. *Ann Thorac Surg* 1976;21:337–340.

24. Simeone JF, Deren MM, Cagle F. The value of the left apical cap in the diagnosis of aortic rupture. *Radiology* 1981;139:35–37.

25. Williams DM, Dake MD, Bolling SF, Deeb GM. The role of intravascular ultrasound in acute traumatic aortic rupture. *Semin Ultrasound CT MRI* 1993;14:85–90.

26. Williams DM, Simon HJ, Marx MV, Starkey TD. Acute traumatic aortic rupture: intravascular US findings. *Radiology* 1992;182:247–249.

27. Williams DM, Andrews JC, Chee SS, Marx MV, Abrams GD. Canine model of acute aortic rupture: treatment with percutaneous delivery of a covered Z stent—work in progress. *J Vasc Intervent Radiol* 1994;5:797–803.

28. Lande A, Berkman YM. Aortitis: pathologic, clinical and arteriographic review. *Radiol Clin North Am* 1976;14:219–240.

29. Ueda H, Morooka S, Ito I, Yamaguchi H, Takeda T, Saito Y. Clinical observation of 52 cases of aortitis syndrome. *Jpn* 1969;10:277–288.

30. Lupi-Herrera E, Sanchez-Torres G, Marcushamer J, Mispireta J, Horwitz S, Espino-Vela J. Takayasu's arteritis: clinical study of 107 cases. *Am Heart J* 1977;93:94–103.

31. Anjos R, Qureshi SA, Rosenthal E, et al. Determinants of hemodynamic results of balloon dilation of aortic recoarctation. *Am J Cardiol* 1992;69:665–671.

32. O'Laughlin MP, Perry SB, Lock JE, Mullins CE. Use of endovascular stents in congenital heart disease. *Circulation* 1991;83:1923–1939.

17

Thoracic Outlet and Upper Extremities

SAMUEL I. WAHL AND PHILLIP S. LAKRITZ

■ Indications for Arteriography and Venography of the Thoracic Outlet and Upper Extremities

Indications for arteriography of the thoracic outlet and upper extremities include the evaluation of upper extremity ischemia, trauma, aneurysms, vasculitides, and arteriovenous malformations. Venography of the thoracic outlet and upper extremities are used routinely in the evaluation of thoracic outlet obstruction, superior vena cava (SVC) syndrome, and hemodialysis access shunts.

Techniques of upper-extremity arteriography

Vascular access for upper-extremity arteriography can be achieved by using a 4 or 5 Fr diagnostic catheter using the Seldinger technique via a transfemoral approach. Additionally, access can be achieved either from an axillary or from a brachial artery approach if the transfemoral approach is not technically feasible. The axillary approach has fallen out of favor because of the potential for brachial plexus injury caused by an access site hematoma. The reported frequency of brachial plexus injury has been between 0.4 and 9.5%. The axillary approach has been replaced by the brachial artery approach.[1] A Headhunter-type catheter may be used to catheterize the brachiocephalic vessels in younger patients, but catheterization may be accomplished more easily by using a Simmons-type catheter in older patients who have tortuous vessels.

The examination should begin with thoracic arch aortography. A complete arteriographic examination of the upper extremities necessitates evaluation of the entire vasculature from the origins of the brachiocephalic and left subclavian arteries to the level of the digital arteries. It is imperative that the arteries of the entire extremity be evaluated thoroughly because abnormalities of the inflow arteries may result in distal clinical symptoms. Furthermore, as many as 15% of patients have an aberrantly high origin of the radial artery arising from the axillary artery, a finding that may be overlooked if evaluation of the more proximal vessels is neglected (Fig. 17-1). Less frequently, the ulnar artery has an aberrantly high origin arising from the brachial artery.[2]

Arterial spasm may be encountered during arteriography of the upper extremity but usually subsides spontaneously or after the intraarterial injection of medications such as tolazoline, phentolamine, or nitroglycerin. These vasodilators also enhance blood flow to the distal extremity, improving digital artery visualization.[3] The temperature of the upper extremity is a critical factor influencing vascular tone and blood flow to the hand and digits. Decreased skin temperature may result in spastic narrowing of blood vessels, whereas temperature elevation improves blood flow. It is well known that artificial temperature elevation with the use of heating pads or warm water improves visualization of distal arteries of the upper extremity and hand.[4] Older techniques of promoting vasodilatation, such as general anesthesia, stellate ganglion blockade, and oral alcohol, have fallen into disuse.[5]

Attention must be given to secondary signs that indicate the presence of vascular disease such as opacification of collateral vessels or retrograde filling of the vertebral artery as a result of a proximal subclavian artery or brachiocephalic artery stenosis. These secondary findings

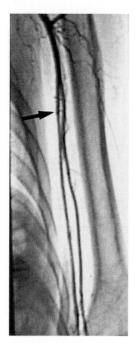

FIGURE 17-1. High origin of the left radial artery (arrow) from the brachial artery.

are important because less complete views of the upper extremities may fail to uncover significant underlying disease.

Upper-extremity arterial contrast injections can be quite painful; however, the degree of discomfort has been decreased since the introduction of digital subtraction angiography (DSA), which allows for the use of more dilute and lower volumes of contrast media compared with cut-film angiography. Newer, low-osmolar contrast agents tend to be better tolerated than the standard high-osmolar agents.[6]

Disease entities

Conditions resulting in upper-extremity arterial insufficiency may be attributable to abnormalities extending from the inominate or subclavian arteries to the digital arteries. The etiologies of critical ischemia of the upper extremity are quite variable, involving both small- and large-vessel arteridites, trauma, atherosclerosis, and vascular complications secondary to thoracic outlet obstruction.[7]

Atherosclerosis

Manifestations of atherosclerosis of the upper extremities vary widely and usually involve proximal rather than distal arteries.[1] Symptoms include claudication, ulcers, and Raynaud's phenomenon. The left upper extremity is more commonly the symptomatic extremity. This is at-

tributed to the perpendicular origin of the left subclavian artery from the aortic arch.[8]

In upper-extremity claudication, multiple segmental occlusions may be identified (Fig. 17-2). Less frequently, embolization may occur, resulting in distal ischemia of the upper extremity.[9] Most emboli arise from a cardiac source, such as emboli resulting from atrial fibrillation or endocarditis.[3,10–12] Emboli may be secondary to atherosclerosis, frequently within the subclavian artery, or as the result of arterial injury secondary to trauma (Fig. 17-3). In up to one third of cases, digital ischemia may be due to embolic occlusion and may mimic primary distal disease of the upper extremities. Therefore, evaluation of the proximal vessels during angiography is imperative.[3]

The goal of arteriography in the setting of embolic occlusion is to demonstrate arterial reconstitution distal to the site of occlusion so that proper management may be planned, such as surgical embolectomy, surgical bypass, or transcatheter thrombolysis. Catheter-directed thrombolysis is frequently the initial treatment of choice.[13]

Trauma

Indications for arteriography for the evaluation of trauma include diminished or absent distal pulses, the presence of a bruit, pulsatile or expanding hematoma, hemothorax, electrical trauma. Trauma to the vessels of the thoracic outlet and upper extremities is classified by the mechanism of injury as *penetrating* or *nonpenetrating*. Both types of injuries are potentially limb threatening.

Penetrating trauma from either gunshot or knife wounds is frequently encountered in the emergency setting. Penetrating trauma may lead to direct intimal injury, vessel transection with or without extravasation of blood and formation of pseudoaneurysms (Fig. 17-4), dissection, occlusion, spasm, arteriovenous fistula formation (Fig. 17-5), and arterial displacement by hematoma. Slow antegrade flow of blood may be identified angiographically and is often due to spasm induced by the trauma itself or to compartment syndrome.[14]

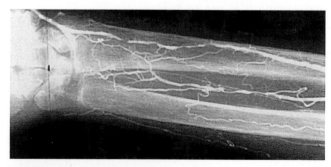

FIGURE 17-2. Atherosclerosis in long-standing diabetes; extensive stenotic and occlusive disease of the medium and small vessels of the forearm and wrist.

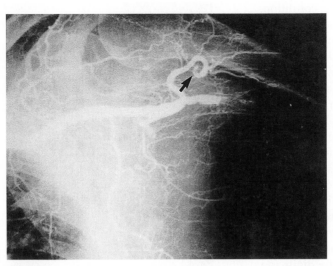
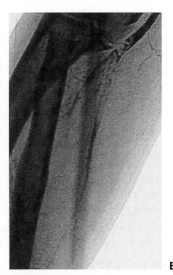

FIGURE 17-3. A: High brachial artery embolic occlusion in a patient with atrial fibrillation and acute onset of ischemic left upper extremity pain. Note the smaller filling defect in the humeral circumflex branch (arrow). **B:** Distal emboli in the proximal right radial and ulnar arteries evident by "tram track" filling defects. Patency was reestablished after transcatheter thrombolysis.

Repetitive blunt trauma may result in pathologic changes in the vessel, including intimal tears or pseudoaneurysms with mural thrombus formation. In turn, this thrombus may result in distal embolization and consequent ischemia. Therefore, prompt diagnosis is critical to minimize morbidity.[15] This type of injury is seen in athletes in whom repetitive motion is the underlying cause of injury. These patients may develop signs and symptoms of acute ischemia of the hand and digits. Some may progress to tissue breakdown evident by skin ulceration and gangrene.[8] The angiographic appearance may be similar to that seen in atherosclerosis with multiple segmental arterial occlusions.[12]

Raynaud's phenomenon

Raynaud's phenomenon is an idiopathic vasospastic condition of the small vessels of the extremities characterized by episodic digital ischemia provoked by cold, emotion, and

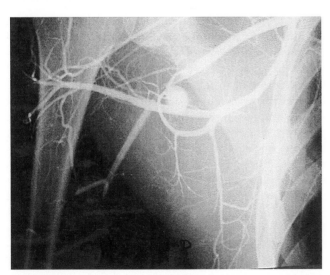

FIGURE 17-4. Stab wound to the axilla with transection and pseudoaneurysm of the proximal right brachial artery but with continued distal flow.

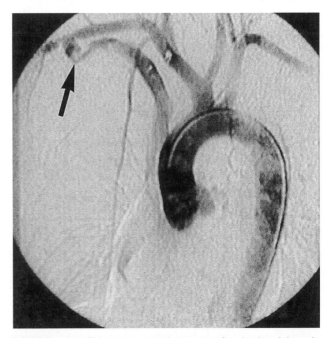

FIGURE 17-5. Traumatic arteriovenous fistula involving the right sublavian artery and brachiocephalic vein following a gunshot wound. Note the bullet fragments.

other sympathetic stimuli.[16] Patients with this condition, most frequently women, develop trophic changes as a result of microcirculatory damage and prolonged local ischemia.[17] It is more often symptomatic in the upper extremities than in the lower.[1] Raynaud-type symptoms are common in the general population, and in a minority of these patients, it may be attributable to an underlying, often reversible cause (*primary* Raynaud's phenomenon or Raynaud's disease), or it may be attributable to a known underlying systemic illness (*secondary* Raynaud's phenomenon) such as systemic lupus erythematosis, scleroderma, or rheumatoid arthritis. Other associated conditions include drug or chemical injury, occupational injury, occlusive arterial disease, and hyperviscosity diseases.[16,18]

Symptoms of Raynaud's phenomenon include pain, paresthesias, pallor, cyanosis, and rubor. Small digital ulceration and or fissuring over the pads of the digits can be seen in severe or recurrent attacks. Gangrene only rarely occurs.[17,18]

Primary Raynaud's phenomenon typically presents during the teenaged years in women who are otherwise healthy, but symptoms may develop as late as the fourth decade. It has been suggested that persons with this condition have a higher incidence of other vascular complications, such as migraine headache, hypertension, and atypical angina.[18]

Although angiography is not particularly useful in the diagnosis or distinction of the various causes of Raynaud's phenomenon, it does, however, have a role in the evaluation of patients presenting with unilateral symptoms. Patients with unilateral symptoms frequently have identifiable underlying upper-extremity pathology of either the major or smaller vessels. An arteriographic finding is stenosis of the subclavian artery. This is usually a result of an extraluminal abnormality. Stenosis can lead to poststenotic aneurysmal dilatation, which may in turn lead to the development of mural thrombus and subsequent embolization with distal ischemic changes.[19]

The typical angiographic findings of Raynaud's phenomenon are those of spasm with slow antegrade flow (Fig. 17-6) and poor opacification of the distal small vessels. Angiography following the injection of vasodilators can lead to dramatic improvements in visualization of small distal arteries.[1]

Vasculitides

All the several categories of vasculitides are relatively rare and affect the upper extremities. These conditions may affect the arteries primarily or relate to a systemic disease process; however, they all share the characteristic of arterial wall inflammation and often necrosis. Differentiation of these vasculitides is best accomplished by a thorough review of the clinical history, with particular attention to the distribution of vessel involvement as well as the rapid-

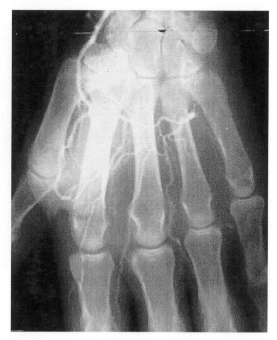

FIGURE 17-6. Raynaud's disease with slow antegrade flow. Late angiographic exposure approximately 28 seconds after contrast was injected in the midbrachial artery via transfemoral catheterization after an intraarterial injection of 60 mg of papvarine. No spasm is seen secondary to artificial vasodilatation, but occlusive disease of the digital arteries remains evident.

ity of onset. The pathogenesis and etiologies of these vasculitides are poorly understood, but most investigators agree that a relationship to immune complex and cell-mediated mechanisms exists.[20]

Buerger's disease (thromboangiitis obliterans)

Buerger's disease is an inflammatory disorder characterized by nonspecific inflammation and cellular infiltration occurring within the vessel wall. There is no direct association with atherosclerosis. Buerger's disease is a painful vasoocclusive disorder of young men in the third and fourth decades of life involving predominately the small and medium-sized arteries of the extremities. The disease process typically begins in the smaller peripheral vessels but may occur proximal to the level of the elbow. Additionally, veins and sometimes the adjacent nerves can become involved in the disease process.[21] Clinically, those afflicted present with signs and symptoms of distal arterial ischemia or migratory superficial thrombophlebitis.[8,21] Peculiar to this disease is the clear association with tobacco use. With the cessation of smoking, signs and symptoms of the disease usually remit or become quiescent. If smoking continues, however, the condition may progress, necessitating amputation.[21] More commonly, however, the disease tends to follow a self-limited course.[22]

Angiography classically demonstrates the abrupt cutoff of small arteries and the appearance of a dense network of "corkscrew-" like collaterals. Although it is commonly confused with atherosclerosis, its angiographic recognition depends on the absence of calcification and a distal rather than a proximal distribution with segmental occlusions of the radial and ulnar arteries with preservation of the interosseous artery.[8]

Takayasu's arteritis

Takayasu's arteritis, also known as *pulseless disease,* is chronic inflammatory obliterative arteritis and is seen predominately in young women.[8] The initial presentation of Takayasu's arteritis commonly involves systemic complaints of night sweats, arthralgias, fever, malaise, and weight loss. Although its cause remains unknown, it may have some relationship to giant cell arteritis.[20] If progression of the disease occurs, symptoms are referable to the involved vascular territory. The brachiocephalic vessels are primarily affected but the aorta and its branches also may be affected.

Although Takayasu's disease predominately results in arterial stenoses, dilatation may be seen as well.[23] The first angiographic changes of the disease may be localized narrowing or irregularity. Although the appearance is nonspecific, the distribution of disease is highly specific. The left subclavian artery is the most commonly involved branch vessel of the aorta in about 45% of patients. Arterial occlusion is the second most common finding, and often a characteristic "flame-shaped" appearance of the occluded vessel is seen (Fig. 17-7). Occlusions of the main branches of the aortic arch usually are associated with extensive collateral circulation.[23] Similar angiographic findings may be seen in temporal arteritis.[24]

Subclavian steal

Subclavian steal is defined as the reversal of flow in the vertebral artery secondary to a stenosis or occlusion of the subclavian artery proximal to the origin of the vertebral artery or brachiocephalic artery. The stenosis or occlusion results in decreased blood flow to the vessel distal to the lesion. Blood flow to the affected extremity may occur from the contralateral vertebral artery, via the basilar artery, and then in a retrograde direction through the ipsilateral vertebral artery and into the subclavian artery distal to the stenosis (Fig. 17-8). Blood is therefore "stolen" from the basilar circulation, resulting in basilar insufficiency and subsequently the subclavian steal syndrome. Symptoms include vertigo, syncope, and extremity paresthesia.

A subclavian artery stenosis may cause myocardial ischemia if it is located proximal to an internal mammary artery used for coronary artery bypass graft. A stenosis or occlusion of the subclavian artery also may jeopardize an

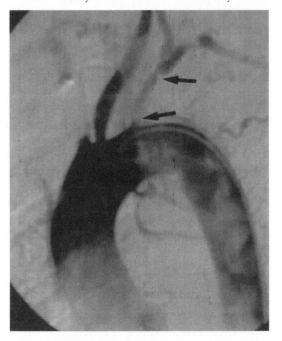

A

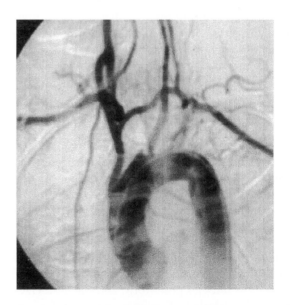

B

FIGURE 17-7. Takayasu's arteritis in a young woman with severe bilateral upper extremity claudication. **A:** Abrupt occlusion of the right brachiocephalic trunk with faint reconstitution of the right subclavian artery via collateral circulation. Additionally, there are at least two high-grade focal stenoses of the left subclavian artery proximal to the origin of the left vertebral artery (arrows) as well as a mild stenosis at the origin of the left common carotid. Note sparing of the aorta; atherosclerosis, in contrast, would involve the aorta as well as its proximal branches. **B:** Same patient after extensive vascular resonstration.

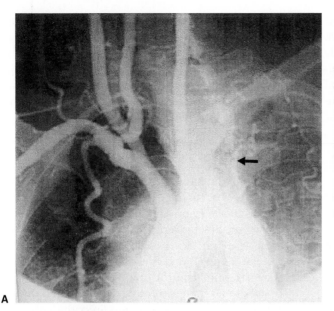 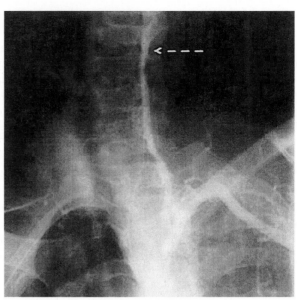

FIGURE 17-8. Subclavian steal syndrome. **A:** Arch aortogram reveals an occlusion of the proximal left subclavian artery (arrow). **B:** Late-phase of arteriogram shows retrograde flow down the left vertebral artery into the left subclavian artery (arrow).

axillofemoral bypass graft. The offending lesion of the proximal subclavian artery or brachiocephalic artery is often amenable to percutaneous transluminal angioplasty or stenting.[25] Potential complications of subclavian and axillary artery angioplasty include distal embolization and stroke.

The most common cause of subclavian steal is atherosclerotic disease. Other causes include trauma, arteritis, vascular obstruction by tumor, radiation therapy, and congenital malformation associated with congenital heart disease.

Thoracic outlet obstruction

The term *thoracic outlet syndrome* refers to a group of disorders resulting in vascular or neurologic compromise at the thoracic outlet, where the neurovascular bundle exits the chest. Only 1% of the cases of thoracic outlet syndrome involve the subclavian artery; a slightly greater percent are venous related, and 97% have a neurologic basis.[26,27]

The thoracic outlet is anatomically defined as a region bounded by the first rib inferiorly, the clavicle superiorly, the scalenus muscles posteriorly, and the costoclavicular ligament anteriorly.[28] The anatomic basis for vascular compromise is most often compression of the subclavian artery between a cervicle rib and the clavicle. Other sites of compression may be between the scalenus anticus and the scalenus medius tendons or at the costoclavicular space due to a prominent subclavius muscle. The axillary artery may course between the coracoid process and the pectoralis tendon.[1,29]

Arterial thoracic outlet syndrome

Angiography plays an important role in the diagnosis and treatment of arterial thoracic outlet syndrome and is indicated in patients with suspected arterial thoracic outlet syndrome when ischemia or embolism is suspected. Angiographic findings include stenoses or occlusions of the subclavian, axillary, or brachiocephlic arteries or their branches; extrinsic compression of vessels between the clavicle and first rib; poststenotic dilatation, increased collateral circulation; mural thrombus or embolization; and retrograde filling of the subclavian artery via the vertebral artery.[30] Frequently, the arterial stenosis is not in the plane of view and is unseen; its presence is indicated only by visualization of the poststenotic dilatation.

It can be difficult to separate an arterial cause of symptoms of the upper extremity and hand from a neurologic etiology. It also can be difficult to determine the significance of a subclavian artery narrowing seen on an angiogram with the extremity stressed as some degree of narrowing can be induced in an asymptomatic patient with the arm hyperextended (Fig. 17-9).

In addition to symptoms produced by direct vascular compression, subclavian artery compression can lead to poststenotic aneurysm formation. The aneurysm walls can be lined with thrombus that can potentially embolize distally. Arteriography is performed with the upper extremity in adduction or in a neutral position and then

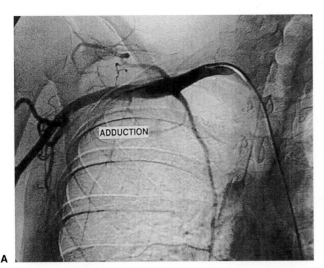
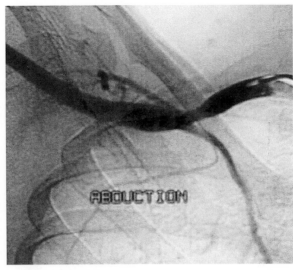

FIGURE 17-9. Thoracic outlet syndrome. **A:** A right subclavian arteriogram in adduction is essentially normal. **B:** Repeat arteriogram with the right arm abducted in a position that produced the patient's symptoms shows an obvious narrowing of the sublcavian artery and poststenotic dilatation (arrow).

in a position that elicits the described symptoms. Despite first rib resection and scalenectomy, 15 to 20% of patients will develop recurrence of symptoms.[31] Today, considerable confusion and disagreement remain over the anatomic basis of thoracic outlet obstruction, the implications of its angiographic findings, and the indications and results of surgical correction.[26,27]

Venous thoracic outlet syndrome

Venous outlet syndrome is synonomous with *axillosubclavian vein obstruction,* and the problems related to venous thoracic syndrome remain more confusing than those of arterial or neurologic obstruction. Deep venous thrombosis of the upper extremities is exceedingly uncommon compared with that occurring in the lower extremities.[32,33]

The etiology of upper-extremity venous thrombosis is variable and includes trauma, SVC syndrome, intrathoracic tumors, foreign bodies, polycythemia, thrombocytosis, cor pulmonale, congestive heart disease, and coagulopathies.[34,35]

Primary or effort thrombosis of the axillosubclavian veins, also known as *Paget-Schoeder's syndrome,* is a distinct clinical entity leading to disabling arm swelling that can be distinguished from other causes of axillosubclavian vein thrombosis. This condition is seen primarily in young men 40 years of age or younger who are otherwise healthy. Axillosubclavian vein occlusion typically occurs following repetitive trauma. Frequently, there is a history of vigorous or unusual exercise preceding the onset of symptoms.[36]

The two major radiographic patterns identified in primary thrombosis of the axillosubclavian veins are localized obstruction of the axillosubclavian veins at the level of the junction of the first rib and clavicle (Fig. 17-10) and a long segment of occlusion of the axillary vein.[36]

Although the diagnosis of axillosubclavian venous thrombosis is much easier to make than neurologic thoracic outlet syndrome, the decisions regarding treatment are more complex. Catheter-directed intravenous thrombolysis may be effective in patients who have acute symptoms of axillosubclavian venous thrombosis. With less acute or chronic occlusions, the incidence of complete lysis is of little or no benefit because rethrombosis is virtually inevitable. Some investigators advocate balloon angioplasty for underlying residual venous stenoses after thrombolysis.[37]

Protection against rethrombosis after complete lysis with long-term warfarin therapy has not proven effective in most patients, even over the short term, when awaiting surgical decompression of the thoracic outlet to prevent rethrombosis after initial lysis. Most agree that surgical decompression to remove external anomalies and outlet compression should be performed immediately following thrombolysis.[26]

Superior vena cava syndrome

The SVC syndrome consists of a constellation of findings that are the result of SVC or bilateral brachiocephalic vein obstruction. The classic presentation of SVC syndrome is the development of head, neck, and upper body edema and cyanosis. Patients frequently complain of chest discomfort, headache, and dizziness. More severe symptoms

A

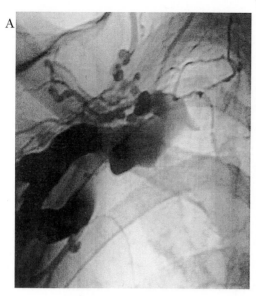

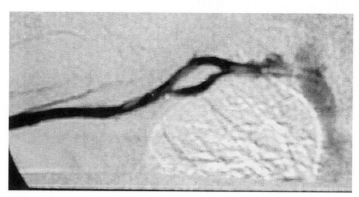

B

FIGURE 17-10. Paget-Schroeder syndrome. Young male weightlifter with acute onset of disabling right arm swelling. **A:** Right upper-extremity venogram demonstrates occlusion of the axillary and subclavian veins at the junction of the first rib and clavicle with an extensive network of venous collaterals. **B:** Follow-up venography 24 hours after direct urokinase infusion shows near complete thrombolysis with only minimal irregularity of the brachiocephalic vein. The patient underwent surgical decompression directly after lysis.

can include changes in mentation, and laryngeal edema with upper airway obstruction. Symptoms may be subacute and slowly progressive, or they may have an acute onset.[38]

The SVC is a relatively thin-walled vessel lying within a nondistensible space in the mediastinum, making it susceptible to extrinsic compression by primary tumors or lymphadenopathy.

The SVC syndrome most commonly is secondary to an underlying malignancy of the mediastinum and has been shown to be responsible for 85 to 97% of all cases.[39,40] Furthermore, SVC syndrome may occur in up to 10% of all patients with a right-sided intrathoracic mass lesion.[41] Prior to the onset of antibiotic therapy, infectious etiologies of the chest and mediastinum were commonly the source of SVC obstruction. Nevertheless, with the increase in the number of immunosuppressed patients secondary to human immunodeficiency virus (HIV) infection with an associated increased incidence of tuberculosis, histoplasmosis, and syphilis, infectious processes remain in the differential diagnosis of SVC syndrome.[39] Rare causes of SVC obstruction result from goiters, benign idiopathic mediastinal fibrosis, and aortic valve replacement.[42–44] Additionally, indwelling central catheters and transvenous pacemaker leads may result in iatrogenic SVC obstruction and should be considered in the differential diagnosis.[45,46]

Radiologic evaluation of suspected SVC syndrome includes conventional chest x-ray, computed tomography

(CT), magnetic resonance imaging (MRI), conventional contrast venography, and radionuclide imaging. CT is the modality of choice because it is readily available, relatively noninvasive, and is useful in accurately localizing the site and often the etiology of the obstruction as well as potential collateral veins. The surrounding lung and mediastinal structures can be evaluated with CT.[39]

Radionuclide imaging using technetium-99m (Tc99m)-labeled sulfur colloid is a valuable screening tool for suspected SVC obstruction. Serial radionuclide examinations can be obtained to evaluate for possible recanalization of the central veins or the restoration of flow following therapy.[47]

Patients with SVC syndrome often gain significant symptomatic improvement from conservative treatment measures, including head elevation and supplemental oxygen. Underlying malignant neoplasms of the chest, predominately small-cell lung carcinoma and lymphoma, may be managed initially with chemotherapeutic agents.[48,49] Additionally, radiotherapy is an effective treatment modality for most underlying causes of SVC syndrome and leads to symptomatic improvement in most patients.[50] Thrombolytic therapy may be required for patients who have demonstrable intraluminal thrombus within the SVC.[51,52] Surgical bypass for SVC obstruction with either autologous vein or synthetic material may be a useful way to palliate symptoms in selected patients.[53] Catheter- directed thrombolysis in conjunction with endovascular stent placement has been shown to be a safe and effective treatment for SVC syndrome.[54]

REFERENCES

1. Gomes A. Diagnostic and interventional angiography. In: Machleder HI, ed. *Vascular Disorders of the Upper Extremity.* 2nd rev. ed. Mt. Kisco, NY: Futura; 1989:59–99.

2. Keller FS, Rosch J, Dotter CT, et al. Proximal origin of radial artery: potential pitfall in hand angiography. *AJR Am J Roentgenol* 1980; 134:169–170.

3. Maiman MH, Bookstein JJ, Bernstein EF. Digital ischemia: angiographic differentiation of embolism from primary arterial disease. *AJR Am J Roentgenol* 1981;137:1183–1187.

4. Rosch J, Antovic R, Porter J. The importance of temperature in angiography of the hand. *Radiology* 1997;123:323–326.

5. Chait A. Abram's angiography: vascular and interventional radiology In: Baum S, ed. *Angiography of the Upper Extremity.* 4th ed. New York, NY: Little, Brown and Company; 1997:1755–1766.

6. Picus D, Hicks ME, Darcy MD, et al. Comparison of nonsubtracted digital angiography and conventional screen-film angiography for the evaluation of patients with peripheral vascular disease. *J Vasc Interv Radiol* 1991;2:359–364.

7. Quraishy MS, Cawthorn SJ, Giddings AE. Critical ischemia of the upper limb. *J R Soc Med* 1992;85:269–273.

8. Fuchs J. The pathology of upper extremity arterial disease. In: *Hand Clinics.* Vol 9. Philadelphia: W.B. Sauders; 1–4.

9. Champion HR, Gill W. Arterial embolus to the upper limb. *Br J Surg* 1973;113–115.

10. Kofoed H, Hansen HJB. Arterial embolism in the upper limb. *Acta Chir Scand Suppl* 1976;472:113–115.

11. Dick R. Arteriography in neurovascular compression at the thoracic outlet with special reference to embolic patterns. *AJR Am J Roentgenol* 1970;110:141–147.

12. Erlandson EE, Forrest ME, Shields JJ, et al. Discriminant arteriographic criteria in the management of forearm and hand ischemia. *Surgery* 1981;90:1025–1036.

13. Wildus DM, Venbrux AC, Benenati JF, et al. Fibrinolytic therapy for upper extremity occlusions. *Radiology* 1990;175:393–399.

14. Schwartz MR, Weaver FA, Bauer M, et al. Refining the indications for arteriography in penetrating extremity trauma: a prospective analysis. *J Vasc Surg* 1993;17:116–122.

15. Modrall JG, Weaver FA, Yellin AE. Vascular considerations in extremity trauma. *Orthop Clin North Am* 1993;24:557–563.

16. Belch JJ. Raynaud's phenomenon. *Curr Opin Rheumatol* 1991;3: 960–966.

17. Isenberg DA, Black C. ABC of rheumatology: Raynaud's phenomenon, scleroderma, and overlap syndromes. *BMJ* 1995;310:795–798.

18. Klippel JH. Raynaud's phenomenon, the french tricolor. *Arch Intern Med* 1991;151:2389–2393.

19. Bouhoutos J, Morris T, Martin P, et al. Unilateral Raynaud's phenomenon in the hand and its significance. *Surgery* 1997;82:547–551.

20. Somer T. Thromboembolic and vascular complications in vasculitis syndromes. *Eur Heart J* 1993;(suppl K):24–29.

21. Olin JW. Thromboagiitis obliterans. *Curr Opin Rheumatol* 1994;6: 44–49.

22. Shionoya S. Buerger's disease: diagnosis and management. *Cardiovasc Surg* 1993;1:207–214.

23. Cho YD, Lee K. Angiographic characteristics of Takayasu's arteritis. *Heart Vessels* 1992;7:97–101.

24. Stanson AW, Klein RG, Hunder GG. Extracranial angiographic findings in giant cell (temporal) arteritis. *AJR Am J Roentgenol* 1976; 116:179–186.

25. Reivich M, Holling HE, Roberts B, et al. Reversal of blood flow through the vertebral artery and its effect on cerebral circulation. *N Engl J Med* 1961;265:878–885.

26. Roos DB. Thoracic outlet syndrome: update 1987. *Am J Surg* 1987; 154:568–573.

27. Roos DB. Overview of thoracic outlet syndromes. In: Machleder HI, ed. *Vascular Disorders of the Upper Extremity.* 2nd rev. ed. Mt. Kisco, NY: Futura; 1989:155–177.

28. Wojtowycz M. Upper extremity angiography. In: Wojtowycz M, ed. *Handbook of Interventional Radiology and Angiography.* 2nd ed. St. Louis, MO: Mosby; 1995:155.

29. Makhoul RG, Machleder HI. Developmental anomalies at the thoracic outlet: an analysis of 200 consecutive cases. *J Vasc Surg* 1992; 16:534–545.

30. Lang EK. Thoracic outlet syndrome. In: Teplick JG, Haskin ME, eds. *Surgical Radiology.* Philadelphia: WB Saunders; 1981:1269–1278.

31. Saunders RJ, Haug CE, Pearse WH. Recurrent thoracic outlet syndrome. *J Vasc Surg* 1990;12:390–400.

32. Oshner A, et al. Thromboembolism: analysis of cases at Charity Hospital in New Orleans over a twelve year period. *Ann Surg* 1951; 134:405–xxx.

33. Barker NW, Nygaard KK, Walters W, et al. Statistical study of prospective venous thrombosis and pulmonary embolism: location of thrombosis: relation of thrombosis and embolism. *Proc Staff Meet Mayo Clin* 1941;16:33.

34. Smith-Behn J, Althar R, Katz W. Primary thrombosis of the axillary/subclavian vein. *South Med J* 1986;79:1176–1178.

35. Demeter S, Pritchard J, Piedad O, et al. Upper extremity thrombosis etiology and prognosis. *Angiology* 1992;33:743–755.

36. Becker GJ, Holden RW, Rabe FE, et al. Local thrombolytic therapy for subclavian and axillary vein thrombosis. *Radiology* 1983;149: 419–423.

37. Drury EM, Trout III HH, Giordano JM, et al. Lytic therapy in the treatment of axillary and subclavian vein thrombosis. *J Vasc Surg* 1985;2:821–827.

38. Stanford W, Doty DB. The role of venography and surgery in the management of patients with superior vena cava obstruction. *Ann Thorac Surg* 1986;41:158–163.

39. Abner A. Approach to the patient who presents with superior vena cava obstruction. *Chest* 1993;103:394–397.

40. Perez CA, Presant CA, Van Amberg AL III. Management of superior vena cava syndrome. *Semin Oncol* 1978;5:123–134.

41. Baker Gl, Barnes HJ. Superior vena cava syndrome: etiology, diagnosis, and treatment. *Am J Crit Care* 1992;1:54–64.

42. Cengiz K, Aykin A, Demrici A, et al. Intrathoracic goiter with hyperthyroidism, tracheal compression, superior vena cava syndrome, and Horner's syndrome. *Chest* 1990;97:1005–1006.

43. Weiss KS, Zidar BL, Wang S, et al. Radiation-induced leiomyosarcoma of the great vessels presenting as superior vena cava syndrome. *Cancer* 1987;60:1238–1242.

44. Davis SR, King HS, Le RI, et al. Superior vena cava syndrome caused by intrathoracic plasmacytoma. *Cancer* 1991;68:1376–1379.

45. Patel V, Igwebe T, Mast H, et al. Superior vena cava syndrome: current concepts of management. *N J Med* 1995;92:245–248.

46. Parish JM, Marschke RF Jr, Dines DE, et al. Etiologic considerations in superior vena cava syndrome. *Mayo Clin Proc* 1981;56:407–413.

47. Conte FA, Orzel JA. Superior vena cava syndrome and bilateral subclavian vein thrombosis: CT and radionuclide venography correlation. *Clin Nucl Med* 1986;11:698–700.

48. Sculier JP, Evans WK, Feld R, et al. Superior vena cava syndrome in small lung cancer. *Cancer* 1986;57:847–851.

49. Perez-Soler R, McLaughlin P, Velasquez WS, et al. Clinical features and results of management of superior vena cava syndrome secondary to lymphoma. *J Clin Oncol* 1984;2:260–266.

50. Armstrong BA, Perez CA, Simpson JR, et al. Role of irradiation in

the management of superior vena cava syndrome. *Int J Radiat Oncol Biol Phys* 1987;13:531–539.

51. Gray BH, Olin JW, Graor RA, et al. Safety and efficacy of thrombolytic therapy for superior vena cava syndrome. *Chest* 1991;99: 54–59.

52. Greenberg S, Kosinski R, Daniels J. Treatment of superior vena cava thrombosis with recombinant tissue plasminogen activator. *Chest* 1991;99:1298–1301.

53. Gloviczki P, Pairoler PC, Cherry KJ, et al. Reconstruction of the vena cava and of its primary tributaries: a preliminary report. *J Vasc Surg* 1990;11:373–381.

54. Kee ST, Kinoshita L, Razavi MK, et al. Superior vena cava syndrome: treatment with catheter-directed thrombolysis and endovascular stent placement. *Radiology* 1998;206:187–193.

18

Carotid, Vertebral, and Spinal Arteriography

JACQUELINE A. BELLO AND BRUCE BERKOWITZ

Although usually they are managed by neuroradiologists, especially in academic institutions, the head, neck, and spine are of interest to the vascular and interventional radiologist, who also may perform diagnostic and interventional procedures in these anatomic areas. This chapter provides a brief, overview of this vascular anatomy and pathology of these regions.

■ Anatomy

Arteries of the neck

Within the superior mediastinum, the aortic arch normally gives rise to three major arteries that supply the upper extremities, head, and neck. The first branch is the brachiocephalic trunk, also called the innominate artery. This vessel courses superiorly for a short distance before bifurcating into the right subclavian and right common carotid arteries (Fig. 18-1). The right subclavian artery (RSCA) courses superiorly, gives off the right vertebral artery, and then turns laterally to supply the right upper extremity. The right common carotid artery (RCCA) courses superiorly to bifurcate into the right internal and external carotid arteries The second vessel off the aortic arch is the left common carotid artery, which travels cephalad and bifurcates into the left internal and external carotid arteries. The left subclavian artery is normally the final arch vessel. It courses superiorly before turning sharply laterally to supply the left upper extremity. The common carotid arteries are paired vessels located anteriorly within the neck. Each common carotid artery courses superiorly, along with the

vagus nerve and internal jugular vein, without branching, and then it bifurcates into the internal carotid artery (ICA) and external carotid artery (ECA) (Figs. 18-2 and 18-3). The bifurcation of the common carotid artery is generally at the level of C3–4, but it may occur anywhere from C1–T2.[1]

The ICA supplies the anterior circulation of the brain as well as a portion of the skull base and is divided into four segments: cervical, petrous, cavernous, and supraclinoid. Only the cervical segment is extracranial. The most proximal portion of the ICA is posterolateral in relation to the ECA and then courses medially to enter the skull base through the carotid canal. The cervical ICA has no named branches. The remaining three segments of the ICA are named as to their location; the petrous and cavernous portions lie within the petrous bone and cavernous sinus, respectively, and the supraclinoid segment runs above the level of the anterior clinoid. The major arteries of the anterior circulation of the brain are branches of the supraclinoid ICA (Fig. 18-4).

The ECA is the smaller of the two branches of the common carotid artery. At its origin, the ECA is anteromedial to the ICA. The branches of the ECA are the superior thyroid, ascending pharyngeal, lingual, facial, occipital, and posterior auricular arteries. The ECA then bifurcates into the internal maxillary and superficial temporal arteries. Certain branches of the ECA may serve as important collaterals to the intracranial circulation in the setting of ICA stenosis or occlusion. These include the distal branches of the internal maxillary artery and the facial artery, both of which may fill the supraclinoid ICA by anastomosing with the ophthalmic artery. Less commonly, the ascending pharyngeal artery and the middle

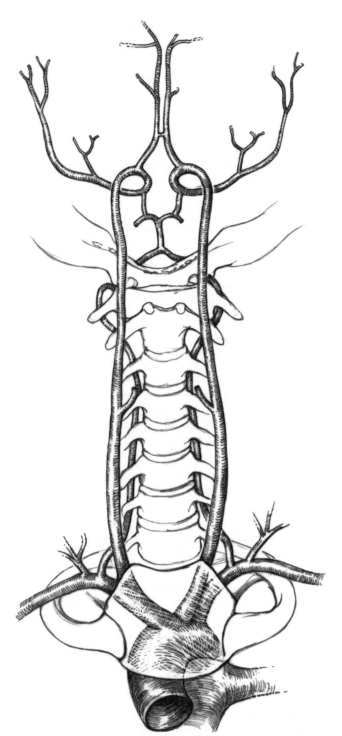

FIGURE 18-1. The aortic arch and its major branches (antero-posterior view).

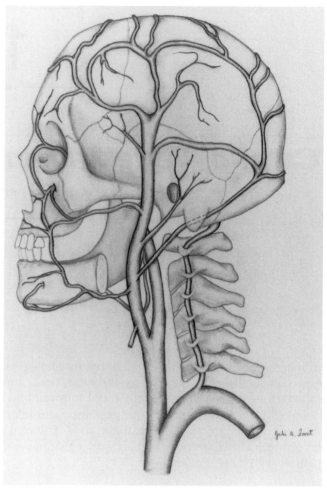

FIGURE 18-2. The external carotid artery and its branches.

the foramina transversaria of the C6 vertebra and then run within bony canals, exiting at the C2 foramena. The artery then turns sharply laterally to course around the lateral mass of C1 before returning medially to ascend through the foramen magnum to join and form the basilar artery. The occipital artery and ascending pharyngeal artery may serve as collateral supply to the vertebral arteries and posterior circulation.

Veins of the neck

The interal jugular veins (IJV), formed by the confluence of the sigmoid sinuses and the inferior petrosal sinuses, drain most of the blood from the brain (Fig. 18-5). The IJVs are paired structures that course inferiorly, lateral to the carotid arteries and deep to the sternocleidomastoid muscle (SCM) in the neck, to join the ipsilateral subclavian vein. The external jugular veins (EJV) drain portions of the face and neck; they course superficial to the SCM to join the subclavian veins. The vertebral veins arise in the occipital region from multiple small veins and

meningeal branch of the internal maxillary artery may serve as collaterals.

The vertebral arteries arise as the first and largest branches of the subclavian arteries and supply the posterior circulation of the brain, spinal cord, and muscles of the neck. The vertebral arteries travel superiorly to enter

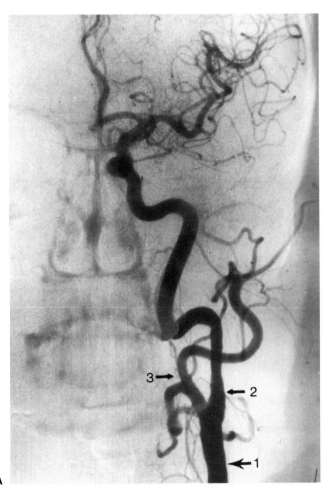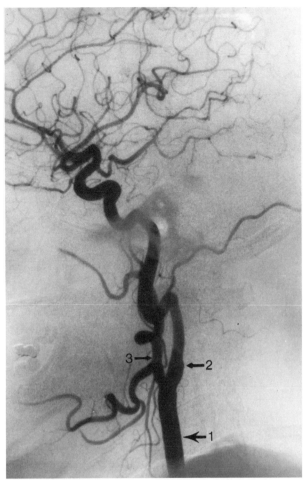

FIGURE 18-3. Film subtraction angiography of the left common carotid artery bifurcation in anteroposterior (A) and lateral (B) views demonstrate the normal branching pattern of the common carotid artery (1) into the internal (2) and external (3) carotid arteries.

travel inferiorly adjacent to the vertebral arteries within the foraminae transversaria to empty into the innominate veins.

■ Pathologic Processes of the Arteries of the Neck

Atherosclerosis

Atherosclerosis is by far the most common disease process to involve the arteries of the neck. Caused by the formation of fibrofatty intimal plaques, its various manifestations include intimal calcification, vessel tortuosity, and ectasia. This process may progress to stenosis, occlusion, and dolichoectasia and aneurysm formation (Fig. 18-6). The most common sites of atherosclerotic stenoses within the neck are, in order of frequency, the common carotid bifurcation, origins of the ICA and ECA, the origins of the vertebral arteries, and the proximal subclavian arteries.[2] Angiography has an important role in this dis-

ease: Several large-scale prospective studies found that carotid endarterectomy is effective in the long-term prevention of stroke in certain patients with moderate to severe stenosis.[3,4]

Fibromuscular dysplasia

Fibromuscular dysplasia (FMD) is an idiopathic process that leads to stenoses of medium to small arteries as a result of segmental overgrowth of fibrous and muscular elements of the arterial media and, to a lesser extent, the adventitia (Fig. 18-7). Originally described in renal arteries, FMD most commonly affects the cervical ICA, but it may involve any of the major arteries of the neck.[2] FMD is often bilateral and is associated with spontaneous arterial dissection as well as intracranial aneurysms. It is more common in women and tends to occur in patients younger than the expected age distribution for atherosclerosis. Radiographically, FMD usually appears as alternating segments of stenosis and dilatation, producing a so-called "string of beads" appearance.

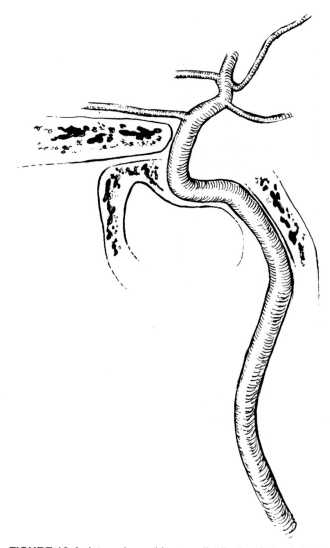

FIGURE 18-4. Internal carotid artery distribution (lateral view).

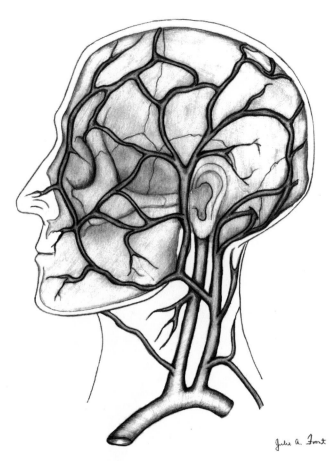

FIGURE 18-5. The draining veins of the cranium and neck.

Takayasu arteritis

Takayasu arteritis, also known as pulseless disease, is characterized by long-segment, smooth stenoses of the proximal arch vessels, although any of the branches of the aorta may be involved (Fig. 18-8). The left subclavian is the artery that is most often involved, although typically several vessels are involved.[5] The process often leads to complete occlusions of vessels. The disease typically affects females aged 15 to 45 years. The pathogenesis of this disease is unknown.

Giant cell arteritis

Giant cell arteritis is an idiopathic process manifested by focal granulomatous inflammation of medium and small arteries. This disease usually affects smaller vessels, such as the superficial temporal artery, but it may involve the larger vessels of the neck. The most common radio-graphic pattern in giant cell arteritis is multiple discrete stenoses.[1]

Subclavian steal

In some cases, collateral pathways are already present but do not manifest until normal hemodynamics are altered, as in the case of subclavian steal syndrome. Subclavian steal syndrome occurs when the subclavian artery, most commonly the left, becomes occluded proximal to the origin of the vertebral artery. In this setting, the distal subclavian artery "steals" blood from the posterior circulation of the brain by means of retrograde flow through the ipsilateral vertebral artery (Fig. 18-9). The decreased blood flow to the posterior circulation of the brain may result in ischemia, from which patients often become symptomatic when exercising the affected upper extremity.

Trauma

Traumatic injury to the neck is a common indication for performing angiography, especially in the setting of penetrating trauma to regions where physical examination is

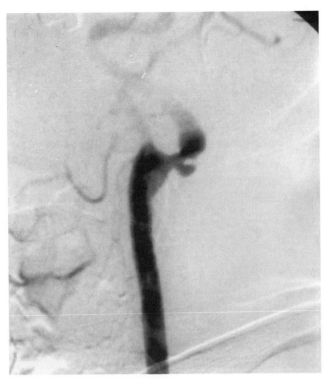

FIGURE 18-6. Digital subtraction angiography of left common carotid artery in anteroposterior oblique projection demonstrates stenosis involving the carotid bulb with a focal collection of contrast projecting posteriorly. The appearance is typical of an ulcerated atherosclerotic plaque.

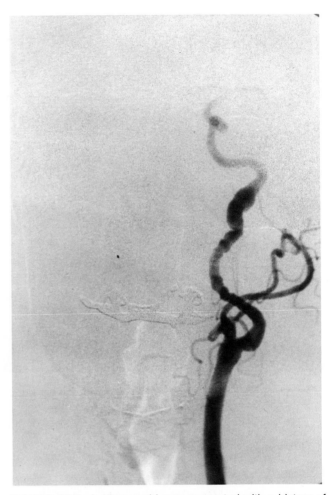

FIGURE 18-7. A 40-year-old man presented with a history of recent stroke. Digital subtraction angiography of left common carotid artery (anteroposterior view) demonstrates a long segment of alternating areas of stenosis and dilatation in the left internal carotid artery distal to the normal bifurcation. This is typical of fibromuscular dysplasia and is commonly referred to as a "string of beads" appearance. (Case courtesy of Dr. Deborah Shatzkes.)

difficult. By convention, the neck is divided into three zones:

- Zone 1 extends from the thoracic inlet to the cricoid cartilage
- Zone 2 extends from the cricoid to the angle of the mandible
- Zone 3 extends from the mandibular angle to the skull base.

Traditionally, penetrating trauma to zones 1 and 3 calls for an angiogram in most surgical algorithms, although angiographic studies for these "proximity" injuries have notoriously low yields.[6] Zone 2 injuries are not usually examined by angiography because damage to the artery is assessed relatively easily clinically because of the superficial position of the artery in this zone. Damage to the cervical vessels may be caused by penetrating or blunt trauma and may manifest as spasm, thrombosis, partial or complete transection, dissection, arteriovenous fistula (AVF), or pseudoaneurysm (Fig. 18-10). As a general rule, wounds cephalad to the angle of the mandible are more likely to result in damage to the vessels, and stab wounds are associated with vascular injury less frequently than gunshot wounds.[6]

These criteria pertain mainly to the carotid circulation, because the vertebral artery is relatively well protected within its bony canal. Clinical indicators of vascular injury include expanding hematoma, absent pulses, bruit, and altered neurological status.

Neoplasms and other disease processes

Although multiplanar imaging modalities have mostly replaced angiography in the evaluation of lesions that do not directly involve the normal vessels of the neck, the ability to facilitate therapy by embolization secures the role of angiography in a select set of disease processes, both neoplastic and nonneoplastic. In the neoplastic category, paraganglioma, juvenile angiofibroma, and meningioma are the tumors most commonly considered for embolization and, hence, for angiography.

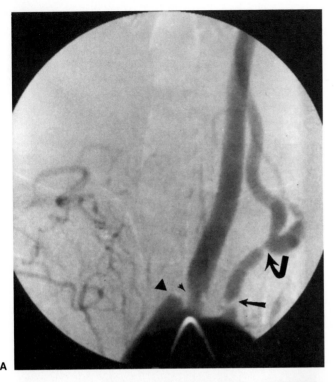

A

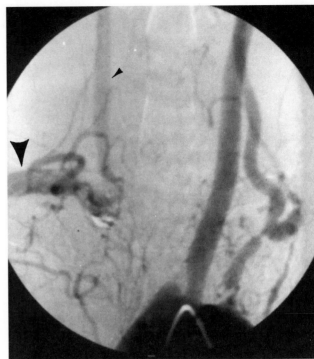

B

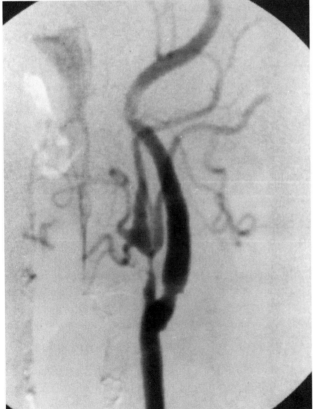

C

FIGURE 18-8. A: Digital subtraction angiography of the aortic arch (anteroposterior projection) of an early arterial phase demonstrates multiple smooth stenoses of the great vessels, including the origins of the left common carotid artery (*small arrowhead*) and left subclavian artery (*straight arrow*) in addition to stenosis more distally in the left subclavian artery (*curved arrow*). Note the occlusion of proximal innominate artery (*large arrowhead*). **B:** Later in the arterial phase of the arch injection, reconstitution of the right subclavian artery (*large arrowhead*) and right common carotid artery (*small arrowhead*) is demonstrated. **C:** Digital subtraction angiography of the left common carotid artery in the lateral projection demonstrates stenoses of the proximal left internal and external carotid arteries.

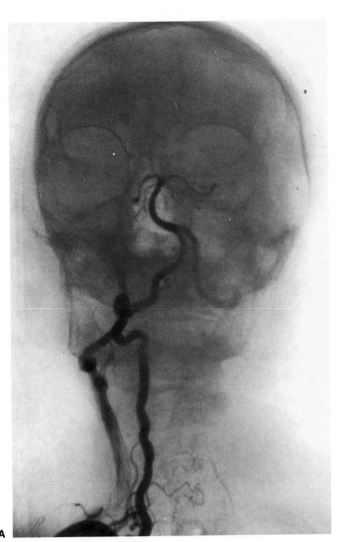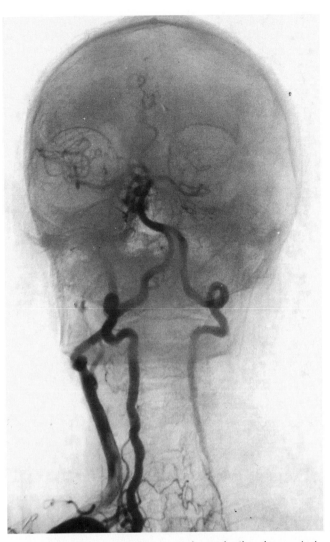

A   B

FIGURE 18-9. **A** and **B**: Anteroposterior, sequential digital subtraction angiograms in the anteroposterior projection demonstrate retrograde flow of contrast into the left vertebral artery **(B)** from the right vertebral artery, which fills antegrade from a right subclavian artery injection. Note reflux filling of the right common carotid artery. (Courtesy of Dr. Paul Sane.)

Paragangliomas

Paragangliomas, of which chemodectomas are a subset, are locally invasive, highly vascular tumors that arise from paraganglion cells.[7] Typically, they are located at the bifurcation of the carotid artery, along the vagus nerve within the jugular vein or within the middle ear along Jacobson's nerve, but they may occur in other locations (Fig. 18-11). Paragangliomas are more prevalent in women (3:1) and have a peak incidence in the fourth to fifth decade of life. These lesions usually are supplied by the branches of the ECA, but may recruit blood supply from other vessels. As a result of their hypervascularity and propensity to bleed profusely at surgery, preoperative angiography with embolization is often performed, especially for glomus jugulare tumors.

Juvenile angiofibroma

Juvenile angiofibroma is a highly vascular nasopharyngeal neoplasm that affects adolescent males. Although the tumor is histologically benign, it may be extremely aggressive and invade surrounding structures.[8] Patients with this tumor are at high risk for life-threatening hemorrhage. Angiography is performed to discern the extent of the tumor and for preoperative embolization. During an episode of uncontrolled bleeding, embolization may be life saving. The blood supply of these tumors originates from the distal internal maxillary artery in most cases; as the tumor grows, any vessel in its vicinity may be parasitized, including branches of the internal carotid artery. Before embolization of these tumors, careful examination of the ICAs must be made to safeguard

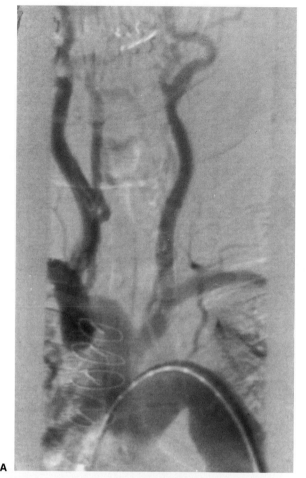

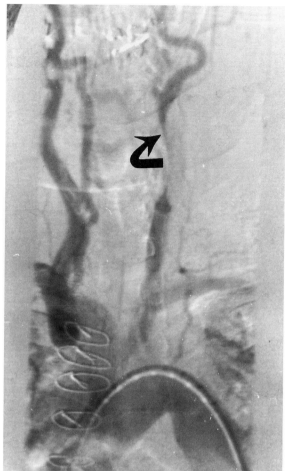

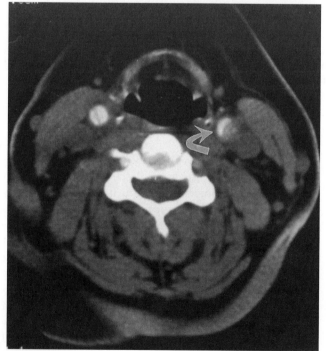

FIGURE18-10. Digital subtraction injection of the aortic arch in the anteroposterior projection in early arterial **(A)** and midarterial **(B)** phases demonstrates filling of the false and true lumen (*curved arrow*) in a hypertensive patient status post spontaneous left common carotid dissection. Axial contrast enhanced dynamic computed tomography (CT) scan through the neck demonstrates bilateral common carotid artery dissections. **(C).** Note the differential filling of the false and true lumen (*curved arrow*) of the left common carotid artery. There is differential opacification of the right and left vertebral arteries as well (also apparent in the arch injection [A,B]).

against refluxing embolic material into the ICA circulation.

Meningioma

Most meningiomas occur in a supratentorial location; however, they may involve the skull base and spinal cord. Meningiomas are typically vascular, exhibiting a dense contrast stain that appears in the early phase of the injection and lingers until late into the venous phase (Fig. 18-12). Preoperative embolization is performed if the blood supply to the lesion is judged to be potentially difficult to control surgically.

Arteriovenous malformations

Arteriovenous malformations (AVMs) constitute the bulk of nonneoplastic lesions for which angiography is routinely obtained. AVMs are congenital lesions that are thought to result from abnormal embryological development of the vascular system. They are high-velocity arteriovenous shunts that consist of a tangle of abnormal

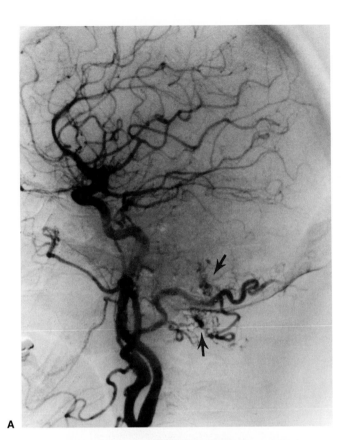

A

B

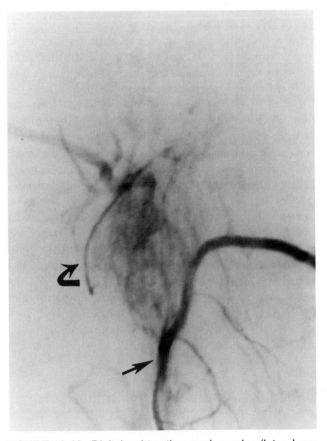

FIGURE 18-11. A: Right common carotid angiogram demonstrates paraganglioma tumor vascularity (*arrows*) supplied by branches of the enlarged occipital artery. **B:** Digital subtraction angiography of the right vertebral artery in the lateral projection demonstrates that the tumor also is supplied by the vertebral artery.

FIGURE 18-12. Digital subtraction angiography (lateral projection) of selective left occipital artery injection (*straight arrow*) shows extensive tumor blush supplied by the left occipital branches. Note the transtumoral filling of the anteriorly bowed ascending pharyngeal artery (*curved arrow*), which also supplied the meningioma.

vessels with arterial feeders and enlarged draining veins. Although most of these lesions are intracranial, AVMs of the neck, scalp, and face do occur.[7] As with the other processes already mentioned, angiography of these lesions is undertaken to define the extent of the lesion and for preoperative embolization. In traumatic AVFs and pseudoaneurysms, embolization may be curative.[9]

Hemangioma

Cavernous hemangiomas, or cavernous venous malformations, are relatively common and may occur in the head and neck region. Composed of large, cavernous vascular spaces, these malformations may grow to a large size. These lesions generally are removed for cosmetic reasons, but they may become symptomatic as a result of thrombosis or mass effect on adjacent structures. Cavernous venous malformations are not associated with arteriovenous shunting. Angiographic study usually demonstrates a normal arterial phase with puddling of contrast within enlarged venous spaces (Fig. 18-13). Arterial embolization is usually not indicated, unless as a preoperative measure.

Refractory epistaxis

Refractory epistaxis is an important indication for angiography. In most episodes of epistaxis, the bleeding point occurs in the anterior portion of the nasal cavity and is easily controlled by packing or cauterization. Bleeds that originate in the posterior or superior nasal cavity are more difficult to manage and often require posterior packs or ligation of the internal maxillary artery. Posterior packs have a significant failure rate and are associated with complications such as pressure-induced necrosis and life-treatening hypoxia.[10] Selective embolization and superselective embolization have emerged as alternatives to surgical management of uncontrolled epistaxis. The distal branches of the internal maxillary artery usually supply the bleeding site, but branches of the facial artery, and less commonly the internl carotid artery, may be involved. As is the case with juvenile angiofibroma, the ICA as well as the ECA must be studied before embolization is done to define the source of the bleeding accurately and to prevent inadvertent embolization of the ICA circulation.

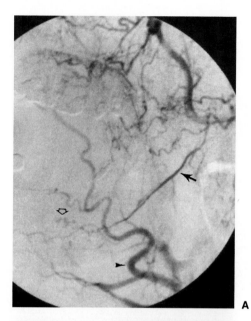

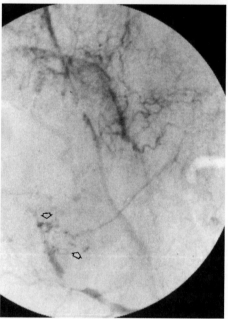

FIGURE 18-13. Lateral projection of left external carotid arterial injection in early arterial **(A)** and capillary **(B)** phases demonstrates contrast puddling characteristic of hemangioma (*open arrows*) supplied by the inferior alveolar branch of the internal maxillary artery (*closed arrow*). Note in **A**, facial artery (*arrowhead*), which is best seen in the arterial phase.

■ Vascular Anatomy of the Spinal Cord

The vascular supply of the spinal cord is provided by the anterior spinal artery and paired posterior spinal arteries (Fig. 18-14A). These arteries arise from the vertebral arteries. The anterior spinal artery originates as paired branches of the vertebral artery that then fuse. The anterior spinal artery runs within the anterior median fissure and supplies the anterior two-thirds to four-fifths of the cord. The posterior spinal arteries course along the posterolateral surface of the spinal cord in the region of the dorsal root entry zone. The volume of blood provided by the vertebral arteries is not sufficient to supply the entire cord, and below the level of C4–C5, the spinal arteries

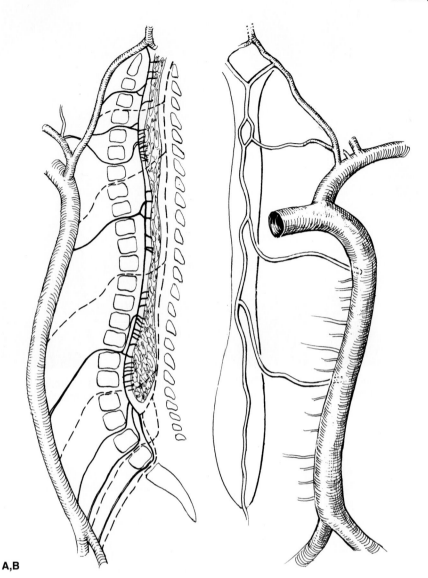

FIGURE 18-14. Spinal cord arterial supply. Lateral (**A**) and anterior (**B**) views.

A,B

rely on anastomoses from radiculomedullary arteries (Fig. 18-14B). The origins of the radiculomedullary arteries vary and may arise from the vertebral, ascending cervical, intercostal, and lumbar arteries (Fig. 18-15). The artery of Adamkiewicz, or arteria radicularis magna, is the largest of the radiculomedullary arteries and generally arises from a left-sided intercostal artery between the levels of T9–12. This artery has a characteristic hairpin curve when seen on anteroposterior angiography (Fig. 18-16). The artery of Adamkiewicz is the main source of blood for the lower cord, and cross-clamping of the aorta above the level of this artery may result in catastrophic neurological deficit.[11]

Venous drainage of the spinal cord is accomplished by intramedullary veins that empty into an extensive venous plexus within the meninges and finally into the external venous plexus or Batson's plexus.

■ Angiography of the Spine, Head, and Neck

Indications for spinal angiography

Angiography is generally not an indicated examination in the evaluation of most disease processes of the spinal cord. Angiography of the spinal cord is performed most commonly for the delineation and treatment of spinal AVMs and for vascular primary and metastatic neoplasms of the bony canal. One of the crucial indications for spinal cord arteriography is to locate the artery of Adamkiewicz before treatment begins, in cases where interruption of the thoracic aortic blood flow may be necessary or where endovascular embolization is being contemplated.[12] Given the reliance of the spinal cord on anastomatic arteries for its blood supply, meticulous technique must be

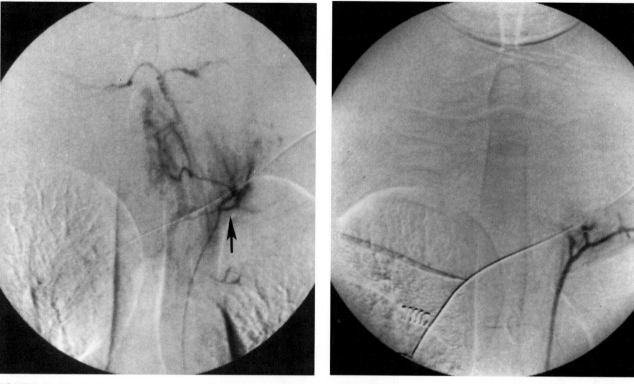

FIGURE 18-15. A: Preembolization digital subtraction anteroposterior (AP) projection of selective left T3 intercostal artery (*arrow*) demonstrates tumor vascularity. **B:** Postembolization digital subtraction AP projection of the left T3 intercostal artery.

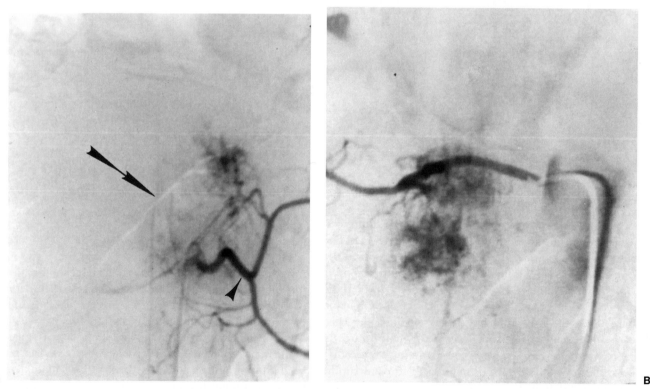

FIGURE 18-16. A: Anteroposterior (AP) projection of selective left intercostal arterial injection demonstrates filling of the left T10 and T11 intercostal arteries from a common trunk (*arrowhead*). In addition, filling of the artery of Adamkiewicz is critical to note (*arrow*). **B:** AP projection digital subtraction angiography of a selective right T9 intercostal artery injection illustrates extensive paraspinal tumor neovascularity. This represents surgically proven nodal metastasis from renal cell carcinoma.

used when performing spinal angiography to avoid embolization or thrombosis of these vessels. There are no absolute contraindications to spinal angiography.

Indications for head and neck angiography

With the advent of multiplanar imaging, the role of angiography in pathological processes of the neck has diminished, although there are multiple indications for which angiography is still performed. It is routinely performed in conjunction with cerebral arteriography. Trauma to the neck in which vascular injury is suspected or cannot be excluded is a common indication for angiography. As previously noted, the percent of positive findings in patients stable enough to undergo angiography is low, and controversy exists as to whether angiography should be performed unless there is a strong suspicion of vascular injury.[13] Evaluation of extracranial carotid disease in both symptomatic and asymptomatic patients with duplex evidence of carotid stenosis is a common indication for angiography. Although recent large-scale studies in both symptomatic and asymptomatic patients have affirmed the efficacy of carotid endarterectomy in the prevention of stroke,[3,4] the need for preoperative angiography versus duplex alone or duplex in conjunction with magnetic resonance angiography (MRA) has been questioned. The Asymptomatic Carotid Artery Stenosis (ACAS) study used both arteriography and ultrasound as separate admitting criteria and stated that the complication rate of carotid angiography significantly added to the morbidity of endarterectomy in the surgical cohort.[3] With this in mind, the indications for angiography of the neck, as in other parts of the body, must be weighed in consideration of the risk-benefit ratio. Angiography should be considered in cases of known trauma to vascular structures, assessment of vascular pathology and malformations, preoperative "road mapping," and in preparation for interventional endovascular procedures such as embolization.

Contraindications for angiography of the spine, head, and neck

There is no absolute contraindication to angiography of the head and neck, although there are a few relative contraindications that are not specific to angiography of this region of the body, including bleeding diatheses, contrast allergy, and compromised renal function. Concurrent migraine headache is thought to be a relative contraindication, because the increased potential for vasospasm in these patients may lead to serious complications, most of which pertain to the posterior circulation (i.e., cortical blindness),[1] which occurs more specifically in relation to selective cerebral angiography.

Angiography versus other modalities

Recently, other imaging modalities have evolved that are able to assess the vascular structures in the neck, including duplex Doppler ultrasound, MRA, and computed tomographic angiography (CTA). Ultrasound is the most frequently used modality in the assessment of carotid disease and has the advantages of being noninvasive, easily tolerated, and relatively inexpensive. Its disadvantages include being operator dependent and, to a certain extent, anatomy dependent in that some vascular structures are inaccessible and that heavily calcified or tortuous vessels may render the study difficult to interpret.[14] MRA is noninvasive and less affected by vessel tortuosity or position, and multiplanar/three-dimensional reconstruction can be obtained. MRA shares the disadvantage of being adversely affected by heavily calcified vessel (field inhomogeneity effects) and being relatively expensive and susceptible to motion artifact. In addition, it is more difficult to monitor the patient while he or she is in the magnet.[14] CTA has become readily available with the advent of spiral CT and fast computer reconstruction. The advantages of CTA include the ability to view the images in any plane, its relatively low cost, and minimal invasiveness. The disadvantages include long postprocessing times, the necessity for iodinated contrast, and the fact that heavily calcified vessels significantly add to the difficulty of postprocessing, thus affecting the accuracy of the study.[15] In comparative studies between modalities, angiography is most accurate in the assessment of stenotic lesions. In a recent study,[13] ultrasound and MRA have been shown to have 65% and 52% exact correlation with angiography, respectively, with both modalities tending to exaggerate stenoses. CTA has been shown to compare favorably with ultrasound and MRA, but it is not as accurate as angiography.[15] In summary, with the superiority of angiography in the assessment of stenotic lesions as well as its versatility, it will continue to be performed until other modalities are proven superior or the discrepancy rates of these other modalities become insignificant compared with the complication rate of angiography.

References

1. Osborne AO. *Introduction to Cerebral Angiography.* Philadelphia: Harper & Row, 1980.
2. Kilgore BB, Fields WS. Arterial occlusive disease in adults. In: Newton, TH, and Potts DG, eds. *Radiology of the Skull and Brain,* vol 4, 1974:2310–2343.
3. Endarterectomy for asymptomatic carotid artery stenosis. *JAMA* 1995;273:1421–1428.
4. North American Symptomatic Carotid Endarterectomy Trial collaborators. *N Engl J Med* 1991;325:445–453.
5. Hall S, Barr W, Lie JT, et al. Takayasu arteritis: a study of 32 North American patients. *Medicine* 1985;64:89–99.
6. North CM, Ahmadi J, Segall HD, et al. Penetrating vascular injuries

of th
J Roe
7. Hurs
Neur
8. Mou
bron
grou
1995
9. Schv
bifu
10. Elde
tion
Hea
11. Anso
ogy.

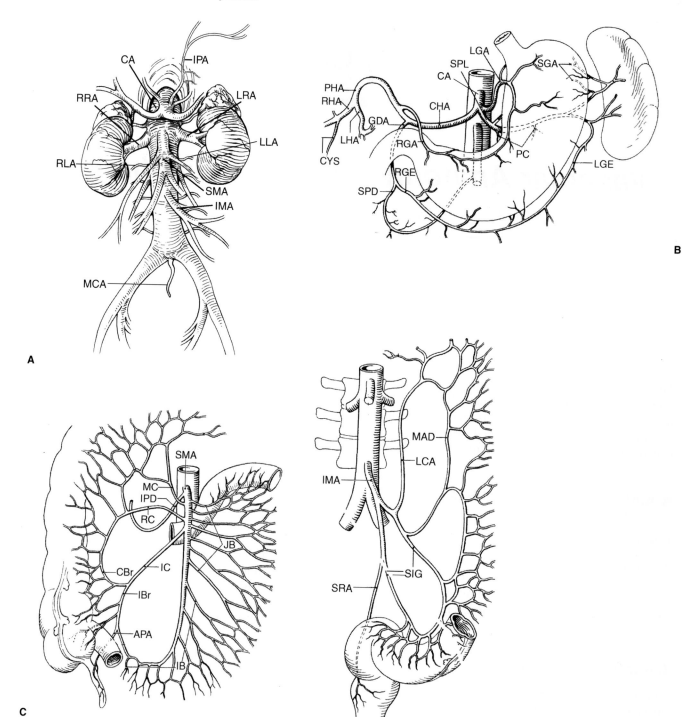

FIGURE 19-1. (A). Abdominal aorta and branches include the inferior phrenic arteries (IPA), celiac artery (CA), superior mesenteric artery (SMA), right and left renal arteries (RRA, LRA), and inferior mesenteric artery (IMA). **(B).** Celiac artery (CA) and branches include: common hepatic artery (CHA), splenic artery (SPL), left gastric artery (LGA), proper hepatic artery (PHA), right hepatic artery (RHA), left hepatic artery (LHA), cystic artery (CYS), right gastric artery (RGA), gastroduodenal artery (GDA), right gastroepiploic artery (RGE), and superior pancreaticoduodenal artery (SPD). Splenic branches include pancreatic (PC), short gastric artery (SGA), and left gastroepiploic arteries (LGE). **(C).** Superior mesenteric artery (SMA) and branches include inferior pancreaticoduodenal artery (IPD), jejunal branches (JB), ileal branches (IB), ileocolic artery (IC), right colic artery (RC), middle colic artery (MC). Branches of the ileocolic artery include the appendicular artery (APA), ileal branch (IBr), and colic branch (CBr). **(D).** Inferior mesenteric artery (IMA) and branches include left colic artery (LCA), sigmoid arteries (SIG), superior rectal artery (SRA), and marginal artery of Drummond (MAD).

typically a terminal branch of the SMA that continues the inferior course of the vessel. The ileocolic typically arises at a 45-degree angle from the main trunk of the SMA and provides flow to the cecum and anastomotic branches to the right colic. Ileal branches and the appendicular artery arise from this vessel as well. The right colic artery arises between the middle and ileo colic origins. Its branches anastomose with both of these vessels. The right colic supplies the right colon and proximal transverse colon.

Inferior mesenteric artery (Fig. 19-1D)

The inferior mesenteric artery (IMA) arises from the left anterolateral surface of the aorta, on the left at about the L3 level. It supplies the distal transverse colon, left colon, and sigmoid and superior rectum. The left colic is the first branch, which divides into ascending and descending branches. The ascending branch joins the left branch of the middle colic to form the important arc of Riolan. This anastomosis is important because there is a high incidence of IMA origin occlusion in elderly patients. A similar anastomosis is the marginal artery of Drummond. This vessel lies within bowel mesentery and is present along the mesenteric border of the large bowel. The marginal artery of Drummond is formed by the arcades of the ileocolic, right colic, middle colic, and left colic branches. There are usually two or three sigmoid branches arising from the IMA. The final branch of the IMA is the superior hemorrhoidal, which divides to supply both sides of the superior rectum. The superior hemorrhoidal forms an important anastomotic network with middle hemorrhoidal branches. The superior hemorrhoidal is a branch of the internal iliac, and therefore these vascular systems are joined here.

Renal arteries

The renal arteries originate just inferior to the SMA origin at about the L1–2 level. The left renal artery orifice is typically lateral or slightly anterolateral in location, and the right renal artery origin is positioned more anterolaterally. There is variant renal artery anatomy in about one third of individuals. About 70% of the population have single renal arteries, and the remainder have multiple renal arteries or an early bifurcation of the renal artery. The early bifurcation usually gives rise to an upper pole, the polar branch. The remaining variations include two large renal arteries on the same side, an upper-pole accesory vessel, a lower-pole accesory vessel, both an upper and lower pole vessel, three renal arteries, or more than three vessels.

The renal artery divides into anterior and posterior divisions at the renal hilus, which divide into lobar arteries. The lobar arteries divide into interlobar branches at the level of the renal pyramids. The terminal branches are the arcuate arteries, which are at the corticomedullary junction. In addition to the renal branches, the renal arteries give off inferior adrenal branches, capsular branches, branches to the renal pelvis, and proximal ureter and gonadal arteries.

Lumbar arteries

There are typically five pairs of lumbar arteries. They have a typical appearance as they initially have a cranial route over the vertebral body pedicle and descend with an ultimate posterolateral branching pattern. They arise from the posterior aspect of the aorta. The last pair arise just at the aortic bifurcation and can give off a middle sacral branch.

Iliac arteries (Fig. 19-2)

The aorta bifurcates into common iliac arteries (CIA) at the L4 or L5 level. The anatomic landmark is the umbilicus. The division is into common iliac arteries (CIA). The CIAs can give rise to renal arteries in ectopic kidneys or horseshoe kidneys. The CIA divides into the internal (IIA) and external (EIA) iliac arteries; another name for the IIA is the hypogastric artery. The distal EIAs give off important branches: the inferior epigastric and deep circumflex iliac. The inferior epigastric forms an anastomosis with the superior epigastric, which is a branch of the internal mammary artery (see Chapter 13). The inferior epigastric is recognizable because it has a truly cephalad and medial course from the EIA. The deep circimflex iliac arises and

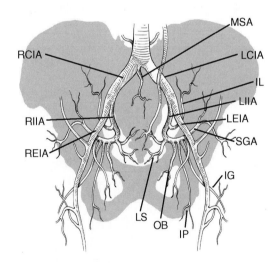

FIGURE 19-2. Arteries of the pelvis include the right and left common iliac arteries (RCIA, LCIA); each divide into an external iliac artery (REIA, LEIA) and an internal iliac artery (RIIA, LIIA). Posterior internal iliac branches include superior gluteal (SGA), iliolumbar (IL), and lateral sacral arteries (LS). Anterior branches include obturator (OB), inferior gluteal (IG), and internal pudendal (IP). The middle sacral artery (MSA) arises as a terminal branch of the aorta.

courses laterally and superiorly. These vessels mark the boundary of the EIA and the common femoral artery.

Internal iliac artery

In most people, the internal iliac artery divides into two main trunks: the posterior and anterior divisions. The posterior division gives off the superior gluteal, iliolumbar, and lateral sacral branches. The anterior division gives rise to the obturator, inferior gluteal, and internal pudendal branches as well as smaller visceral branches. The obturator artery terminates, as its name suggests, in the obturator foramen. The inferior gluteal, in its course to supply the gluteus muscle, gives off branches to the sciatic nerve. The internal pudendal gives off the inferior hemorrhoidal branch before giving rise to the penile arteries, the dorsal artery of the penis, and the cavernosal artery (also called *deep*). Visceral branches of the internal iliac include the middle hemorrhoidal, branches to the bladder (superior and inferior vesical arteries), and genital branches (prostate and seminal vesicles in men, the uterine arteries in women).

3A). The profunda femoris varies in size. It courses lateral and posteriorly, hence its other name is the *deep femoral artery*. Less frequently, the profunda may arise immediately posteriorly or medial to the common femoral artery. The medial and lateral femoral circumflex arteries most commonly arise from the profunda femoris.

The superficial femoral artery (SFA) courses within the medial thigh until it dives posteriorly at the level of the adductor canal. This fenestration in the adductor magnus muscle is also known as the *Hunter's canal*. The canal is the anatomic boundary of the SFA and popliteal artery. Near the level of the adductor canal, the popliteal artery gives off important branches: descending genicular, superior genicular, and supreme geniculate. These are important collateral vessels in popliteal artery occlusive disease. About two thirds of the popliteal artery is superior to the knee joint; the remaining third is inferior. Inferior to the knee joint inferior geniculate branches arise. The popliteal artery demonstrates variation in its division. Most frequently, there is division into the anterior tibial artery and the tibioperoneal trunk (Fig. 19-3B). The anterior tibial artery courses anteriorly to perforate the in-

■ Lower Extremity

The anatomic boundary of the external iliac artery and common femoral artery is the inguinal ligament. The common femoral artery divides into the superficial femoral artery and the profunda femoris artery (Figure 19-

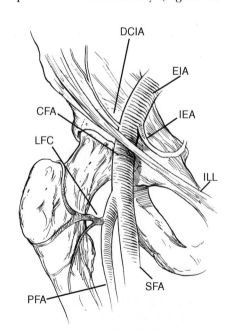

A

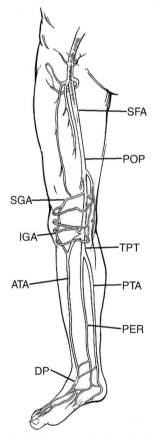

B

FIGURE 19-3. (A). The distal external iliac (EIA) becomes the common femoral (CFA) at the inguinal ligament, the superficial femoral (SFA), deep femoral (PFA) and lateral femoral circumflex (LFC) arteries. Note also the relationship of the deep circumflex iliac (DCIA) and the interior epigastric (IEA) arteries to the inguinal ligament (ILL). **(B).** Lower extremity arteries include superficial femoral artery (SFA) popliteal artery (POP), superior and inferior geniculate arteries (SGA, IGA), tibial peroneal trunk (TPT), anterior tibial artery (ATA), peroneal artery (PER), posterior tibial artery (PTA), dorsalis pedis artery (DP)

terosseous membrane and continue inferiorly, overlying the tibia to terminate as the dorsalis pedis artery in the foot. The tibioperoneal trunk is a short vessel. The peroneal artery has a medial course posterior to the interosseous membrane of the tibia and fibula. The peroneal artery terminates with a posterior communicating branch and an anterior perforating branch. These can act as important collaterals in the reconstitution of foot vessels in tibial occlusive disease. The posterior tibial artery continues medially to pass posterior to the medial malleolus. It then courses anteriorly and inferiorly as a plantar branch. Together with branches of the dorsalis pedis branch, a pedal arch is formed.

■ Venous Anatomy

Two important axioms that all medical students have learned are that veins follow their respective arteries and that veins vary. True to form, we will attempt to stay with this teaching.

Inferior vena cava (Fig. 19-4)

The confluence of iliac veins forms the inferior vena cava (IVC) at approximately the L5 level. It is a retroperitoneal structure that lies anterior and slightly to the right of the spine. It courses through the liver along the posterior surface of the caudate lobe. It then has a short segment between the liver and heart, where it pierces the

diaphragm. It drains into the posterior aspect of the right atrium. Along its retroperitoneal course, it drains lumbar branches, renal veins, right adrenal veins, and hepatic veins. The caudate lobe of the liver drains directly into the intrahepatic segment of the IVC. Duplication of the IVC, left-sided IVC, or absence of the IVC with azygos or hemiazygos continuation is seen in 0.5 to 2% of individuals.

Renal and adrenal veins (Fig. 19-5)

The right renal vein typically enters the IVC at approximately the L1 level. It is usually single; however, supranumerary right renal veins have been noted as well as drainage of adrenal and gonadal veins. The left renal vein is single and anterior (preaortic) in about 80% of individuals. A circumaortic ring of veins is seen in about 20%, a single retroaortic vein (posterior to aorta) in about 3%. The left adrenal vein and gonadal vein typically drain into the left renal vein. The right adrenal vein most commonly drains directly into the IVC just superior to the right renal vein insertion. Rarely, there can be drainage into a hepatic vein as well.

Hepatic and portal veins (Fig. 19-6A and B)

Typically, there are three hepatic veins: right, middle, and left. The middle and left commonly form a single trunk, and the right hepatic vein drains directly into the IVC. As stated, the caudate lobe of the liver drains directly into the IVC. This explains its frequently encountered "hypertrophy" noted in cirrhosis.

The portal vein runs in the hepatoduodenal ligament

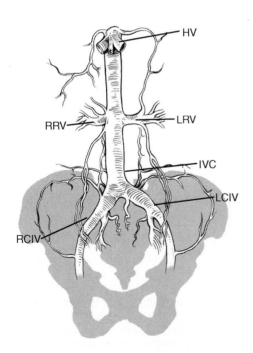

FIGURE 19-4. Inferior vena cava (IVC). Major tributaries include bepatic vein (HV), left renal vein (LRV), right renal vein (RRV), right and left common iliac veins (RCIV, LCIV).

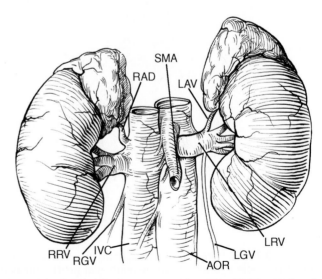

FIGURE 19-5. Renal and adrenal veins. Right renal vein (RRV), right gonadal vein (RGV) and right adrenal vein (RAD). Left renal vein (LRV), left gonadal (LGV) and left adrenal vein (LAV). Note the relationship of the aorta (AOR), the superior mesenteric artery (SMA) and the inferior vena cava (IVC).

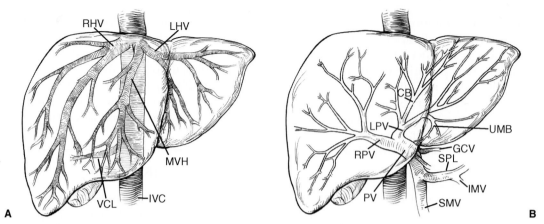

FIGURE 19-6. (A). Hepatic veins. Left (LHV), middle (MHV), and right (RHV). Veins from the caudate lobe of the liver (VCL) drain separately into the inferior vena cava (IVC). **(B).** Portal venous system includes superior mesenteric vein (SMV), splenic vein (SPL), inferior mesenteric vein (IMV), and gastrocoronary vein (GCV). Main portal vein (PV), right and left branches (RPV, LPV), umbilical (UMB) and caudate (CB) branches of LPV are noted.

posterior to the common bile duct and the hepatic artery; however it is usually flanked by the common bile duct to its right and the hepatic artery to its left. The portal vein forms where the superior mesenteric vein and splenic vein conjoin at approximately the L1–2 level. The splenic vein has a horizontal course, posterior to the pancreas, much less tortuous than the typical appearance of the splenic artery. The inferior mesenteric vein drains the IMA territory and empties into the splenic vein. Within the hepatic parenchyma, the portal vein divides into left and right branches. The left branch maintains its

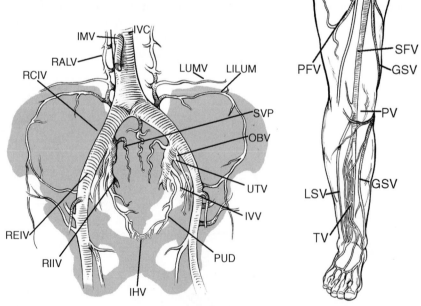

FIGURE 19-7. (A). Pelvic veins include right external, common and internal iliac veins (REIV, RCIV, RIIV). Branches of the left internal iliac vein shown: inferior hemorrhoidal (IHV), pudendal (PUD), inferior vesical (IVV), uterine (UTV), obturator (OBV) veins. Note also sacral venous plexus (SVP), left lumbar and iliac lumbar veins (LUMV, LILUM), right ascending lumbar vein (RALV), as well as inferior mesenteric vein (IMV) and inferior vena cava (IVC). **(B).** Veins of the lower extremity include the superficial venous system, which includes the greater saphenous vein (GSV) and lesser saphenous (LSV). Deep venous system includes paired anterior tibial, posterior tibial, and peroneal veins (TV), popliteal vein (PV), superficial femoral vein (SFV), and profunda femoris veins (PFV).

embryonic connections to the umbilical vein and ductus venosus. Once obliterated, these are termed the *ligamentum teres* and *ligamentum venosum,* respectively. These vessels can recannulate with portal hypertension. It is important to recognize that numerous gastric and pancreatic veins are present, and these veins drain into the portal vein; however these are frequently not seen in patients with normal portal vein pressures. Their recognition is vital in studies for portal hypertension.

Pelvis and lower extremity

The external iliac veins and common iliac veins are direct conduits for the return of blood from the lower extremity (Fig. 19-7A). The internal iliac (or hypogastric veins) are conveniently divided into three components, as described by Kadir: (1) The veins arising external to the pelvis, such as the gluteal veins (superior and inferior), the pudendal veins (prostatic plexus in the male or uterovaginal plexus in the female), and the obturator veins, which typically follow their respective arteries; (2) posterior pelvic veins, which arise from the sacral venous plexus, and have important connections with the paravertebral veins; and (3) the internal pelvic veins, which drain the pelvic viscera, and are the hemorrhoidal, vesicular, external pudendal, and uterine veins.

The veins of the lower extremity comprise both superficial and deep systems (Fig. 19-7B). The superficial system is dominated by the greater saphenous vein, which arises along the medial and anterior aspect of the foot. A deep system arises at the popliteal vein, which is the confluence of smaller leg veins. Like their so-named arteries, the superficial femoral vein starts at the adductor hiatus and continues into the common femoral vein. These drain directly into the external iliac veins, as described previously herein. The deep and superficial systems communicate via perforating veins. These veins contain valves that direct flow toward the deep system. Failure of this valve system can result in varicosities. Accessory saphenous veins aid in draining the thigh, and a lesser saphenous vein begins drainage of the lateral aspect of the foot and ultimately empties into the deep system.

SUGGESTED READINGS

1. Abrams HL, Baum S, Pentecost MJ. *Abrams' Angiography: Vascular and Interventional Radiology,* 4th ed. Boston: Little, Brown; 1997.
2. Clemente C. *Anatomy: A Regional Atlas of the Human Body.* 2nd ed. Baltimore: Urban & Schwarzenberg; 1981.
3. Kadir S. *Diagnostic Angiography.* Philadelphia: WB Saunders; 1986.
4. Kadir S. *Atlas of Normal and Variant Angiographic Anatomy.* Philadelphia: WB Saunders; 1991.
5. Moore KL. *Clinically Oriented Anatomy.* 2nd ed. Baltimore: Williams & Wilkins; 1985.
6. Moore KL. *The Developing Human: Clinically Oriented Embryology.* 3rd ed. Philadelphia: WB Saunders; 1982.
7. Strandness E, van Breda A. *Vascular Diseases: Surgical and Interventional Therapy.* New York: Churchill Livingstone; 1994.

20

Atherosclerotic Disease of the Aorta, Pelvis, and Lower Extremities

CURTIS W. BAKAL and JACOB CYNAMON

Diagnostic arteriography for atherosclerotic disease of the aorta, pelvis, and lower extremities is performed after the decision to treat has been made. Clinical history and noninvasive studies that precede the angiogram almost always can make the diagnosis of chronic atherosclerotic occlusive disease and often will be able to define the levels at which critical stenoses occur. The purpose of the angiogram is to define specifically the anatomy to plan interventional or surgical therapy. Multiple views are often necessary to define the anatomy clearly (Fig. 20-1). Thus, a thorough knowledge of potential available therapies is important to obtain an adequate study.

Traditional vascular surgical techniques require that three things be defined. The first is the status of the "inflow," that is, the arteries upstream of the target lesion. (Because atheroocclusive disease is almost always infrarenal, the infrarenal aorta and the common iliac and external iliac arteries serve as the inflow for the infrainguinal arteries, as an example.) The second is the status of the "outflow," the vascular segment or segments downstream of the occlusive lesion. (For example, for popliteal occlusion at Hunter's canal, the outflow is the popliteal artery and trifurcation vessels.) These two vessel sets define where the proximal anastomosis and distal anastomosis of a bypass graft are placed. The third parameter is the type of conduit, for example, autologous vein versus polytetrafluoroethylene (PTFE). Synthetic conduits are used exclusively in the aortoiliac distribution, whereas an autologous vein is much preferred for bypass to the tibial and pedal vessels. For femoropopliteal bypass grafts, if vein is available, most vascular surgeons will use it, especially if the graft has to cross the knee joint; otherwise, PTFE is used (surgical bypasses are usually named by their proximal and distal anastomoses; see Table 20-1.)

■ Chronic Occlusive Disease

Arteriosclerosis obliterans

Arteriosclerosis is a chronic disease that is progressive and usually symmetric. Patients present with gradual onset or worsening of symptoms. Most patients with arteriosclerosis obliterans present with claudication. Risk factors for arteriosclerosis obliterans include advanced age, hypertension, smoking, diabetes, hypercholesterolemia, hypertriglyceridemia, and male sex. In the United States, the most commonly accepted categorization of chronic limb ischemia is the Rutherford Criteria, which is listed in Table 20-2.[1]

Rutherford criteria

Category 0
Asymptomatic patients in this category include those with occlusive disease and congenital variants. The dorsal pedal pulse can be absent in about 12% of patients, although the posterior tibial pulse is rarely absent in normal patients. Asymmetric pulse decrement alone is not an indication for intervention in chronic disease.

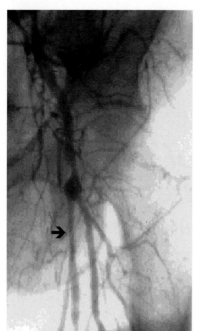 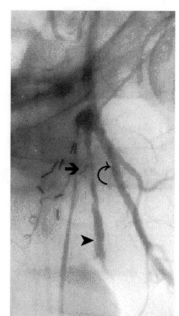 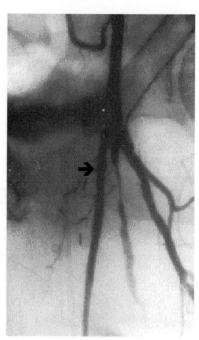

A–C

FIGURE 20-1. (A). An arteriogram was performed to evaluate a failing left common femoral to peroneal artery vein graft. The proximal portion of the graft is not seen secondary to the overlapping superficial femoral artery (*arrow*). **(B).** An oblique view demonstrates severe narrowing of the proximal portion of the vein graft (*straight arrow*). The superficial femoral artery (*arrowhead*) is seen better; the left deep femoral artery is visualized (*curved arrow*). **(C).** After balloon angioplasty of the proximal graft, flow and lumenal patency (arrow) are improved.

Categories 1–3

Patients with intermittent claudication usually have single-segment stenosis or occlusion (80% of cases). In these patients, the level of claudication usually develops distal to the level of stenosis. Claudication is a reproducible pain or soreness brought on by a defined amount of exercise and relieved by rest. (The term is derived from (Latin "to limp," after the Roman Emperor Claudius, who limped across Europe as his armies conquered the continent). These patients usually should be treated conservatively. Claudication must be differentiated from pseudoclaudication caused by spinal stenosis. Pseudoclaudication presents with variable onset relieved by a change in position and with normal peripheral pulses. Claudication and pseudoclaudication can coexist. The prevalence of intermittent claudication increases with age and is present in 3% of the population under 60 years of age and in 20% of the population older than 75 years of age. It is relatively stable in 60% of patients, with 15% actually improving with conservative therapy such as exercise and cessation of smoking. Twenty-five percent of claudicators progress to critical ischemia. Amputation is done in only 5 to 6% of patients within 10 years of presentation of peripheral vascular disease (PVD); the amputation rate is higher in smokers and diabetics. Intervention should be reserved for patients with debilitating or lifestyle-limiting claudication

TABLE 20-1. Typical Surgical Procedures

Operation	Indication
Aortoaortic bypass	Abdominal aortic aneurysm, without iliac extension
Aortoiliac bypass	Abdominal aortic aneurysm extending to common iliac arteries
Aorto bifemoral bypass	Aortoiliac occlusive disease involving both iliac arteries
Femoral–femoral bypass ("cross-femoral" bypass)	Unilateral severe iliac disease ipsilateral to symptoms; needs intact donor iliac artery contralateral to symptomatic side
Axillofemoral bypass	Used in high-risk patients with bilateral severe iliac disease; generally, axillary artery to femoral artery bypass (ipsilateral side), combined with cross-femoral bypass
Femoropopliteal bypass	Long-segment superficial femoral artery stenosis/occlusion; typically, common femoral artery serves as proximal anastomosis
Femorotibial bypass ("fem-distal" bypass)	Combined superficial femoral and popliteal artery stenosis/occlusion; occlusive disease frequently extends into proximal/midtibial arteries
Profundaplasty	Surgical revision of focal profunda femoris origin stenosis; often done in conjunction with femoropopliteal bypass
Iliac endarterectomy	Rarely used

TABLE 20-2. Clinical Categories of Chronic Limb Ischemia

Grade	Category	Clinical Description	Objective Criteria
0	0	Asymptomatic: no hemodynamically significant occlusive disease	Normal treadmill or reactive hyperemia test[b]
	1	Mild claudication	Completes treadmill exercise, AP after exercise > 50 mm Hg but at least 20 mm Hg lower than resting value
I	2	Moderate claudication	Between categories 1 and 3
II	3	Severe claudication	Cannot complete standard treadmill exercise and AP after exercise < 50 mm Hg
II[a]	4	Ischemic rest pain	Resting AP < 40 mm Hg, flat or barely pulsatile ankle or metatarsal PVR; TP < 30 mm Hg
III[a]	5	Minor tissue loss: nonhealing ulcer, focal gangrene with diffuse pedal ischemia	Resting AP < 60 mm Hg, ankle or metatarsal PVR flat or barely pulsatile; TP < 40 mm Hg
	6	Major tissue loss extending above TM level, functional foot no longer salvageable	Same as category 5

AP, ankle pressure; PVR, pulse volume recording; TP, toe pressure; TM, transmetatarsal.

[a]Grades II and III, categories 4, 5, and 6, are embraced by the term *chronic critical ischemia*.

[b]Five minutes at 3 mph on 12% incline.

From Rutherford RB, Baker JD, Ernest C, et al. Recommended Standards for reports dealing with lower extremity ischemia: revised version. *J Vasc Surg* 1997;26:517–538. With permission.

and for patients with critical ischemia. It is important to remember that claudication is a marker for coronary artery disease, which is prevalent in nearly all PVD patients.

Categories 4–6

Patients with critical ischemia have a threatened extremity that requires intervention. Diagnostic studies such as angiography should be performed to plan treatment. Percutaneous and surgical interventions generally are directed at restoring continuous or "straight-line" flow to the foot. The purpose of such intervention is to maintain a functional foot and allow ambulation. Critically ischemic patients usually have multilevel occlusive disease. Symptoms from perfusion deficit develop in the end organ, that is, the skin of the foot. Ischemic rest pain (category 4) usually develops in the forefoot because resting-limb blood flow is insufficient to meet basal metabolic demand, causing pain in the cutaneous nerves. It is often nocturnal, aggravated by elevation and relieved by dependency. Dependent rubor is characteristic.

Category 5 patients present with ischemic ulcers. The lesions usually are located distally on the toes, but they also may be noted on the malleoli or shins. They may result from minor trauma that fails to heal secondary to chronically inadequate circulation. In diabetics, peripheral neuropathy allows repeated minor trauma, for example, from ill fitting shoes, to persist without being noted by the patient. Superimposed infection can put the limb at risk; gangrene may develop. These patients need to be treated aggressively. A limb with major tissue loss (category 6) does not have a salvageable foot; however, an angiogram and intervention may be indicated to pre-

serve as much of the lower limb as possible because amputation sites may not heal in the face of vascular insufficiency.

Angiographic findings

Atherosclerotic plaque is usually irregular and eccentric but may also be smooth and concentric (Fig. 20-2). Plaques may be ulcerated. Rarely, they are weblike. Collateral development is the hallmark of chronic arterial occlusive disease, developing over time (weeks to months) (Fig. 20-3). Collateral arteries can partially compensate for occlusion of major vessels. Acute occlusion of normal vessels generally yields rapid, profound, limb-threatening ischemia. This typically occurs with trauma or arterial emboli in young patients. In patients with underlying occlusive disease, chronic collaterals may reduce the effect of an acute occlusion. (Fig. 20-4).

PVD can occur in focal and diffuse patterns. A critical stenosis can undergo in situ thrombosis and convert to a total occlusion. A superior convex meniscus usually marks the proximal edge of the thrombosis. The occurrence of acute in situ thrombosis may be marked by a sudden increase in the level of symptoms, for example, sudden progression from claudication to rest pain or by new onset claudication. With time, there is retrograde propagation to the nearest large collateral and organization of the thrombus by fibrin.

Arteriosclerosis obliterans is progressive and generally symmetric (Fig. 20-5). Significant atherosclerosis of the abdominal aorta is usually infrarenal. In adult patients, the adductor canal is usually the site of earliest plaque. In young patients with a smoking history who develop premature PVD, aortoiliac disease may be manifest first. The

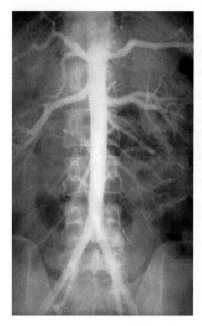
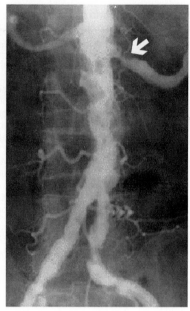

A,B

FIGURE 20-2. (A). Normal aortogram is seen. Note the smooth contour and slight tapering distally. **(B).** Aortogram demonstrating severe aortoiliac atherosclerosis. There also is a proximal left renal artery stenosis (*straight arrow*).

Leriche syndrome occurs in men and is characterized by absent or severely diminished femoral pulses, thigh and buttock claudication, and impotence. Anatomically, the Leriche syndrome consists of severe atherosclerotic narrowing of the distal aorta and common iliac arteries. Nonsmoking diabetic patients generally develop occlusions of the tibioperoneal arteries in addition to femoropopliteal lesions; aortoiliac involvement is seen much less frequently. Thus, diabetic patients presenting for limb salvage will have multilevel disease, which is generally infrainguinal and more difficult to treat than disease in the larger, more proximal vessels (Fig. 20-6).

Lower-extremity ischemia has a differential diagnosis that is extensive and includes arteriosclerosis obliterans, thromboembolic disease, dissection, thrombosis of an aneurysm, and in situ thrombosis. Classically, patients with the "blue toe" syndrome present with ischemic toes with intact pedal pulses. This disease is due to cholesterol microembolization from aortic, iliac, and femoral artery plaques. Angiography is performed to find the source. Blue toe syndrome may be treated by angioplasty stents, atherectomy, or surgical means.

Treatment for chronic atheroocclusive disease

As noted, patients with claudication usually should be treated by managing risk factors such as hyperlipidimia and smoking; an exercise program in which walking through claudication is probably of value. In patients with critical limb ischemia (Rutherford categories 4 to 6),

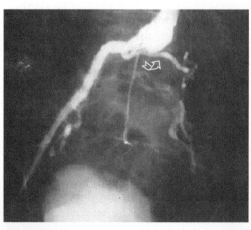
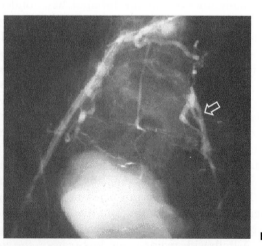

A

B

FIGURE 20-3. (A). An early phase of a pelvic arteriogram. There is diffuse narrowing of the right common and external iliac artery. The left common iliac artery is occluded, and an L4 collateral (*curved arrow*) is noted. **(B).** Reconstitution of the external iliac artery (*arrow*).

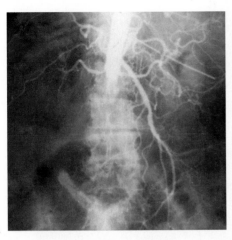
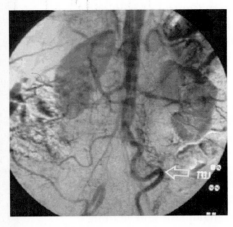

A   B

FIGURE 20-4. **(A).** Acute aortic occlusion, studied via translumbar aortogram. There are atherosclerotic renal arteries and a normal superior mesenteric artery. **(B).** Another patient demonstrates chronic aortic occlusion. There is a markedly enlarged and tortuous inferior mesenteric artery providing collateral flow.

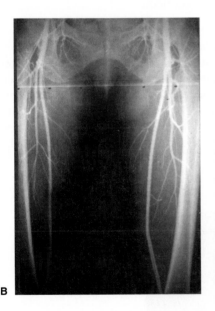
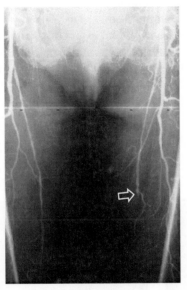

A,B

FIGURE 20-5. (A). Normal femoral arteriogram showing widely patent common, superficial, and deep femoral arteries bilaterally. **(B).** Arteriogram from another patient shows patent profunda femoral arteries and diffuse atherosclerosis of the superficial femoral arteries which occlude at the adductor canal on the right and just above the adductor canal on the left (arrow). Note the rear symmetry.

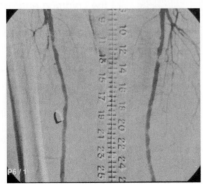
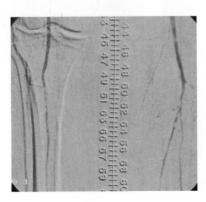

A, B

FIGURE 20-6. Severe bilateral multilevel infrainguinal disease in a male patient with diabetes mellitus. **(A).** Severe bilateral superficial femoral and popliteal artery occlusive disease. (The bullet in the soft tissues is old.) **(B).** Marked severe bilateral tibial disease.

however, intervention is indicated. Control of pain and infection related to the ischemic limb and optimization of cardiorespiratory function are important. The primary aim of endovascular or open surgical techniques is relief of rest pain and healing of ischemic skin lesions. The choice between a percutaneous interventional procedure and open surgery generally depends on the exact level and extent of the obstructive disease. In a large series of limb salvage patients, about one third underwent angioplasty alone or angioplasty combined with open surgery to treat multisegment disease.[2]

Combinations of percutaneous and open procedures and surgery can be used to treat multisegment disease.[2] For example, donor iliac artery angioplasty and stenting may be used to improve inflow for a cross-femoral graft. The presence of a pressure gradient across an iliac stenosis indicates the need for dilatation (Figs. 20-7 through 20-9).[3]

Some interventional radiologists prefer primary stenting of all iliac artery occlusions and stenoses; however, there is evidence to suggest that the first-line treatment for a focal, simple iliac stenosis should be angioplasty, with stenting reserved for percutaneous transluminal angioplasty (PTA) failure or complex lesion morphology such as occlusion, ulceration, or grossly irregular plaque (Fig. 20-10).[4,5] Immediate PTA failure is defined by the presence of residual pressure gradient, flow limiting dissection, thrombosis, or elastic recoil with residual lumenal narrowing.[6]

Many interventional radiologists prefer primary stent-

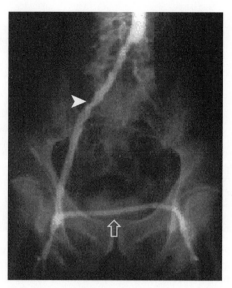

FIGURE 20-7. Cross-femoral bypass graft (*vertical arrow*). The donor right common iliac artery is moderately narrowed (*arrowhead*) but demonstrated no pressure gradient. The right internal iliac artery is occluded.

ing (i.e., stent placement without preceding PTA) of all external iliac artery lesions, believing that the external iliac artery is more susceptible to PTA-related dissection, occlusion, or perforation (Figs. 20-11 and 20-12). The use of PTA with stenting has resulted in patency rates in the iliac segments of 90% and 80% at 1 and 3 years respectively. Angioplasty alone is generally applied to focal, simple stenoses of the common iliac arteries (Figs. 20-13

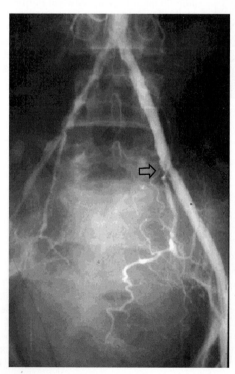
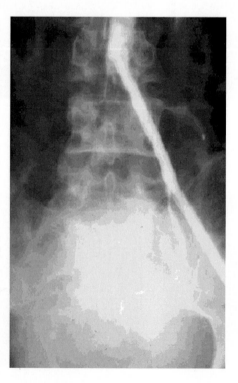

A,B

FIGURE 20-8. (A). There is a focal lesion at the junction of the common and external iliac artery (arrow). No gradient was demonstrated without pharmacologic enhancement. After a 60 mg intra-arterial bolus of papaverine, a gradient of 25 mmHg was measured. **(B).** After angioplasty, luminal is widely patent, and the gradient was resolved. The left iliac artery was used as a donor for a left-to-right cross-femoral bypass graft.

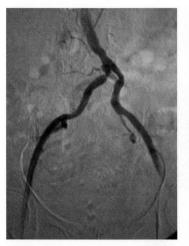
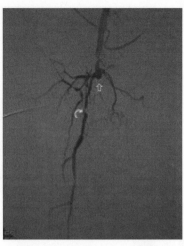
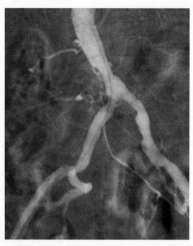

A–C

FIGURE 20-9. (A). Right common iliac artery stenosis with poststenotic dilatation in 77-year-old woman with end-stage renal disease, chronic critical lower limb ischemia, and femoropopliteal occlusion. The poststenotic dilatation infers hemodynamic significance. **(B).** Superficial femoral artery occlusion (*vertical arrow*) and marked diffuse disease of the profunda femoris artery (*curved arrow*). This virtually occluded outflow from the iliac segments precluded generation of an effective pressure gradient across the lesion. **(C).** A primary stent was placed with luminal restoration prior to planned right femoropopliteal bypass surgery.

through 20-15). The use of stents in conjunction with a PTA in the aortoiliac segments has improved immediate technical success and durability. Technical success for all occlusions and stenoses ranges from 85 to 99%, with primary patency and clinical success rates at 2 to 3 years of up to 80 to 82%.[6–9] With secondary interventions, patency rates can be improved even further.[10] Procedural complications range from 4 to 7% (Fig. 20-16).

It is important to note that many patient-related and anatomy-related factors will affect the outcome of a PTA and stenting. In general, focal disease responds well to

percutaneous therapy, whereas diffuse disease does not. Proximal lesions (e.g., aortoiliac segments) respond better to either percutaneous techniques or surgery than do distal ones (e.g., tibial segments). Stenoses historically fare better than occlusions, primarily because some occlusions cannot be crossed. With current technology, virtually all femoropopliteal artery stenoses and occlusions now can be crossed and dilated. The status of runoff below the angioplasty site is an extremely important predictor of patency. Patients presenting with critical limb ischemia rather than claudication generally fare less well

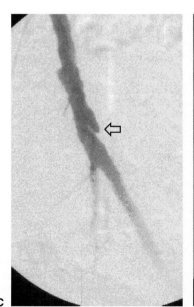
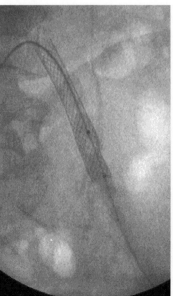
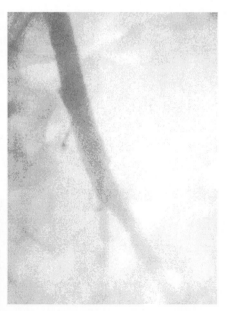

A–C

FIGURE 20-10. (A). Left common iliac artery atherosclerotic plaque with ulceration (*arrow*). **(B).** This was treated by primary stenting from the contralateral approach. **(C).** Follow-up arteriogram demonstrates excellent results.

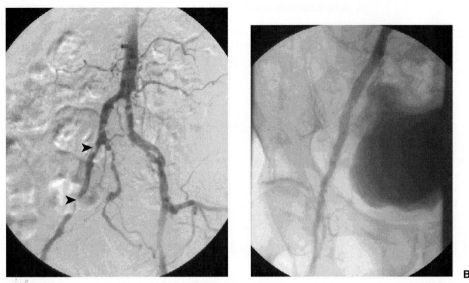

FIGURE 20-11. (A). Moderate diffuse disease of the right external artery is noted. Two focal stenoses are noted by the arrowheads. **(B).** The patency of the external iliac artery is restored after primary stenting.

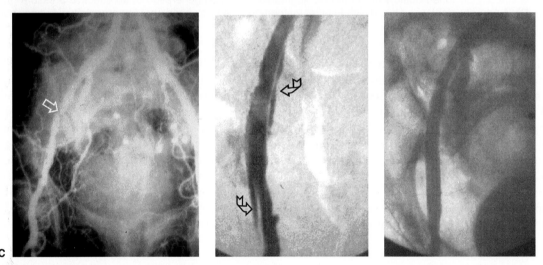

FIGURE 20-12. (A). Tight focal right external iliac artery lesion is noted (*arrowhead*) in a patient with severe multilevel occlusive disease and critical ischemia. Right femoropopliteal bypass graft was planned after percutaneous restoration of iliac inflow. **(B).** Post angioplasty dissection is noted (*curved arrows*). This was partially occlusive. **(C).** A self-expanding stent was placed to tack this dissection down, with restoration of the lumen.

FIGURE 20-13. (A). Concentric tight focal right iliac artery stenosis (*horizontal arrow*). There is a large right L-4 collateral (*vertical arrow*). Note is also made of severe stenoses of the left external iliac (*curved arrow*) and internal iliac (*arrowhead*) arteries. The patient had markedly diminished femoral pulses bilaterally. **(B).** After an angioplasty of the right iliac artery that was performed around the aortic bifurcation, the sheath was placed in the left iliac artery to perform the right iliac angioplasty. There is excellent lumenal restoration (*horizontal arrow*) with return of a normal right femoral pulse. The left iliac catheter is highly occlusive in the diseased external iliac artery segment with essentially no flow down the external iliac artery (*curved arrow*); the patient was heparinized to prevent left iliac thrombosis. The arrowhead highlights the left internal iliac artery.

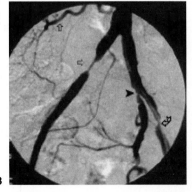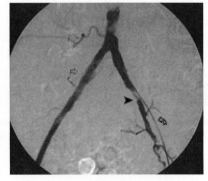

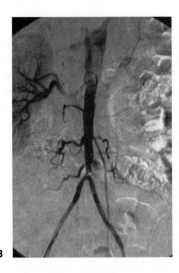
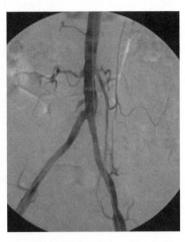

FIGURE 20-14. (A). Focal stenosis of the aortic bifurcation in a patient with Leriche's syndrome. **(B).** Excellent result after angioplasty with (bilateral) "kissing balloon."

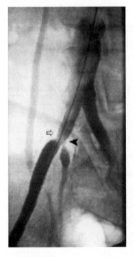
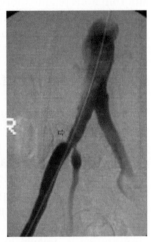

FIGURE 20-15. (A). Focal stenosis of the junction of the right common and external iliac arteries (*arrow*). In addition to the narrowing seen on this single left anterior oblique view, the lesion appears gray, indicating significantly decreased luminal diameter in the axis of the x-ray beam. There is a tight stenosis of the internal iliac artery origin (*arrowhead*). **(B).** After balloon angioplasty, there is luminal restoration (*arrow*).

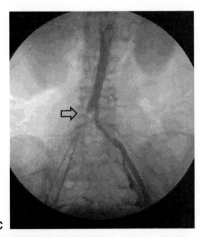
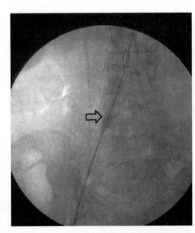
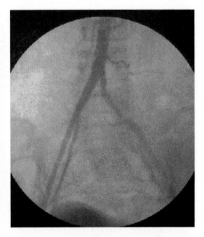

FIGURE 20-16. (A). Right common iliac artery occlusion (*arrow*). The diagnostic catheterization is from the left common femoral artery. **(B).** Right common femoral artery puncture with placement of a second catheter through the occlusion. A balloon expandable stent is placed across the lesion and dilated (*arrow*). **(C).** Follow-up arteriogram demonstrates wide patency of the stent placement.

with percutaneous techniques, primarily because they have more diffuse disease. Similarly, diabetic patients have been reported to fare worse than nondiabetics with infrainguinal PTA, but this is probably statistically confounded by runoff status and extent of disease.[11]

Femoropopliteal artery angioplasty has a technical success rate of 85 to 95%, 62 to 86% primary patency at 1 year, and 45 to 60% primary patency at 3 years (Fig. 20-17). The prognosis for durability in the femoropopliteal distribution is highly dependent on lesion site, length, and runoff status as well as clinical presentation. Claudicators with proximal focal lesions and good runoff fare best; conversely, limb-salvage patients with diffuse disease do poorly. Lesions 10 cm or longer usually should be treated surgically.[12–20] Stents are effective in salvaging acute failed PTA (due to elastic recoil, dissection, or thrombosis) but not as a primary therapy or in treating late restenoses.[21–23]

PTA of infrapopliteal arteries is reserved for patients with limb-threatening critical ischemia (Rutherford categories 4 through 6.) Infrapopliteal PTA is associated with a limb salvage rate of 60 to 80%, and a technical success rate greater than 90%. It is most effective in selected patients with focal lesions, and good runoff distal to the PTA site. It is ineffective in diffuse disease. It may be performed in conjunction with femoropopliteal PTA (Fig. 20-18).[24–30] Adjunctive mechanical techniques (e.g., rotoblator, atherectomy) may be helpful in selected patients, but they are not a first-line therapy or widely used.

It is difficult to compare the results of surgery and PTA in patients with peripheral arterial disease. In patients with anatomically favorable lesions who were predominantly claudicators, one randomized study found about equal effectiveness, that a failed PTA did not place the patient at higher risk for limb loss or surgical failure, and

that survival was improved in the PTA group.[31,32] Another demonstrated a significant decrease in the length of hospital stay[33] for the PTA group compared with the surgery group and comparable medium-term results in both patient groups. One recent cost-effectiveness study demonstrated that for claudicators, femoropopliteal angioplasty is more cost effective as a first strategy for stenosis and occlusion, but for patients with chronic limb ischemia, femoropopliteal occlusions should be bypassed, whereas patients with stenoses should undergo PTA first.[34]

It is likely that surveillance and repeat intervention would improve the assisted primary patency rates of PTA.[25,35] The use of intravascular metallic stents to rescue failed angioplasties has proven beneficial in the femoropopliteal distribution, but not as a primary therapy. Some researchers believe that lysis of the organized fibrin thrombus in a long chronic iliac or femoropopliteal artery occlusion will unmask a shorter underlying critical atheromatous plaque more amenable to PTA. The role of thrombolysis for "debulking" chronic iliac occlusions prior to PTA is controversial.

■ Acute Ischemia of the Lower Extremities

Patients with acute ischemia of the lower extremities typically present with the five P's on physical examination: pain, pulse deficit, pallor, paresthesia, and paralysis. Urgent arteriography is indicated. The pain is often more diffuse than in chronic critical ischemia, extending from the foot up the calf. Pedal pulses are usually absent. Pallor may be seen early, but cyanosis may supervene with time (Table 20-3). A cool or cold extremity, especially if the opposite leg is normal in temperature, is important to note; transition levels for cooler temperature may be

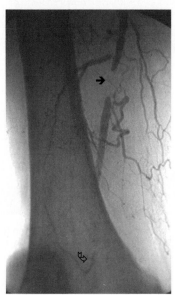 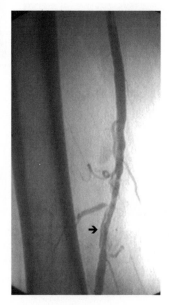

A, B

FIGURE 20-17. (A). Right femoral arteriogram demonstrates focal occlusion of the right popliteal artery (*straight arrow*). This is an early film with underfilling of the distal popliteal segment via collaterals (*curved arrow*). **(B).** After angioplasty there is luminal recanalization with a small nonobstructive intimal flap (*arrow*). There was restoration of the popliteal pulse.

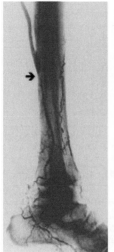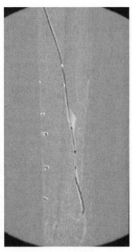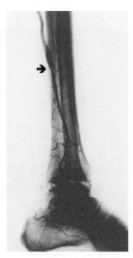

A–C

FIGURE 20-18. (A). Tight focal stenosis in the peroneal artery just distal to the anastomosis of a femoral–peroneal artery bypass graft. Close postoperative surveillance in this failing graft uncovered poor flow. **(B).** Placement of a low-profile balloon and guidewire across the stenosis. **(C).** There is luminal restoration. Marked increase in flow in the graft was noted postangioplasty.

present and are generally one limb segment below the level of arterial occlusion. Patients may complain of numbness or paresthesias, which may be subtle and should be differentiated from underlying diabetic neuropathy. The presence of paralysis or even a partial motor deficit is an indication of advanced limb-threatening ischemia; in such cases, where a delay could cause further deterioration, the patient may be taken directly to the operating room. With newer and quicker lytic techniques these patients may also benefit from angiography and percutaneous intervention.

Nonatherosclerotic causes of acute limb ischemia or acute pulse loss include thromboembolism, dissection (Fig. 20-19) trauma, arteritis, hypercoagulable state with thrombosis, vasospasm (e.g., ergotism), cardiogenic "low-flow" state, and popliteal cyst or entrapment with thrombosis and distal embolism. In atherosclerotic patients, in situ thrombosis of a critical athrosclerotic plaque may engender acute limb ischemia. Abdominal or popliteal aneurysm thrombosis or thrombosis of a surgical bypass graft also can cause acute limb ischemia in patients with

atherosclerosis. Acute deep venous thrombosis, low-flow states in patients with heart failure, or acute compressive neuropathy occasionally may mimic acute limb ischemia. The blue toe syndrome results from microembolism off proximal athrosclerotic sites, resulting in a painful and cool cyanotic toe. In this syndrome, pedal pulses are preserved.[36]

Thromboembolic disease

Patients with lower-extremity emboli present with sudden profound ischemia if the underlying vessels are normal and there are no large collaterals. These patients may have bilateral or multilevel occlusion. The emboli usually lodge at branch points, where vessels change caliber, occluding both main and collateral vessels. Fifty-eight percent of peripheral emboli are found in the lower extremities distal to the inguinal ligament, and 38% of lower-extremity emboli lodge at the common femoral artery bifurcation. Risk factors include cardiac arrythmias (e.g., atrial fibrillation) and endocarditis (e.g., intra-

TABLE 20-3. Clinical Categories of Acute Limb Ischemia

Category	Description or Prognosis	Findings		Doppler signals	
		Sensory loss	Muscle weakness	Arterial	Venous
I. Viable	Not immediately threatened	None	None	Audible	Audible
II. Threatened					
a. Marginally	Salvageable if promptly treated	Minimal (toes) or none	None	Inaudible	Audible
b. Immediately	Salvageable with immediate revascularization	More than toes, associated with rest pain	Mild, moderate	Inaudible	Audible
III. Irreversible	Major tissue loss or permanent nerve damage inevitable	Profound, anesthetic	Profound, paralysis (rigor)	Inaudible	Inaudible

From Rutherford RB, Baker JD, Ernest C, et al. Recommended Standards for reports dealing with lower extremity ischemia: revised version. *J Vasc Surg* 1997;26:517–538. With permission.

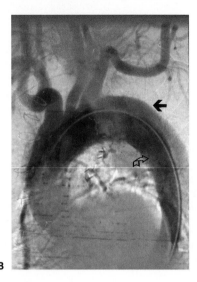
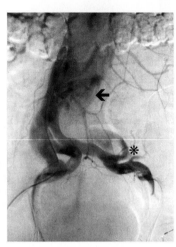

FIGURE 20-19. (A). Arch aortogram showing type B dissection. False lumen noted by straight arrow. The true lumen (*curved arrow*) has been catheterized. **(B).** Distal aortic extension of false lumen (*straight arrow*). Reentry point is noted (*asterisk*). The left femoral pulse was diminished.

venous drug abuse). The heart is the most common source of emboli, and workup should include echocardiography. Aortic or peripheral aneurysms, mural aortic thrombi, and iatrogenic causes also must be considered. Rarely, paradoxical emboli through a patent foramen ovale can present with peripheral arterial emboli and pulmonary emboli. Emboli to the renal and mesenteric arteries can occur with peripheral emboli. Angiography should be directed toward defining the levels of occlusion, distal runoff, and defining the vascular source, if possible. Angiographically, there are occlusions of minimally diseased vessels, intraluminal filling defects, and poorly developed arterial collaterals (Fig. 20-20). Branch-point occlusions and superior convex menisci are seen. Multiplicity is the hallmark of peripheral emboli (Fig. 20-21). There may be associated vasospasm.

The differentiation of acute thromboembolic disease versus thrombosis in situ may be straightforward, given the clinical history and the angiogram. In elderly patients with underlying atherosclerosis, however, there may be some difficulty in narrowing the diagnosis. A superior convex meniscus alone may be seen with both entities

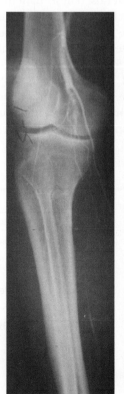
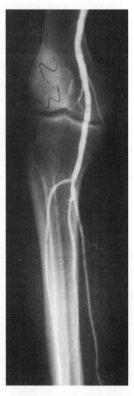

FIGURE 20-20. (A). This patient presented with acute ischemia of the right lower extremity as a result of a popliteal artery embolus. There is an acute cutoff of the popliteal artery with poor collateralization and virtually absent distal flow. **(B).** Perfusion has been restored after overnight regional thrombolysis.

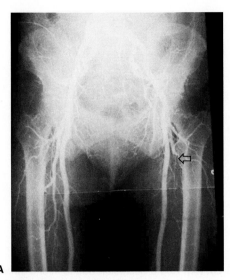
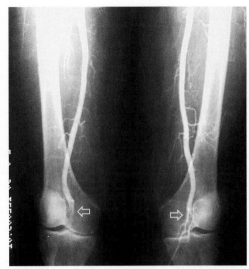

A   B

FIGURE 20-21. Multiple emboli in a patient with atrial fibrillation **(A).** There is acute occlusion of the left profunda femoris artery (*arrow*). **(B).** Bilateral popliteal artery occlusions are seen (*arrowheads*). The femoropopliteal arteries are otherwise widely patent without significant atherosclerosis.

and represents the most proximal extent of thrombus after retrograde propagation from the focal embolic nidus or thrombosed focal plaque (Fig. 20-22.) Retrograde thrombosis usually extends back to a well-developed collateral branch. Thus, multiple concurrent sites of acute occlusion are needed to make the angiographic diagnosis of emboli with absolute certainty.

Treatment for acute limb ischemia

Amputation rates are proportional to the interval from the onset of acute limb ischemia to treatment; urgent angiography is warranted. Immediate management is directed toward administering therapeutic levels of heparin, which will minimize thrombus propagation and decrease the incidence of additional emboli.[37,38] Treating associated congested heart failure or cardiac arrythmias is also important, and pain control is usually necessary. Acute limb ishemia continues to be associated with substantial limb loss and mortality from coexistent cardiac disease. Clinical categories of acute ischemia are noted in Table 20-3.

In patients in whom the degree of limb ischemia allows time for aortofemoral arteriography, catheter-directed "regional" thrombolysis is often the initial treatment of choice.

The lytic agents are delivered intraarterially, directly into the clot. The location and anatomy of the target lesions as well as patient and surgery-related risk factors must be considered. Catheter-directed thrombolysis has advantages over surgical thromboembolectomy in decreasing the manipulation of and trauma to the endothelium during dissolution of thrombus, uncovering the underlying lesion, and visualizing the runoff vessels.[39] Successful recanalization is possible in most patients who

are appropriately selected. Ability to pass a Bentson guidewire through the thrombosed segment is predictive of success[40] in both grafts and native arteries. Correction of the underlying lesion by the most appropriate percu-

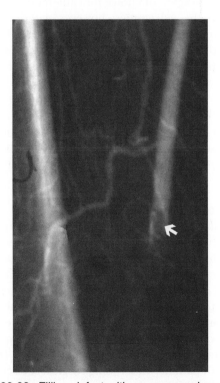

FIGURE 20-22. Filling defect with convex meniscus (*arrow*). Although often associated with thromboembolus, a single defect such as this one could represent any acute occlusion, including embolus, in situ thrombosis, or trauma. In narrowing the diagnosis, one must consider other anatomic factors (e.g., multiplicity, the presence or absence of collaterals, associated atherosclerotic change) and the clinical setting (e.g., arrythmias, trauma).

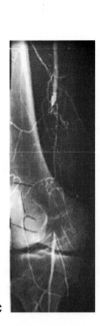
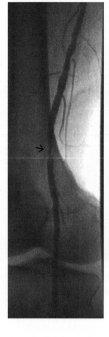
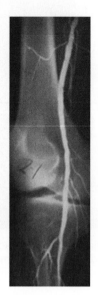

A–C

FIGURE 20-23. **(A).** Acute occlusion due to in situ thrombosis of the right popliteal artery. **(B).** After an overnight transcatheter intrathrombic thrombolytic infusion, a tight underlying critical stenosis is identified. **(C).** This was dilated with a 5 mm balloon.

taneous or surgical technique is necessary to preserve long-term patency (Fig. 20-23).[41] Until recently, urokinase was the agent of choice for catheter-directed thrombolysis in the extremities; however, withdrawal of this agent from the market in late 1998 and early 1999 saw increased use of tissue plasminogen activators in the periphery (Activase rt-PA, and retavase, r-PA).

Absolute contraindications to thrombolysis include recent gastrointestinal bleeding, recent neurosurgery or intracranial trauma, active bleeding diathesis, or recent transient ischemia attack or stroke. Relative contraindications include recent history of major nonvascular surgery or trauma, uncontrolled hypertension, and intracranial tumor.

Results of thrombolysis

Randomized trials comparing catheter-directed thrombolysis and surgical revascularization have been published and included hundreds of patients. These trials are not directly comparable because of differences in inclusion and exclusion criteria as well as in endpoints. There appears to be no significant difference in limb salvage at 6 to 12 months, reported at 81 to 89%. Patients having catheter-directed thrombolysis as initial therapy, however, appear to have decreased mortality (6.5 to 16%) compared with patients undergoing surgical revascularization (8.5 to 42%). Many interpret these findings to suggest that catheter-directed therapy may be safer for high-risk patients, with lysis appearing beneficial to the myocardium as well as the periphery. Furthermore, lysis appears to reduce the magnitude of the surgical procedure needed to restore perfusion. These trials used both tPA and urokinase.[42–44] It is important to remember that the ultimate result of thrombolysis is highly dependent on treating the underlying lesion. Treatment of a diffusely diseased native vessel or bypass graft is unlikely to yield a durable result. Catheter-directed lysis is best when the duration of ischemia is 14 days or less.

If there is an embolic complication during lysis, the catheter can be advanced into the clot and lysis can be continued or a percutaneous aspiration can be performed using nontapered, large-diameter catheters attached to a 50-mL suction syringe. Thrombectomy devices such as the AngioJet by Possis Medical Inc. (Minneapolis, MN) can be used to augment thrombolysis and decrease infusion time.[45] A variety of percutaneous mechanical thrombectomy devices have been used in Europe.

Miscellaneous conditions with vascular narrowing

Giant cell arteritis generally affects the upper extremities, but it occasionally can affect the femoral artery segments and is typically a disease of the medium-sized arteries. Takayasu's disease is of gradual onset and rarely affects the lower extremities; however, Takayasu's disease can involve the midabdominal aorta and renal arteries. Renal artery involvement is seen in about 35% of patients; the celiomesenteric arteries also can be involved. These patients can present with claudication (upper and lower extremity), renovascular hypertension, and abdominal angina (Fig. 20-24). Abdominal aortic coarctation ("mid-aortic" syndrome) can occur without the typical aortic arch lesions of Takayasu's disease and generally is seen in younger patients; there is controversy over whether mid-aortic syndrome is a subtype of Takayasu's disease or

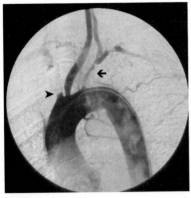
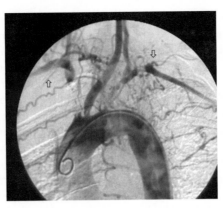
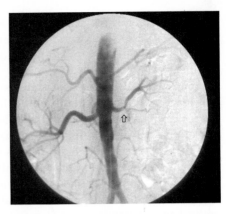

A–C

FIGURE 20-24 A 43-year-old woman with Takayasu's disease who presented with arm claudication. **(A).** There is a smooth, nonatherosclerotic aortic arch. There is occulusion of the innominate artery (*arrowhead*) and marked disease of the left subclavian artery (*arrows*). **(B).** The late-phase film demonstrates reconstitution of the right subclavian artery (*arrow*) via retrograde filling of the vertebral artery. **(C).** Abdominal aortogram demonstrates very minimal atheroscleroses of the infrarenal aorta and mild left renal artery stenosis (*arrow*).

whether it is a distinct entity. Neurofibromatosis also must be considered in the differential diagnoses of renal or abdominal aortic narrowing.

Buerger's disease

Buerger's disease (thromboangiitis obliterans) is found in male smokers aged 25 to 45 years.[46] It is a rare vasculitis and characteriscally presents with focal gangrene or ischemic ulcers. Angiographically, there are abrupt occlusions and stenoses of the tibial arteries with small corkscrew collaterals. There may be thrombotic occlusion; there is proximal sparing. Buerger's disease also can affect the upper extremities and can present as an acute ischemia.

Ergot disease

Ingestion of ergot compounds, typically for headache, may cause arterial spasm that can progress to thrombosis if untreated. The lesions are usually smooth, asymmetric, and atypical for atherosclerosis (Fig. 20-25). Withdrawal of the offending drug will clear the symptoms.[47]

Aneurysm disease

An *aneurysm* is a focal dilation of an artery greater than 1.5 times normal caliber. When diffuse, it is termed *arteriomegaly*. Aneurysm disease traditionally was considered a manifestation of atherosclerosis, but recent evidence suggests it to be a heritable autoimmune process resulting in inflammation and degradation of the medica and adventitia of the wall vessel.[48–51] Aneurysmal disease is also thought to be a deficiency in collagen elastase; there is an association between aortic aneurysm disease and pulmonary emphysema.

Abdominal aortic aneurysm

The aorta is the most common site of aneurysm formation; 90 to 95% of abdominal aortic aneurysms (AAAs) are infrarenal. AAA disease predominates strongly in

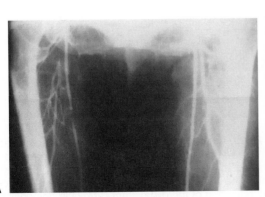
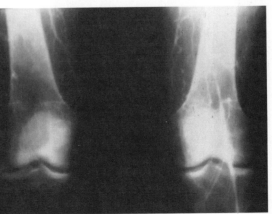

A
B

FIGURE 20-25. Ergotism. A 40-year-old woman presented with painful lower extremities and decreased pedal pulses. She had a history of café ergot ingestion for headaches. **(A,B).** Smooth stenoses in asymmetric, atypical locations. There is occlusion of the right popliteal artery. After withdrawal of her headache medication, the pedal pulses reappeared, and symptoms resolved.

men. Iliac aneurysms usually occur as an extension of AAAs or are associated with femoral and popliteal aneurysms. Iliac aneurysms generally do not occur as isolated findings.

Abdominal aortic aneurysms are associated with complications that can be catastrophic if left untreated. The most feared complication of an AAA is rupture. The risk of rupture increases with aneurysm size. Generally, elective repair is recommended for AAAs greater than 5 cm in diameter. AAAs also can thrombose or embolize thrombus peripherally. Inflammatory aneurysms have an added component of perianeurysmal fibrosis that can entrap or obstruct ureters; inflammation is best depicted by computed tomography (CT). The surgical procedure for AAA depends on the extent of the disease. Aorto–aorto grafts (tube grafts) are placed when there is a good cuff above the aortic bifurcation; if there is no cuff and the aneurysm extends down to the bifurcation or into the common iliac arteries, an aortobiiliac bypass usually is performed.

Imaging of abdominal aortic aneurysms has undergone change over the past few years. Previously, most patients with AAAs underwent aortography. Now most uncomplicated aneurysms are imaged by CT, with aortography reserved for problem cases. These problem cases may include aneurysms in which there is less than 1.5 cm infrarenal neck or in which the aneurysm extends to the suprarenal aorta. Patients with suspected stenosis of the renal, mesenteric, or celiac arteries also may undergo aortography. Angiography is indicated if there is associated iliac stenosis because the usual aorto–aorto or aortoiliac bypass graft may need to be modified to an aorto–bifemoral bypass graft. The aortogram also may depict the status of the inferior mesenteric artery and the presence or absence of large lumbar arteries, which can cause problems with bleeding at surgery. Other problems encountered during surgery include unsuspected retroaortic or circumaortic renal veins, and these must be searched for on preoperative CT. Endovascular grafting for AAA is currently under active investigation, with two devices recently approved for market use: These devices typically need mapping angiography prior to placement. These patients are followed by interval CT after placement. Angiography is usually necessary to plan treatment for postimplant complications such as endoleaks, which can be seen in up to 22% of patients (Fig. 20-26).

Aortography performed for abdominal aortic aneurysms must include biplane views with a pigtail above the celiac artery. The lateral view is essential to demonstrate the presence or absence of an infrarenal neck because the aorta usually buckles forward at this level, underestimating the neck length on the frontal projection. The celiac axis and proximal aorta are demonstrated best on the lateral view. Pelvic arteriography is performed to demonstrate the distal extent of the AAA. In patients who have lower-extremity pulse decrements or a history of claudication or critical ischemia, associated runoff studies are obtained. The slow flow within an aneurysm may mandate decreasing the injection rate and lengthening the film series timing. Unstable patients with suspected rupture should not undergo CT or angiography but should be brought directly to surgery. Angiograms will not show a leak and may delay getting the patient to the operating room. In stable patients with suspected rupture, an emergency CT should be obtained to confirm the leak and demonstrate anatomy prior to repair.

Angiographic findings in AAA include a focal widening of the aortic lumen greater than 3 cm; this is typically fusiform but may be saccular. This focal widening occasionally may be absent because contrast may progress

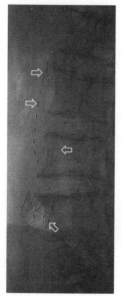
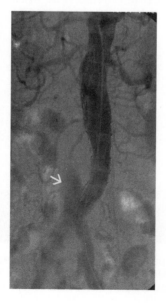

A,B

FIGURE 20-26. An tube endovascular graft has been placed for treatment of an abdominal aortic aneurysm. **(A).** Opaque markers which line the graft material (*straight arrows*). The arrowheads show the distal anchoring stent. **(B).** A distal endoleak caused by retraction of the distal stent (*arrow*) is demonstrated. Due to the difficulty in anchoring a stent-graft in the distal aorta, most physicians are placing bifurcated stent-grafts even when the distal aorta may be normal.

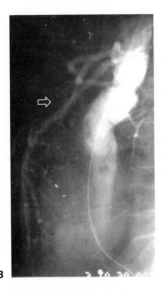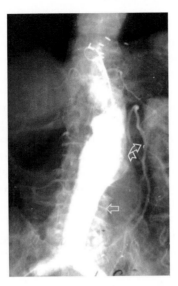

A, B

FIGURE 20-27. (A). Lateral aortogram of abdominal aortic aneurysm. This demonstrates large, soft tissue mass; mild forward angulation of the neck; and draping of the superior mesenteric artery over the aneurysm mass (*arrow*). **(B).** AP aortogram shows paradoxical smoothness of the aorta due to laminated thrombus and absence of lumbar arteries (*arrow*). The inferior mesenteric artery is occluded, with marginal artery collaterals from the superior mesenteric artery (*curved arrow*).

down a nondilated luminal channel surrounded by thrombus. (The distance between the contrast column and intimal calcium will be increased.) A "bald" aorta with absent lumbar arteries, inferior mesenteric artery occlusion, slow flow, and draping of the superior mesenteric artery over the aneurysm are all angiographic findings associated with the presence of AAA (Fig. 20-27). Paradoxic smoothness of the lumen as a result of laminated thrombus also may be present.

If the aneurysm is unusually shaped (e.g., saccular) or in an unusual location, a mycotic aneurysm should be considered. *Salmonella* species and *Staphylococcus aureus* are usually responsible for mycotic aneurysms. Mycotic aneurysms also include syphilitic aneurysms; these are rare but are more frequently suprarenal and may be multiple.

Lower-extremity aneurysms

Aneurysms in the lower extremities may be multiple. Extremity aneurysms are usually due to atherosclerosis. Lower-extremity aneurysms are associated with aortic, common iliac, and internal iliac artery aneurysm; thus, aortography and pelvic arteriography also should be obtained.

Common femoral artery aneurysms are defined as having a diameter larger than 150% of the external iliac artery diameter. There is a high incidence of bilaterality and an association with popliteal aneurysms. These aneurysms can rupture, occlude, or embolize. The differential diagnosis must include pseudoaneurysm. Common femoral artery pseudoaneurysms usually have a neck and usually are related to previous catheterizations; these may be treated by ultrasound compression if of recent origin and small.[52]

Popliteal aneurysms are focal dilatation of the popliteal artery, with a diameter greater than 150% the di-

ameter of the distal superficial femoral artery. The popliteal artery is most frequently the lower-extremity site for the development of an aneurysm. Popliteal aneurysms typically occur above the knee joint, starting just distal to Hunter's canal (Fig. 20-28). More than 50% of popliteal aneurysms are bilateral, and bilaterality is associated with the presence of aortic, iliac, and femoral aneurysms. Only 25% of popliteal aneurysms are solitary; thus, it is essential to invoke a search for other sites when a popliteal aneurysm is seen.

AAAs occur in one third of patients with popliteal aneurysms. Abdominal ultrasound should be obtained.

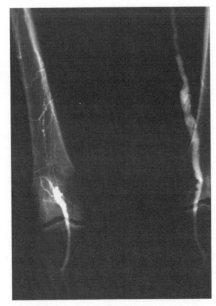

FIGURE 20-28. Right lower-extremity ischemia as the result of a thrombosed popliteal artery aneurysm. A patent left popliteal aneurysm is noted; the left leg was asymptomatic.

There is a high association of popliteal aneurysms with diffuse pelvic and lower extremity arteriomegaly. In cases of popliteal artery thrombosis or in other cases where popliteal aneurysms are suspected, the arteriographer should search for calcium or mass effect as evidenced by draping of collaterals. Ultrasound is essential if a suspect popliteal aneurysm cannot be seen on angiography. Complications of popliteal aneurysms include thrombotic occlusion and distal embolization. There is a high incidence of limb loss (33 to 50%) if a popliteal aneurysm is missed. Rupture is rare, occurring in fewer than 4% of cases. These patients present with limb ischemia from embolization or thrombosis, but rarely they present with deep venous thrombosis from aneurysmal compression of the popliteal vein. Popliteal aneurysms are treated by excluding them from the circulation by a surgical bypass. Catheter-directed thrombolysis may be used to restore distal popliteal and trifurcation runoff after acute thrombotic or thromboembolic occlusion to improve the results of bypass.

Other vascular abnormalities in the popliteal fossa

Cystic adventitial disease of the popliteal artery is a rare cause of popliteal occlusion or stenosis, typically occurring in young men. Cysts develop in the media and adventitia and compress the lumen. Calf pain is the usual presenting symptom. On angiography, there may be segmental popliteal artery stenosis or occlusion with normal caliber proximally and distally. Ultrasound can be used to make a definitive diagnosis. The popliteal artery maintains a normal course.

Popliteal entrapment syndrome is another rare cause of peripheral ischemia and is due to an aberrant attachment of the gastrocnemius or popliteus muscle. Usually, medial deviation of the popliteal artery occurs, although the artery may have a normal course or lateral deviation, depending on the type of entrapment. Aneurysm formation and thrombosis may develop. Narrowing is elicited by forced plantar flexion (Fig. 20-29).

■ Extremity Trauma

Emergency angiography is indicated for enlarging hematoma, pulse deficit, or neurologic abnormality. Angiography is also usually obtained if there is knee dislocation or if the patient has suffered a shotgun wound, even if there are no immediate symptoms. Proximity injury without physical findings has a low angiographic yield (1 to 5%), and most now agree that emergency angiography is not needed.[53] With trauma, the angiogram may show pseudoaneurysm or extravasation, with or without arteriovenous fistula occlusion; dissection; intimal flap; mural hematoma; or distal embolization. Whereas street or vehicular incidents are prominent causes of arterial trauma, iatrogenic trauma from needle punctures or catheterization is another increasingly important etiology (Figs. 20-30 through 20-33). Arterial standing waves (Fig.

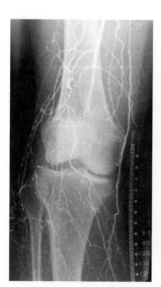 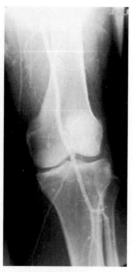 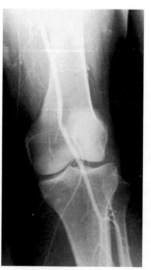 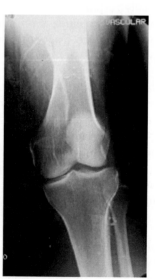

A,B   **C,D**

FIGURE 20-29. Popliteal entrapment. A 46-year-old woman presented with subacute disabling right lower-extremity claudication and an absence of the right popliteal pulse. **(A).** The right lower extremity arteriogram demonstrates occlusion of the popliteal artery at the patella. The presentation and level of occlusion are atypical for atherosclerotic disease. **(B).** Arteriogram of the left lower extremity in the same patient demonstrates slight medial deviation of the popliteal artery in the popliteal fossa. This extremity was asymptomatic. **(C).** Active plantar flexion during arteriography of the left lower extremity demonstrated increased angulation of the vessel and lumen narrowing. **(D).** Further plantar flexion lead to occlusion.

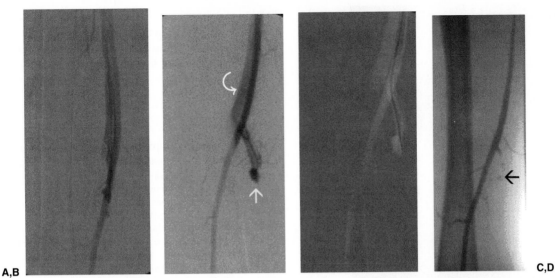

A,B   C,D

FIGURE 20-30. A 17-year-old patient with expanding hematoma in the left thigh after a knife wound. **(A).** Anteroposterior arteriogram demonstrates a small collection of contrast overlying the superficial femoral artery. **(B).** Oblique view better demonstrates a small pseudoaneurysm (*arrow*) from a muscular perforating branch of the superficial femoral artery. There is an associated arteriovenous fistula, with prominent early venous drainage (*curved arrow*). **(C).** A catheter guidewire system is used to enter the pseudoaneurysm and its branch feeder. **(D).** Coils (*arrow*) have been placed to embolize the pseudoaneurysm and its solitary feeder. The hematoma resolved over several days.

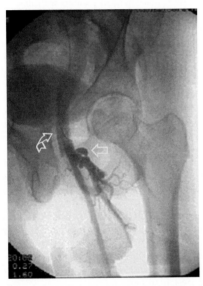

FIGURE 20-31. Pseudoaneurysm (*arrow*) of the left common femoral deep femoral artery junction with arteriovenous fistula (*vein, curved arrow*) after cardiac catheterization. The position precluded treatment by a covered stent or coils; it was repaired surgically.

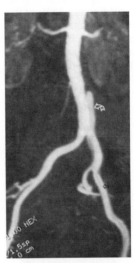

FIGURE 20-32. Iatrogenic retrograde dissection. Magnetic resonance angiogram of a patient who previously underwent attempted cardiac catheterization from the left femoral approach. An intimal flap is seen in the left iliac artery (*straight arrow*), and a false lumen is also seen (*curved arrow*), with decreased signal intensity relative to the true lumen.

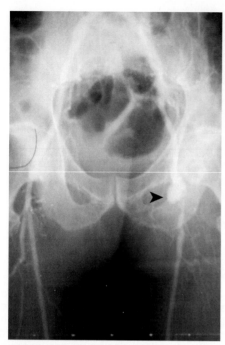

FIGURE 20-33. Translumbar aortogram of a 70-year-old man with an ongoing history of chronic intravenous drug abuse. He presented with acute profound lower-extremity ischemia and pulsatile masses in both groins. The arrowhead demonstrates a pseudoaneurysm of the left common femoral artery, which resulted from a direct needle injury and was responsible for distal embolization to the trifucation vessels (not shown), the cause of his acute ischemia. Note also the absence of the left deep femoral artery, due to needle related trauma. The right common femoral artery also had a smaller pseudoaneurysm, which is not seen well in this single view.

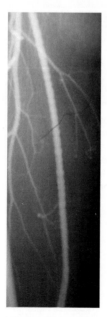

FIGURE 20-34. Arterial standing waves.

20-34), which are seen in compliant vessels in young patients, or early atheromatous lesions can be sources of confusion. Thus, some angiographers prefer to perform bilateral angiograms for extremity trauma so that the uninvolved leg can serve as a comparison.

REFERENCES

1. Rutherford RB, Baker JD, Ernst C, et al. Recommended standards for reports dealing with lower extremity ischemia: revised version. *J Vasc Surg* 1997;26:517–538.
2. Veith FJ, Gupta SK, Wengerter KR, et al. Changing arteriosclerotic disease patterns and management strategies in lower-limb-threatening ischemia. *Ann Surg* 1990;212:402–414.
3. Perler BA, Williams GM. Does donor iliac artery percutaneous transluminal angioplasty or stent placement influence the results of femorofemoral bypass? Analysis of 70 consecutive cases with long term follow-up. *J Vasc Surg* 1996;24:363–370.
4. Bosch JL, Hunink MGM. Metaanalysis of the results of percutaneous transluminal angioplasty and stent placement for aortoiliac occlusive disease. *Radiology* 1997;207:87–96.
5. Bosch JL, Tetteroo E, Mali WP, et al. Iliac arterial occlusive disease: cost-effectiveness analysis of stent placement versus percutaneous transluminal angioplasty. Dutch Iliac Stent Trial Study Group. *Radiology* 1998;208:641–648.
6. Tetteroo E, van der Graaf Y, Bosch JL, et al. Randomized comparison of primary stent placement versus primary angioplasty followed by selective stent placement in patients with iliac-artery occlusive disease. Dutch Iliac Stent Trial Study Group. *Lancet* 1998;351: 1153–1159.
7. Vorwerk D, Gunther RW, Schurman K, et al. Aortic and iliac stenoses: follow-up results of stent placement after insufficient balloon angioplasty in 118 cases. *Radiology* 1996;198:45–48.
8. Blum U, Gabelmann A, Redecker M, et al. Percutaneous recanalization of iliac artery occlusions: results of a prospective study. *Radiology* 1993;189:536–540.
9. Vorwerk D, Gunther RW, Schurman K, et al. Primary stent placement for chronic iliac artery occlusions: follow-up results in 103 patients. *Radiology* 1995;194:745–750.
10. Murphy TP, Webb MS, Lambiase RE, et al. Percutaneous revascularization of complex iliac artery stenoses and occlusions with use of Wallstent: three-year experience. *J Vasc Interv Radiol* 1996;7:21–27.
11. Stokes KR, Strunk HM, Campbell DR, et al. Five-year results of iliac and femoropopliteal angioplasty in diabetic patients. *Radiology* 1990;174:977–982
12. Gallino A, Mahler F, Probst P, et al. Percutaneous transluminal angioplasty of the arteries of the lower limbs: a 5-year follow-up. *Circulation* 1984;70:619–623.
13. Krepel VM, van Andel GJ, van Erp WF, Breslau PJ. Percutaneous transluminal angioplasty of the femoropopliteal artery: initial and long term results. *Radiology* 1985;156:325–328.
14. Jeans WD, Armstrong S, Cole SEA, et al. Fate of patients undergoing transluminal angioplasty for lower-limb ischemia. *Radiology* 1990;177:559–564.
15. Capek P, Mclean GK, Berkowitz HD. Femoropopliteal angioplasty: factors influencing long-term success. *Circulation* 1991;83:I-7–I-80.
16. Johnston KW. Femoral and popliteal arteries: reanalysis of results of balloon angioplasty. *Radiology* 1992;183:767–771.
17. Hunink MG, Donaldson MC, Meyerovitz MF, et al. Risks and benefits of femoropopliteal percutaneous balloon angioplasty. *J Vasc Surg* 1993;17:183–192.
18. Matsi PJ, Manninen HI, Vanninen RL, et al. Femoropopliteal angioplasty in patients with claudication: primary and secondary

patency in 140 limbs with 1–3 year follow-up. *Radiology* 1994;191:727–733.

19. Murray JG, Apthorp LA, Wilkins RA. Long segment (>10 cm) femoropopliteal angioplasty: improved technical success and long-term patency. *Radiology* 1995;195:158–162.

20. Currie JC, et al. Femoropopliteal angioplasty for severe limb ischemia. *Br J Surg* 1994;81:191–193.

21. Sapoval MR, Long AL, Raynaud AC, et al. Femoropopliteal stent placement: long-term results. *Radiology* 1992;184:844–840.

22. Do DD, Triller J, Walpoth BH, et al. A comparison study of self-expandable stents vs. balloon angioplasty alone in femoropopliteal artery occlusions. *Cardiovasc Interv Radiol* 1992;15:306–312.

23. Rousseau HP, Raillat CR, Joffre, et al. Treatment of femoropopliteal stenoses by means of self-expandable endoprostheses: midterm results. *Radiology* 1989;172:961–964.

24. Bakal CW, Sprayregen S, Scheinbaum K, et al. Percutaneous transluminal angioplasty of the infrapopliteal arteries: results in 53 patients. *AJR Am J Roentgenol* 1990;154–171.

25. Bakal CW, Cynamon J, Sprayregen S. Infrapopliteal percutaneous transluminal angioplasty: what we know. *Radiology* 1996;200–236.

26. Schwarten DE, Cutcliff WB. Arterial occlusive disease below the knee: treatment with percutaneous transluminal angioplasty performed with low-profile catheters and steerable guide wires. *Radiology* 1988;169:71–74.

27. Schwarten DE. Clinical and anatomic considerations for nonoperative therapy in tibial disease and the results of angioplasty. *Circulation* 1991;83(suppl I):I-86–I-90.

28. Brown KT, Morre ED, Gertrajdman GI, et al. Infrapopliteal angioplasty: long-term follow up. *J Vasc Interv Radiol* 1993;4:139–144

29. Brown KT, Schoenberg NY, Moore ED, et al. Percutaneous transluminal angioplasty of infrapopliteal vessels: preliminary results and technical considerations. *Radiology* 1988;169:75–78.

30. Horvath W, Oertl M, Haidinger D. Percutaneous transluminal angioplasty of crural arteries. *Radiology* 1990;177:565–569.

31. Wilson SE, Wolf GL, Cross AP, et al. Percutaneous transluminal angioplasty vs. operation for peripheral arterial sclerosis: report of a prospective randomized trial and selected group of patients. *J Vasc Surg* 1989;9:1–9.

32. Wolf GL, Wilson SE, Cross AP, et al, for the principal investigators and their associates of Veterans Administration Cooperative Study Number 199. Surgery or balloon angioplasty for peripheral vascular disease: a randomized clinical trial. *J Vasc Interv Radiol* 1993;4:639–648

33. Holm J, Arfvidsson B, Lennart J, et al. Chronic lower limb ischemia: a prospective randomised controlled study comparing the 1-year results of vascular surgery and percutaneous transluminal angioplasty (PTA). *Eur J Vasc Surg* 1991;5:517–522.

34. Hunink MGM, Wong JB, Donaldson MC, et al. Revascularization for femoropopliteal disease: a decision and cost-effectiveness analysis. *JAMA* 1995;274:165–171.

35. Varty K, Bolia A, Naylor AR, et al. Infrapopliteal percutaneous transluminal angioplasty: a safe and successful procedure. *Eur J Vasc Endovasc Surg* 1995;9:341–345.

36. Kaufman JL, Shah DM, Leather RP. Atheroembolism and microembolic syndromes (blue toe syndrome and disseminated atheroembolism). In: Rutherford RB, ed. *Vascular Surgery*. 4th ed. Philadelphia: WB Saunders; 1995:669–677.

37. Panetta T, Thompson JE, Talkington CM, et al. Arterial embolectomy: 34-year experience with 400 cases. *Surg Clin North Am* 1986;66:339–353.

38. Blaisdell FW, Steele M, Allen RE. Management of acute lower extremity ischemia due to embolism and thrombosis. *Surgery* 1978;84:822–834.

39. Verstatrate M, Belch JJ, Dormandy JA, et al. Thrombolysis in the management of lower limb peripheral arterial occlusion: a consensus document. *Am J Cardiol* 1998;81:207–218.

40. McNamara TO, Bomberger RA. Factors affecting initial and six month patency rates after intra-arterial thrombolysis with high dose urokinase. *Am J Surg* 1986;152:709–712.

41. Gardiner GA, Harrington DP, Koltun W, et al. Salvage of occluded bypass grafts by means of thrombolysis. *J Vasc Surg* 1989;9:426–431.

42. The STILE Investigators. Results of a prospective randomized trial evaluating surgery versus thrombolysis for ischemia of the lower extremity. *Ann Surg* 1994;220:251–266.

43. Ouriel K, Shortell CK, De Weese JA, et al. A comparison of thrombolytic therapy with operative vascularization in the initial treatment of acute peripheral arterial ischemia. *J Vasc Surg* 1994;19:1021–1030.

44. Ouriel K, Veith FJ, Sasahara AA. A comparison of recombinant urokinase as initial treatment for acute arterial occlusion of the legs: thrombolysis or peripheral arterial Surgery (TOPAS) Investigators *N Engl J Med* 1998;338:1105–1011.

45. Starck EE, McDermott JC, Crummy AB, et al. Percutaneous aspiration thromboembolectomy. *Radiology* 1985;156:61–66.

46. Shionoya S. Buerger's disease: pathology, diagnosis and treatment. Nagoya, Japan: The University of Nagoya Press; 1990:101–116.

47. Wells KE, Steed DL, Zajko AB, et al. Recognition and treatment of arterial insufficiency from Cafergot. *J Vasc Surg* 1986;4:8.

48. Hirose H, Takagi M, Miyagawa N, et al. Genetic risk factor for abdominal aortic aneurysm: HLA-DR2(15), a Japanese study. *J Vasc Surg* 1998;27:500–503.

49. Gregory AK, Yin NX, Capella J, et al. Features of autoimmunity in the abdominal aortic aneurysm. *Arch Surg* 1996;131:85–88.

50. Newman KM, Jean-Claude J, Li H, et al. Cellular localization of matrix metalloproteinases in the abdominalaortic aneurysm wall. *J Vasc Surg* 1994;20:814–820.

51. Newman KM, Jean-Claude J, Ramey WG, et al. Cytokines that activate proteolysis are increased in abdominal aortic aneurysms. *Circulation* 1994;90(5 Pt 2):II224–II227.

52. Fellmeth BD, Roberts AC, Bookstein JJ, et al. Postangiographic femoral artery injuries: nonsurgical repair with US- guided compression. *Radiology* 1991;178:671–675.

53. Katz MD, Hanks S. Arteriography and transcatheter treatment of extremity trauma. In: Baums S, Pentecost MJ, eds. *Abram's Angiography: Interventional Radiology*. Boston: Little Brown & Co; 1997:857–868.

21

Venous Thromboembolic Disease and Vena Cava Filters

TIMOTHY P. MURPHY

■ Epidemiology

Lower-extremity deep-vein thrombosis (DVT) is a common condition that is seen in 34% of unselected medical patients and in 60% of unselected surgical patients by autopsy series.[1] Of the patients presenting with lower-extremity DVT, 35% to 51% have evidence of pulmonary embolism (PE) by ventilation perfusion scan, indicating that these two disease processes should be thought of as a continuum of the same process rather than as two separate conditions.[2–4] PE has been stated to be the third leading cause of death in this country[5] and is the third most common disease of the cardiovascular system, after myocardial infarction and stroke.[6]

The incidence of PE in the United States has been estimated to be as high as 750,000 to 900,000 cases per year, with a mortality of 120,000 to 150,000 cases annually.[7,8] Untreated, proximal DVT or PE has a 30.5 to 50% chance of developing into recurrent PE, with a mortality rate of 18 to 26%.[9–11] Of pulmonary emboli, 85 to 95% arise from the iliofemoral veins,[12,13] with most of the other 5 to 15% arising from thrombi in the vena cava, ovarian veins, right atrium, or upper extremities.[12,14,15]

Asymptomatic thrombus formation in the veins of the calf, particularly the soleal sinuses, is probably a normal process that occurs throughout life in all persons. It is only when thrombus is not lysed by the body but rather propagates to a large central vein that a pathological condition exists. The propensity for progression to this pathological state has been observed for several groups of hospitalized patients, including those with recent surgery or trauma, heart disease, neoplastic disease, and systemic diseases.[6] Ultrasound examinations of the lower

extremities often demonstrate asymptomatic DVT in many of these patients. For example, routine ultrasound examination of the lower-extremity veins in 542 asymptomatic intensive care unit (ICU) patients demonstrated previously unsuspected DVT in 11.4% of patients.[16] Unsuspected proximal DVT has been reported in 13 to 16% of patients presenting with acute hip fracture in two series using ultrasound;[17,18] the incidence of proximal DVT has been reported as even higher (32%) in one series using ascending venography.[19] Recently, the incidence of postoperative DVT in 50 patients who underwent abdominal aortic aneurysm repair was reported as 18%, although involvement was limited to the calf veins in 78% of these patients.[20] Unfortunately, in 70% of patients, the diagnosis of PE is not made before the patient dies.[21]

■ Diagnosis of DVT

Before the arrival of real-time ultrasound, the standard method of documenting lower-extremity DVT was contrast venography (Fig. 21-1). Contrast venography possesses several disadvantages relative to ultrasound that have led to replacement of venography by ultrasound as the initial imaging method for diagnosing this disease. First, contrast venography cannot be performed at the bedside. Patients must be transported to the radiology department to be evaluated by this technique and additionally must be able to tolerate the changes in position required for optimal performance of this examination. Also, contrast introduced into the lower-extremity veins has been associated with an increased incidence of postvenography thrombophlebitis. This condition is sus-

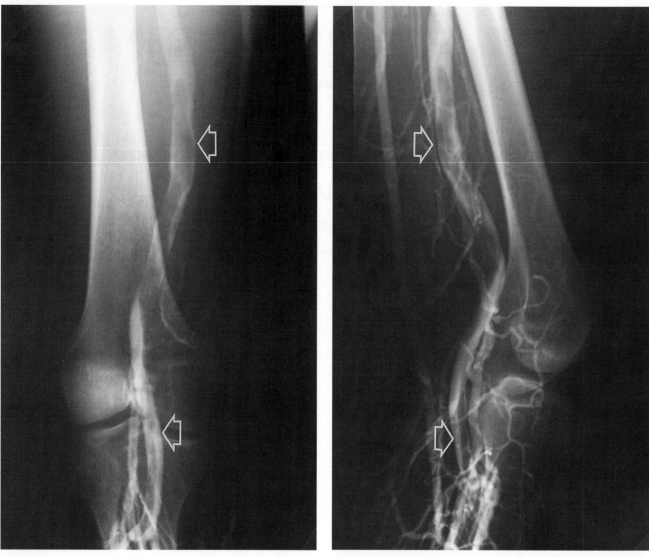

A   B

FIGURE 21-1. Anterior **(A)** and lateral **(B)** views from a contrast venogram of the left lower extremity, showing an intraluminal filling defect in the popliteal and superficial femoral veins (*arrows*). A filling defect is the most specific sign of deep vein thrombosis on contrast venograms.

pected to result from osmotic injury to the venous endothelium, which causes local inflammation and pain,[22,23] and is seen in up to 24% of patients studied with full-strength contrast medium.[22] Some authors believe that contrast venography occasionally can result in occlusive thrombosis of the vein.[24] It also has been reported that up to 4.6% of attempts to perform lower-extremity venography are unsuccessful because of an inability to cannulate a suitable vein or because of inadequate opacification of the femoral or iliac veins.[25] Contrast venography is still useful in patients who undergo nondiagnostic or technically inadequate examinations (e.g., obese patients).

Other noninvasive imaging methods for evaluating lower-extremity veins include impedance plethysmography (IPG), radionuclide venography, magnetic resonance venography, and ultrasound. IPG is inaccurate in assessing the popliteal and calf veins and requires patient cooperation to prevent false-positive results.[26,27] Radionuclide venography is inaccurate and insensitive to isolated thrombus below the knee and to nonocclusive thrombus above the knee.[28] Iodine-125 labeled fibrinogen leg scanning is insensitive to thrombus above the midthigh, is expensive, and requires 24 to 48 hr to complete.[28] Magnetic resonance venography has demonstrated a sensitivity of 90 to 100% and a specificity of 95 to 100% in four published series with a total of 325 patients.[29–32] At present, magnetic resonance angiography does not have a role in the diagnosis of DVT in most patients because of its lack of demonstrated benefit over ultrasound, which is less expensive. D-dimer assays of whole blood have demonstrated excellent negative predictive value and may be useful in excluding DVT without imaging tests; however, the specificity of an elevated D-dimer level is poor, and this test cannot reliably establish the diagnosis of DVT.[33]

Ultrasound is the imaging method of choice for the initial evaluation of DVT. The standard ultrasound lower-extremity examination for deep venous thrombosis includes real-time compression of the vein (Fig. 21-2), Doppler analysis at rest and during compression of the calf, and color Doppler assessment of the vein. Examination of the calf veins often is performed if proximal thrombi are not detected, and reflux studies often are done if all the preceding are normal and there is suspicion of chronic venous insufficiency. Ultrasound also can allow the diagnosis of chronic venous changes to be made by visualization of thickening of the vein wall.

Review of the literature since the advent of venous ultra-

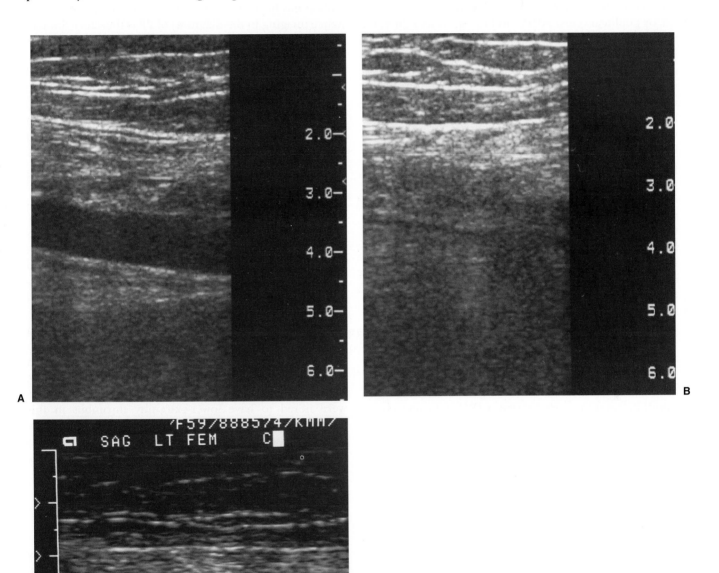

FIGURE 21-2. A: Sagittal view of the superficial femoral vein by real-time ultrasound. **B:** After compression, the vein collapses and the lumen is obliterated, indicating absence of thrombus. **C:** Sagittal compression view of the superficial femoral vein from another patient demonstrates lack of compression, consistent with thrombosis of the vein.

sound reveals 20 studies in which compression ultrasound and Doppler interrogation of the veins or compression ultrasound alone was compared with contrast venography for the detection of symptomatic DVT.[34] Some controlled studies included venograms and ultrasound examinations performed on consecutive patients, whereas others had venographic confirmation performed only for abnormal ultrasound studies; however, the cumulative sensitivity of the technique for proximal thrombus (in the iliac, femoral, or popliteal veins) is 97% and the specificity 96%, for an accuracy of 97% in a total of 1,660 patients who had venographic control of ultrasound studies. Although specific examination of calf veins was not performed in these series, inclusion of isolated calf clot accounting for false-negative ultrasound studies yields only eight additional false-negative examinations in a total of 754 patients with symptomatic lower extremity DVT, which reduces sensitivity to 94%.[34] Although examination of calf veins can be performed accurately by ultrasound, to do so will lengthen examination time significantly and is operator dependent. It is also of dubious clinical use because patients with clinically significant pulmonary embolus usually do not have thrombi limited to the calf veins, and when they do, it is likely that emboli arose proximal to the calf veins.[35,36] Rather than treating calf thrombus detected on ultrasound, repeat studies at 3- to 5-day intervals can search for the estimated 5 to 20% of clots that will propagate upward into the femoropopliteal system.[35,36] Interobserver variability in the interpretation of lower-extremity venograms has been reported to be 10%,[37] and venography has been reported to be as low as 89% sensitive and 97% specific compared with autopsy findings, including calf vein thrombosis.[38] The overall clinical performance of ultrasound in assessing lower extremity DVT appears to be at least equal to that of contrast venography.

■ Diagnosis of PE

Pulmonary angiography is the gold standard for the evaluation of PE; however, this test is invasive, and major complications occur in 3.2%, and 0.2% of patients die.[39] Most deaths occur in patients with elevated pulmonary artery pressures.[39] Pulmonary angiography is also expensive. Although radioisotope lung scanning is established as the best screening test for patients with suspected PE and is highly specific in the proper clinical setting, this test suffers from lack of sensitivity. The Prospective Investigation of Pulmonary Embolism Diagnosis (PIOPED) investigators noted that of 755 patients undergoing pulmonary angiography and radioisotope lung scanning, only 41% of patients with angiographically proved pulmonary embolus had high-probability ventilation–perfusion scans.[40] The incidence of angiographically proved pulmonary embolus in those patients with low-probability ventilation-perfusion scans was 16%.[41]

Noninvasive tests have been proposed to improve the sensitivity of ventilation/perfusion scanning for pulmonary embolus in hopes of obviating pulmonary angiography. Magnetic resonance angiography has been used for the diagnosis of acute and chronic PE with mixed results.[40,42,43] These studies demonstrate a sensitivity of 85% to 90% for emboli greater than 1 cm in diameter,[40,41,44] and a specificity of 77%.[42,44] Insensitivity for peripheral emboli has been noted,[40] and the role of magnetic resonance imaging in the diagnosis of PE is therefore limited. Quantitative D-dimer levels possess excellent negative predictive value, although specificity is low.[45]

Ultrasound of the lower-extremity veins has a limited role in the evaluation of the patient with suspected PE. Previous work has demonstrated a 29% incidence of negative bilateral lower-extremity venograms in patients with proven PE by pulmonary angiography.[46] Ultrasound would be expected to be similarly insensitive and therefore should not be used to exclude pulmonary embolus. Radionuclide ventilation–perfusion scanning is the initial recommended evaluation in patients with suspected PE; however, in patients with low- or indeterminate-probability ventilation–perfusion scans, ultrasound represents a noninvasive alternative test.[47] In one report, 15% of patients with this presentation will demonstrate DVT on ultrasound examination.[48] Although it may appear to increase costs to incorporate lower-extremity ultrasound into the workup of PE, this report noted a decrease of 9% in overall costs by avoiding pulmonary angiograms in some patients.[49] In a second report, 19% of patients with low- or intermediate-probability ventilation–perfusion scans had abnormal ultrasound studies.[50] Interestingly, 21% of patients with normal ventilation–perfusion scans were noted to have lower-extremity thrombus in this study.[50] As noted, if lower-extremity ultrasound is negative, thromboembolic disease cannot confidently be excluded and further evaluation with pulmonary angiography is necessary.

■ Medical Management of DVT and PE

Anticoagulation is the standard treatment for pulmonary deep venous thromboembolic disease in most patients. This is usually achieved by beginning intravenous heparin and oral coumadin simultaneously, with maintenance of intravenous anticoagulation for 5 days to allow for depletion of circulating vitamin K–dependent clotting factors II, V, VII, IX, and X.[51–53] Low-molecular-weight heparin, which has a long half-life and can be administered subcutaneously once daily, has been shown to be at least equally effective as continuous intravenous unfractionated heparin in preventing pulmonary embolus in patients with proximal deep venous thrombi, with a lower incidence of bleeding complications.[54]

Thrombolysis has been used in selective patients with

DVT and PE. In general, thrombolysis in the lower extremities is reserved for patients with phlegmasia cerulea dolens, or painful swelling with cyanosis. These patients are at risk for venous gangrene and systemic hypotension; 25 to 32% of patients die.[55,56] Clinical improvement with catheter-directed thrombolysis has been reported in this condition.[57] Recently, less selective criteria for thrombolytic therapy in patients with lower-extremity DVT have been applied. In one series, 21 consecutive patients with iliofemoral DVT underwent catheter- directed thrombolysis.[58] Technical and clinical success was achieved in 85%, with 92% 3-month patency (11 of 12) by ultrasound.[58] No major complications were seen. No control group was present, only a few patients were treated, and follow-up was brief.[58] It should be noted that the doses of urokinase (Abbokinase, Abbott Laboratories, North Chicago, IL) used to treat acute DVT are high,[58] and further data are needed. There is currently an ongoing registry of patients treated in this manner. In a preliminary report from this registry, complete or partial success of thrombolysis was achieved in 48% and 38% of 73 limbs, respectively.[59] The mean urokinase dose for patients treated with intrathrombic infusion was 7.4 million units.[59] Technical success was greatest in patients who received intrathrombic infusion and in those with iliac vein involvement.[59] Stents were used in 47% for abnormalities in iliac veins after thrombolysis.[59] Major bleeding complications were observed in seven (10%) patients and remain a concern,[59] especially because the effectiveness of this therapy in reducing the incidence of postphlebitic syndrome will not be known for many years. A decision analysis of the best treatment strategy for DVT based on patients' responses to a questionnaire regarding the relative value of potential outcomes, including postphlebitic syndrome, intracerebral hemorrhage, and death, found that no patient surveyed was willing to incur the risk of thrombolysis to reduce the risk of postphlebitic syndrome.[60] At present, thrombolysis for DVT should be reserved for patients with thrombosis that includes the iliac vein or inferior vena cava (IVC), whose symptoms are severe, who have reasonably long life expectancies, and no contraindication to thrombolysis. Conversely, most patients with spontaneous upper-extremity thrombosis (*Paget-Schroetter syndrome*) are believed to experience optimal long-term outcome by undergoing thrombolysis in the acute period.[61]

■ History of Venous Interruption

Virchow's triad was originally postulated in 1860.[62] Just 8 years later, mechanical obstruction as a method to prevent lower-extremity thrombi from traveling to the lungs was conceived.[63] Homans recognized in 1944 that most symptomatic pulmonary emboli arise from the lower-extremity and pelvic veins and that these proximal thrombi usually originate in the deep veins of the calf.[63] Homans,

Debakey, and Ochsner advocated early femoral interruption in patients who had experienced PE.[63] Ligation of the IVC became popular because of the venous stasis sequelae of common femoral vein ligation.[64,65] Although mortality rates for IVC ligation as low as 2% were reported,[66] most series had mortality rates in the 8 to 15% range.[67–71] Immediate and severe leg swelling remained a frequent debilitating sequela, occurring in 10 to 16% of patients.[68,71] Because heparin did not become available for clinical use until 1935[72] and warfarin was not synthesized and available for widespread clinical use until 1948,[73,74] the use of anticoagulation paralleled vein interruption in the treatment of this disease process.

Methods of partial interruption of the IVC were developed in the late 1960s in an attempt to preserve flow through the IVC while trapping or filtering out potentially harmful emboli. These methods include suture plication[75] and various designs of clips used to narrow the lumen of the IVC (Moretz) or compartmentalize the lumen into several smaller channels (Miles, Adams-DeWeese) (Fig. 21-3).[71,75] Comparison of partial versus complete interruption of the IVC demonstrated similar procedure-related mortality and recurrent PE rates but a significantly lower incidence of lower-extremity morbidity in the patients treated with partial caval interruption (46 versus 76%).[67] Clips and suture plication of the vena cava were associated with 30 to 40% incidence of IVC occlusion.[67,71] It is interesting to note that IVC ligation was associated with immediate shock in only approximately 5% of patients[67] despite causing significant transient hemodynamic alterations in experimental animals.[76]

In 1967, Mobin-Uddin introduced the first transvenous device for caval interruption, the Mobin-Uddin umbrella (Edwards Laboratories, Santa Ana, CA) (Fig. 21-4).[77] This device was placed through the right internal jugular vein after surgical exposure, through a catheter-based carrier system with an inner diameter of 9 mm (27 Fr). The device was deployed in the IVC using fluoroscopic guidance, and the procedures therefore usually were performed in the angiography suite. The jugular approach was used to avoid potential iliocaval thrombus; a femoral carrier for the Mobin-Uddin umbrella did not exist. The superiority of the transvenous method of IVC interruption compared with surgical methods was established by marked improvement in procedure-related mortality, which was negligible for transvenous placement.[77–82]

The Mobin-Uddin umbrella was designed as an adjunct to anticoagulation in patients who experienced recurrent PE during adequate anticoagulation. Broad use of devices for caval interruption in patients with contraindications to anticoagulation, currently the most frequent indication for filter placement, was an infrequent indication when the Mobin-Uddin umbrella was introduced. The original version of this device was imperforate, but the design was modified to include multiple holes, which were intended to permit delayed occlusion of the IVC to allow time for

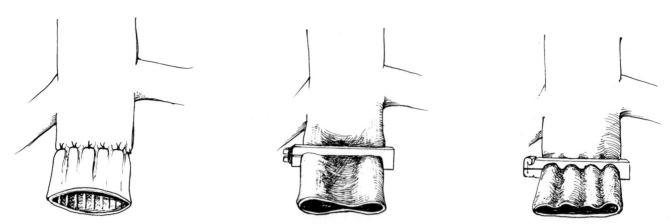

FIGURE 21-3. Line drawings of early surgical approaches to partitioning of the vena cava. **A:** The "harp-string" grid method of surgical plication popularized by Spencer. **B:** Moretz vena cava clip. **C:** Miles vena cava clip. (After Adams JT, Feingold BE, DeWeese JA. Comparative evaluation of ligation and partial interruption of the inferior vena cava. Arch Surg 1971; 03:272–276).

collaterals to develop,[77] theoretically reducing the risk of hypotension associated with acute caval occlusion.[76] As experience with this device accumulated, it became evident that approximately one third of patients maintained patency of the vena cava after umbrella placement, with no increase in the incidence of recurrent PE, which was reported as 3.6% in a review of 2,215 patients.[78] The silicone membrane of this device was subsequently heparin bonded in an attempt to improve caval patency rates. The diameter of the Mobin-Uddin umbrella was increased from 23 to 28 mm in the mid-1970s secondary to occasional proximal migration.[78]

The observation that patients with Mobin-Uddin umbrellas who maintained patency of the IVC had no in-

creased incidence of recurrent PE[80,83] and a lower incidence of lower extremity sequelae[80,83] led to the subsequent development of new devices designed to maintain caval patency and to the demise of the Mobin-Uddin umbrella, which was removed from the market in 1986. Methods of caval interruption resulting in a high incidence of caval occlusion are performed infrequently in favor of devices designed to preserve patency of the IVC while trapping clinically significant pulmonary emboli. The first such device to be introduced was the Kimray-Greenfield filter, now known as the Greenfield filter.

The Greenfield filter (Boston Scientific, Watertown, MA) was introduced in 1973. Despite the proliferation of many small-profile filter systems, the Greenfield filter

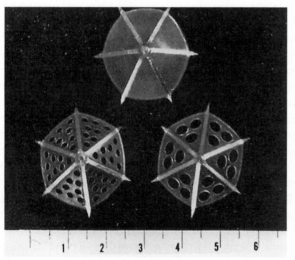

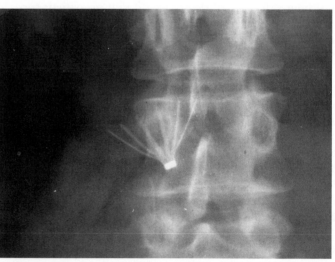

FIGURE 21-4. A: Axial view of three configurations of the Mobin-Uddin umbrella. The initial configuration consisted of six radial struts with a solid silicone membrane. Subsequently, the filter was modified to contain fenestrations of 1.5 mm or 3 mm in the silicone membrane. (Reprinted with permission from Mobin Uddin K, McLean R, Bolooki H, Jude JR. Caval interruption for prevention of pulmonary embolism: long-term results of a new method. Arch Surg 1969;99:711–715). **B:** A radiograph of a Mobin-Uddin umbrella demonstrates the caudal orientation of the filter apex.

remains one of the most popular vena cava filters in use today. Because the original Greenfield had a large profile, it was initially placed by surgical cut-down, usually of the right internal jugular vein, but also occasionally by the right common femoral vein. Percutaneous placement was first described by Tadavarthy in 1984.[84]

■ Indications for Vena Cava Filter Placement

DVT or PE and a contraindication to anticoagulation, noted in 38 to 77% of patients, are currently the most frequent indications for vena cava filter placement.[85–90] Absolute contraindications to anticoagulation include recent (within 2 months) stroke or neurosurgical procedure, recent major surgery or trauma (within 2 weeks), active internal bleeding, intracranial neoplasm, recent ocular surgery, and heparin-induced thrombocytopenia.[91–95] Coumadin is contraindicated in pregnancy because it crosses the placenta and potentially can cause fetal anomalies.[94] Relative contraindications include recent trauma (within 2 weeks), hematuria, occult blood in the stools, peptic ulcer disease, pericarditis, bacterial endocarditis, and unstable gait. Less frequent indications for vena cava filter placement include complications of anticoagulation, which occur in 5 to 50% of patients and include bleeding, thrombocytopenia secondary to heparin therapy, and warfarin-induced skin necrosis.[91–95] Long-term anticoagulation is associated with 5 to 12% mortality rate.[91–95] Complications of anticoagulation are the indication for filter placement in 6 to 17% of patients.[85–90] In 3 to 27% of patients, the indication for filter placement is recurrent PE or proximal propagation of lower-extremity thrombus while adequately anticoagulated.[85,87–90] High-risk of PE is seen in patients with free-floating iliofemoral or caval thrombus, occuring in 27 to 60% of these patients despite adequate anticoagulation.[96–99] These situations also warrant placement of a vena cava filter, ideally as an adjunct to anticoagulation.[87]

In the era when filters were placed surgically, filter placement was reserved for the most severely affected patients. Patients with recurrent PE constituted a disproportionately large percentage of patients receiving vena cava filters. Although PE is rare when patients are adequately anticoagulated (usually < 5%),[10,53] such patients were seen in up to 31% of those who underwent surgical placement of vena cava filters.[98] After introduction of the percutaneous method of vena cava filter placement, the mortality of filter placement was recognized to be negligible and clinically significant complications rare. The number of patients having filters placed subsequently increased at most institutions,[99] and the threshold for filter placement was lowered. This approach resulted in broadening the indications for vena cava filter placement, including routine use of vena cava filters at some institutions in high-risk trauma patients without DVT or PE or in patients with cancer as primary therapy for DVT or PE so that anticoagulation can be avoided.

The considerations for the treatment or prophylaxis of deep venous thromboembolic disease in patients with advanced cancer are multifaceted and complex. First, many patients demonstrate a high risk of developing thromboembolic disease, known as *migratory thrombophlebitis*, or *Trousseau syndrome*,[99–103] often seen in patients with mucinous adenocarcinomas or pancreatic and gastrointestinal origin as well as in patients with lung, breast, ovary, and prostate carcinoma. The mechanism is poorly understood but abnormalities of coagulation are seen in up to 92% of these patients.[104] Possible causes include increased coagulation factors produced in response to chronic low-grade disseminated intravascular coagulation, circulating cancer-produced procoagulants, tumor-associated thrombocytosis, and effects of cancer cells exposed to circulating blood.[105–107] Hypercoagulability seen in migratory thrombophlebitis in cancer patients is best treated with heparin rather than coumadin.[108]

Despite the frequent presence of hypercoagulability, patients with cancer have a high incidence of hemorrhagic complications when treated with anticoagulants; the prevalence ranges from 20 to 50%.[109–112] Patients with malignancies who are treated with anticoagulation have a significantly higher risk of major complications than those treated with vena cava filter placement,[113] which led to the approach of using vena cava filters as the primary therapy in cancer patients with DVT or PE.[108,113,114]

It has been claimed that vena cava filter placement as primary therapy in patients with cancer and DVT or PE is less expensive than anticoagulation due to the cost of treating hemorrhagic complications during anticoagulation therapy;[104] however, the relative benefits of vena cava filter placement depend on expected survival after filter placement. One series reported a 43% in-hospital mortality in patients with advanced cancer and multisystem organ failure who had vena cava filters placed, and benefits of filter placement were considered dubious.[115] Others have reported better survival, with in-hospital mortality of 18% in one series[116] and 26% in another, which reported that 21 of 61 patients with malignancies who had vena cava filters placed expired within 59 days of filter placement.[117] This experience led to the recommendation that patients should be treated while considering the expected longevity and the likelihood of the patient leaving the hospital alive.[104,114] In patients who do not have multisystem failure but do have a risk of severe adverse outcome of hemorrhagic complications, such as patients with metastatic disease to the brain or pericardium, filter placement should be the primary treatment of choice for deep venous thromboembolic disease.[104] Adjuvant therapy using heparin in patients with tumor-associated hypercoagulability who undergo vena cava filter placement should be considered.[117]

In contrast to patients with metastatic cancer, most patients admitted for trauma are young and have little or no significant medical history. Therefore, if they survive the initial event, the potential exists for long-term survival and excellent quality of life.

Although fatal pulmonary embolus is rare in trauma patients, occuring in approximately 1% of patients,[118,119] PE has been implicated in 11 to 20% of deaths in hospitalized trauma patients.[120–122] Prolonged immobility, advanced age, surgical procedures, and extremity and pelvic fractures all contribute to the relatively frequent occurence of DVT in these patients.[119–124] The risk of proximal DVT in such patients is approximately 7% with DVT prophylaxis and 18% without DVT prophylaxis.[119,123] In these patients, aggressive prophylaxis for pulmonary thromboembolic disease may be warranted.

Prophylactic use of vena cava filters in high-risk trauma patients has been evaluated in two large series.[118,122] The overall prevalence of fatal PE in consecutive admitted trauma patients was 0.25%, a significant reduction compared with the 1% rate before the use of prophylactic vena cava filters in high-risk patients.[118] The benefits of prophylactic filter placement in high-risk trauma patients was supported in the other large series.[122] The disadvantages of prophylactic use of vena cava filters in high-risk patients is minimal, with virtually no mortality, minimal morbidity,[122] and low cost. It has been estimated that in high-risk patients without DVT or PE, the cost of this approach is $80,000 per prevented death,[125] which, considering the yield in number of quality life-years in a mostly young patient population, seems a reasonable expense.

■ Technique of Vena Cava Filter Placement

Optimum technique for placement of vena cava filters includes thorough venography of the vena cava, including a search for venous anomalies, as well as venography of the iliofemoral system if the vena cava filter is to be introduced through the femoral vein. Contrast should be injected into the femoral vein immediately after it is accessed, through the access needle or catheter placed peripherally in the external iliac vein, to ensure absence of the thrombus in the vein selected for filter placement (Fig. 21-5). This step should be done regardless of the results of noninvasive studies because it is a quick maneuver with low morbidity, and periprocedural deaths resulting from PE have been reported as occurring after filter placement through iliac thrombus.[87] A catheter then can be placed safely into the infrarenal IVC cephalad to the confluence of the iliac veins, and a venacavagram can be

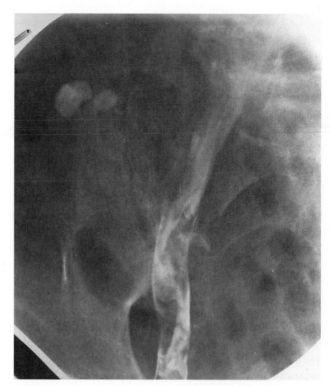

FIGURE 21-5. Contrast injection in the right common femoral vein in a patient with a high-probability ventilation/perfusion scan referred for vena cava filter placement shows thrombus in the right iliac system. Subsequently, the filter was placed using right jugular access. Confirmation of patency of the access vein is important to prevent potentially fatal pulmonary embolism caused by the filter introducer system.

obtained by using digital or cut-film techniques. The vena cavagram is done to show caval diameter, intracaval extension of thrombus, and venous anomalies. A ruler or marked catheter should be used to standardize for magnification to enable measurement of the caval diameter. If a venous anomaly is evident on the vena cavagram, appropriate modification of the filter placement technique should be made. Such important information is found on 15% of vena cavagrams.[126] The normal IVC is formed at the L5 level by the confluence of the common iliac veins. The renal veins are usually singular and enter the IVC at approximately L2. Above this level, the hepatic veins join, before emptying into the right atrium. In patients without IVC anomalies, placement of the filter in the upper part of the infrarenal segment is suggested. If the filter is placed in the caudal IVC, filter occlusion may be associated with a higher incidence of clot propagation in the remaining blind segment of the infrarenal IVC, with increased risk of subsequent PE, compared with high infrarenal placement.

Well-recognized venous anomalies that may affect the vena cava filter placement technique include duplicated renal veins, seen in up to 30% of patients when selective catheter techniques are employed;[127] circumaortic renal vein, seen in 6% of patients;[127,128] duplication of the IVC (2%); and transposition of the IVC (1%) (Fig. 21-6).[129] Modification of filter placement indicated by such findings includes placement of the filter below the caudal circumaortic limb to eliminate a major collateral route should the filter become occluded when placed between the circumaortic limbs, placement of a filter in each duplicated vena cava,[130] and placement of the filter in the left vena cava[129] rather than in the right renal vein or right gonadal vein in patients with this anomaly. Of course, a suprarenal filter will be effective in patients with these anomalies but adds the theoretical (although unreported) risk of renal failure should the filter become occluded.[131]

■ Evaluation and Comparison of Vena Cava Filters

Currently, five intracaval filters are approved for use in the United States. All are permanent: the stainless steel Greenfield filter (Boston Scientific, Watertown, MA), the titanium Greenfield filter (Medi-tech, Watertown, MA), the LGM (Vena Tech) filter (Vena Tech, Evanston, IL), the bird's nest filter (Cook, Bloomington, IN), and the Simon-Nitinol filter (Nitinol Medical Technologies, Woburn, MA). The Gunther filter and Amplatz filters

have undergone clinical trials, most of which were conducted in Europe. Filters differ in size, design, composition, and size of introducer. Criteria used to assess filters include rates of recurrent PE after filter placement, rates of death resulting from PE after filter placement, occlusion of the filter and IVC, thrombosis of the insertion site, incidence of filter angulation, filter migration, and ease of placement. An ideal vena cava filter should effectively filter all clinically significant emboli, be biocompatible and nonthrombogenic, result in minimal flow disturbance, be stable within the vena cava, result in no injury to adjacent structures, be simply and safely placed, and be low cost.[132,133] Retrievability is a debatable attribute.[133]

Most published series include data obtained by clinical follow-up; few studies have assessed filters objectively with imaging studies to document outcome according to the above criteria. In addition to available clinical data to assess effectiveness of filters, the ability of vena cava filters to trap experimental thrombi has been tested with in vitro models of the vena cava and in animal models.[134–137] In Katsamouris's study, the Greenfield filter was relatively ineffective at trapping small emboli (<3 mm in diameter), whereas the Mobin-Uddin, Amplatz, Gunther, Simon nitinol, and bird's nest filters were effective in filtering most of even the smallest emboli (2 mm diameter).[134] In tilted or eccentric position or with prolapse or elongation of the filaments of the bird's nest

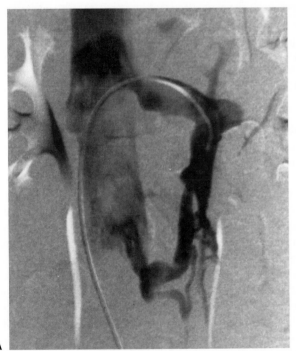
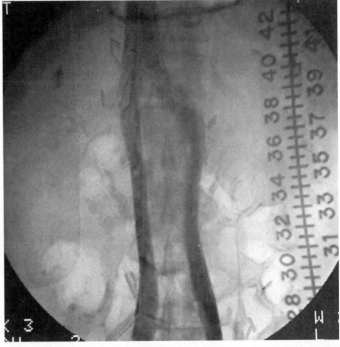

FIGURE 21-6. A: Selective left renal vein injection demonstrating a circumaortic renal vein. In such patients, vena cava filters should not be placed between the circumaortic limb and the renal vein, because occlusion of the filter by emboli could result in additional emboli being transmitted through the circumaortic conduit, bypassing the filter. **B:** Contrast venogram performed with simultaneous injections into catheters in left and right vena cavae. This anomaly may require placement of filters in each vena cava or, alternatively, in the suprarenal inferior vena cava.

filter, the Amplatz, Gunther, and Simon nitinol filters maintained their effectiveness in filtering emboli of all sizes.[134] The Mobin-Uddin umbrella and the Greenfield were significantly less effective in filtering even large thrombi (7 mm diameter) when not oriented properly.[134] This finding was not confirmed, however, in an animal experiment where thrombi were injected into the vena cava of sheep.[135] In this study, the Greenfield filter removed 89% of emboli of either 4 or 8 mm diameter, with failures limited to smaller emboli. No significant decrease in clot filtration was seen in four animals in which the filter tilted so that the apex was against the wall of the vena cava.[135] Another animal model was used to study the LGM and titanium Greenfield filters.[136] In this study, two sizes of thrombi, 5 × 5 mm or 5 × 10 mm, were injected into eight adult sheep.[136] The LGM filter trapped 70% of the smaller and 100% of the larger thrombi, and the titanium Greenfield trapped 26% of the smaller and 34% of the larger thrombi.[136] Additionally, the titanium Greenfield trapped only 37% of 5 × 30 mm emboli.[136] The only consistent conclusion is that the Greenfield filter appears relatively ineffective at filtering small emboli;[134–136] however, the clinical significance of this finding is dubious, as these small emboli may not be clinically significant, and the filter may have a higher patency rate because of fewer trapped emboli.[136] Furthermore, none of these models duplicates the physiology of the IVC in humans. The filters that are most effective at filtering small emboli (such as the bird's nest or Simon-Nitinol filters) probably have a higher incidence of IVC occlusion. The Greenfield design demonstrated adequate filtration ability based on large clinical experience, and whereas filtration is probably adversely affected by improper orientation, the potential benefit of improved IVC patency with clinical effectiveness resulted in this filter design dominating the filter market.

Stainless steel Greenfield filter

The stainless steel Greenfield filter consists of six radiating struts, projecting downward and outward from a central point, making the shape of a cone (Fig. 21-7). The apex of the cone is directed toward the head. The filter is 4.4 cm high. Each of the six legs of the filter is angled, taking a zigzag course from apex to base. At the base, each strut has a single barb or tine that anchors the filter within the vena cava. The filter is self-expanding and is deposited from the jugular or femoral vein, either by percutaneous puncture or via cutdown. A hole in the apex of the filter permits placement over a guidewire. The original version of the filter required a 24 Fr (29.5 Fr outer diameter) introducer. This filter has been reconfigured, and the new version can be placed through a 14 Fr sheath (Fig. 21-8). Although the larger version of the

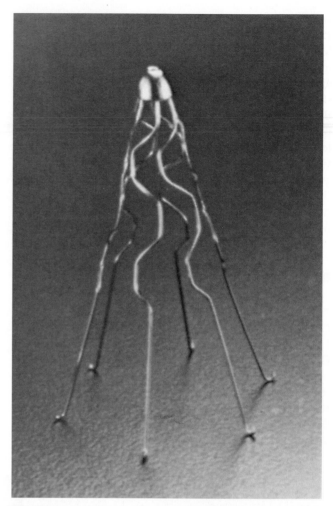

FIGURE 21-7. Photograph of the stainless steel Greenfield filter. (Reprinted with permission. Greenfield LJ, Cho KJ, Pais SO, Van Aman M. Preliminary clinical experience with the titanium Greenfield vena cava filter. Arch Surg 1989;124:657–659.)

stainless steel Greenfield has been stockpiled by the manufacturer, it is no longer being produced.

The original stainless steel Greenfield filter has been used since 1973.[137] The incidence of recurrent PE in patients not treated with anticoagulation is approximately 30%,[9] and the mortality rate in patients with PE not treated with anticoagulation in 6 months is 25%.[10] By contrast, in Greenfield's review of his first 12 years of experience with this device, he reported a 4% clinically suspected or confirmed rate of recurrent PE in 469 patients,[85] demonstrating the effectiveness of this device in preventing clinically significant PE. Because 258 patients in this series had a contraindication or a complication of anticoagulation, this number is likely a reliable indicator of filter effectiveness because it is assumed that at least this many patients were treated with filter placement alone, without adjunctive anticoagulation. A separate report by Greenfield documented a 95% patency rate of the IVC in 59 patients using contrast and radioisotope

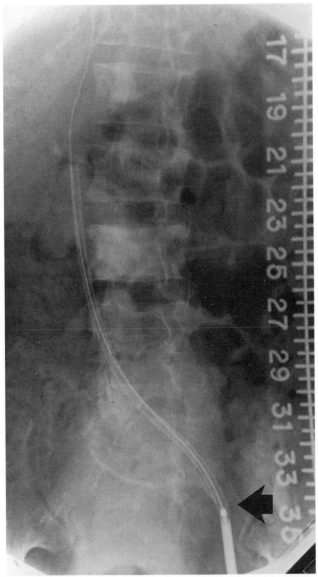

FIGURE 21-8. Radiograph obtained during insertion of the 14 Fr stainless steel Greenfield filter through the left common femoral vein. Despite over-the-wire placement, the sheath is kinked (*arrow*) and the filter could not be placed. Redesign of the filter carrier has reduced many of the problems with inability to pass this filter in tortuous left iliac veins. It is our practice to attempt left femoral vein placement prior to right jugular placement if the right common femoral or iliac veins are thrombosed, because successful placement usually can be achieved and potential life-threatening complications such as carotid or vertebral artery injury are avoided.

vena cavography;[138] similar findings also have been reported by other investigators.[137,139] Periprocedure mortality is rare.[85,137–139]

The necessity of coordinating the vascular surgeon, operating instruments, the radiologist, and angiography equipment in the angiography suite in a combined procedure has resulted in delays and frustration.[140] Radiologists therefore began to use dilators originally designed

for creation of large tracts for renal calculi removal to gain suitable access to the deep central veins. Percutaneous placement of the Greenfield filter was first reported in 1984[84] and was achieved by puncture of either the jugular or femoral vein, placement of a guidewire in the vein through the needle, and subsequent dilatation of the tract using serial dilators, up to 24 Fr (inner diameter) size, which was required to accommodate the delivery system.[140] Hemostasis after removal of the delivery system was achieved by manual compression within 15 to 30 min.[137,138] With the radiologist acting independently, placement of a vena cava filter lengthened the procedure time by only approximately 10 min after performance of an inferior vena cavogram.[140] Tract dilatation subsequently was performed using an angioplasty balloon, which saved time and was less traumatic to the vein than multiple dilators.[141,142] The new 14 Fr system has considerably simplified delivery.

Bird's nest filter

The bird's nest filter has been in use since 1982 (Fig. 21-9).[88] Its design is unique. Filtration is achieved by a network of four 25-cm-long filaments 0.18 mm in diameter, which during deployment are wound in such a way so that their relationship is fairly compact.[88] These filaments are anchored to the vena cava by two sets of V-shaped struts, each composed of two legs connected to each other at one end with an acute angle at their junction. The legs have barbs and loops at their ends opposite their junction point to prevent movement within the vena cava and to limit penetration of the vena cava wall. One set of struts is deposited first, with the apex directed caudally. After these are anchored firmly within the vena cava, the filaments are deployed. The filaments are not visible fluoroscopically and only occasionally are seen with plain radiography. Manipulation of the introducer sheath, which is rotated 90 degrees four times during filament deployment, minimizes prolapse of the filaments beyond the anchoring struts.[88] Finally, the second set of anchoring struts is deployed, with the apex or junction point of the legs directed cephalad, overlapping the first set of struts by at least 50%. The filter is placed through a 12 Fr introducer.[88] Because the maximum expansion diameter between the free ends of the legs of the anchoring struts is 60 mm, this filter has been particularly useful in patients with vena cavae larger than 28 mm in diameter, which is the maximum acceptable diameter for placement of the Greenfield filter and other currently available filters of similar design.[143] This filter has been placed in vena cavae up to 42 mm in diameter and has demonstrated equal clot trapping efficiency in an in vitro oversized vena cava model with less flow disturbance compared with bilateral iliac placement of other filters.[144] The prevalence of

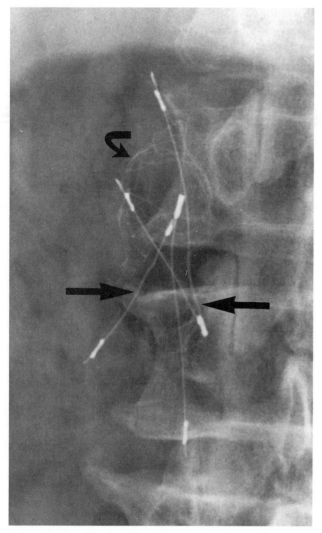

FIGURE 21-9. Radiograph of the bird's nest filter, which clearly demonstrates the stabilizing struts (*straight arrows*). The nest of filaments is less visible (*curved arrow*).

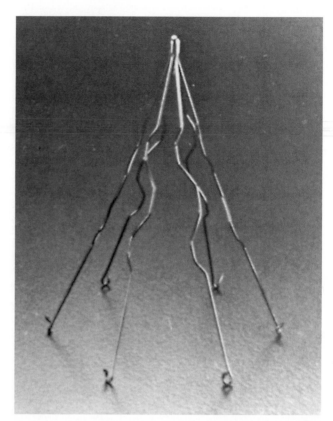

FIGURE 21-10. Photograph of the titanium Greenfield filter. (Reprinted with permission. Greenfield LJ, Cho KJ, Pais SO, Van Aman M. Preliminary clinical experience with the titanium Greenfield vena caval filter. Arch Surg 1989;124:657–659.)

megacavae (> 28 mm diameter) has been reported as 3%.[145]

Results obtained with use of the bird's nest filter were reported in the largest series of filter patients published to date, comprising 568 patients.[88] Unfortunately, follow-up was almost exclusively clinical, with few imaging studies performed to document outcome, and duration of follow-up was short, with minimum required follow-up of 6 months and maximum of 5 years.[88] Twelve of 440 patients (2.7%) on whom 6-month follow-up information was available demonstrated clinically suspected recurrent PE, and 13 patients (2.9%) had clinical evidence of IVC thrombosis.[88] Recurrent PE was confirmed in only two patients and thrombosis of the IVC in seven patients. Of 27 follow-up vena cavograms performed, six demonstrated thrombosis; this report does not state whether all these vena cavograms were obtained for symptoms.

Two configurations of the bird's nest filter have been used. Significant migration of the original filter was seen in five of the first 422 patients.[88] Subsequently, the struts were modified to become more rigid. This change required increasing the diameter of the insertion sheath from 8 Fr to 12 Fr. No migrations were reported in the next 147 patients treated with the modified filter,[88] although rare migrations subsequently were described.[146]

Titanium Greenfield filter

The titanium Greenfield filter is similar in design to the stainless Greenfield filter, but it is slightly larger, with a length of 4.7 cm and a width at the filter base of 38 mm (Fig. 21-10).[90,147] It is approximately half the weight of the stainless steel Greenfield filter and is designed to be placed using a 12 Fr carrier through a 14 Fr sheath. Unlike the stainless steel Greenfield filter, the filter is not placed over a guidewire. Titanium has demonstrated biocompatibility comparable to stainless steel.[147]

The original version of the titanium Greenfield filter was plagued by a high incidence of filter migration (27%)[90,147–149] as well as by reports of penetration of the wall of the vena cava and adjacent structures in up to 13% (Fig. 21-11).[148,149] Therefore, the filter hooks were modi-

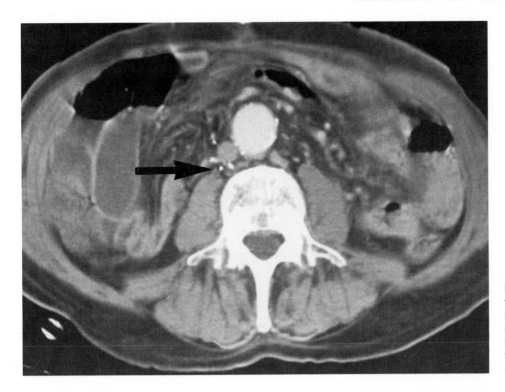

FIGURE 21-11. Penetration of the wall of the inferior vena cava by several legs of the titanium Greenfield filter (*arrow*) as seen by computed tomography performed for abdominal aortic aneurysm.

fied by curving them to limit penetration and angling them 80 degrees to minimize migration.[90] The modified filter design demonstrated an improved rate of migration 1 cm or greater in 11% in a follow-up study.[90] Caval penetration was assessed by splaying of the filter base

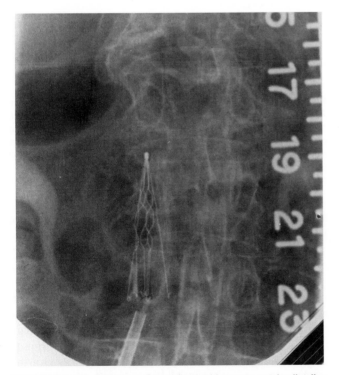

FIGURE 21-12. Titanium Greenfield with asymmetric distribution of legs. Two of the legs are crossed.

more than 5 mm in 17 of 121 patients; further evaluation with computed tomography confirmed filter penetration of the vena cava in one patient (0.8%).[90]

The titanium Greenfield filter often demonstrates crossing one or more pairs of the filter struts after deployment, which was reported in a total of 7.4% of 181 cases[90] (Fig. 21-12) and results in uneven segmentation of the vena cava, which in some cases may be unsatisfactory, requiring placement of an additional filter. Alternatively, the filter can be manipulated in an attempt to separate crossed legs or reposition a tilted filter, but this can be difficult and is not recommended by the manufacturer (Fig. 21-13). In our experience, crossing the legs is seen less frequently with jugular placement, possibly because of the presentation of the filter struts on deployment as opposed to the apical presentation with femoral placement.

The titanium Greenfield demonstrated similar clot trapping effectiveness as the stainless steel Greenfield filter in clinical trials.[90,147] Post-filter placement PE rates have been clinically suspected in 3% of 181 patients in one series.[90] In this series, thrombosis of the IVC was not clinically suspected in any patients, although follow-up was only 30 days in this study.[90] Thrombosis of the insertion site has been reported in 3 to 8.7% of patients.[90,147]

Simon-Nitinol filter

The Simon-Nitinol filter is composed of a nickel-titanium alloy that has thermal memory (Fig. 21-14). This filter is molded into a predetermined shape at high temperature.

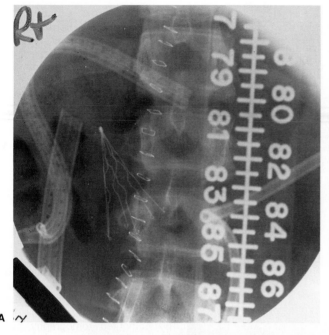

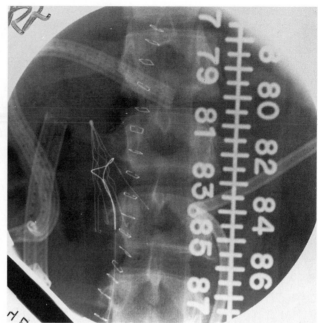

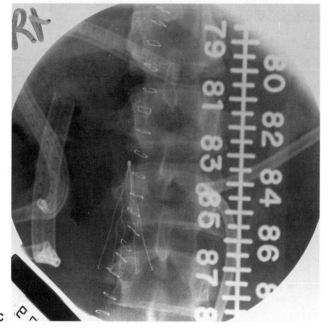

FIGURE 21-13. Repositioning of the titanium Greenfield filter. **A:** The filter is tilted after initial deployment. **B:** The filter is captured with a nitinol snare. **C:** The filter is repositioned slightly caudally in a more axial orientation. Repositioning of the filter in a satisfactory orientation in this way can be difficult and is not recommended as a routine maneuver.

When cooled, the filaments become pliable, and the filter can be straightened for introduction. The filter is cooled with iced saline as it is introduced. As it is warmed on contact with blood, it assumes its molded configuration within seconds. The filter is 3.8 cm long, and the filter dome has a diameter of 28 mm.[150] The filter is placed through a 7 Fr introducer (9 Fr outer diameter). It has six radiating legs projected from the center of the filter, each with a hook designed to minimize motion of the filter within the vena cava. Additionally, the filter has a second tier of struts that are designed for filtration, are located cranially to the anchoring struts, and consist of

seven wire loops arranged in the configuration of the petals of a flower.

In preliminary data from 103 patients with Simon nitinol filters placed at 17 centers, recurrent PE was confirmed in two patients and suspected in a third, for a recurrent PE rate of 3%.[150] Occlusion of the IVC was reported in six of 44 patients (14%) and insertion site thrombosis in five of 44 patients (11%).[150] No significant filter migration was observed in this series, although three cases of migration to the heart or pulmonary arteries have been published.[151,152] Although tilting of the dome of the filter was observed in 55% of 44 patients, it

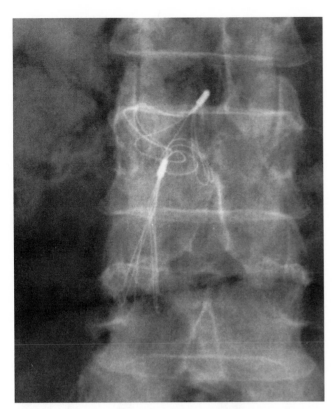

FIGURE 21-14. Radiograph of the Simon nitinol filter. The film demonstrates slight tilting of the filter petals compared with the longitudinal axis of the vena cava, which has been shown experimentally not to reduce filtration effectiveness.

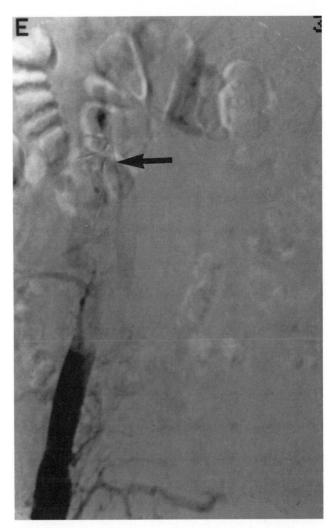

FIGURE 21-15. Digital subtraction vena cavogram from a patient who had a Simon nitinol filter placed 1 month previously demonstrates thrombosis of the vena cava at the level of the filter (*arrow*) with a patent lumen in the caudal inferior vena cava.

has been stated that this does not affect filter effectiveness.[150] In the largest series published to date, the number of patients undergoing objective testing for each of these outcomes is not specified, and it must be presumed that all patients did not undergo such testing.

Thrombosis of the vena cava after filter placement has been the major disadvantage of the Simon nitinol filter (Fig. 21-15). In one series in which this was assessed, occlusion of the vena cava was seen in 21% of 24 patients.[153] The possibility of more frequent occurrence of vena caval occlusion in patients with malignancies has been raised, although this conclusion was based on a small number of patients.[153] Filter penetration was documented by imaging studies in five patients of 20 (25%), including penetration of the aorta in two patients.[151] Observation of tilting of the cephalad cluster of loops in undersized vena cavas was observed, and it was postulated that this may impart excessive torque on the filter anchoring struts that may increase the likelihood of penetration of the vena cava,[151] although this has not been proved. This series confirmed the ability of this filter to prevent PE, with no clinically suspected postfilter emboli seen in 20 patients with mean follow-up of 14 months.[151]

Problems such as occlusion of the vena cava and penetration of the vena cava have limited acceptance of this filter. However, the Simon nitinol vena cava filter has one clear advantage over other currently available devices: the filter's low profile and flexible delivery system allow placement from virtually any access site, including the antecubital and left jugular veins (Fig. 21-16).

LGM Vena Tech filter

The LGM Vena Tech filter is cone-shaped, with six radiating struts, and originally measured 4.5 cm high in its initial configuration, with a base width of 28 mm (Fig. 21-17). The filter is composed of a stainless steel alloy called Elgiloy and is stamped and point welded. The filter has six longitudinal side rails attached to the struts at the base of the filter, parallel to the wall of the vena cava, designed to contact the wall of the vena cava throughout their length, providing transverse stability.[87] The side rails were 34 mm long in the original design and therefore

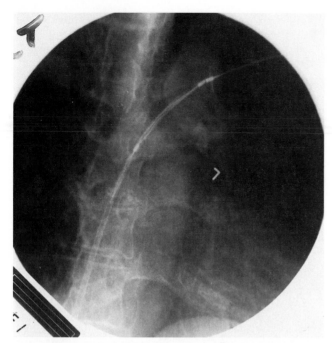

FIGURE 21-16. Spot film obtained during placement of a Simon nitinol filter through left basilic vein access in a patient with no other suitable route for filter introduction.

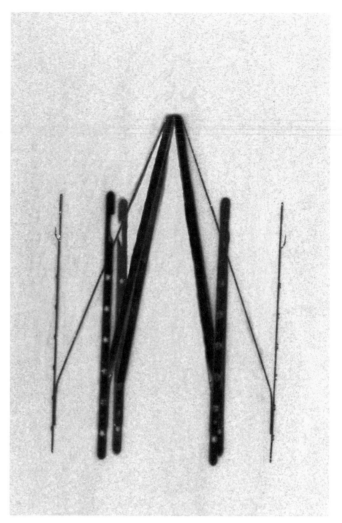

FIGURE 21-17. Lateral photograph of the LGM Vena Tech filter.

shorter than the diagonal struts. Hooks are punched from the metal at the cephalad ends of the side rails to provide longitudinal stability. This filter is designed for rapid deployment; indeed, slow deployment may result in incomplete opening of the filter.[87] Because incomplete opening of the filter was reported in up to 42% of filters placed by the jugular approach,[154] the filter was modified so that the side rails are now nearly equal in height to the filter when deployed. This modification was done to minimize crossing of the side rails with the diagonal struts upon filter deployment, which can result in incomplete opening of the filter.[87]

The LGM filter has been used in Europe since 1985;[155] use in the United States began in 1989.[87] This filter is the most thoroughly and objectively evaluated filter to date, with four large studies reporting mostly imaging-based follow-up.[87,155–157] The filter is effective in preventing recurrent PE, with recurrent PE rates of 0 to 3.5% reported in five large series with a cumulative total of 482 patients.[87,151–158]

Occlusion of the IVC was studied using imaging tests in two series and is approximately 92% at 6 months to 1 year.[87,155] A significantly higher rate of thrombotic occlusion of the vena cava was reported in another series, seen in 14 of 64 patients by sonography or autopsy, for an IVC occlusion rate of 22%.[157] This result is considerably higher than those in other reports of short follow-up[87,155] but was not confirmed in another series in which a rate of IVC occlusion of 8% of 39 patients was reported.[156]

In a recently published series with 2- to 6-year follow-up, patency of the IVC as documented by transabdominal Doppler ultrasound was 92% after 2 years, but this rate continued to decrease by approximately 5% annually thereafter to 70% after 6 years.[158] This rate is lower than those reported for the stainless steel Greenfield filter; however, imaging studies were not done to document the long-term patency of the stainless steel Greenfield filter. Therefore, the difference may be attributable to closer scrutiny of the LGM filter. The observation that the patency rate of the vena cava with the LGM filter continued to decline at a consistent rate up to 6 years raises the possibility that the filter causes thrombosis of the vena cava in the absence of embolized or propagating thrombosis. Because the material that the filter is composed of is biologically stable and the normal vena cava is a high-flow vessel, spontaneous thrombosis seems unlikely without constriction of the vein lumen.[151] Indeed, narrowing of the filter base was highly correlated with thrombosis of the vena cava in this series.[158] Whereas in previous experience this was considered attributable to retraction of thrombus, it is possible that the filter side rails incite a hyperplastic or fibrotic response in the vein wall that results in narrowing and occlusion.[158] Whether this feature is unique to the LGM filter awaits further study.

Thrombosis of the insertion site following placement of the LGM Vena Tech filter has been reported in 6% and 23% of patients in the two series in which this was evaluated.[87,157] Significant filter migration ($\geq$1 cm) was seen in 14% of 65 patients in one series, with a maximum migration of 3 cm,[87] and in 13% in another series.[156] Similar results were supported in one other series.[155] When assessing filter stability 1 cm is assumed to be the minimum for significant migration, because shorter migration cannot be distinguished reliably from perceived change due to parallax. As a result of its self-centering design, filter migration is rarely a problem.[87,156,157]

As mentioned, incomplete opening of the LGM Vena Tech filter has been its only significant problem and most frequently is encountered with jugular placement (Fig. 21-18). This problem was reported in between 9% and 42% of cases when the jugular approach is used.[87,154,156,157] It is interesting, however, to note that in the two largest series reporting significant numbers of jugular filter placements in which incomplete opening of the filter was encountered (22% and 42% rates of incomplete filter opening),[87,154] two institutions contributed patients to both reports in the same period, presumably the same patients, which will skew the results from both reports toward those achieved at these institutions. Results obtained with the new configuration are not yet available.

Amplatz filter

Although not currently available in the United States, discussion of the Amplatz filter (William Cook, Europe; Bjaerverskov, Denmark) is warranted because it represents a new generation of filters that is designed to be retrievable. To facilitate transfemoral removal of the filter, a hook is present at the apex of the cone, and the filter is deposited with the apex directed caudally.[89] This feature may be desirable in the patient who has a transient contraindication to anticoagulation, such as a recent trauma or recent or impending surgery. It is also a feature with intuitive appeal, because deep venous and pulmonary thromboembolic disease is usually time-limited. Organization of thrombus is complete within 3 to 6 months.[159] Patients who can be protected from potentially fatal pulmonary emboli during this acute period by medication or filter placement usually will not require either of these treatments after that time.

Percutaneous removal of the Amplatz filter was reported in one series in six patients.[89] Removals were complicated by incorporation of the filter struts in the endothelium of the vein and occasional incorporation of the

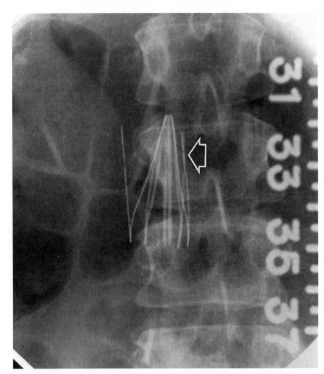

FIGURE 21-18. Incomplete opening LGM filter. Two of the side rails are crossed (*arrow*), and the filter is slightly angulated.

filter hook. Filter removal was fairly traumatic, resulting in intramural hemorrhage in two patients, which did not result in acute symptoms.[89] Three filter retrievals were described as "difficult" as a result of the filter's adherence to the vein wall, which takes approximately 2 to 3 weeks to occur.[89,160–162] Because two retrievals were performed within 24 hours, three of the four more delayed retrievals probably were complicated.[89] Removability in this context therefore does not justify the little benefit that it provides.

■ Conclusions

The high mortality of untreated pulmonary embolism or DVT makes mechanical interruption of the IVC necessary in patients with this condition who cannot be treated medically with anticoagulation, who suffer PE, or who demonstrate proximal propagation of thrombus while adequately anticoagulated. Additionally, high-risk situations exist, such as free-floating iliac or vena cava thrombus, that warrant caval interruption in addition to anticoagulation. Partial interruption of the vena cava by percutaneous placement of a vena cava filter is the method of choice, optimally performed using fluoroscopic guidance following vena cavography.

Five vena cava filters are available in the United States: the stainless steel Greenfield filter, the bird's nest filter, the titanium Greenfield filter, the Simon nitinol filter, and the LGM filter. Of these, the Greenfield filter design is slightly less effective in removing small emboli from the bloodstream than the bird's nest or Simon nitinol filters; however, it is equally effective in preventing clinically significant PE and has a better rate of patency of the vena cava after placement. This filter design is suitable for most patients. The bird's nest or Simon nitinol filters may be useful in patients unable to tolerate small pulmonary emboli, such as those with cor pulmonale or chronic lung disease. The bird's nest filter is ideal in patients with mega vena cava (>28 mm diameter), and the Simon nitinol filter is useful in patients without traditional routes of access for filter placement. Because no significant differences in clinical outcome have proved the superiority of one filter design over the others, it is likely that the differences are minor, and no filter is ideal for all patients. Rather, the choice of which filter to use should be made on an individual basis until a randomized clinical trial clearly elucidates the relative benefits of each of these devices.

REFERENCES

1. Le Quesne LP. Diagnosis and prevention of postoperative deep-vein thrombosis. *Annu Rev Med* 1975;26:63.
2. Huisman MV, Vuller HR, ten Cate JW, et al. Unexpected high prevalence of silent pulmonary embolism in patients with deep venous thrombosis. *Chest* 1989;95:498–502.
3. Dorfman GS, Cronan JJ, Tupper TB, et al. Occult PE: a common occurrence in deep venous thrombosis. *AJR Am J Roentgenol* 1987;148:263–266
4. Moser KM, Fedullo PF, LittleJohn JK, et al. Frequent asymptomatic pulmonary embolism in patients with deep venous thrombosis. *JAMA* 1994;271:223–225
5. Evans AJ, Sostman HD, Knelson MH, et al. Detection of deep venous thrombosis: prospective comparison of MR imaging with contrast venography. *AJR Am J Roentgenol* 1993;161:131–139.
6. Giuntini C, Di Ricco G, Mrini C, et al. Pulmonary embolism: epidemiology. *Chest* 1995;107(Suppl 1):3S–9S.
7. Ferris EJ. Deep venous thrombosis and pulmonary embolism: correlative evaluation and therapeutic implications. *AJR Am J Roentgenol* 1992;159:1149–1155.
8. Harmon B. Deep vein thrombosis: a perspective on anatomy and venographic analysis. *J Thorac Imaging* 1989;4:15–19.
9. Barker NW, Nygaard KK, Walters W, et al. Statistical study of post-operative venous thrombosis and pulmonary embolism: time of occurrence during post-operative period. Proc Staff Meet Mayo Clin 1941;16:17–23.
10. Barritt DW, Jordan SC. Anticoagulant drugs in the treatment of pulmonary embolism: a controlled trial. *Lancet* 1960;1:1309–1312.
11. Rohrer MJ, Scheidler MG, Wheeler HB, et al. Extended indications for placement of an inferior vena cava filter. *J Vasc Surg* 1989;10:44–50.
12. Homans J. Deep quiet venous thrombosis in the lower limb: preferred levels for interruption of veins; iliac sector or ligation. *Surg Gynecol Obstet* 1944;79:70–82.
13. Moser KM. Pulmonary embolism. *Am Rev Respir Dis* 1977;115:829–852.
14. Horattas MC, Wright DJ, Fenton AH, et al. Changing concepts of deep venous thrombosis of the upper extremity: report of a series and review of the literature. *Surgery* 1988;104:561–567.
15. Monreal M, Lafoz E, Ruiz J, et al. Upper-extremity deep venous thrombosis and pulmonary embolism: a prospective study. *Chest* 1991;99:280–283.
16. Habscheid W, Stratmann A, Dammrich J. Compression sonography as a screening method in thrombosis diagnosis. *Dtsch Med Wochenschr* 1990;115:1003–1008.
17. Cronan JJ, Froehlich JA, Dorfman GS. Image-directed Doppler ultrasound: a screening technique for patients at high risk to develop deep vein thrombosis. *J Clin Ultrasound* 1991;19:133–138.
18. Woolson ST, McCrory DW, Walter JF, et al. B-mode ultrasound scanning in the detection of proximal venous thrombosis after total hip replacement. *J Bone Joint Surg* 1990;72:983–987.
19. Leyvraz PR, Richard J, Bachmann F, et al. Adjusted versus fixed-dose subcutaneous heparin in the prevention of deep-vein thrombosis after total hip replacement. *N Engl J Med* 1983:309:954–958.
20. Olin JW, Graor RA, O'Hara P, et al. The incidence of deep venous thrombosis in patients undergoing abdominal aortic aneurysm resection. *J Vasc Surg* 1993;18:1037–1041.
21. Rosenow EC. Venous and pulmonary thromboembolism: an algorithmic approach to diagnosis and management. *Mayo Clinic Proc* 1995;70:45–49.
22. Bettmann MA, Paulin S. Leg phlebography: the incidence, nature and modification of undersirable side effects. *Radiology* 1977;122:101–104.
23. Thomas L, McAllister V, Tonge K. Simplified phlebography in deep venous thrombosis. *Clin Radiol* 1971;22:490–494.
24. Albrechtsson U, Olsson C. Thrombotic side-effects of lower-limb phlebography. *Lancet* 1976;723–724.
25. Naidich JB, Feinberg AW, Karp-Harman H, et al. Contrast venography: reassessment of its role. *Radiology* 1988;168:97–100.
26. Ramchandani P, Soulen RL, Fedullo LM, et al. Deep vein thrombosis: significant limitations of noninvasive tests. *Radiology* 1985;156(1):47–49.
27. Holden RW, Klatte EC, Park HM, et al. Efficacy of noninvasive modalities for diagnosis of thrombophlebitis. *Radiology* 1981;141:63–66.
28. Barnes RW. Current status of noninvasive tests in the diagnosis of venous disease. *Surg Clin North Am* 1982:62:489–500.
29. Erdman WA, Jayson JT, Redman HC, et al. Deep venous thrombosis of extremities: role of MR imaging in the diagnosis. *Radiology* 1990;174:425–431.
30. Evans AJ, Sostman HD, Knelson MH, et al. Detection of deep venous thrombosis: prospective comparison of MR imaging with contrast venography. *AJR Am J Roentgenol* 1993;161:131–139.
31. Carpenter JP, Holland GA, Baum RA, et al. Magnetic resonance venography for the detection of deep venous thrombosis: comparison with contrast venography and duplex Doppler ultrasonography. *J Vasc Surg* 1993;18:734–741.
32. Spritzer CE, Norconk JJ, Sostman HD, et al. Detection of deep venous thrombosis by magnetic resonance imaging. *Chest* 1993;104:54–60.
33. Wells PS, Brill-Edwards P, Stevens P, et al. A novel and rapid whole-blood assay for D-dimer in patients with clinically suspected deep vein thrombosis. *Circulation* 1995;91:2184–2187.
34. Cronan JJ, Murphy TP. A comprehensive review of vascular ultrasound for the intensivist. *J Intensive Care Med* 1993;8:188–201.
35. Philbrick JT, Becker DM. Calf deep venous thrombosis: a wolf in sheep's clothing? *Arch Intern Med* 1988;148:2131–2138.
36. Moser KM, LeMoine JR. Is embolic risk conditioned by location of deep venous thrombosis? *Ann Intern Med* 1981;94:439–444.
37. McLachlan MSF, Thomson JG, Taylor DW, et al. Observer variation in the interpretation of lower limb venograms. *AJR Am J Roentgenol* 1979;132:227–229.
38. Lund F, Diener L, Ericson J. Postmortem intraosseous phlebogra-

phy as an aid in studies of venous thromboembolism. *Angiology* 1969;20:155–176.

39. Mills SR, Jackson DC, Older RA, et al. The incidence, etiologies and avoidance of complications of pulmonary angiography in a large series. *Radiology* 1980;136:295–299.

40. The PIOPED Investigators. Value of the ventilation/perfusion scan in acute pulmonary embolism: results of the prospective investigation of pulmonary embolism diagnosis (PIOPED). *JAMA* 1990;263: 2753–2759.

41. Erdman WA, Peshock RM, Redman HC, et al. Pulmonary embolism: comparison of MR images with radionuclide and angiographic studies. *Radiology* 1994;190:499–508.

42. Schiebler, ML, Holland GA, Hatabu H, et al. Suspected pulmonary embolism: prospective evaluation with pulmonary MR angiography. *Radiology* 1993;189:125–131.

43. Hatabu H, Gefter WB, Axel L, et al. MR imaging with spatial modulation of magnetization in the evaluation of chronic central pulmonary thromboemboli. *Radiology* 1994;190:791–796.

44. Loubeyre P, Revel D, Douek P, et al. Dynamic contrast-enhanced MR angiography of pulmonary embolism: comparison with pulmonary angiography. *AJR Am J Roentgenal* 1994;162: 1035–1039.

45. Goldhaber SZ, Simons GR, Elliot CG, et al. Quantitative plasma D-dimer levels among patients undergoing pulmonary angiography for suspected pulmonary embolism. *JAMA* 1993;270:2819–2822.

46. Hull RD, Hirsh J, Carter CJ, et al. Pulmonary angiography, ventilation lung scanning, and venography for clinically suspected pulmonary embolism with abnormal perfusion lung scan. *Ann Intern Med* 1983;98:891–899.

47. Cronan JJ. Contemporary venous imaging. *Cardiovasc Intervent Radiol* 1991;14:87–97.

48. Smith LL, Iber C. Venous duplex ultrasound in the diagnosis of pulmonary embolism. *J Vasc Tech* 1989;13:227–230.

49. Beecham RP, Dorfman GS, Cronan JJ, et al. Is bilateral lower-extremity compression sonography useful and cost-effective in the evaluation with suspected pulmonary embolism. *AJR Am J Roentgenol* 1993;161:1289–1292.

50. Smith LL, Iber C, Sirr S. Pulmonary embolism: confirmation with venous duplex US as adjunct to lung scanning. *Radiology* 1994; 191:143–147.

51. Gallus AS, Jackaman J, Tillet J, et al. Safety and efficacy of warfarin started early after submassive venous thrombosis or pulmonary embolis. *Lancet* 1986;2:1293–1296.

52. Hull RD, Raskob GE, Rosenbloom D, et al. Heparin for 5 days as compared with 10 days in the initial treatment of proximal venous thrombosis. *N Engl J Med* 1990;322:1260–1264.

53. Brandjes DPM, Meigboer H, Buller HR, et al. Acenocoumarol and heparin compared with acenocoumarol alone in the initial treatment of proximal-vein thrombosis. *N Engl J Med* 1992;327:1485–1489.

54. Hull RD, Raskob GE, Pineo GF, et al. Subcutaneous low-molecular-weight heparin compared with continuous intravenous heparin in the treatment of proximal-vein thrombosis. *N Engl J Med* 1992; 326:975–982.

55. Brockman SK, Vasko JS. Phlegmasia cerulea dolens. *Surg Gynecol Obstet* 1965;121:1347–1356.

56. Elliot MS, Immelman EJ, Jeffery P, et al. The role of thrombolytic therapy in the management of phlegmasia cerulea dolens. *Br J Surg* 1979;66:422–424.

57. Robinson DL, Teitelbaum GP. Phlegmasia cerulea dolens: treatment by pulse-spray and infusion thrombolysis. *AJR Am J Roentgenol* 1993;160(6):1288–1290.

58. Semba CP, Dake MD. Iliofemoral deep venous thrombosis: aggressive therapy with catheter-directed thrombolysis. *Radiology* 1994; 191:487–494.

59. Mewissen M. Interim report from the data collection center. *J Vasc Interv Radiol* 1997;8(1Part 2):50–52.

60. O'Meara JJ, McNutt RA, Evans AT, et al. A decision analysis of streptokinase plus heparin as compared with heparin alone for deep-vein thrombosis. *N Engl J Med* 1994;330:1864–1869.

61. Machleder HI. Evaluation of a new treatment strategy for Paget-Schroetter syndrome: spontaneous thrombosis of the axillary-subclavian vein. *J Vasc Surg* 1993;17:305–317.

62. Virchow R, Chance F, trans. Cellular pathology. New York: Dewitt, 1860.

63. Greenfield LJ, DeLucia A. Endovascular therapy of venous thromboembolic disease. *Surg Clin North Am* 1992;72:969–989.

64. Crane C. Femoral vs. caval interruption for venous thromboembolism. *N Engl J Med* 1964;270:819–821.

65. Mozes M, Adar R, Bogokowsky H, et al. Vein ligation in the treatment of pulmonary embolism. *Surgery* 1964;55:621–629.

66. Nasbeth DC, Moran JM. Reassessment of the role of inferior vena cava ligation in venous thromboembolism. *N Engl J Med* 1965;273: 1250–1253.

67. Adams JT, Feingold BE, DeWeese JA. Comparative evaluation of ligation and partial interruption of the inferior vena cava. *Arch Surg* 1971;103:272–276.

68. Amador E, Kai T, Crane C. Ligation of inferior vena cava for thromboembolism: clinical and autopsy correlations in 119 cases. *JAMA* 1968;206:1758–1760.

69. McConnel D, Mulder D, Buckberg G. The placement of vena cava umbrella filters: the value of phlebography. *Arch Surg* 1974;108: 789–791.

70. Bernstein E. The place of venous interruption in the treatment of pulmonary thromboembolism. In: Moser K, Stein, eds. *Pulmonary thromboembolism.* Chicago: Year Book Medical Publishers, 1973: 312–323.

71. Miles RM, Elsea PW. Clinical evaluation of the serrated vena caval clip. *Surg Gynecol Obstet* 1971;132:581–587.

72. McLean J. The thromboplastic action of cephalia. *Am J Physiol* 1916;41:250–257.

73. Allen EV, Barker NW, Waugh JM. A preparation from spoiled sweet clover. *JAMA* 1942;120:1009–1015.

74. Seidman M, Robertson DN, Link KP. Studies on 4-hydroxycoumarins: X. Acylation of 3-(alpha-phenyl-beta-acetylethyl)-4-hydrocycoumarin. *J Am Chem Soc* 1950;72:5193–5195.

75. Spencer FC, Quattlebaum JK, Quattlebaum JK, et al. Plication of the IVC for pulmonary embolism; a report of 20 cases. *Ann Surg* 1962;155:827.

76. Maraan BM, Taber RE. The effects of inferior vena caval ligation on cardiac output. An experimental study. *Surgery* 1968;63:966–969.

77. Mobin-Uddin K, McLean R, Bolooki H, et al. Caval interruption for prevention of pulmonary embolism. *Arch Surg* 1969;99: 711–715.

78. Mobin-Uddin K, Utley JR, Bryant LR. The inferior vena cava umbrella filter. *Prog Cardiovasc Dis* 1975;17:391–399.

79. McIntyre AB, McCready RA, Hyde GL, et al. A ten year follow-up study of the Mobin-Uddin filter for vena cava interruption. *Surg Gynecol Obstet* 1984;158:513–516.

80. Wingerd M, Bernhard VM, Maddison F, et al. Comparison of caval filters in the management of venous thromboembolism. *Arch Surg* 1978;113:1264–1271.

81. Cimochowski GE, Evans RH, Zarins CK, et al. Greenfield filter versus Mobin-Uddin umbrella. *J Thorac Cardiovasc Surg* 1980;79:358–365.

82. Menzoian JO, LoGerfo FW, Weitzman AF, et al. Clinical experience with the Mobin-Uddin vena cava umbrella filter. *Arch Surg* 1980;115:1179–1181.

83. Gomez GA, Cutler BS, Wheeler HB. Transvenous interruption of the inferior vena cava. *Surgery* 1983;93:612–619.

84. Tadavarthy SM, Castaneda-Zuniga W, Salomonowitz E, et al. Kim-

ray-Greenfield vena cava filter: percutaneous introduction. *Radiology* 1984;151:525–526.

85. Greenfield LJ, Michna BA. Twelve-year clinical experience with the Greenfield vena caval filter. *Surgery* 1988;104:706–712.

86. Dorfman GS. Percutaneous inferior vena caval filters. *Radiology* 1990;174:987–992.

87. Murphy TP, Dorfman GS, Yedlicka JW, et al. LGM vena cava filter: objective evaluation of early results. *J Vasc Interv Radiol* 1991;2: 107–115.

88. Roehm JOF, Johnsrude IS, Barth MH, et al. The bird's nest inferior vena cava filter: progress report. *Radiology* 1988;168: 745–749.

89. Epstein DH, Darcy MD, Hunter DW, et al. Experience with the Amplatz retrievable vena cava filter. *Radiology* 1989;172:105–110.

90. Greenfield LJ, Cho KJ, Proctor M, et al. Results of a multicenter study of the modified hook-titanum Greenfield filter. *J Vasc Surg* 1991;14:253–257.

91. Hirsh J. Treatment of pulmonary embolism. *Annu Rev Med* 1987; 38:91105.

92. Hayes SP, Bone RC. Pulmonary emboli with respiratory failure. *MCN Am J Matern Child Nurs* 1983;67:1179–1191.

93. Carter BL, Jones ME, Waickman LA. Pathophysiology and treatment of deep-vein thrombosis and pulmonary embolism. *Clin Pharmacokinet* 1985;4: 279–296.

94. Wessler S, Gitel SN. Warfarin from bedside to bench. *N Engl J Med* 1984;311:645–652.

95. Mant MJ, O'Brien BD, Thong KL, et al. Haemorrhagic complications of heparin therapy. *Lancet* 1977;1:1133–1135.

96. Norris CS, Greenfield LJ, Herrmann JB. Free-floating iliofemoral thrombus. *Arch Surg* 1985;120:806–808.

97. Radomski JS, Jarrell BE, Carabasi RA, et al. Risk of pulmonary embolus with inferior vena cava thrombosis. *Am Surg* 1987;53:97–101.

98. Greenfield LJ. Current indications for and results of Greenfield filter placement. *J Vasc Surg* 1984;1:502–504.

99. Tobin KD, Pais SO, Austin CB. Reevaluation of indications for percutaneous placement of the Greenfield filter. *Invest Radiol* 1989;24:115–118.

100. Sack GH, Levin J. Trousseau's syndrome and other manifestations of chronic disseminated coagulopathy in patients with neoplasms. *Medicine* 1977;56:814–828.

101. Schafer AI. The hypercoagulable states. *Ann Intern Med* 1985;102: 814–828.

102. Luzzato G, Schafer AI. The prethrombotic state in cancer. *Semin Oncol* 1990;17:147–159.

103. Oster M. Thrombophlebitis and cancer. *Angiology* 1976;27:557–567.

104. Sarasin FP, Eckman MH. Management and prevention of thromboembolic events in patients with cancer-related hypercoagulable states. *J Gen Intern Med* 1993;8:476–486.

105. Rickles FR, Edwards LR. Activation of blood coagulation in cancer: trousseau's syndrome revisited. *Blood* 1983;62:14–31.

106. Kitchens CS. Concept of hypercoagulability: a review of its development, clinical application, and recent progress. *Semin Thromb Hemost* 1985;11:293–315.

107. Colman RW, Rubin RN. Disseminated intravascular coagulation due to malignancy. *Semin Oncol* 1990;17:172–186.

108. Calligaro KD, Bergen WS, Haut MJ, et al. Thromboembolic complications in patients with advanced cancer: anticoagulation versus Greenfield filter placement. *Ann Vasc Surg* 1991;5:186–189.

109. Clarke-Pearson DL, Synam IS, Creasman WT. Anticoagulation therapy for venous thromboembolism in patients with gynecologic malignancy. *Am J Obstet Gynecol* 1983;147:369–375.

110. Krauth D, Holden A, Knapic N, et al. Safety and efficacy of long-term oral anticoagulation in cancer patients. *Cancer* 1987;59: 983–985.

111. Menzoian JO, Sequeira JC, Doyle JE, et al. Therapeutic and clinical course of deep venous thrombosis. *Am J Surg* 1983;146:581–585.

112. Erricheti AM, Holden A, Ansell J. Management of oral anticoagulation therapy: experience with an anticoagulation clinic. *Arch Intern Med* 1984;144:1966–1968.

113. Cohen JR, Tenenbaum N, Citron M. Greenfield filter as primary therapy for deep venous thrombosis and/or pulmonary embolism in patients with cancer. *Surgery* 1991;109:12–15.

114. Hubbard KP, Roehm JO, Abbruzzese JL. The bird's nest filter: an alternative to long-term oral anticoagulation in patients with advanced malignancies. *Am J Clin Oncol* 1994;17:115–117.

115. Magnant JG, Walsh DB, Juravsky Ll, et al. Current use of inferior vena cava filters. *J Vasc Surg* 1992;16:701–706.

116. Lossef SV, Barth KH. Outcome of patients with advanced neoplastic disease receiving vena caval filters. *J Vasc Interv Radiol* 1995;6: 273–277.

117. Rosen MP, Porter DH, Kim D. Reassessment of vena caval filter use in patients with cancer. *J Vasc Interv Radiol* 1994;5:501–506.

118. Rogers FB, Shackford SR, Wilson J, et al. Prophylactic vena cava filter insertion in severely injured trauma patients: indications and preliminary results. *J Trauma* 1993;35:637–642.

119. Geerts WH, Code KI, Jay RM, et al. A prospective study of venous thromboembolism after major trauma. *N Engl J Med* 1994;331: 1601–1606.

120. Sevitt S, Gallagher N. Venous thrombosis and pulmonary embolism: a clinico-pathological study in injured and burned patients. *Br J Surg* 1961; 48:475–489.

121. Sevitt S. Fatal road accidents: injuries, complications, and causes of death in 250 subjects. *Br J Surg* 1968;55:481–505.

122. Leach TA, Pastena JA, Swan KG, et al. Surgical prophylaxis for pulmonary embolism. *Am Surg* 1994;60:292–295.

123. Schackford SR, Davis JW, Hollingsworth-Fridlund P, et al. Venous thromboembolism in patients with major trauma. *Am J Surg* 1990; 159:365–369.

124. Knudson MM, Collins JA, Goodman SB, et al. Thromboembolism following multiple trauma. *J Trauma* 1992;32:2–11.

125. Rohrer MJ, Scheidler MG, Wheeler B, et al. Extended indications for placement of an inferior vena cava filter. *J Vasc Surg* 1989; 10:44–50.

126. Martin KD, Kempczinski RF, Fowl RJ. Are routine interior vena cavograms necessary before Greenfield filter placement? *Surgery* 1989;106:647–651.

127. Hicks ME, Malden ES, Vesely TM, et al. Prospective anatomic study of the inferior vena cava and renal veins: comparison of selective renal venography with cavography and relevance in filter placement. *J Vasc Interv Radiol* 1995;6:721–729.

128. Layton BT, Shaff MI, Mazer M, et al. Major venous anomalies of the inferior vena cava and renal veins: a radiographic and pictorial essay. *Semin Interv Radiol* 1990;7:86–92.

129. Sardi A, Minken SL. The placement of intracaval filters in an anomalous (left-sided) vena cava. *J Vasc Surg* 1987;6:84–86.

130. Rohrer MJ, Cutler BS. Placement of two Greenfield filters in a duplicated vena cava. *Surgery* 1988;104:572–574.

131. Stewart JR, Peyton JWR, Crute SL, et al. Clinical results of suprarenal placement of the Greenfield vena cava filter. *Surgery* 1982;92:1–4

132. Yune HY. Inferior vena cava filter: search for an ideal device. *Radiology* 1989;172:15–16.

133. Grassi CJ. Inferior vena caval filters: analysis of five currently available devices. *AJR Am J Radiol* 1991;156:813–821.

134. Katsamouris AA, Waltman AC, Delichatsios MA, et al. Inferior vena cava filters: in vitro comparison of clot trapping and flow dynamics. *Radiology* 1988;166:361–366.

135. Thompson BH, Cragg AH, Smith TP, et al. Thrombus-trapping efficiency of the Greenfield filter in vivo. *Radiology* 1989; 172:979–981.

136. Millward SF, Marsh JI, Pon C, et al. Thrombus-trapping efficiency of the LGM (Vena Tech) and titanium Greenfield filters in vivo. *J Vasc Interv Radiol* 1992;3:103–106.

137. Pais SO, Tobin KD, Austin CB, et al. Percutaneous insertion of the Greenfield inferior vena cava filter: experience with ninety-six patients. *J Vasc Surg* 1988;8:460–464.

138. Greenfield LJ, Peyton R, Crute S, et al. Greenfield vena caval filter experience: late results in 156 patients. *Arch Surg* 1981;116: 1451–1456.

139. Rose BS, Simon DC, Hess ML, et al. Percutaneous transfemoral placement of the Kimray-Greenfield vena cava filter. *Radiology* 1987;165:373–376.

140. Denny DF, Cronan JJ, Dorfman GS, et al. Percutaneous Kimray-Greenfield filter placement by femoral vein puncture. *AJR Am J Roentgenol* 1985;145:827–829.

141. Shetty PC, Bok LR, Sharma RP. Balloon dilation of the femoral vein expediting percutaneous Greenfield vena caval filter placement. *Radiology* 1986;161:275.

142. Dorfman GS, Cronan JJ, Paolella LP, et al. Iatrogenic changes at the venotomy site after percutaneous placement of the Greenfield filter. *Radiology* 1989;173:159–162.

143. Reed RA, Teitelbaum GP, Taylor FC, et al. Use of the bird's nest filter in oversized inferior venae cavae. *J Vasc Interv Radiol* 1991;2:447–450.

144. Korbin CD, Reed RA, Taylor FC, et al. Comparison of filters in an oversized vena caval phantom: intracaval placement of a bird's nest filter versus biiliac placement of Greenfield, Vena Tech-LGM, and Simon nitinol filters. *J Vasc Interv Radiol* 1992;3:559–564.

145. Prince MR, Novelline RA, Athanasoulis CA, et al. The diameter of the IVC and its implication for the use of vena cava filters. *Radiology* 1983;149:687–689.

146. Rogoff PA, Hilgenberg AD, Miller SL, et al. Cephalic migration of the bird's nest inferior vena caval filter: report of two cases. *Radiology* 1992;184:819–822.

147. Greenfield LJ, Cho KJ, Pais SO, et al. Preliminary clinical experience with the titanium Greenfield vena cava filter. *Arch Surg* 1989;124:657–659.

148. Teitelbaum GP, Jones DL, van Breda A, et al. Vena caval filter splaying: potential complication of use of the titanium Greenfield filter. *Radiology* 1989;173:809–814.

149. Ramchandani P, Koolpe HA, Zeit RM. Splaying of titanium Green-field inferior vena caval filter. *AJR Am J Roentgenol* 1990;155: 1103–1104.

150. Simon M, Athanasoulis CA, Kim D, et al. Simon nitinol inferior vena cava filter: initial clinical experience. *Radiology* 1989;172: 99–103.

151. McCowan TC, Ferris EJ, Carver DK, et al. Complications of the nitinol vena caval filter. *J Vasc Interv Radiol* 1992;3:401–408.

152. LaPlante JS, Contractor FM, Kiproff PM, et al. Migration of the Simon nitinol vena cava filter to the chest. *AJR Am J Roentgenol* 1993;160:385–386.

153. Grassi CJ, Matsumoto AH, Teitelbaum GP. Vena caval occlusion after Simon nitinol filter placement: identification with MR imaging in patients with malignancy. *J Vasc Interv Radiol* 1992;3:535–539.

154. Reed RA, Teitelbaum GP, Taylor FC, et al. Incomplete opening of LGM (Vena Tech) filters inserted via the transjugular approach. *J Vasc Interv Radiol* 1991;2:441–445.

155. Ricco JB, Crochet D, Sebilotte P, et al. Percutaneous transvenous caval interruption with the "LGM" filter: early results of a multicenter trial. *Ann Vasc Surg* 1988;2:242–247.

156. Taylor FC, Awh MH, Kahn CE, et al. Vena tech vena cava filter: experience and early follow-up. *J Vasc Interv Radiol* 1991;2:435–440.

157. Millward SF, Marsh JI, Peterson RA, et al. LGM (Vena Tech) vena cava filter: clinical experience in 64 patients. *J Vasc Interv Radiol* 1991;2:429–433.

158. Crochet DP, Stora O, Ferry D, et al. Vena Tech-LGM filter: long-term results of a prospective study. *Radiology* 1993;188:857–860.

159. Murphy TP, Cronan JJ. Evolution of deep venous thrombosis: a prospective evaluation with US. *Radiology* 1990;177:543–548.

160. Lund G, Rysavy J, Hunter DW, et al. Retrievable vena cava filter percutaneously introduced. *Radiology* 1985;155:831.

161. Darcy MD, Smith TP, Hunter DW, et al. Short-term prophylaxis of pulmonary embolism by using a retrievable vena cava filter. *AJR Am J Roentgenol* 1986;147: 836–838.

162. Hunter DW, Lund G, Rysavy JA, et al. Retrieving the Amplatz retrievable vena cava filter. *Cardiovasc Intervent Radiol* 1987;10: 32–36.

22

Anatomy of the Kidneys and Genitourinary Tract

ANDREI FROST

The urinary system comprises the upper urinary tracts (kidneys and ureters), the urinary bladder, and the urethra. The genital system consists of the testes, epididymides, deferent ducts, seminal vesicles, ejaculatory ducts, the prostate, and the penis in males; and the ovaries, uterine tubes, uterus, and vagina in females. A complete review of the embryology and anatomy is beyond the scope of this book; instead, an overview is given from the perspective of the vascular and interventional radiologist (VIR). The emphasis, therefore, is on the urinary system and the uterine tubes, which provide a fertile ground for interventional procedures. Anatomy of the penis is more appropriately discussed in Chapter 2. Embryology is presented for a better understanding of the anatomy and of the more frequently encountered variants and anomalies.

■ Embryology

The urinary tract develops in three overlapping stages: the pronephros, the mesonephros, and the metanephros (Fig. 22-1).[1] Development progresses from the cranial aspect toward the cloaca. As the more caudal segments develop, the earlier, cranial ones involute. The pronephros does not have an excretory function in the human and involutes completely. The mesonephros is constituted by a pair of medially located mesonephric ducts (wolffian ducts) and laterally located nephrogenic cords. The nephrogenic cords form a collection of glomeruli and primitive tubules connected to the mesonephric ducts. The mesonephric duct eventually extends caudally and establishes a communication with the cloaca, allowing excretion of urine. Unlike the pronephros, some of the mesonephric remnants participate in the formation of the adult male genital tract (efferent ductules, epididymis, paradidymis, vas deferent, seminal vesicles, and ejaculatory ducts). The metanephros develops from two separate components: the metanephric duct (ureteral bud) and the metanephric blastema. The ureteral bud is a small outpouching that arises from the caudal aspect of the mesonephric (wolffian) duct in approximately the 5-week-old embryo. This bud grows ventrally and superiorly, forming a long tube with a dilated cranial blind end, called the *ampulla*. Surrounding the ampulla of the metanephric duct on each side is a cellular mass called the *metanephric blastema*. As the metanephric ducts elongate, they also divide and penetrate the blastema, inducing differentiation.

As the ureteral bud lengthens, the lumbosacral region of the embryo undergoes accelerated growth. The combination of these processes results in an apparent ascension of the kidneys from the initial caudal origin toward their final position in the midabdomen. Concomitant with this apparent cranial migration, the kidneys also rotate medially, which results in the final position at birth, with the excretory portion of the kidney being lateral and the renal pelvis located medially. Failure of these processes results in a variety of abnormalities of size, shape, position, and number of the kidneys. Frequently, these anomalies coexist. For example, in the *horseshoe kidney* (the most frequent fusion anomaly, where the lower poles of the kidneys are fused across the midline), the renal pelves are ventral because of the absence of normal rotation, the kidney is lower than normal (ectopic), and the arterial supply is commonly aberrant (multiple renal arteries originating from the

255

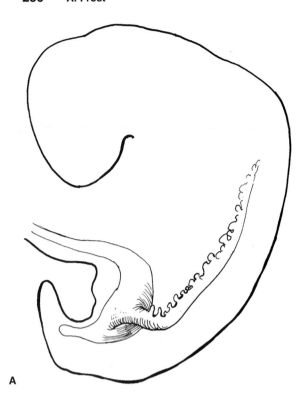

A

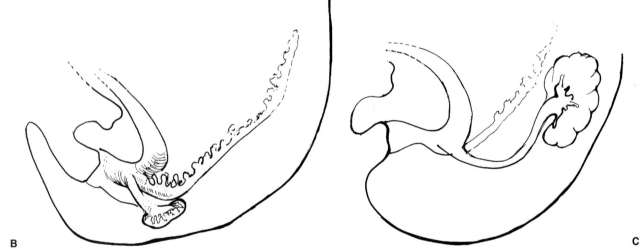

B   C

FIGURE 22-1. A: Pronephros (2nd through 6th somites) and early mesonephros; approximately 3 weeks. **B:** Mesonephros (9th through 16th somites) and early metanephros; 3+ weeks. **C:** Metanephros and apparent renal migration; 5 weeks to term. Note the complete degeneration of the pronephros and partial degeneration of the mesonephros.

distal aorta and the iliac arteries). During ascension, the kidneys are supplied with blood by paired mesonephric branches of the aorta. As kidneys ascend, branches arising at lower levels involute and more cranial branches substitute for them. Failure of this involution results in accessory or aberrant renal arteries (25% of normal); these arteries are usually lower and of smaller caliber than the main renal arteries and supply the polar regions.

Renal ontogenesis concludes with the process of *maturation,* which entails the overall growth of the organ and variable degree of fusion of the approximately 14 initial lobes (seven ventral, seven dorsal) (Fig. 22-2A).[2] A result of this lobar fusion is the smoothing of the renal surface with effacement of interlobar septations (Fig. 22-2B). This process is more pronounced at the poles than at the interpolar region (Fig. 22-3). Another consequence of the lobar fusion is the formation of compound calyces. This process is also more pronounced in the polar regions; therefore, the upper and lower pole calyces tend to be compound, whereas the interpolar calyces usually maintain their original ventral and dorsal distribution. The implications of lobar fusion for the VIR will be further discussed in the subsection on renal anatomy.

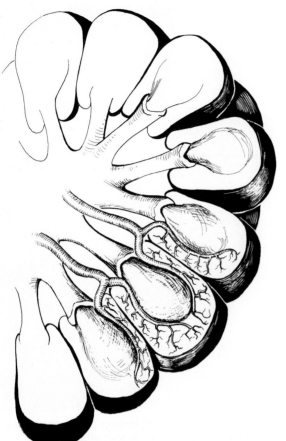

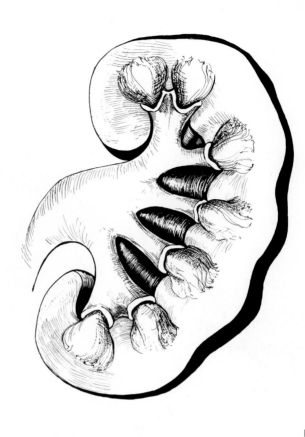

A

B

FIGURE 22-2. **A:** Diagram of the fetal kidney at approximately 28 weeks (coronal section). On average, there are 14 lobes (7 ventral and 7 dorsal), each irrigated by at least two interlobar arteries. The lobes are separated by connective tissue planes and demarcated by deep grooves on the surface of the kidney. **B:** Fetal kidney at term (coronal section). Variable degree of lobar fusion results in compound calices and effacement of the surface grooves.

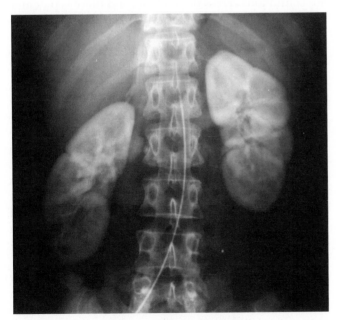

FIGURE 22-3. Marked bilateral fetal lobulation of the kidneys (left greater than right); abdominal aortogram, late venous phase. Note the predominance in the interpolar area (right).

■ Anatomy

Kidneys

Good knowledge of renal anatomy is a prerequisite for percutaneous access to the renal collecting system, a well-established procedure performed for relief of obstruction or as a preamble for other diagnostic or therapeutic procedures (biopsy, diversion of the urinary stream, stricture treatment, ureteral occlusion, or percutaneous stone extraction).

The mature kidneys are paired organs. The left is usually slightly larger than the right, and there is significant individual variation in size; however, as an overall rule, kidney size is relatively symmetric (Fig. 22-4). The kidneys are bean shaped with a medial indentation called *hilum*. The contours are variably smooth, depending on the degree of lobar fusion. Contours can be deformed by indentation by adjacent organs, most frequently in the left kidney, secondary to splenic impression (Fig. 22-5). Normally, the kidneys are located at the level of the twelfth thoracic to the third lumbar vertebrae. The left

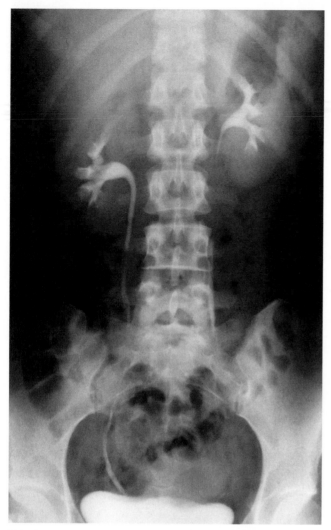

FIGURE 22-4. Normal urogram. Note the symmetry of the shape and size of the kidneys, the higher position of the left kidney, and the compound calices in the polar areas. Some asymmetry can be seen in the morphology of the pelves.

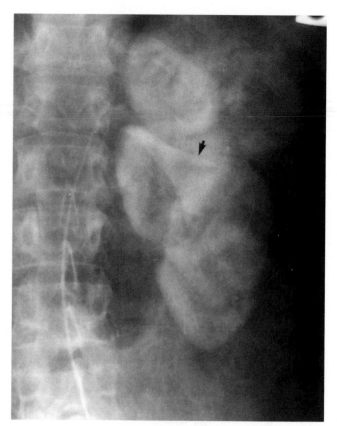

FIGURE 22-5. Splenic impression on the left kidney (*arrow*); abdominal aortogram, late venous phase.

kidney is usually slightly higher than the right. Both kidneys are mobile and can change position significantly, both with the phase of respiration and with change in position of the patient.[3] This mobility can be used to the advantage of the VIR because a needle inserted percutaneously into the kidney will swing characteristically with respiratory motion, whereas an extrarenal needle will not change position appreciably with respiratory motion.

Both kidneys are retroperitoneal organs. The retroperitoneal space is delineated anteriorly by the parietal peritoneum, posteriorly by the fascia transversalis, superiorly by the diaphragm, and inferiorly by the pelvic brim. The retroperitoneal space is subdivided in three important compartments (Fig. 22-6).[4] The anterior pararenal space is delineated by the parietal peritoneum and posteriorly by the anterior renal fascia (Gerota's fascia). This space contains the ascending and descending colon, the

pancreas, duodenum, and a small amount of retroperitoneal fat. The two sides of the anterior pararenal space are continuous across the midline, and there is potential communication with the posterior pararenal space inferiorly.

The perirenal space is delineated anteriorly by the anterior renal fascia and posteriorly by the posterior renal fascia (fascia of Zuckerkandl). It contains the kidneys, adrenal glands, ureters, abundant perirenal fat, and the great vessels (aorta and the inferior vena cava). The perirenal fat is continuous with the renal sinuses. The perirenal space does not communicate across the midline and therefore has two separate compartments (right and left). A strong, fibrous, nonadherent capsule envelopes each kidney, separating it from the perirenal fat. This capsule and the thoracolumbar fascia (aponeurosis of transverse abdominal muscle) are the points where a needle meets resistance during percutaneous puncture of the renal collecting system.[2]

The posterior pararenal space is bordered anteriorly by the posterior renal fascia and posteriorly by the fascia transversalis. This space contains only fat. It communicates potentially with the anterior pararenal space at the pelvic rim and with the mediastinum superiorly through the paravertebral space. The importance of the retroperi-

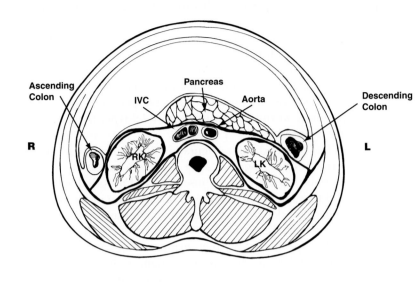

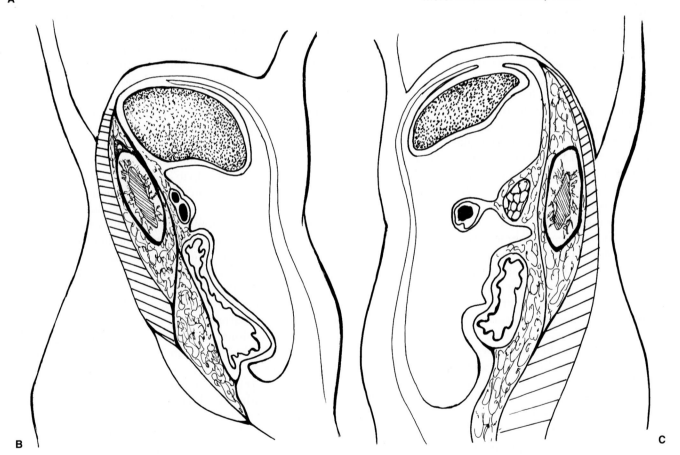

FIGURE 22-6. Axial (**A**) and right (**B**) and left (**C**) parasagittal diagramatic sections through the abdomen, illustrating the retroperitoneal compartments. The anterior pararenal space contains the pancreas, ascending and descending colon and the duodenum. The perirenal space contains the kidneys, ureters and adrenal glands. The posterior pararenal space contains fat. Note rotation of the kidneys about the longitudinal and transverse axes. From Castaneda-Zuniga, WR, Tadavarty, SM, eds. Interventional radiology, 2nd ed. Baltimore: William & Wilkins, 1992.

toneal space divisions lies in the characteristic radiological findings of fluid or gas collections within each of these compartments.

Posterior relationships of the kidneys within the renal fossa are important for the understanding and planning of percutaneous procedures.[5] Superficially, a muscle layer formed by the quadratus lumborum muscle laterally and the psoas muscle medially extends from the costal margin to the iliac crest. Superiorly, the posterior aspect of the diaphragm comes in relationship with the upper poles of the kidneys. The aponeurosis of the transverse abdominal muscle completes the posterior wall of the abdomen. Because of the slightly higher position of the left kidney, it is crossed posteriorly by the eleventh and the twelfth ribs, whereas usually the right kidney comes in posterior contract with only the twelfth rib. As mentioned, the position of the kidneys and their mobility with respiratory motion will vary significantly. As a result, the posterior pleural space may be traversed during an attempted upper pole (intercostal) percutaneous puncture. Because such punctures sometimes are required by the clinical situation, care must be taken to ensure an extrapleural tract by careful fluoroscopic examination with steep oblique or lateral projections or by cross-sectional studies [computed tomography (CT) scan].[2] Transpleural punctures can result in significant complications such as pneumothorax, hydrothorax, or hemothorax. Also noteworthy is the need to avoid the intercostal vessels, which course along the inferior groove of the ribs. Therefore, intercostal punctures should be performed with the needle hugging the superior aspect of the rib.

The lateral relationships of the kidneys are also relevant to the VIR because of the potential injury to adjacent organs during performance of percutaneous nephrostomy. On the right side, the most important relationships are to the liver and to the hepatic flexure of the colon; on the left side, the important relationships are with the spleen and the splenic flexure of the colon. Both the spleen and the liver are bulkier in their cranial aspects, which makes for a more medial relationship with the upper poles of the kidneys. More inferiorly, as the spleen and liver decrease in bulk, their relationship with the kidneys becomes more lateral. As a consequence, the lower the percutaneous puncture (subcostal, lower pole caliceal puncture versus supracostal, upper pole puncture), the more lateral the skin puncture site can be while still avoiding injury to the adjacent organs. A more lateral puncture will allow for a straighter tract into the collecting system, which in turn ensures easier manipulations during subsequent procedures, such as percutaneous stone extraction or antegrade ureteral stenting. This concept will be better understood after discussion of the orientation of the kidneys and collecting systems.

The kidneys are obliqued in reference to the sagittal, coronal, and axial planes of the body.[2] The upper poles are most medial and posterior; lower poles are most lateral and anterior. In the axial plane, the lateral borders of the kidneys are rotated approximately 30 degrees posterior to the coronal plane (Fig. 22-6). The hilum points anteromedially and the lateral border posterolaterally. Because of the embryological development of anterior and posterior renal lobes, the mature collecting system has two rows of calyces, one anterior and one posterior. Lobar fusion leads to the formation of compound calyces, particularly at the poles. The nonfused calyces, predominantly in the interpolar segment, are oriented at a 90-degree angle to each other. The disposition of the calyces follows one of the two extreme configurations (Hodson's or Brodel's) or an in-between variation (Fig. 22-7). The Hodson type is more common and has the ventral calyces positioned at a shallow 20-degree angle anterior to the coronal plane of the kidney, whereas the dorsal calyces are positioned at a steeper 70-degree angle posterior to this plane. In the Brodel type, these angles are reversed.[1,2]

The perpendicular orientation of the anterior and posterior calyces, together with the overall rotation of the kidneys, has important consequences for both diagnostic and therapeutic procedures. Opacification of the collecting system depends on the type of contrast used and the position of the patient. Iodinated contrast, which has a higher specific gravity than urine, accumulates in the dependent regions. In a prone patient, iodinated contrast preferentially will opacify the anterior and lower pole calyces. Air or carbon dioxide, which are gases, on the other hand will preferentially opacify the posterior and upper pole calyces in a prone patient. Carbon dioxide occasionally is used as a contrast agent in patients who are allergic to iodinated contrast. Drainage of calyces into the renal pelvis is also influenced by gravity and patient position. For example, with the patient prone, the upper pole and posterior calyces will empty of iodinated contrast first while the remainder of the collecting system may retain some contrast. Knowledge of the anatomy and understanding of preferential filling and emptying with the contrast medium used will help to identify and select the most appropriate calyx for puncture. The straightest possible tract is desirable for a successful percutaneous intervention (e.g., nephrostomy, antegrade ureteral stenting, stone extraction). The trajectory of the needle must be planned in such a way as to minimize the angle with the calyx, infundibulum, and pelvis while also avoiding injury to the adjacent organs (liver, spleen, colon, intercostal arteries, and lungs). Fluoroscopy at various oblique angulations, using a C-arm or turning the patient, and occasionally cross-sectional studies are used for this purpose.

The arterial blood supply and the venous drainage are also important considerations in performing percutaneous renal interventions. Usually, there are single right and left renal arteries, which are direct branches of the abdominal aorta. These branches originate at the upper level of the second lumbar vertebra. The left renal artery is straighter and shorter than the right renal artery and has a posterolateral course, whereas the right renal artery is longer and has an anterolateral proximal course. On an angiogram, therefore, the origins of the renal arteries are best visualized on the left anterior oblique projection. The renal arteries have a variable branching pattern. The most frequent pattern shows a ventral division, which usually has four segmental branches and supplies the

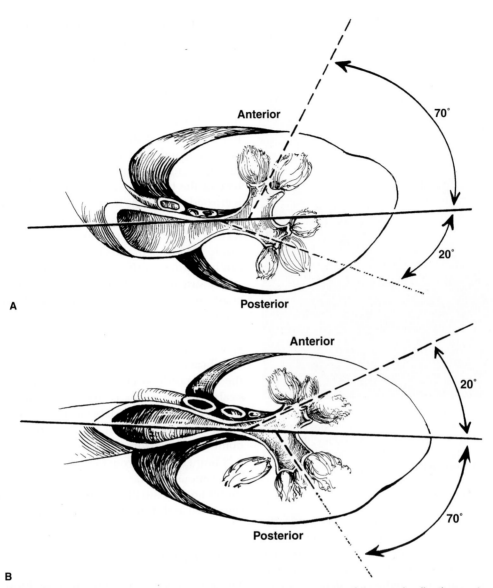

FIGURE 22-7. Diagramatic cross-sectional representation of the two basic types of the renal collecting system: **A:** Brodel type (dorsal calyces are positioned at a 20-degree angle posterior to the coronal plane and ventral calyces at a 70-degree angle anterior to the coronal plane of the kidney) and **B:** Hodson type (dorsal clayces are at 70-degree angle posterior to the coronal plane and ventral calyces at a 20-degree angle anterior to the coronal plane). From Castaneda-Zuniga WR, Tadavarty SM, eds. Interventional radiology, 2nd ed. Baltimore: Williams & Wilkins, 1992.

upper pole and the ventral aspect of the kidney and a dorsal division, which usually has a single segmental branch and supplies the lower pole and dorsal aspect of the kidney (Fig. 22-8). The five segmental arteries mentioned already are "end" arteries. They branch into interlobar arteries, which further branch into arcuate arteries at the level of the corticomedullary junction. Interlobular arteries branch from the arcuate arteries into the renal cortex. Renal blood flow is distributed about 80% to the cortex and 20% to the medulla. A relatively hypovascular area is located along the lateral-posterior aspect of the kidney, between the territories of distribution of the ventral and dorsal divisions of the renal artery. This hypovas-

cular area is the ideal site for percutaneous punctures because it minimizes chances of injury to a large sized vessel (Fig. 22-9).[2]

The intrarenal venous drainage of the kidney is constituted by stellate, arcuate, and interlobar veins, which parallel the arteries; unlike the arterial circulation, however, the venous drainage is highly anastomosed (Fig. 22-10). Eventually, single right and left renal veins usually form and drain directly into the inferior vena cava at approximately the level of the second lumbar vertebra. The left renal vein courses anteriorly to the aorta and posteriorly to the superior mesenteric artery and is longer than the right renal vein. The left adrenal vein

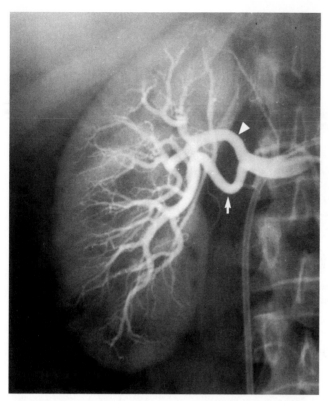

FIGURE 22-8. Normal renal artery: selective right renal angiogram, arterial phase. The ventral division (*arrowhead*) supplies the upper pole and the ventral aspect of the kidney; the dorsal division (*arrow*) supplies the lower pole and the dorsal aspect. (Courtesy of Andrew Kerr, M.D.)

and gonadal vein are its tributaries. On the right side, the gonadal and adrenal veins drain directly into the inferior vena cava. This anatomic distribution is of obvious interest when sampling venous blood for evidence of adrenal adenomas and explains the higher incidence and increased severity of left-sided varicocele caused by valvular incompetence of the testicular vein. This subject is discussed further in Chapter 26.

Ureters

The ureters are paired muscular tubes. They connect the right and left renal pelves to the urinary bladder. At the level of the bladder, each ureter penetrates the thick wall of the bladder in an oblique anteromedial course, which constitutes the intramural segment. Ureters are approximately 25 to 30 cm long, are distensible, and have a largest diameter of approximately 8 mm. At the entrance into the true pelvis, both ureters cross anteriorly to the common iliac vessels, which frequently cause extrinsic impression upon the ureters. The ureteropelvic junction, the ureterovesical junction, and the crossing of the common iliac vessels are the three most common sites for stone impaction. The most important relationship of ure-

ters in their abdominal portion, in the perirenal space, is to retroperitoneal lymph nodes: Because of this relationship, ureters can be involved and obstructed by metastatic adenopathy. Relationships in the pelvic course are different in males and females. In males, the pelvic ureter is related to the ipsilateral deferent duct, seminal vesicle, internal iliac vessels, and iliac lymph nodes. The distalmost segment of the ureter is lateral and cranial to the prostate gland, as it approaches the trigone. In females, the pelvic ureter crosses posteriorly to the ovary, in the base of the broad ligament of the uterus. At this level, it is crossed posteriorly by the uterine artery. More caudally, the pelvic ureter is crossed anteriorly by the uterine artery, as it lies lateral and anterior to the cervix and superior to the fornix of the vagina. In this location, the ureter can be injured during obstetric or gynecologic surgery.

The vascular supply of the ureter is variable and highly anastomosed. The arterial supply usually consists of a *superior ureteric artery*, which is a branch of the renal artery, and an *inferior ureteric artery*, which is a branch of the middle vesical artery. The *middle vesical artery* is a branch of the umbilical artery, which is one of the ventral branches of the hypogastric artery. Another name for the middle vesical artery in males is the *vesiculodeferential artery*. Less common and more variable arterial supply for the ureter derives from peritoneal arteries, directly from the abdominal aorta, from the external and common iliac artery branches, and from branches of the gonadal arteries. The venous drainage of the ureter follows the arterial supply and eventually drains into the renal veins, inferior vena cava, and its tributaries.

Urinary bladder

The *urinary bladder* is a muscular sac located in the true pelvis, posterior to the pubic symphysis. Inferiorly, the male urinary bladder lies atop the prostate, which separates it from the floor of the perineum. In females, the bladder lies directly on the muscular perineum.

The arterial supply of the urinary bladder is variable. It is supplied by branches of the anterior division of the internal iliac arteries. The three most constant such branches are the superior, middle, and inferior vesical arteries. The *superior vesical artery* is a terminal branch of the umbilical artery. The *middle vesical artery* (also called vesiculodeferential in males) can be a branch of the umbilical artery or of the uterine artery in females. The *inferior vesical artery* is a branch of the internal iliac artery. There are extensive anastomoses between the right and left internal iliac arteries and between the ventral and posterior division branches of the ipsilateral internal iliac artery, resulting in a perivesical plexus. This arrangement explains the need to perform bilateral embolization of the hypogastric arteries to control hemorrhage of the

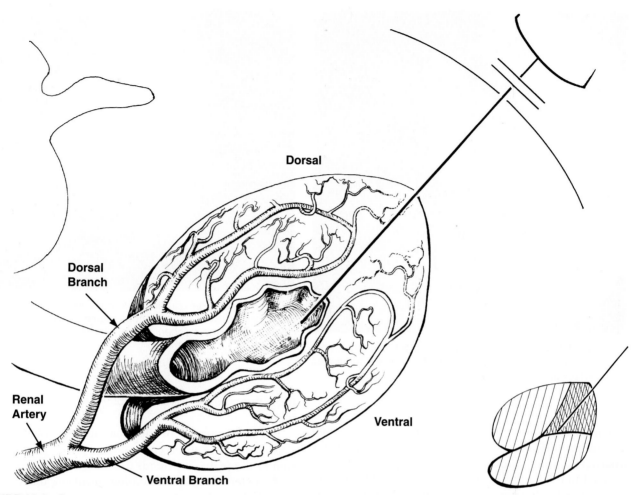

FIGURE 22-9. Cross-section through the interpolar aspect of the kidney, in prone position, showing ventral and dorsal distribution of the renal vessels. The hypovascular, peripheral area of the kidney (diagram) is the preferred site for percutaneous punctures, since it is least likely to contain large caliber vessels. From Castaneda-Zuniga, WR, Tadavarty, SM (eds): Interventional radiology, 2nd ed. Baltimore: Williams & Wilkins, 1992.

urinary bladder. The high degree of anastomosis also prevents bladder ischemia following such embolization.

The venous drainage of the urinary bladder is through the perivesical plexus, which is highly anastomosed with the dorsal vein of the penis/clitoris, parietal pelvic veins, and veins of the thigh and buttock. The vesical plexus drains into the right and left internal iliac veins.

Urethra

The urethra, the lowest component of the lower urinary tract, differs in females and males. The female urethra is a straight conduit, approximately 4 cm long, which stretches from the bladder neck to the external meatus (Fig. 22-11). It is susceptible to traumatic injuries, particularly related to childbirth. The male urethra is longer and more complex. It is usually divided into three segments (Fig. 22-12): the most cranial is the prostatic urethra, which measures approximately 3 cm long, and ex-

tends from the bladder neck to the level of the external sphincter (the floor of the perineum). This segment is enveloped completely by the prostate gland. On its posterior wall, a contour defect is formed by an elongated cranial portion termed the *urethral crest* and a rounded caudal portion called the *verumontanum*. Multiple prostatic ducts open in the region of the urethral crest, whereas the utricle and the two ejaculatory ducts open at the level of the verumontanum. This segment of the urethra can be stenosed by tumors or benign prostatic hyperplasia, conditions that are targets of recent developments in interventional radiology, such as balloon prostatic urethroplasty, hyperthermic ablation, and prostatic stents.[6,7]

The second segment of the male urethra is the membranous urethra, which is approximately 1 cm long, and is the segment of the urethra that pierces the floor of the perineum. It is circled by muscle fibers that form the external sphincter. This segment of the urethra is believed to play a

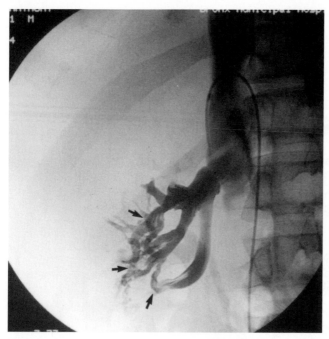

FIGURE 22-10. Normal renal vein: selective right renal venogram. Note the anastomoses of the venous tributaries (*arrows*). (Courtesy of Andrew Kerr, M.D.)

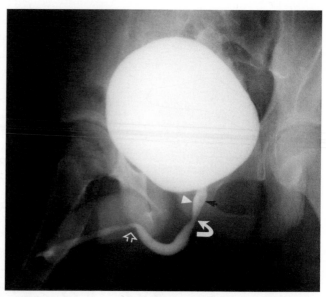

FIGURE 22-12. Retrograde male urethrogram: prostatic segment (*arrowhead*), membranous segment (*curved arrow*), cavernous segment (*open arrow*), and verumontanum (*black arrow*).

role in dysmotility conditions of the urinary bladder seen in patients with spinal cord injury ("detrusor-sphincter dyssynergia"). An investigational technique is being developed to relieve this condition by balloon dilatation of the external sphincter.[7] The membranous urethra, because of its location immediately posterior and inferior to

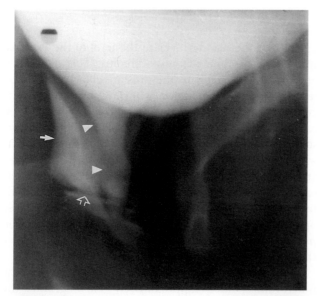

FIGURE 22-11. Normal female urethra: voiding cystogram, oblique projection; urethra (*arrowheads*), vaginal reflux (*arrow*), and hymen (*open arrow*).

the pubic symphysis is susceptible to injury in pelvic fractures.

The third portion of the male urethra is termed the *cavernous urethra* and is contained in the corpus spongiosum of the penis. It extends from the external sphincter to the external meatus. Pathology involving this segment is related mostly to strictures of various etiologies (posttraumatic, infectious, congenital, or iatrogenic). Classically, the urethral strictures are treated by repeated dilatations or by surgery. More recently, balloon dilatation and stenting of such strictures have been performed with good results up to 2 years posttreatment.[7]

Uterus

The uterus is a pear-shaped, muscular organ located in the female pelvis. It is attached inferiorly to the fornix of the vagina and lies between the urinary bladder anteriorly and the rectum posteriorly.[8]

The arterial supply to the uterus is constituted by the *uterine arteries,* which are branches of the right and left internal iliac arteries. The uterine arteries divide into ascending and descending branches, which course alongside the lateral aspect of the uterus, within the myometrium. The *ovarian arteries,* which are direct branches of the abdominal aorta, also supply the uterus and anastomose with the branches of the uterine arteries. The venous drainage of the uterus originates in a plexus around the cervix from which branches paralleling the uterine arteries extend into the broad ligament and drain into the iliac veins. Anastomoses between the uterine venous plexus and the superior rectal vein contribute to porto-systemic anastomoses.

Uterine tubes

The uterine (fallopian) tubes are paired, approximately 10 cm long tubular structures, located on the right and left sides of the uterus. Each tube extends from the level of its respective uterine cornu to the pelvic peritoneum in the vicinity of the ipsilateral ovary. A direct communication is thus established between the peritoneal cavity and the exterior, through the endometrial cavity, the cervical canal, and the vagina (Fig. 22-13).[9]

On hysterosalpingography, the uterine tube has four segments.[8] The intramural segment is the part of the tube contained within the myometrium and extending from the uterine ostium to the lateral aspect of the wall of the uterus. The isthmus is the narrowest segment of the tube and has the thickest wall. It extends for a length of 2 to 5 cm laterally to the intramural segment and is continued by the ampulla, which is the widest and longest segment of the tube and the site where fertilization of the oocyte takes place. The infundibulum, the funnel-shaped lateral segment of the tube, contains the abdominal ostium, which is surrounded by digitations called *fimbriae.* The uterine tubes are intraperitoneal (being contained in the cranial edge of the broad ligament) and therefore are

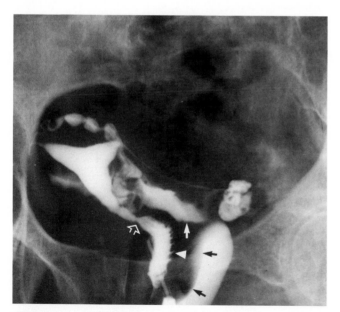

FIGURE 22-13. Normal hysterosalpingogram, left anterior projection; note the plicae palmatae of the cervix (*arrowhead*), the internal cervical os (*open arrow*), anteverted and anteflexed uterine body with triangular appearance of the endometrial cavity, and patency of both uterine tubes with pooling of contrast in the peritoneal cul-de-sac (*white arrow*). Contrast refluxed into the formix of the vagina, outlining the vaginal segment of the cervix (*black arrow*).

relatively mobile. The arterial supply and the venous drainage derive from anastomoses between uterine and ovarian vessels.

Female infertility can be caused by tubal occlusion. A promising development in interventional radiology is the selective retrograde catheterization of the tubes, for both diagnostic and therapeutic purposes (see Chapter 27).[10]

■ Congenital Anomalies of Relevance to the VIR

A full discussion of urological and reproductive congenital anomalies is beyond the scope of this chapter. The following is a brief analysis of the relevance of some of these anomalies to the VIR.

Many of the congenital anomalies result in urinary obstruction and infections, with or without renal failure, especially in the pediatric age group. In older patients, stone formation can complicate many of these conditions. Uroradiologic interventions are required for the diagnosis and treatment of these conditions and their secondary complications; these interventions are detailed in Chapter 24. Examples of such congenital anomalies are: ureteral multiplications (sometimes associated with ectopic implantation of the ureter and ureterocele), various forms of renal fusion (most frequent of which is the horseshoe kidney), renal ectopia (particularly the pelvic kidney), retrocaval ureter, megaloureter, ureteral stenosis, diverticula (caliceal, ureteral, or urethral), and urethral valves.

Other congenital anomalies present with hematuria and require diagnostic or therapeutic radiological renovascular procedures. Examples of such conditions are congenital aneurysms, congenital arteriovenous fistulae, and the "nutcracker syndrome" (i.e., compression of the left renal vein between the aorta and the mesenteric vessels, with increased pressure in the left renal vein and formation of peripelvic and periureteral varices) (see Chapter 23).

A causal relationship was proved between varicocele and male infertility. Varicoceles are related to developmental abnormalities of spermatic vein valves. Transcatheter embolization of varicocele is now an established procedure (Chapter 27).[11–12]

Certain congenital anomalies impede interventional access or require modification of standard interventional techniques. For example, percutaneous nephrostomy access can be difficult in horseshoe, ectopic (crossed or uncrossed, fused or unfused), or malrotated kidneys. Percutanous insertion and positioning of inferior vena cava filters, venous catheterization, and blood sampling may be influenced by the presence of anomalies such as multiple renal veins, circumaortic renal veins, and double or left-sided inferior vena cava (see Chapters 19 and 27).[13]

Finally the presence of certain anomalies or normal variants must be documented before surgical interventions are performed. For example, aberrant or accessory renal arteries must be identified before repair of abdominal aortic aneurysm or renal transplant donor nephrectomy. The preoperative evaluation of the renal transplant donor is discussed in Chapter 23.

REFERENCES

1. Davidson AJ. Radiologic anatomy of the kidney. In: *Radiology of the kidney.* Philadelphia: WB Sauders, 1985;71–88.

2. Castaneda-Zuniga WR, Tadavarthy SM, Hunter DW. Percutaneous uroradiologic techniques. In: Castaneda-Zuniga WR, Tadavarty SM, eds. *Interventional radiology,* 2nd ed. Baltimore: Williams & Wilkins, 1992:777–787.

3. Preminger GM, Schulz S, Clayman RV, et al. Cephalad renal movement during percutaneous nephrostolithotomy. *J Urol* 1987;137: 623.

4. Meyers M. The extraperitoneal spaces; normal and pathologic anatomy. In: *Dynamic radiology of the abdomen: normal and pathologic anatomy.* New York: Springer-Verlag, 1976:113.

5. Netter FH. Kidneys, ureters and urinary bladder. In: Shapter RK, Youkman FF, eds. *The CIBA collection of medical illustrations,* 4th ed. West Caldwell: CIBA, 1987:2–4.

6. Castaneda F, Hunter DW, Amplatz K, et al. Retrograde transurethral prostatic urethroplasty with balloon catheter. In: Castaneda-Zuniga WR, Tadavarty SM, eds. *Interventional radiology,* 2nd ed. Baltimore: Williams & Wilkins, 1992:1015–1027.

7. Castaneda F, Brady TM, Bertino RE, et al. Other lower urinary tract interventions. In: Castaneda-Zuniga WR, Tadavarty SM, eds. *Interventional radiology,* 2nd ed. Baltimore: Williams & Wilkins, 1992: 1034–1042.

8. Moore KI. The perineum and pelvis. In: Clinically oriented anatomy, 2nd ed. Baltimore: Williams & Wilkins, 1985:373–380.

9. Gray H. The urogenital system. In: Clemente CD, ed. *Anatomy of the human body,* 30th ed. Philadelphia: Lea and Febiger, 1985: 1571–1576.

10. Thurmond AS. Fallopian tube catheterization for improved diagnosis and treatment of proximal tube obstruction. In: Castaneda-Zuniga WR, Tadavarty SM, eds. *Interventional radiology,* 2nd ed. Baltimore: Williams & Wilkins, 1992:1046–1051.

11. Kunnen M, Cornhaire F. Nonsurgical cure of varicocele by transcatheter embolization of the internal spermatic vein(s) with a histoacryl tissue adhesive. In: Castaneda-Zuniga WR, Tadavarty SM, eds. *Interventional radiology,* 2nd ed. Baltimore: Williams & Wilkins, 1992:73.

12. Herrera MA, Di Segui R, Kaye KW, et al. Embolization of the internal spermatic vein with mechanical devices for the treatment of varicocele. In: Castaneda-Zuniga WR, Tadavarty SM, eds. *Interventional radiology,* 2nd ed. Baltimore: Williams & Wilkins, 1992:101.

13. Herrera MA, Tadavarty SM, Yedlicka JW et al. Inferior vena cava filters. In: Castaneda-Zuniga WR, Tadavarty SM, eds. *Interventional radiology,* 2nd ed. Baltimore: Williams & Wilkins, 1992:666.

23

Vascular Manifestations of Renal Disease

JONATHAN J. TRAMBERT

This chapter deals with diseases of the kidneys for which angiography or percutaneous transcatheter vascular interventional procedures play a major role. Nonneoplastic entities are discussed first.

■ Renovascular Hypertension

The interventional radiologist often is called on to help diagnose or treat renovascular hypertension. Renovascular hypertension is hypertension that is caused by arterial inflow reduction, which in turn causes renal ischemia and a secondary increased renin production. The mechanism of renovascular hypertension is believed to be as follows. When blood flow to the kidneys is limited to the point that it causes renal ischemia, glomerular filtration pressure drops, resulting in decreased filtration of blood by the kidney. Cells in the juxtaglomerular apparatus are stimulated to secrete renin, which causes elevation of the blood pressure, increasing the perfusion to the ischemic kidney, correcting the ischemia, and increasing the glomerular filtration pressure. The physiologic mechanism of renovascular hypertension is summarized in Figure 23-1.[1]

It must be kept in mind that hypertension related to excess renin secretion can have other causes. For example, it can be the result of chronic renal inflammation, which results in renal parenchymal insufficiency, or, rarely, a renin secreting tumor (a reninoma or juxtaglomerular tumor).

Etiology of renal artery occlusive disease

Renal artery occlusive disease can result from several disease processes. The two most common causes of renovascular hypertension are atherosclerosis and fibromuscular dysplasia (FMD).

Atherosclerosis is the most common cause of renovascular hypertension, accounting for approximately 60% of such cases.[2] Most patients are older men, usually aged over 50 years. A relatively large percentage (37%) of patients with atherosclerotic renovascular hypertension will have bilateral renal artery stenosis.[3] Most atherosclerotic renal artery stenoses are located in the proximal third of the renal artery and frequently involve the renal artery origin secondary to overhanging aortic mural atherosclerotic plaques (Fig. 23-2). This pattern of disease is relevant to the efficacy of balloon angioplasty in treating atherosclerotic renal artery stenosis.

FMD is the cause of renal artery stenosis in approximately one third of patients with renovascular hypertension.[2] Unlike atherosclerotic stenoses, stenoses of FMD tend to occur in children and young adults, and the lesion tends to affect the mid to distal main renal artery and in some cases its branches. Branch vessel disease is quite common in FMD-induced renovascular hypertension in children. There are several types of FMD based on their pathology (Table 23-1).[2] The most common variety encountered in practice is medial fibroplasia, which is caused by areas of circumferential medial thickening alternating with areas of aneurysm formation. Angiographically, this type manifests as a "string of beads" appearance (Fig. 23-3).

Other less common causes of renovascular hypertension include chronic aortic dissection with impingement on the renal artery ostium by the intimal flap, aortoarteritis such as Takayasu's disease, neurofibromatosis, renal artery aneurysm, atheromatous and cholesterol emboli, postoperative stenosis at a previous bypass graft anast-

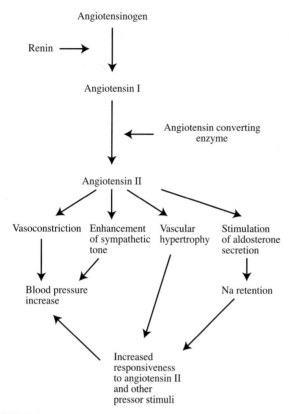

FIGURE 23-1. Physiologic mechanism of hypertension.

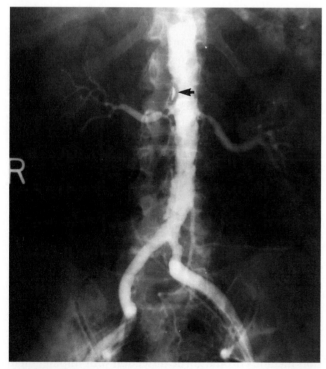

FIGURE 23-2. Bilateral atherosclerotic proximal renal artery stenoses: moderate on left, severe on right. Note the diffusely diseased abdominal aorta and prominent plaque immediately superior to right renal artery ostium (*arrow*).

TABLE 23-1. Categories of fibromuscular dysplasia

Type	Prevalence (%)	Angiographic findings
Medial fibroplasia	60–70	"String of beads" caused by focal stenosis alternating with aneurysmal dilatation
Perimedial fibroplasia	15–25	Chain of irregular stenoses without aneurysms
Medial hyperplasia	5–15	Long, smooth narrowing
Medial dissection	5	False channel, aneurysm
Intimal fibroplasia	1–2	Short, focal stenosis
Adventitial fibroplasia	<1	Long, segmental stenosis

From Kadir S. Diagnostic angiography. Philadelphia: WB Saunders, 1986:459.

omosis or renal transplant artery anastomotic stenosis, and coarctation of the aorta with renal artery stenosis.[4]

Diagnosis

Of the entire hypertensive population, fewer than 5% will have renovascular hypertension. The remaining 95% have essential hypertension, which is not attributable to any specific anatomic abnormality and thus is treatable only by long-term medication. Long-term medication for hypertension often involves multiple medications that have possible side effects. For this reason, detection of a correctable anatomic abnormality is a desirable goal.

Initially there was a great deal of enthusiasm for screening all hypertensive patients for renovascular hypertension, but, given the low prevalence of renovascular hypertension, even with a test of moderately good sensitivity and specificity, the frequency of false-positives equals or exceeds the frequency of true-positives.[5] Invasive examinations, although capable of diagnosing renal artery stenosis as the cause of a patient's hypertension with a higher degree of certainty, are not appropriate as screening examinations because of their cost and morbidity. These problems led to the abandonment of indiscriminate screening for renovascular hypertension.

The current approach to screening patients for renovascular hypertension involves screening only those hypertensive patients who, based on clinical parameters, are most likely to have renoocclusive disease as an etiology. These parameters include abrupt onset of hypertension before age 30 or after age 55, severe hypertension (diastolic blood pressure greater than 120 mm Hg), accelerated or malignant hypertension with retinopathy, hypertension refractory to triple-drug therapy, epigastric bruit, moderate hypertension with unexplained azotemia, and azotemia induced by angiotensin-converting enzyme (ACE) inhibitors.[6]

Radionuclide renography, Doppler ultrasound velocity measurements, and Doppler renal-resistive index measurements are among the noninvasive modalities used in the diagnosis of renovascular hypertension. Each modal-

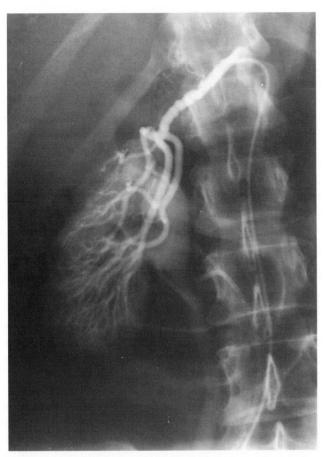

FIGURE 23-3. Fibromuscular dysplasia, medial fibroplasia type, of right renal artery. Note the "string of beads" appearance of the main artery.

ity has its limitations, but each also has some value in screening carefully selected persons.[7–9]

Magnetic resonance angiography

Magnetic resonance angiography (MRA) shows great promise as a noninvasive modality for visually depicting the renal arteries and aorta. The available types of image acquisition techniques include two-dimensional (2-D) time-of-flight (TOF), 2-D or 3-D phase-contrast, and 3-D TOF, with or without intravenous gadolinium. The goal of MRA acquisition is to suppress signal from surrounding nonvascular structures and either to enhance or at least limit the suppression of flowing blood signal, which, in effect, produces a "subtraction arteriogram." The resultant image data set can be reconstructed in a 3-D image depiction that can be rotated and viewed from multiple angles.

MRA is reasonably sensitive and specific in depicting the aorta and proximal renal arteries. It is less sensitive for defining the distal main renal artery or beyond the division points of the main renal artery.[10,11] Renal MRA has proved extremely valuable in the evaluation of the patient in whom there is a reasonable clinical suspicion of renovascular hypertension but in whom renal insufficiency poses a relative contraindication to contrast arteriography. A negative MRA virtually excludes a central renal artery lesion as the cause of the hypertension or the cause of acute onset of renal insufficiency (Fig. 23-4).

Spiral CT angiography

Spiral computed tomagraphy angiography (CTA) also holds promise as a modality for evaluating the renal ar-

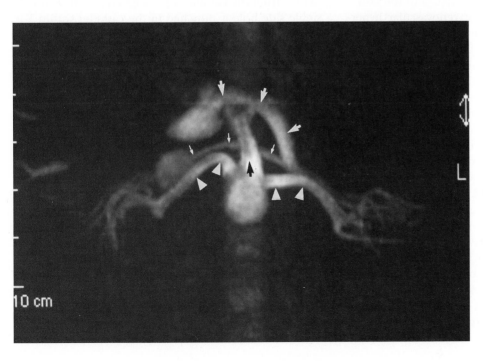

FIGURE 23-4. Magnetic resonance angiogram (MRA) of normal proximal renal arteries (*white arrowheads*). Axial maximum intensity projection (MIP) constructed from a three-dimensional phase-contrast intravenous MRA using gadolinium. Other structures depicted on this MIP are the superior mesenteric artery (SMA) (*black arrow*), left renal vein joining the inferior vena cava (IVC) (*small white arrows*), and splenic vein joining the portal vein (*large white arrows*).

teries because of its relative noninvasiveness compared with catheter arteriography. The premise behind CTA is the rapid acquisition of axial images in the areas of interest in a single breath-hold, made possible by slip ring technology. The axial images can be reconstructed into a 3-D model of the arterial system that can be viewed from different angles.[12] The disadvantage of CTA is the need for intravenous iodinated contrast, which limits its usefulness in certain patient populations, especially in patients with renal insufficiency or renal transplant artery stenosis. Often the amount of contrast needed for CTA far exceeds that required for a properly performed catheter arteriogram.

Contrast arteriography

Contrast arteriography is still the gold standard when it comes to anatomic detection of a renal artery stenosis; however, finding a renal artery stenosis in a hypertensive patient does not necessarily mean that the patient has renovascular hypertension. The renal artery arteriosclerotic lesion may be a consequence of the long-standing essential hypertension rather than a cause of it, or it may be totally unrelated. Furthermore, a significant percentage of patients who were found to have a renal artery stenosis at autopsy had been normotensive.[13]

Renal arteriography technique

When performing renal arteriography, a nonselective aortogram almost always is obtained first. The aortogram discloses the number of renal arteries supplying each kidney, the relative location of the renal arteries and kidneys, the origins of the renal arteries, and the aorta. When considering intervention for renovascular hypertension, the aortogram should be tailored to assess the celiac artery and its branches; in the event that surgical bypass is needed for treatment, these arteries frequently are used for inflow. The information on the aortogram facilitates the performance of selective renal arteriography and interventions, because without it, locating the renal artery orifice for selection may be more difficult and time consuming, accessory renal arteries may be missed, and renal artery origin disease may go undetected by a more distal selective catheter injection. Indeed, selective renal arteriography may not be needed in the evaluation of suspected renovascular hypertension if the aortogram clearly discloses a proximal renal artery stenosis or renal artery occlusion.

If the aortogram fails to disclose a lesion in a patient in whom there is a high suspicion of renovascular hypertension based on clinical history and noninvasive studies, selective renal arteriography must be performed. Transcatheter pressure gradient measurements can be helpful. Branch artery stenosis can be the cause of renovascular hypertension especially in children, and can be difficult to detect on nonselective aortography. Renovascular hypertension secondary to a distal branch artery stenosis can occur in FMD and less commonly in atherosclerotic disease. Specifics regarding technique and performance of aortography, selective vessel catheterization, angiographic contrast injections, and image acquisition are discussed in Chapter 2.

If arteriography discloses a significant renal artery stenosis, corroborated by clinical history, laboratory findings, and noninvasive studies, percutaneous transcatheter therapy can be initiated in the same session in selected patients.

Renal vein renin assay

Renal vein renin assay directly measures and compares the renin output of each kidney. It reflects the pathophysiology of renovascular hypertension. Combined with noninvasive modalities or angiographic detection of renal artery stenosis, renal vein renin assay increases the likelihood of confirming the presence of a lesion whose treatment will cure or improve the hypertension.

Blood samples are drawn from each renal vein and from the inferior vena cava below and above the renal veins. Care should be taken to ascertain whether any accessory renal veins are in the area. Also, whenever possible, the left renal vein sample is drawn peripheral to the gonadal vein to minimize dilution by nonrenal blood. Usually, a cobra-shaped catheter is used to select the renal veins. Peripheral selection of the left renal vein can be facilitated by the use of a tip deflector wire when necessary. To minimize the risk of blood aspiration impedance from the catheter tip invaginating the vein wall, a single side hole is punched in the catheter within 1 to 2 mm of the tip. Contrast injection is minimized because it can adversely affect the renin output measurements. Before blood samples are drawn, approximately 3 to 4 mL of blood in the catheter should be aspirated and discarded. Then approximately 5 mL of blood is *slowly* aspirated (to avoid causing excess turbulence in the blood flow during aspiration), and samples are placed on ice immediately to preserve them on route to the radioimmunoassay laboratory. Each sample must be meticulously labeled, and each sample location should be indicated on a vein diagram to allow exact correlation between assay levels and vein location.

The accuracy of renal vein renin sampling is diminished in patients with renal insufficiency, long-standing hypertension, and bilateral renal artery stenosis and also by the administration of antihypertensive medications during the assay. The ratio of renin levels of the two renal veins must be greater than 1.5:1 to be considered significant. A more complicated but more specific method for the use of renin levels in predicting the therapeutic response to the treatment of renal artery stenosis has been reported.[14]

Treatment

Before the advent of percutaneous transluminal balloon angioplasty (PTA), surgical bypass and endarterectomy were the only treatment options for renovascular hypertension. PTA has revolutionized the treatment of renal artery stenosis. Surgical bypass is still indicated in some patients with relative contraindications to renal PTA. Furthermore, surgical bypass is still an option for patients who fail to respond to renal PTA or who develop complications of PTA that are not correctable with percutaneous transcatheter measures.

In addition to the risk of general anesthesia, potential surgical morbidity includes renal failure, with a significant risk of cholesterol emboli related to cross clamping of a severely calcified atherosclerotically diseased aorta. The perioperative mortality rate is 2 to 4%.[15] Successful surgical reconstructions have a somewhat better long-term primary patency than renal PTA, but the far greater morbidity and mortality of operative repair mitigate in favor of using PTA as the initial treatment, with surgery reserved for those patients who fail renal PTA or who have relatively strong contraindications to PTA.[16]

Percutaneous transluminal angioplasty

Pharmacologic aspects

Because of the chance of therapeutic benefit of post-renal PTA with a resultant precipitous drop in blood pressure, the patient's antihypertensive medications must be appropriately adjusted. Long-acting antihypertensive medication must be discontinued prior to renal PTA; short-acting drugs (e.g., intravenous nitroprusside) should be substituted. One must be prepared to administer vigorous intravenous hydration to increase vascular volume in the event of a significant post-renal PTA blood pressure drop.

Risks of renal PTA include thrombosis and small artery branch spasm induced by catheter-guidewire manipulations. The risk of vasospasm can be minimized by administering an antispamodic drug at the outset of the procedure, such as a calcium channel blocker (e.g., nifedipine 10 mL sublingual). It is also essential to heparinize the patient therapeutically to minimize the risk of thrombosis. Doses for heparin range from 3,000 to 10,000 units, and adequacy of anticoagulation can be monitored by obtaining activated clotting times in the angiography suite. Low-dose aspirin (325 mg/day), beginning the day before and continuing for 6 months following PTA, also is advised by most practitioners to decrease the risk of post-PTA thrombosis and possibly the risk of restenosis.

Technique

After suitable angiographic evaluation of the renal artery stenosis, the affected renal artery is selected. Renal artery PTA necessitates the advancement of a guidewire well into the periphery of the renal arterial tree to ensure secure access across the stenosis for balloon advancement, which usually can be accomplished by using conventional selective catheters such as the cobra or simple C-shaped curve. In situations where the affected renal artery possesses a caudal angulation or where there is a very tight stenosis, conventional selective catheter shapes may not permit guidewire advancement across the stenosis or sufficiently peripheral guidewire advancement to allow catheter exchanges and balloon placement. In such a situation, use of a downward curving catheter such as a sidewinder, Simmons, or "shepherd's crook" shape often can facilitate superselective secure catheterization. The advantage of the sidewinder curve in this circumstance is that withdrawing the catheter at the femoral puncture site will advance the catheter tip across the tight stenosis or into the downward angling renal artery with a force that is not obtainable with conventional cobra or simple C-shaped catheters.[17,18] To minimize the risk of arterial dissection, it is important that catheter advancement across the renal artery stenosis be performed using a soft-tipped guidewire such as a Bentson (Cook Incorporated, Bloomington, IN) or TAD II (Mallinckrodt, St. Louis, MO) or during simultaneous contrast injection that will keep the tip off of the wall. A less commonly used approach for downward angling renal arteries is the axillary puncture.

After a catheter has been advanced securely into the renal artery, a guidewire must be advanced sufficiently peripherally into the renal arterial tree to permit safe catheter exchange and balloon advancement. The ideal guidewire has a short, floppy atraumatic end with rapid transition to a robust stiff section. The short soft tip is important to minimize the risk of trauma in the renal artery branch in which the wire is anchored, but it is important that the section of wire bridging the stenosis be stiff enough to guide the balloon successfully. A commonly used wire is the Rosen wire, which possesses these properties. There is controversy as to whether the guidewire tip should possess a tight 1.5 mm radius "J" or be straight. The advantage of the "J" tip is that the tip presents a blunt end that is less likely to perforate a peripheral renal artery branch. The disadvantage of the "J" tip wire is that when it is wedged into an artery branch smaller in diameter than the radius of the "J," it can induce vasospasm, a problem that is avoided when using a straight tip.

Intraarterial nitroglycerine should be administered immediately prior to superselective catheterization of the peripheral renal artery branches to minimize the risk of vasospasm. Nitroglycerine is effective and has a short half-life, allowing for administration of repeat doses (50 to 200 μg).

After the guidewire has been advanced into a peripheral renal artery branch, the balloon is advanced across the stenosis (Fig. 23-5). Balloon size is chosen based on the measured size of the adjacent "normal" renal artery on the angiogram. The balloon used for renal PTA should

have a short length and short distance between the balloon's distal end and the catheter tip. This configuration will minimize "torquing" of the renal artery with respect to the aorta as the balloon inflates and tries to straighten.

Other catheter guidewire combinations that can be

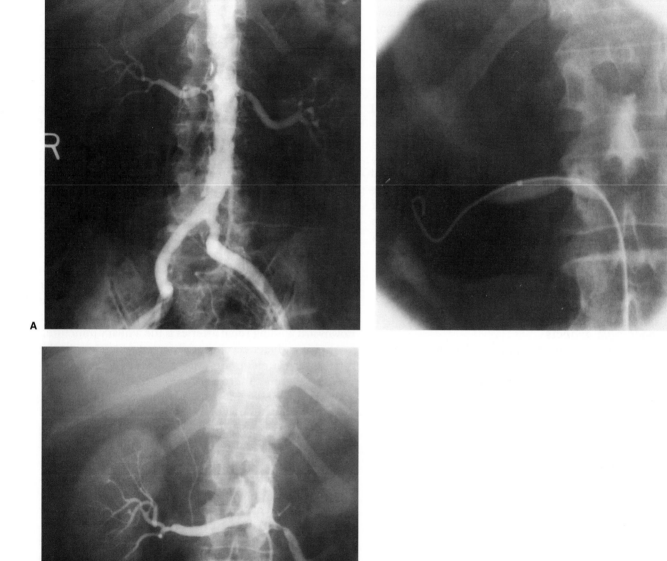

FIGURE 23-5. Renal artery angioplasty. **A:** Aortogram showing severe proximal right renal artery atherosclerotic stenosis (same patient as in Fig. 23-1) before angioplasty. **B:** Balloon being inflated across stenosis (note waist). **C:** Right renal arteriogram after angioplasty using sidehole catheter demonstrating good lumen response to angioplasty.

used to facilitate successful treatment of difficult renal lesions include hydrophilic balloon catheters to decrease friction, miniature low-profile balloon catheters such as the 3.8 Fr Medi Tech sub-4 balloons, and a balloon mounted on a guidewire (Teg wire, Medi Tech Inc.). The performance of renal PTA also can be facilitated by using an outer guiding catheter positioned at the renal artery orifice through which the balloon is advanced, allowing test injection of contrast with the balloon or guidewire still across the stenosis.

Just as with extremity PTA, it is essential to evaluate the result of renal PTA while access is maintained across the newly treated stenosis. If a guiding catheter is used, contrast can be injected through it. My preference is a straight or simple curve catheter with side holes placed along its distal few centimeters. After renal PTA, this catheter is placed across the treated lesion, allowing contrast injection to opacify the entire renal artery out to the aorta and allowing assessment of the result of renal PTA (see Fig. 23-5). If necessary, the guidewire can be readvanced through the catheter to allow additional manipulations as needed.

Complications

Besides vasospasm and arterial thrombosis, other complications of renal PTA include cholesterol or atheroemboli, renal artery rupture, acute renal artery occlusion resulting from dissection, and renal failure. Cholesterol/atheroemboli is an occasional and feared complication that can cause peripheral end-artery occlusions and potentially segmental or diffuse renal infarction. Unfortunately, anticoagulation cannot prevent this type of embolization, and thrombolysis does not reverse it. The risk is much higher in patients who have extremely diseased aortas with ulcerated and irregular plaques.

Renal artery rupture is an uncommon occurrence, but the risk of rupture is minimized by proper balloon sizing. Angiographic measurements of vessel size result in a 15 to 20% overestimation of vessel size from magnification.[18] This slight overdistenstion is desirable to maximize the chance of successful plaque dehiscence and durable stenosis dilation. Larger balloons should be used with extreme caution, and the onset of severe pain during balloon inflation is probably an indication that the balloon is too large, risking renal artery rupture. Persistence of pain after the balloon is deflated may indicate that rupture has occurred. If rupture is suspected, a quick confirming contrast injection should be performed and the balloon should be inflated across the arterial breach to tamponade it temporarily while awaiting definitive surgical repair. Future availability of covered stents may allow percutaneous treatment of such ruptures. Acute occlusion of the renal artery caused by dissection now can sometimes be treated with renal artery expandable wire mesh stents but occasionally requires urgent reconstructive surgery.

Post-renal PTA renal failure can occur because there is a certain minimum amount of contrast that must be used to guide the procedure and to evaluate the result. For this reason, it is advisable to limit the amount of contrast used to the minimum necessary, to use nonionic contrast, and to wait at least 2 days between diagnostic arteriography and arterial intervention in patients with renal insufficiency to minimize the risk of cumulative contrast load to the kidneys.[19]

Renal PTA should be performed only in situations where skilled vascular surgery backup is available on short notice. The absence of skilled vascular surgery backup should be considered a contraindication to the performance of renal PTA, because some of the potential complications can only be treated surgically and must be done expeditiously. Acute renal artery occlusion secondary to dissection sometimes can be treated by placement of a stent.

Renal artery thrombosis can be treated by intraarterial thrombolysis. Nonetheless, one must be aware that, unlike the arteries of the lower extremities, the renal artery is an end vessel, and hence renal artery occlusion results in renal ischemia that cannot be tolerated for a long period. Another relative contraindication to renal PTA is the presence of an extremely diseased irregular aorta in which the risk of cholesterol or atheroemboli is relatively high.

Results

The ultimate result of renal PTA depends on the successful revascularization of the renal artery and subsequent amelioration of the hypertension and improvement in the renal function. Martin et al.[19] reviewed the renal artery PTA literature and determined that PTA of atherosclerotic lesions results in cure in 13% and improvement in 52%. Renal artery PTA for FMD, on the other hand, results in cure in 44% and improvement in 45% of cases. *Cure* is defined as reduction of diastolic blood pressure to 90 mm Hg or lower, without the need for medications. Improvement is defined as a 15% reduction in diastolic blood pressure to a value between 90 and 110 mm Hg.

The reason why the cure and benefit rate is higher for FMD than for atherosclerotic renal artery stenosis probably relates to demographics and overall clinical status of the patients involved as well as to the usual morphology of the respective lesions. Atherosclerotic renal artery stenosis usually occurs in association with other manifestations of atherosclerosis, such as coronary artery disease, peripheral vascular disease, and cerebral vascular disease. Many of these patients are older, with chronic concomitant essential hypertension and some element of nephrosclerosis related to these factors.

Successful revascularization of the renal artery is thus more likely to partially ameliorate the hypertension than to cure it. In addition, a large percentage of atherosclerotic lesions are ostial lesions related to overhanging aortic atherosclerotic plaque. Therefore, it is more difficult to produce a lasting dilation. It is possible that the results might be improved by the use of stents in ostial lesions.

Fibromuscular dysplasia, on the other hand, tends to occur in younger patients who do not have atherosclerosis or essential hypertension. Successful renal artery revascularization thus intuitively has a greater chance of effecting a cure. Nonetheless, because long-standing hypertension can result in renal damage and acceleration of atherosclerosis, it is important that young patients with renovascular hypertension be diagnosed and treated as early as possible.

Renal PTA also has been evaluated as a measure to improve renal function in patients in whom renal insufficiency is presumed to be due to bilateral renal artery stenosis or to a renal artery stenosis in a unilateral solitary kidney. Miller et al. reported their experience in 44 such patients and noted a significant improvement in glomerular filtration rate that persisted for up to 6 months. Although the improvement may not last indefinitely, the resultant improvement in renal function from PTA may delay the need for placing a patient on dialysis.[20]

Expandable metal stents

Expandable metal stents, which have had extensive evaluation in the iliac arteries, have recently been used in the renal arteries with promising results. There are technical differences between the placement of stents in renal arteries and placing them in the iliac arteries. Placement and positioning of the renal artery stent are more difficult because of the inherent limited margin of error. Renal artery stents are, by necessity, shorter than iliac stents. Because of respiratory motion, the exact position of the renal artery stenosis with respect to bony landmarks is harder to pinpoint than in the iliac arteries; therefore, roadmapping is of more limited use. Treatment of an ostial lesion is more difficult because the stent, must straddle the lesion; therefore, the stent protrudes slightly into the aorta. Excessive stent protrusion into the aortic lumen may increase the risk of a thrombogenic nidus. Nonetheless, metal stents are valuable for treating post-PTA occlusions secondary to dissections and for increasing the revascularization success rate in ostial atherosclerosis renal artery stenosis.

One recent study reported a 19% rate of renovascular hypertension cure and a 60% rate of improvement using Palmaz (Johnson and Johnson Interventional Systems, Warren, NJ) stents.[21] It also described a 6-year primary patency rate of 69% and a secondary patency rate of 90%.

Clearly, expandable stents substantially improve the long-term amelioration of renovascular hypertension, particularly that resulting from atherosclerosis with its high incidence of ostial stenosis.

■ Renal Transplantation

Renal transplantation is increasingly becoming a treatment option for patients with end-stage renal diseases. As surgical techniques of harvesting and transplantation become more refined and immunosuppressive regimens are improved, renal transplants are being performed with greater success, with patient and allograft survival rates at 1 year in the 80 to 95% range.[22] As a result, vascular and interventional radiologists are being consulted more frequently regarding the preoperative evaluation of potential renal donors and to assess the failing renal transplant.

Arteriography prior to transplant

Radiologic evaluation of the prospective kidney donor should ensure that there are two normally functioning kidneys and that the kidneys are free from neoplasm or vascular disease that may disqualify the donor or harm the patient. Clinical screening and preceding noninvasive cross-sectional or nuclear studies are used to assess function and may uncover the presence of renal mass. Whereas aortography, with or without selective renal arteriography, may uncover abnormal parenchymal morphology, its primary role is to map the renal arterial blood supply. The number of renal arteries is of extreme importance to the transplant surgeon. When the number of renal arteries is equal on both sides and both kidneys are functioning equally well, the left kidney is usually harvested because of its longer renal vein;[23] however, the presence of accessory renal arteries on the left side alone usually changes the donor side. The need for multiple anastomoses, yielding longer warm ischemia times, and the smaller vessels involved will increase the technical difficulty of the transplant. Furthermore, the presence of multiple renal artery anastomoses increases the chance for subsequent anastomotic strictures. The aortogram, with selective renal arteriography as necessary, depicts arterial stenoses (e.g., from FMD) and may reveal small arteriovenous malformations not seen on cross-sectional imaging studies (Fig. 23-6).

Arteriography after transplant

Arteriography in the posttransplant recipient is performed to diagnose an anatomically correctable cause of transplant failure or the cause of renovascular hypertension (i.e., a transplant renal artery stenosis). Renal trans-

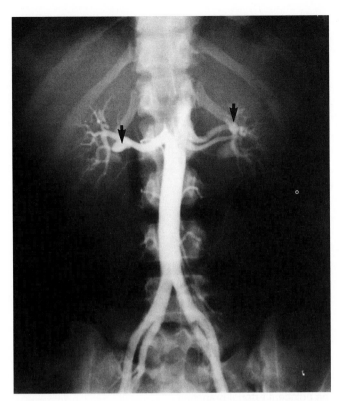

FIGURE 23-6. Aortogram in a prospective kidney donor revealing two left renal arteries as well as fibromuscular dysplasia with bilateral aneurysms (*arrows*).

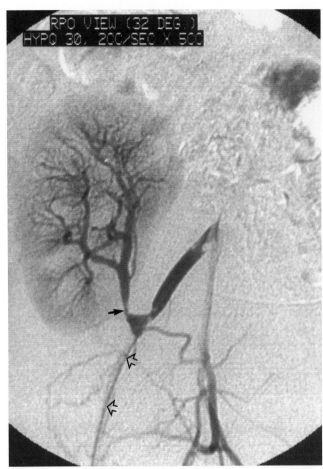

FIGURE 23-7. Right external iliac arteriogram demonstrating an end-to-side renal transplant artery anastomosis to the external iliac artery. Note postanastomotic stenosis (*solid arrow*). Also note the catheter-induced spasm of the external iliac artery distal to the transplant artery (*open arrows*).

plant artery stenosis, usually a consequence of a fibrotic stricture at the anastomosis site, is thus a different disease process from atherosclerosis. Clinical consequences include renovascular hypertension and renal transplant insufficiency. In situations of renal transplant insufficiency, renal transplant malfunction resulting from rejection must be ruled out before embarking on a search for an arterial lesion.

Because contrast load hazards are much higher in this group of patients, the workup and evaluation of suspected transplant renal artery stenosis should favor the use of modalities not dependent on iodinated contrast, such as Doppler ultrasound and MRA. When necessary, angiographic evaluation should be as goal directed as possible, using nonionic contrast, digital subtraction to minimize the overall contrast dose needed for diagnostic arteriography, and directed selective arteriography based on a knowledge of anastomosis anatomy from the operative report. Usual anastomosis sites are either the internal or the external iliac artery (Fig. 23-7). Experience with renal PTA in this subgroup of patients is more limited; however, reported success rates have ranged from a low of 22.7% to a maximum of 80.5%.[19]

Acute transplant rejection presents angiographically as stenosis and occlusions of intrarenal branch vessels as well as rapid tapering and pruning of interlobar branches. In chronic rejection, the kidney appears shrunken, with the number of intrarenal vessels diminished. These intrarenal branches also appear to be pruned.

■ Renal Trauma

Blunt renal trauma results from deceleration type injuries associated with motor-vehicle accidents, sports-related collisions, and external impact as in assault with a blunt weapon. Penetrating trauma usually results from stab or gunshot wounds, renal biopsy, percutaneous nephrostomy, or nephrolithotomy (Fig. 23-8)

Blunt trauma causes impact distributed over a wide area and can have a spectrum of consequences ranging from mild renal contusion (which may result in transient hematuria and resolve spontaneously) fracture of the kidney or dehiscence of the renal pedicle. Severe injuries of this sort usually are associated with injuries to other abdominal viscera.[24]

Penetrating trauma, with the exception of gunshot

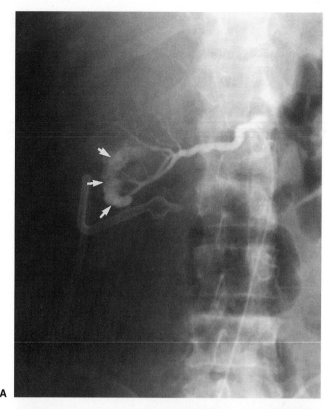

A

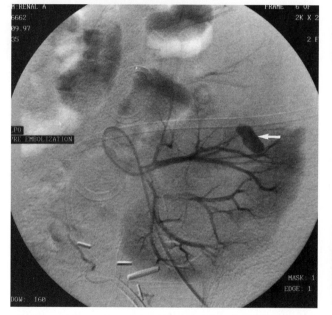

B

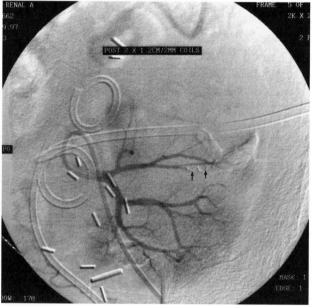

C

FIGURE 23-8. A: Right renal arteriogram demonstrating extravasation (*arrows*) from a branch resulting from trauma during percutaneous nephrolithotomy. **B:** Renal transplant arteriogram demonstrating pseudoaneurysm (*arrow*) of a peripheral arterial branch, a complication of percutaneous nephrostomy. **C:** Renal transplant arteriogram in the same patient as (**B**) following superselective embolization of the pseudoaneurysm with steel coils (*arrows*). Note the sparing of the remainder of the adjacent arterial branches.

wounds, results in a more focal injury, often to a segmental intralobar renal artery branch. The consequence can be active perirenal extravasation and hematoma formation, arteriovenous fistula, and arteriocaliceal fistula. The refinement of selective catheter technique, fluoroscopic equipment, embolization particles, and the development of coaxial microcatheters have made superselective catheterization and embolization of the involved renal artery branch possible, thus allowing the cessation of bleeding or the elimination of an arteriovenous fistula while preserving the kidney.

Renal trauma patients who are hemodynamically unstable should not undergo radiologic imaging or angiography but should proceed straight to surgery. Gunshot wounds involving the kidney generally warrant relatively urgent surgery because of the high likelihood of injury to intraperitoneal viscera as well as the high likelihood of "blast" injury to renal tissue surrounding the bullet's path.

Penetrating trauma in the posterior flank region that is confined to the retroperitoneal tissues may not require surgery. When intraperitoneal injury is excluded by peritoneal lavage, patients can be observed expectantly. If clinical evidence of bleeding is present, such as hematuria, or an expanding flank hematoma, the patient can be evaluated arteriographically and superselective embolotheraphy instituted if an internal bleeding point is identified. Attempts at operative control of hemorrhage from small intrarenal branch vessels is sometimes quite difficult and can result in the loss of renal substance, even nephrectomy. Hemostasis with minimal or no loss of renal parenchyma can be obtained with superselective percutaneous transcatheter embolotherapy.[25-28]

Superselective renal catheterization and embolization

Superselective catheterization of renal artery branches can be accomplished using 5 Fr catheters with or without 2 to 3 Fr coaxial microcatheters. Specifics regarding the technique and equipment needed for superselective catheterization are covered in Chapter 2. The available techniques and equipment now make it possible to expeditiously superselect the arterial branch that is the site of hemorrhage, arteriovenous malformation (AVM), or pseudoaneurysm, and to place embolic materials precisely at that site while sparing the vasculature to the uninvolved portions of the kidney (see Fig. 23-8). The preferred embolic material for treating renal artery hemorrhage is metal coils. The advantage of coils is that they can be deployed precisely, and they can be advanced through coaxial microcatheters. Gelfoam plugs and autologous blood clot can be extremely difficult to inject through the tiny lumen of coaxial microcatheters, and there is a greater risk of unintended nontarget vessel embolization with these agents. In hemodynamically stable patients, success rates of 88 to 100% have been reported for percutaneous transcatheter embolotherapy in renal artery injury from penetrating trauma.[27,28]

Nonneoplastic causes of hematuria

Patients rarely present with gross or microscopic hematuria without any antecedent history of trauma, and neoplasm is excluded on the basis of extensive workup. Other possible etiologies for hematuria include renal artery aneurysm rupture, renal arteriovenous malformations, calculi, renal vein hypertension secondary to the nutcracker syndrome, sickle cell disease, pyelonephritis, and idiopathic causes. The usual cause of single renal artery aneurysms is atherosclerosis. Fibromuscular dysplasia may result in single or multiple renal artery aneurysms (see Fig. 23-6). The differential diagnosis of multiple intrarenal arterial aneurysms includes polyarteritis nodosa (renal microaneurysms in 80%), hypersensitivity necrotizing angiitis, mycotic aneurysms from septic emboli related to bacterial endocarditis, Wegener's granulomatosis, and systemic lupus erythematosus.[29]

Congenital AVMs have been reported as rare causes of hematuria.[30] Superselective embolization (see section on renovascular trauma) can be effective if a distinct arteriovenous communication can be identified and occluded.

Renal vein hypertension is a condition that manifests in the left kidney when the left renal vein is subject to compression between the superior mesenteric artery and aorta (the nutcracker syndrome). This results in increased pressure in the left renal vein and formation of intrarenal, parapelvic and periureteric varices that may cause hematuria.[31] Intrarenal varices secondary to the nutcracker syndrome causing caliceal filling defects mimicking transitional cell carcinoma also have been reported (Fig. 23-9).[32]

Rarely, the cause of a patient's hematuria is never determined, despite careful selective arteriography and venography. Venous communications with the caliceal fornices have been identified on careful sectioning of nephrectomy specimens from some patients with idiopathic hematuria.[33]

■ Renal Neoplasms

Although renal neoplasms can be either benign or malignant, malignant tumors constitute the majority of renal masses encountered in clinical practice probably because, in part, benign tumors rarely cause symptoms; hence, although benign adenomas have been reported in up to 3% of autopsies,[34] they are uncommonly encountered in clinical situations, and, when they are, it is usually as incidental findings. Even though many malignant kidney tumors present as incidental findings without causing symptoms, the overwhelming majority of solid renal masses are malignant.

Benign renal tumors

Adenomas

Adenomas constitute the largest group of the benign renal tumors. There are four types: papillary adenomas (also called *cyst adenomas*) constitute 38%, tubular adenomas another 38%, alveolar adenomas 3%, and mixed-type adenomas 21%.[35]

Arteriographically, the papillary type tends to be hypovascular. The other adenoma types tend to be hypervascular, but their boundaries tend to be better circumscribed than those of renal adenocarcinomas. Oncocytomas represent a specific subset of tubular ade-

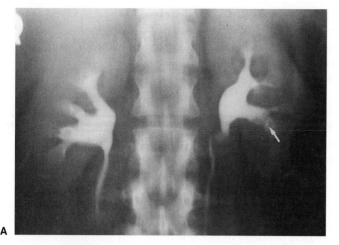

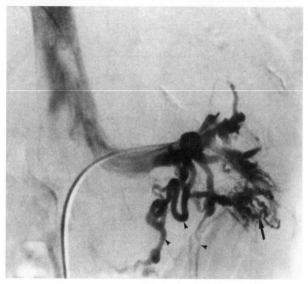

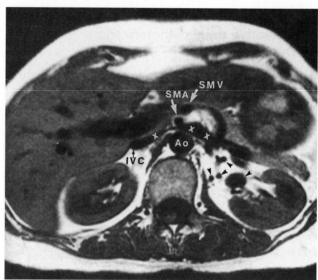

FIGURE 23-9. Intrarenal and retroperitoneal venous varices due to the nutcracker syndrome. **A:** Intravenous pyelogram showing extrinsic impression of varices on the lower pole infundibulum and calix mimicking a urothelial neoplasm (*arrow*). **B:** Left renal venogram demonstrating the intrarenal varices causing the impression (*arrow*) as well as periureteric and other retroperitoneal varices (*arrowheads*). Pressure gradient periureteric and other retroperitoneal varices (*arrowheads*). Pressure gradient between peripheral left renal vein and inferior vena cava (IVC) was 4 mm Hg (normal ≤1 mm Hg). **C:** Magnetic resonance imaging (MRI) demonstrating compression of left renal vein (x) between the superior mesenteric artery (SMA) and aorta (Ao), the nutcracker phenomenon. *Black arrowheads* point to periureteric and other retroperitoneal varices.

nomas. They display a pattern of hypervascularity that can often be described as a "spoke wheel" pattern (Fig. 23-10).[36] On CT and ultrasound, oncocytomas tend to display a central stellate scar.[37]

Although imaging and arteriographic features may suggest renal adenoma, particularly in the case of oncocytoma, these features are not diagnostic, and in no way do they rule out an adenocarcinoma. Surgical resection is mandatory in all solid renal masses in the absence of medical contraindications. Indeed, at pathological examination, it is sometimes difficult to distinguish renal adenoma from a well-differentiated adenocarcinoma. Nonetheless, because renal adenomas can be cured by simple extirpation, preoperative suspicion of a renal adenoma based on imaging studies and arteriography can allow a surgical approach geared toward local tumor excision and sparing of the kidney. The potential of the preservation of the kidney makes it of utmost importance to be aware of the imaging and arteriographic features of renal adenomas.

Angiomyolipoma

Angiomyolipomas are not true neoplasms but are actually hamartomas consisting of fat, muscle, and angioid elements in varying relative amounts. Angiomyolipomas can spontaneously hemorrhage, causing retroperitoneal hematoma, hematuria, or both. There is an association between renal angiomyolipomas and tuberous sclerosis. Tuberous sclerosis syndrome is characterized by mental retardation and epilepsy associated with various cutaneous lesions, retinal phakomas, and cerebral hamartomas. Renal angiomyolipomas have been reported in 40 to 80% of patients with tuberous sclerosis, but the converse is not true: Only a small minority of patients with a renal angiomyolipoma have tuberous sclerosis.[38] Angiomyolipomas occuring as part of the tuberous sclerosis syndrome are often bilateral and multicentric. Lesions not associated with tuberous sclerosis are almost always unilateral and solitary. Angiomyolipomas constitute 0.3 to 3% of renal masses and 1% of surgically resected renal tumors.[39]

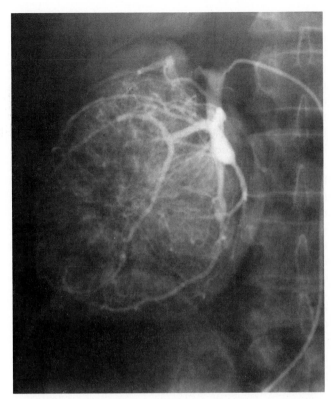

FIGURE 23-10. Oncocytoma. Renal arteriogram demonstrating typical "spoke wheel" distribution of tumor vessels and well-defined boundaries of tumor vascularity.

Angiographically, angiomyolipomas tend to be hypervascular with irregular, tortous vessels, often with aneurysms (Fig. 23-11A). In short, angiographically, angiomyolipomas are often indistinguishable from adenocarcinomas.

Angiomyolipomas possess unique features on ultrasound and CT studies. Because most of these tumors possess a large percentage of fat, they tend to be hyperechoic on ultrasound and hypodense (fat density) on CT (Fig. 23-11B). The CT finding of fat density in a renal mass is virtually diagnostic of angiomyolipoma, with only rare exceptions. As such, surgical resection is not indicated.

Of the angiomyolipomas larger than 4 cm in diameter, 50 to 60% bleed spontaneously, sometimes catastrophically; so prophylactic transcatheter embolotherapy may be indicated. Embolization, as the sole means of treatment, has been reported to be effective in 90% of patients with angiomyolipomas 4 cm or larger.[39] For angiomyolipomas, superselective embolization with absolute ethanol is preferred over coils because ethanol causes devascularization at the capillary level and infarction of the lesion. Proximal embolizations with coils can allow collaterals to develop and revascularize the lesion. As with superselective embolotherapy for renal trauma complications, therapeutic benefit is obtainable while sparing the remaining normal kidney.

Renin-secreting adenomas

Renin-secreting adenomas (reninoma, juxtaglomerular tumor) are rare, histologically benign tumors occurring in the cortical tissue, usually just below the renal capsule. They tend to be small, on average around 2 to 3 cm in diameter, but perhaps as small as a few millimeters. As such, they may be undetectable on imaging studies, including angiography. Nonetheless, they constitute an uncommon cause of renin-mediated hypertension in young patients and may be suspected when lateralizing renal-vein renin levels are obtained, arteriography fails to disclose a renal artery stenosis, and there is no underlying renal parenchymal disease. Tumor extirpation or partial

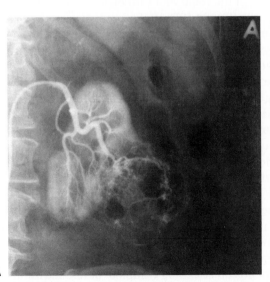

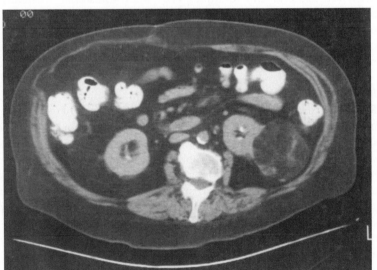

FIGURE 23-11. Angiomyolipoma. **A:** Renal arteriogram displaying irregular neovascularity and some puddling within lesion. **B:** Computed tomography finding of fat within left renal lesion is diagnostic of angiomyolipoma.

nephrectomy of the involved portion of kidney is curative.[40,41]

Malignant tumors

Malignant neoplasms of the kidney include primary renal tumors and secondary or metastatic tumors of the kidney. Metastases are the most common malignant tumor of the kidney, twice as common as primary tumors.[42] Metastases to the kidney are seldom symptomatic, because patients with disseminated malignancies usually die before their renal metastases have a chance to become symptomatic. Breast and lung carcinomas constitute approximately half of the lesions that metastasize to the kidney, followed by lymphoma and metastatic renal cell carcinoma from the contralateral kidney.

Of the primary renal malignancies, adenocarcinoma (also known as *renal cell carcinoma* and *hypernephroma*) constitutes approximately 83%. Carcinoma of the urothelium constitutes approximately 8%, nephroblastoma (Wilms' tumor) 5.5%, and sacromas 3%.[43]

Renal cell carcinoma

Renal cell carcinoma, or hypernephroma, is an adenocarcinoma that arises from renal tubular cells. It has approximately a 2:1 male predilection and tends to occur in the fifth through seventh decades, although it occasionally presents in young adults. Symptoms are classically hematuria, weight loss, anemia, and flank pain. Sometimes the tumor is asymptomatic and is discovered incidentally. Occasionally, this tumor is not detected until it is already large and disseminated.

Most renal cell carcinomas are single, unilateral lesions. In patients with von Hippel-Lindau disease (VHL), renal cell carcinomas occur in 38 to 55%,[44] and such tumors often are bilateral and multiple. VHL is an autosomal dominant disorder comprising retinal, cerebellar, and spinal hemangioblastomas, pheochromocytomas, and renal cell carcinomas. In patients without VHL, renal cell carcinoma can be bilateral in up to 5%.

Imaging

Renal cell carcinoma usually is confirmed on the basis of urography, ultrasound, and CT. CT is most valuable for staging renal cell carcinoma by assessing its level of extension, presence of contralateral renal masses, presence of renal metastases to retroperitoneal nodes or liver, and, at times, venous invasion. As such, preoperative arteriography becomes more of an option when much of the requisite preoperative information is supplied by CT. Arteriography is valuable in clarifying the indeterminate-appearing masses on CT, and many surgeons prefer an anatomic roadmap of the number of arteries supplying the kidney. A 3- to 5-sec-long contrast injection usually allows good visualization of the renal vein as well and allows determination of the presence of tumor extension into the renal vein and inferior vena cava (Fig. 23-12). Such extension is sometimes not apparent on CT or ultrasound and is of vital importance to surgical planning, as the surgeon will know to exercise caution when cross clamping the inferior vena cava to avoid dislodging tumor thrombus causing symptomatic pulmonary embolus or lung metastases. MRA and spiral CTA have excellent potential to provide much of this information, and it is likely that in the future angiography will be performed less frequently in the preoperative evaluation. Nonetheless, angiography presents detailed information about the peripheral vascularity of the mass from a diagnostic standpoint that is not yet attainable by CTA or MRA; these modalities currently are reliable for the central main vasculature. Arteriography is also essential in preoperative planning for renal cell carcinomas in patients with VHL disease, because it may detect additional tumors or contralateral tumors too small to be detected on CT. In such situations, attempts at partial nephrectomies are justified to conserve renal function, and the anatomic information provided by arteriography is essential in planning partial nephrectomies.

Renal cell carcinoma manifests usually, but not universally, as a hypervascular lesion. Approximately 62% are distinctly hypervascular, 16% moderately vascular, 16% minimally vascular, and 6% avascular.[45] Specific angiographic features associated with renal cell carcinoma include random irregular vessel distribution, lack of peripheral tapering of vessels, puddling of contrast or aneurysmal-type vascular spaces, and arteriovenous shunting. Tumor neovascularity often is displayed in renal vein and interior vena cava extensions of tumor, referred to as *tumor thrombus* (Fig. 23-12A,C). Other angiographic features of renal vein involvement on arteriography include nonvisualization of the renal vein with opacification of multiple collaterals (Fig. 23-12B). If doubt exists as to the presence of tumor extension into the vena cava, inferior venacavography must be performed, preferably using a pigtail catheter in the lower inferior vena cava. Care should be exercised to minimize manipulation of catheters and guidewires around a suspected tumor thrombus to avoid the risk of detaching a tumor embolus. If renal vein thrombus is suspected, selective renal vein catheterization is contraindicated. Tumor extension presents on the inferior venacavagram as a distinct constant filling defect within the lumen, in contradistinction to the inconstant striated hypodense appearance caused by unopacified inflowing blood from patent renal veins. (Preoperative embolization of large, hypervascular renal cell carcinomas can decrease intraoperative blood transfusion requirements significantly. The success of embolization depends on achieving complete devascularization, preferably with absolute ethanol, and embolizing any accessory feeding vessels as well.)

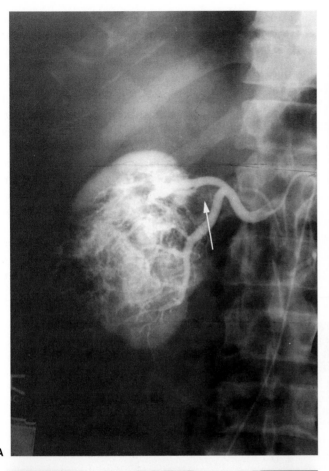

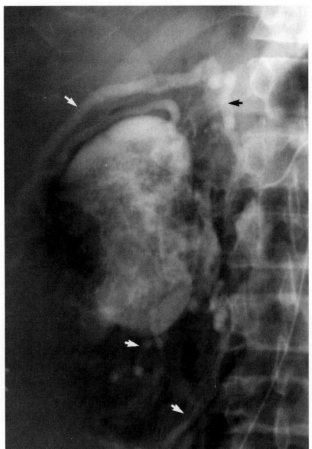

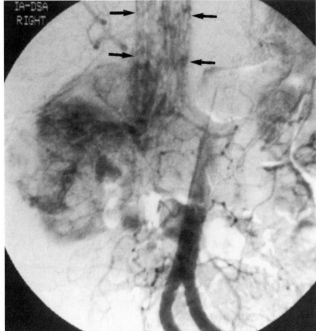

FIGURE 23-12. Hypervascular renal cell carcinoma. **A:** Right renal arteriogram, midarterial phase, showing large tumor with tumor neovascularity extending into the right renal vein (*arrow*). **B:** Late venous phase of arteriogram showing opacification of capsular and other retroperitoneal collateral veins (*arrows*) resulting from renal vein occlusion by tumor thrombus. **C:** Aortogram in another patient demonstrating hypervascular tumor thrombus from a right renal cell carcinoma occupying entire suprarenal inferior vena cava (IVC) (*arrows*).

Angioinfarction

Preoperative embolization of large hypervascular renal cell carcinomas can decrease intraoperative blood transfusion requirements significantly. The success of embolization depends on achieving complete devascularization, preferably with absolute ethanol, and embolizing any accessory feeding vessels.[46] Angioinfarction is also a valuable palliative procedure in patients with advanced renal cell carcinoma causing unremitting hematuria or pain, who, because of metastatic disease, are ineligible for surgical nephrectomy.[47]

Technique

After diagnostic arteriography to assess the blood supply and vascular nature of the renal tumor, an occluding balloon is positioned securely in the renal artery. Estimation of the volume of the vascular space of the kidney and

tumor is done by measuring the volume required to fill the vascular spaces almost to venous reflux with contrast while the occlusion balloon is inflated. This same measured volume of absolute ethanol then is infused after reinflation of the occlusion balloon, allowing it to sit for several minutes. Before deflating the balloon, blood is gently aspirated through the balloon catheter lumen to eliminate the risk of ethanol backflow into the aorta (Fig. 23-13).

Ethanol angioinfarction for ablation is a safe procedure. The risk of abscess formation in the infarcted kidney is slight as long as the procedure is done under strict sterile conditions and patients are protected with prophylactic antibiotics.[48] The risk is further decreased if a nephrectomy is performed within 24 to 48 hr after embolization. Many patients who undergo renal artery embolization will experience a postembolization syndrome

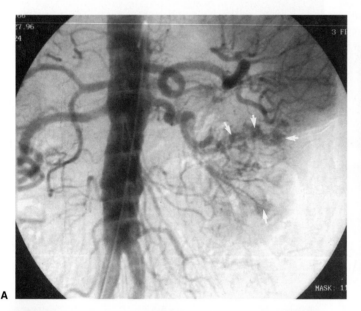

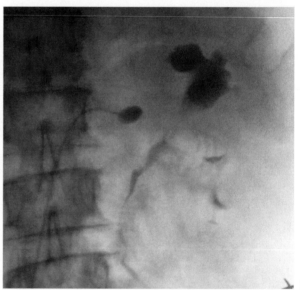

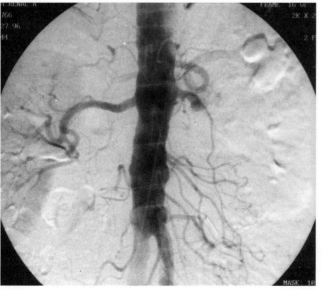

FIGURE 23-13. Ethanol angioinfarction of the left kidney to treat hematuria from an inoperable renal cell carcinoma. **A:** Aortogram demonstrating hypervascular lesion (*arrows*). **B:** Balloon inflated in preparation for anhydrous ethanol infusion. **C:** Aortogram after ethanol embolization showing occluded left renal artery.

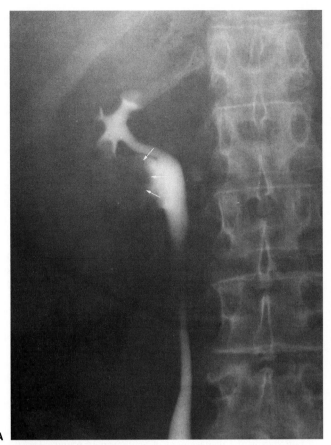
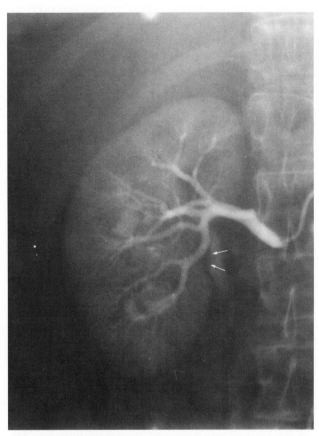

A   B

FIGURE 23-14. Transitional cell carcinoma. **A:** Retrograde pyelogram demonstrating a lesion occupying much of the right renal pelvis (*arrows*). **B:** Right renal arteriogram showing typical lack of arterial abnormality in the region of the tumor (*arrows*).

consisting of pain, fever, and leukocytosis, which is self-limited and amenable to supportive measures. There is evidence that complete renal infarction with absolute ethanol, rather than partial or incomplete embolization with larger particles such as Gelfoam, results in less severe postembolization syndrome.[46,48]

Urothelial neoplasms

Urothelial neoplasms are the second most common primary tumors involving the kidney, and most are transitional cell carcinomas (TCC). Usually TCC is confined to the urothelium and collecting system, and it almost never presents any significant arterial abnormality (Fig. 23-14). When the lesions grow bulky and invade the renal parenchyma, they can appear as hypovascular or, at most, minimally vascular masses.

Wilms' tumor

Wilms' tumor, or nephroblastoma, is the third most common primary renal malignancy. It tends to occur in early childhood, usually before the age of 5 years, although, rarely it does occur in adults. The tumors usually present as a palpable abdominal mass and can be associated with hematuria, anemia, fever, and weight loss, much like renal cell carcinoma. The lesion is usually identified from the history, physical examination, and noninvasive imaging studies. Wilms' tumors are bilateral in approximately 9% of cases.[49] Angiographically, the lesions look similar to renal cell carcinoma.

It must be emphasized that there is no distinguishing angiographic appearance that can give a histologic diag-

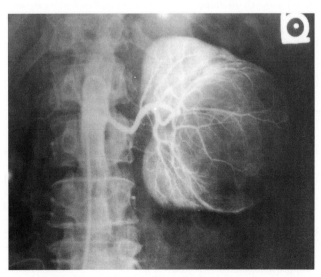

FIGURE 23-15. Avascular renal cell carcinoma.

nosis. Renal cell carcinoma, Wilms' tumor, and even angiomyolipoma and benign renal adenomas can present similar angiographic appearances. In addition, renal cell carcinoma, although usually hypervascular, occasionally is avascular, making angiographic distinction from a simple cyst difficult (Fig. 23-15). Inflammatory infiltrative disease such as xanthogranulomatous pyelonephritis sometimes results in a neovascularity similar to a moderately vascular renal cell carcinoma. Frequently, the correct diagnosis is made by correlating clinical history, noninvasive imaging studies, and angiographic findings; however, the definitive diagnosis is not available until histologic evaluation of the resected surgical specimen is complete.

REFERENCES

1. Waeber B, Nussberger J, Brunner HR. Angiotensin converting enzyme inhibitors in hypertension. In: Laragh JH, Brenner BM, eds. *Hypertension: pathophysiology, diagnosis, and management,* 2nd ed. New York: Raven Press, 199:2862.
2. Kadir, Saadoon. *Diagnostic angiography.* Philadelphia: WB Saunders, 1986:457–458.
3. Bookstein JJ, Maxwell MH, Abrams HL, et al. Cooperative study of the radiologic aspects of renovascular hypertension. *JAMA* 1977; 237:1706–1709.
4. Knutson DW, Abt AB. Pathophysiology, pathology, and clinical features of renovascular hypertension. In: Strandness DE, van Breda A, eds. *Vascular diseases: surgical and interventional therapy.* New York: Churchill Livingstone, 1994.
5. Thornbury JR, Stanley JC, Fryback DG. Hypertensive urogram: a nondiscriminatory test for renovascular hypertension. *AJR Am J Roentgenol* 1982;138:43–49.
6. Nally JV Jr. Provocative captopril testing in the diagnosis of renovascular hypertension. *Urol Clin North Am* 1994;21:227–234.
7. Sfakianakis GN, Bourgoignie JJ, Jaffe D, et al. Single dose captopril scintigraphy in the diagnosis of renovascular hypertension. *J Nucl Med* 1987;28:1383–1392.
8. Berland LL, Koslin DB, Routh WD, et al. Renal artery stenosis: prospective evaluation of diagnosis with color duplex ultrasound compared with angiography. *Radiology* 1990;174:421–423.
9. Schwerk WB, Restrepo IK, Stellway M, et al. Renal artery stenosis: grading with image-directed Doppler ultrasound evaluation of renal resistive index. *Radiology* 1994;190:785–790.
10. Grist TM, Kennell TW, Sprivat IA, et al. Prospective evaluation of renal MR angiography: comparison with conventional angiography in 35 patients. *Radiology* 1993;189(P):190.
11. Kim D, Edelman RR, Kent KC, et al. Abdominal aorta and renal artery stenosis: evaluation with MR angiography. *Radiology* 1990; 174:727–731.
12. Galanski M, Prokop M, Chavan A, et al. Renal arterial stenosis: spiral CT angiography. *Radiology* 1993;189:185–192.
13. Holly KE, Hunt JC, Brown AL, et al. A clinical pathologic study in normotensive and hypertensive patients. *Am J Med* 1964;37:14–22.
14. Pickering TG, Sos TA, Vaughan ED, et al. Predictive value and changes of renin secretion in hypertensive patients with unilateral renovascular disease undergoing successful renal angioplasty. *Am J Med* 1984;76:398–404.
15. Atnip RG, Thiele BL. Surgical management of renovascular hypertension. In: Strandness DE, van Breda A, eds. *Vascular diseases: surgical and interventional therapy.* New York: Churchill Livingstone, 1994:703–720.
16. Weibull H, Bergqvist D, Bergentz SE, et al. Percutaneous transluminal renal angioplasty versus surgical reconstruction of atherosclerotic renal artery stenosis: a prospective randomized study. *J Vasc Surg* 1993;18:841–852.
17. Sos TA, Pickering TG, Saddekni S, et al. The current role of renal angioplasty in the treatment of renovascular hypertension. *Urol Clin North Am* 1984;11:503–512.
18. Tegtmeyer CJ, Sos TA. Techniques of renal angioplasty: state of the art. *Radiology* 1986;161:577–586.
19. Martin LG, Rees CR, O'Bryant T. Percutaneous angioplasty of the renal arteries. In: Strandness DE, van Breda A, eds. *Vascular diseases: surgical and interventional therapy.* New York: Churchill Livingstone, 1994:721–741.
20. Miller RL, Fontaine AB, Nahman NS Jr, et al. Balloon angioplasty improves and stabilizes glomerular filtration rate in patients with bilateral renal artery stenosis or single kidney with renal artery stenosis. SCVIR 21st Annual Scientific Meeting. *J Vasc Interv Radiol* 1996;7(suppl):140.
21. Henry M, Amor M, Henry I, et al. Renal artery stent placement with the Palmaz stent: six year single center experience. SCVIR 21st Annual Scientific Meeting. *J Vasc Interv Radiol* 1996;7(Suppl): 140–141.
22. Flechner SM. Current status of renal transplantation. *Urol Clin North Am* 1994;21:265–282.
23. Orrons PD, Zaiko AB. Angiography and interventional aspects of renal transplantation. *Radial Clin North Am* 1995;33:461–471.
24. McAninch JW, Carroll PR. Renal exploration after trauma: indications and reconstructive techniques. *Urol Clin North Am* 1989; 16:203–212.
25. Peterson NE. Complications of renal trauma. *Urol Clin North Am* 1989;16:224.
26. Kantor A, Sclafani SJA, Scalea T, et al. The role of interventional radiology in the management of genitourinary trauma. *Urol Clin North Am* 1989;16:255–264.
27. Huppert PE, Duda SH, Erley CM, et al. Embolization of renal vascular lesions: clinical experience with microcoils and tracker catheters. *Cardiovasc Interv Radiol* 1993;16:361–367.
28. Eastham JA, Wilson TG, Larsen DW, et al. Angiographic embolization of renal stab wounds. *J Urol* 1992;148:268–270.
29. Longstreth PL, Korobkin M, Palubinskas AJ. Renal microaneurysms in a patient with systemic lupus erythematosus. *Radiology* 1974;113: 65–66.
30. Kopchick JH, Boume NK, Fine SW, et al. Congenital renal arteriovenous malformations. *Urology* 1981;17:13–17.
31. Beinart C, Sniderman KW, Saddekni S, et al. Left renal vein hypertension: a cause of occult hematurial. *Radiology* 1982;145:647–650.
32. Trambert JJ, Rabin AM, Weiss KL, et al. Pericaliceal varices due to the nutcracker phenomenon. *AJR Am J Roentgenol* 1990;154:305–306.
33. Mitty HA, Goldman H. Angiography in unilateral renal bleeding with a negative urogram. *AJR Am J Roentgenol* 1974;121:508–517.
34. Elkin ME. Radiology of the urinary system. Boston: Little, Brown and Company, 1980:297.
35. Bruenton JN, Ballanger P, Ballanger R, et al. Renal adenomas. *Clin Radiol* 1979;30:343–352.
36. Weiner SN, Bernstein RG. Renal oncocytoma: angiographic features of two cases. *Radiology* 1977;125:633–635.
37. Amis ES, Newhouse JH. *Essentials of uroradiology.* Boston: Little, Brown and Company, 1991:127.
38. Elkin ME. *Radiology of the urinary system.* Boston: Little, Brown and Company, 1980:344.
39. Soulen MC, Faykus MH, Shlansky-Goldberg RD, et al. Elective embolization for prevention of hemorrhage from renal angiomyolipomas. *J Vasc Interv Radiol* 1994;5:587–591.
40. Kadir S. *Diagnostic angiography.* Philadelphia: WB Saunders, 1986: 474.

41. Amis ES, Newhouse JH. *Essentials of uroradiology.* Boston: Little, Brown and Company, 1991:128.

42. Newsam JE, Tulloch WS. Metastatic tumors in the kidney. *Br J Urol* 1966;38:1–6.

43. Elkin ME. *Radiology of the Urinary System.* Boston: Little, Brown and Company, 1980:296.

44. Amis ES, Newhouse JH. *Essentials of uroradiology.* Boston: Little, Brown and Company, 1991:142.

45. Abrams HL. *Abram's angiography,* 3rd ed. Boston: Little, Brown and Company, 1983:1136.

46. Bakal CW, Cynamon J, Lakritz PS, et al. Value of preoperative renal artery embolization in reducing blood transfusion requirements during nephrectomy for renal cell carcinoma. *J Vasc Interv Radiol* 1993;4:727–731.

47. Wallace S, Charnsangavej C, Carrasco CH, et al. Interventional radiology in renal neoplasms. *Semin Roentgenol* 1987;22:303–315.

48. Lanigan D, Jurriaans E, Hammonds JC, et al. The current status of embolization in renal cell carcinoma—survey of local and national practice. *Clin Radiol* 1992;46:176–178.

49. Kadir S. *Diagnostic angiography.* Philadelphia: WB Saunders, 1986:484.

24

Obstructive Uropathy and Renal Calculus Disease

MARLENE E. RACKSON

Ureteral obstruction leads to dilation of the proximal ureter and hydronephrosis. This chapter deals with percutaneous nephrostomy (PCN) and ureteral stenting procedures, which are used to relieve obstruction and help in the management of renal calculus disease.[1–3]

■ Clinical Presentation

Many patients presenting with obstructive uropathy have malignancies; the etiology and the obstruction can be bilateral or unilateral. When both kidneys are obstructed, the patient will present in renal failure with elevated blood urea nitrogen (BUN) and creatinine levels. This clinical picture often is seen in patients who have prostate cancer, bladder cancer, or gynecologic malignancies. Because malignancies grow slowly, they cause the kidney to dilate slowly. Thus, malignant obstruction is usually painless. Unilateral obstruction caused by malignancy may be difficult to diagnose clinically if the other kidney is functioning normally, because the obstruction is painless and the BUN and creatinine levels may be normal. Unsuspected unilateral obstruction often is detected during the course of an imaging study such as ultrasound or computed tomography (CT) of the abdomen. The decision to treat an asymptomatic unilateral obstruction caused by malignancy is a clinical one that may be influenced by many factors, such as the need to optimize renal function before administration of chemotherapy with known nephrotoxicity (Fig. 24-1).[4,5]

Patients undergoing PCN for benign causes of obstruction usually have calculi or strictures. Only a small fraction of patients presenting with renal stones require percutaneous decompression. In the acute setting, a patient with pyonephrosis may have severe flank pain, fever, elevated white blood cell (WBC) count, and other signs of infection along with a stone and hydronephrosis identified on an imaging study.[6] In the elective setting, PCN is performed to provide preoperative access to the renal collecting system in patients about to undergo percutaneous nephrolithotomy (PNL).[7]

Ureteral strictures also may be treated by percutaneous methods. Causes of strictures include radiation, retroperitoneal fibrosis, prior instrumentation, and fistulae. These patients may present with one or many signs and symptoms: fever, flank pain, renal failure, hydronephrosis, or urinoma formation on imaging studies.

Patients with renal allografts (transplants) may present with urine leaks, ischemic ureter, and obstruction and may be treated with PCN. Percutaneous procedures also are used to perform *Whitaker tests* (see Chapter 9), which measure the pressure gradient across a ureteral stenosis, to infuse antibiotics for fungal infections, to infuse agents for stone dissolution, and to provide access for removal of encrusted stents.[8–10]

■ Differential Diagnosis

The need for a PCN is generally straightforward. The presence or absence of hydronephrosis can be determined quickly, safely, and with certainty by ultrasound or CT scanning. The proper clinical setting will confirm the need for the procedure. Hydronephrosis can be due to reflux, however, and does not always mean obstruction or translate into a need for a PCN. Furthermore, it is important to

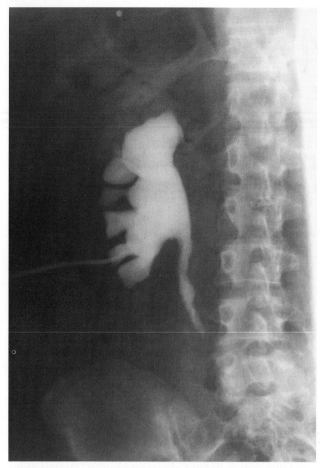

FIGURE 24-1. Percutaneous nephrostomy (PCN) placed to relieve ureteral obstruction resulting from cervical carcinoma. Note that the tube enters the collecting system below the costal margin through a posterior mid–lower pole calyx, which provides safe avascular access and a good "pushing angle" for future attempts at ureteral stent placement. Irregularity of upper ureter is due to ureteritis cystica.

determine when a PCN is elective and when the procedure needs to be performed as an emergency.

Some patients have chronic hydronephrosis (determined from serial imaging studies) with a new elevation of the BUN and creatinine levels. In the patient with a solitary kidney, PCN is certainly indicated to preserve the remaining renal parenchyma. The same is true when one kidney demonstrates cortical atrophy and the other demonstrates relatively normal cortex: The more normal kidney should be decompressed. When bilateral cortical atrophy and hydronephrosis are present, progressive renal failure may not be stabilized or improved by decompression. Sometimes the only way to prove or disprove the value of decompression in preserving renal function is to perform the PCN and then remove the tube if the kidney does not produce urine or if the function on a nuclear medicine scan does not improve.

The opposite situation, in which the BUN and creat-

inine levels are rising but there is minimal hydronephrosis, also can occur. Although the renal failure is most likely due to medical renal disease, there is also the possibility of obstruction without dilation, which occurs when the kidney shuts down before it dilates. This type of obstruction has been reported in patients with prostatic carcinoma.[11] Although this situation is unusual, it should be kept in mind because percutaneous decompression will improve renal function.

PCN should be performed as an emergency procedure[12] in the following situations:

1. In the setting of high fever and elevated WBC count or frank sepsis, when the patient is suspected of having pus in the kidney: This is usually seen in a patient with hydronephrosis and an identifiable obstructing calculus causing urosepsis.
2. Iatrogenic trauma to the ureter that is recognized when it happens: If the urologist calls from the operating room and says that the ureter has been dissected, the patient should have a PCN to divert the urine and to avoid urinoma formation. Stent placement to preserve the integrity of the ureter and avoid stricture formation should be attempted.
3. Severe unmanageable flank pain resulting from an obstructing calculus or steinstrasse from a preceding extracorporeal shock-wave lithotripsy (ESWL) treatment: Decompression via a PCN (antegrade approach) or a ureteral stent placed by the urologist (retrograde approach) will provide pain relief.
4. Acute renal failure resulting from bilateral obstruction or obstruction in a solitary kidney: This procedure should be done urgently to preserve renal parenchyma and to induce a diuresis to correct fluid and electrolyte imbalances.

■ Treatment Alternatives

Whenever possible, the retrograde approach (i.e., opposite the direction of flow of urine) to ureteral stent placement is preferable to the antegrade approach. The retrograde approach, usually performed by the urologist, has the advantage of avoiding creation of an 8 or 10 Fr hole extending from the flank to the kidney, which can be complicated by bleeding and may produce pain. Retrograde ureteral stent placement is also a one-step procedure, whereas antegrade stent placement may require at least two visits to the radiology department: first for the initial nephrostomy and then for placement of the stent. Until the antegrade stent has been placed and the urine is free of blood, the patient must wear an external nephrostomy bag (so that the stent will not occlude from blood clots). Patients who have small ureteral calculi and require stents with normal bladders and visible ureteral

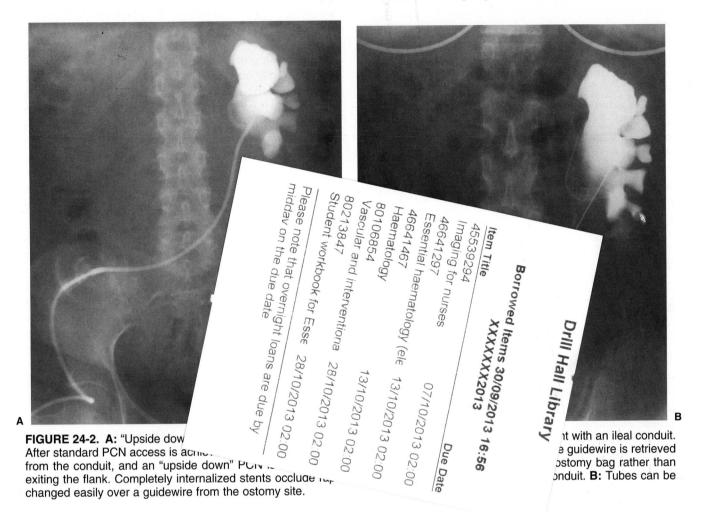

FIGURE 24-2. A: "Upside dow[...] t with an ileal conduit. After standard PCN access is ac[...] [...] e guidewire is retrieved from the conduit, and an "upside down" PCN [...] [...]stomy bag rather than exiting the flank. Completely internalized stents occlude [...][...]onduit. **B:** Tubes can be changed easily over a guidewire from the ostomy site.

orifices and patients undergoing precautionary ureteral stenting prior to bowel or pelvic surgery are examples of two situations in which retrograde ureteral stenting is preferable to the antegrade approach and is usually successful. In patients with malignant obstructions at the level of the ureterovesicle junction, the ureteral orifice often cannot be identified and attempts at retrograde stent placement will usually fail. In fact, many patients undergo percutaneous procedures after failure of the retrograde approach.

Although retrograde approaches usually are performed by the urologist, they also can be performed by the interventional radiologist. This approach is easier in female patients because the urethra is shorter than in male patients. On occasion, the urologist will be able to advance a small catheter from the urethra into the ureter but will not be able to place a true stent. If the patient is transferred to the radiology suite with the catheter still in place, the interventionalist often will succeed in retrograde placement of the stent, thereby avoiding nephrostomy. Retrograde approaches also can be useful in patients with ileal conduits and other diversionary pouches (Fig. 24-2).[13]

Actually, most cases of stone disease that require inter-

vention usually are treated by ESWL rather than by PNL; however, when ESWL is not applicable or has failed, percutaneous approaches are used. Situations in which ESWL is not applicable are stones larger than 3 cm, cysteine stones, lucent or infected stones, large staghorn calculi, and stones trapped in an infected calyx. Open surgery is rarely necessary for the treatment of stone disease.

■ Imaging Workup

When a patient is referred for a PCN to relieve obstruction, an imaging study is needed to prove hydronephrosis. This may be done quickly and easily by using ultrasound, which also will demonstrate cortical thickness and the level of obstruction, as well as the presence of stones and potential technical difficulties such as large cysts, urinomas, and duplicated collecting systems. The ultrasound machine also can be wheeled into the interventional suite and can be very helpful in localizing the kidney. The more costly CT scan gives the same information as the ultrasound, but it also shows the level of the kidney, which, if it is located unexpectedly high or low, could make fluoroscopic localization difficult. Sometimes an excretory urogram is performed just before the PCN (usually in stone cases); if there is contrast in the collecting system of the obstructed kidney, access to the collecting system is facilitated.

PCNs often are performed to provide access to the renal collecting system prior to PNL.[14,15] Excretory urograms and retrograde pyelograms are best for locating the number and size of stones in the intrarenal collecting system before access for removal. When outpatients arrive for procedures, often only a clinical history has been provided but no studies are available. In this situation, good prone scout films with 30-degree obliques before and after contrast is injected should be obtained, either intravenously or through an antegrade pyelogram (direct skinny-needle puncture into the renal pelvis).

■ Interventions: Percutaneous Nephrostomy and Ureteral Stenting

The approach to the PCN could be titled, "Why are we doing this case?" The goal of the procedure will determine how general or specific the puncture into the collecting system needs to be. The main goals of PCN are to relieve obstruction (the simplest approach), to stent the ureter (the more specific approach), and to provide access for stone removal (the approach that requires the most planning and is the most specific).

PCN to relieve obstruction

When the goal of the PCN is to relieve obstruction by providing external drainage without planning any further interventions, a nonspecific approach will suffice. Essentially any access from the flank to the intrarenal collecting system will be sufficient as long as the tube traverses the renal cortex (to anchor the tube) and enters through a calyx (an avascular area that does not have large crossing vessels) and direct pelvic punctures are avoided (see Fig. 24-1). The initial puncture can be made into the renal pelvis from a direct posterior translumbar approach in order to opacify the collecting system; a skinny (21- or 22-gauge) needle should be used. The final entry site into the kidney should be roughly along the posterior axillary line, below the 12th rib. An entry site that is too medial will be too posterior and will be uncomfortable for the patient. An entry site that is too lateral runs the risk of puncturing the colon. A subcostal approach will avoid the risk of pneumothorax and the potential for periosteal pain from a tube placed between the ribs as well as avoiding the liver and spleen.[16,17] Percutaneous access kits such as the Neff set (Cook, Inc., Bloomington, IN) or the Accustick set (Medi-tech, Boston, MA) have been more fully described previously. Establishment of percutaneous access is followed by tract dilatation and placement of the PCN tube.

When frank pus is aspirated from the intrarenal collecting system, only external drainage should be performed. Contrast injections will pressurize the collecting system and increase the risk of sepsis resulting from pyelovenous backflow. These injections should be limited to a few milliliters, just enough to confirm needle placement in the collecting system. Catheter and guidewire manipulations in a grossly infected collecting system also increase the risk of sepsis resulting from pyelovenous backflow and must be minimized. The aspirated material should be sent for Gram's stain and culture and sensitivity.

The initial drainage procedure in a renal transplant patient should be kept simple. Because the allograft is placed anterior to the iliac wing in the pelvis, the procedure is done with the patient in a supine position, not prone (Fig. 24-3). The hydronephrotic renal pelvis is anterior to the calyces and is sometimes palpable under the anterior abdominal wall. Therefore, the initial drainage procedure is often through a puncture directly into the renal pelvis.[8] Ultrasound guidance not only localizes the transplant kidney, it also eliminates the possibility of transgressing an interposed bowel loop.

Ureteral stenting and specific techniques of stent insertion

Internal ureteral drainage through a stent is preferable to external drainage with a leg bag for the urine. Whenever possible, access for the PCN should be planned in anticipation of ureteral stent placement, which entails creating a favorable angle for pushing a catheter across a ureteral lesion. In a normally located kidney, middle-pole calyces are preferable to lower-pole calyces, which require pushing a catheter upward to the renal pelvis and then downward into the ureter. If the kidney is high above the ribs and the patient cannot inspire deeply enough to depress the kidney, only lower-pole calyces will be accessible for puncture. Conversely, if the kidney is ptotic, superior pole calyces may be low enough to puncture and will provide a straight downward line of pushing force into the ureter.

Ureteral stenting is indicated in the presence of benign and malignant strictures, fistulae, some stones, trauma, and iatrogenic complications (Fig. 24-4). The length of time a ureteral stent remains in place depends on why the stent was placed. Stents for strictures and fistulae can be in place anywhere from 3 weeks to 3 months. Stents for malignant strictures are usually permanent. All patients who require long-term stenting should have the stents exchanged every 3 to 6 months to prevent encrustation and occlusion of the stent by urinary sediment. The stent can be inserted at the time of the original PCN or after the kidney has been decompressed at a separate session.[18-20]

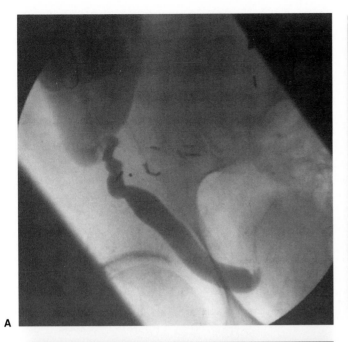

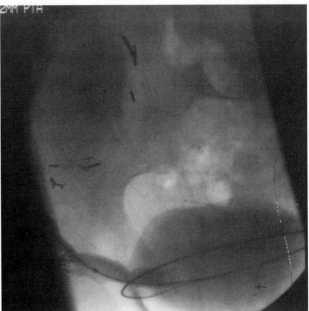

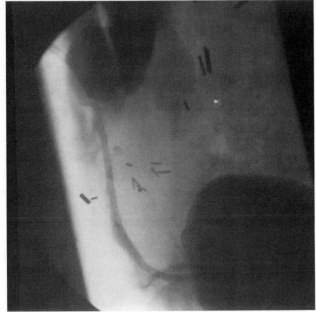

FIGURE 24-3. Distal ureteral stricture in a transplant kidney. **A:** Antegrade nephrostogram demonstrates marked hydronephrosis with a stricture of the distal ureter. Note the position of allograft over the iliac bone and the presence of a J-tip "safety wire" in the renal pelvis. **B:** The stricture was dilated with a 12-mm-high pressure balloon. **C:** An internal–external stent was placed across the stricture for 6 weeks following the procedure.

There are two basic types of stent: the completely internalized ureteral stent and the nephroureteral stent (NU) (Fig. 24-5).

The internalized stent

The internalized ureteral stent lies completely within the body and extends the length of the ureter from the renal pelvis to the bladder. This stent is commonly called a *double pigtail* or *double J* stent, which refers to the shape of the tips of the stent. The proximal pigtail or J-shaped tip anchors the stent in the renal pelvis and prevents it from slipping down into the bladder. The distal pigtail prevents the tip from wedging into the bladder wall and causing discomfort or exiting the urethra. For a patient who requires long-term stenting, a completely internalized stent is preferable because the patient does not have to wear a leg bag with its attendant discomfort and lifestyle inconveniences. Interventional radiologists usually place 8 or 10 Fr stents from the antegrade approach, whereas urologists usually place 5 or 6 Fr stents from the retrograde approach.

The nephroureteral stent

The NU is a one-piece combination of a nephrostomy tube and an internal ureteral stent that extends from the

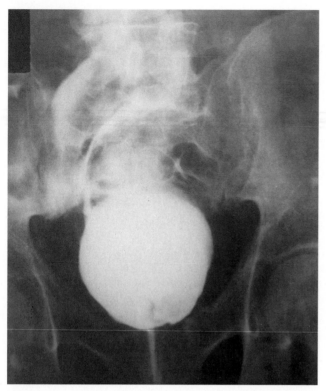
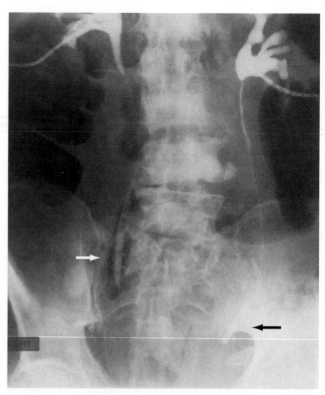

FIGURE 24-4. Bilateral percutaneous nephrostomy (PCN) tubes placed for urinary diversion after attempt at suprapubic cystostomy resulted in an intraperitoneal bladder perforation. **A:** Cystogram demonstrates contrast extravasation superior to the bladder. **B:** Bilateral PCN tubes alongside ureteral occlusion balloons placed to prevent any urine from flowing into the bladder. (*arrows*)

skin into the renal pelvis and descends through the ureter to terminate in the bladder. The NU can be left to external drainage with a leg bag, or it can be capped off to promote internal drainage.

Internalized ureteral stents usually are replaced by using cystoscopy.[21] If the exchange is anticipated to be difficult, an NU tube that is capped off to external drainage is a good solution, because the tube can be simply replaced over a guidewire.

The NU often is placed during the initial PCN procedure when an internal stent is eventually planned. Frequently, the ureteral obstruction can be transversed during the initial PCN, but the procedure is bloody. Placement of a completely internalized ureteral stent in a bloody system will not allow adequate flushing and the stent may clot; therefore, the NU is placed until the urine is clear. Once the urine has cleared, the NU is capped off to external drainage overnight to determine whether the patient can void normally without developing fever, flank pain, or urine leaking around the tube at the skin. If these events occur, the tube should be reopened to external drainage. An NU tube always should be left to external drainage whenever the urine is bloody, the patient is febrile, or the urine is infected. If the patient tolerates capping the tube, the NU can be replaced easily by an internal stent using a stiff guidewire for the exchange. If

the trial of internal drainage fails, the internal portion of the NU may be occluded, or there may also be a bladder outlet obstruction. If an internal stent is placed in the presence of a bladder outlet obstruction, hydronephrosis would persist because the urine in the bladder would reflux up the stent and the patient would still require a Foley catheter to drain the bladder.[22] An NU tube left to external drainage will decompress the kidney and the urinary bladder, which drains the other kidney, without the need for the Foley. Even if the patient has only one kidney and a bladder outlet obstruction, a long NU is less likely than a short PCN tube to fall out inadvertently because it is more firmly anchored.

Specific techniques of stent insertion[23]

The preexisting PCN tube or percutaneous access catheter is removed from the renal pelvis over a stiff guidewire, such as an Amplatz Superstiff (Meditech, Boston, MA) wire, and is replaced for a short directional catheter with a distal curve such as a cobra or hockey stick shape, and the system is opacified with dilute contrast injections. The ureteropelvic junction is engaged with the catheter tip and a floppy-tipped wire (Bentson) or hydrophilic guidewire (Glidewire Meditech, Boston, MA), and the catheter–wire combination is advanced down the ureter to the point of obstruction. With contrast injections and gentle torquing

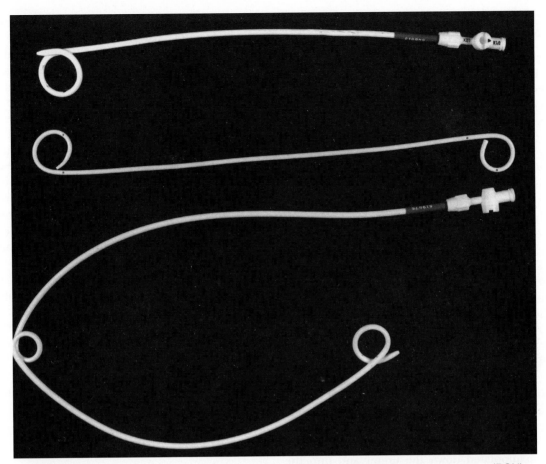

FIGURE 24-5. Examples of percutaneous urinary drainage catheters: **Top:** Percutaneous (PCN) tube. The pigtail lies in the renal pelvis and external portion of the tube connects to a drainage bag. **Middle:** Internal ureteral stent. One pigtail lies in the renal pelvis, and the other pigtail lies in the bladder. The entire tube is inside the patient's body. **Bottom:** Nephroureteral (NU) tube. The pigtail at the end of the tube lies in the bladder, the central pigtail lies in the renal pelvis, and the external portion of the tube can be capped off or connected to a drainage bag.

of the catheter, the guidewire usually can be advanced beyond the obstruction without perforating the ureter, even though the ureter appears to be completely occluded. Once the catheter and guidewire are in the bladder, the initial guidewire is replaced for a stiff guidewire, which will support advancement of the stent. The stiff guidewire must be advanced far into the bladder to allow good "purchase." If the bladder is not full, this maneuver will be painful to the patient. A Foley catheter, if present, should be clamped. The nephrostomy tract is dilated, and the NU or ureteral stent can be inserted over the wire with the distal pigtail positioned in the bladder and the proximal pigtail positioned in the renal pelvis.

When it is difficult to advance the stent over the stiff guidewire, a few techniques will help "inch" the process along. First, the bladder needs to be full, and as much guidewire as possible needs to be in the bladder. The stent will tend to creep downward when there is countertension on the wire, that is, pulling back the wire as the stent is being pushed forward. Second, introducing the stent through a "peel-away" sheath usually corrects the difficulties resulting from a steep pushing angle and tightly strictured distal ureters. The peel-away sheath requires a separate step, a slightly larger hole in the kidney, and an additional piece of equipment. Third, the guidewire tip in the bladder sometimes can be steered out the urethra, more easily in women, or when there is a Foley in the bladder. When the wire extends from the flank, through the kidney, down the ureter, and out the bladder, both wire ends can be held taut, thus easing the stent's advancement down the ureter.

A "safety" wire is also useful to have in position when performing complex manipulations or in less experienced hands. This safety wire is simply a second guidewire placed alongside the first wire, known as the *working wire.* If the working wire is inadvertently removed from the collecting system, access will be preserved by having the safety wire in place.

Providing access for stone removal before PNL[7,24–26]

Renal calculus disease requires the most specific approach to PCN. The particular calyx that must be punctured varies with the size, location, and number of stones; more than one tract may be necessary. It is of paramount importance to discuss the case with the referring urologist to agree on the optimum approach as well as a backup plan. After the system has been accessed and the tract is dilated to 28 to 32 Fr, the urologist will insert a large-bore rigid working sheath into the tract. An endoscope will be placed through this sheath to visualize and extract the stones. If the angle between the endoscope and the stones is too acute or the tract is too long, the likely outcome is hours of operative frustration and an unsuccessful stone retrieval. Complications such as parenchymal damage due to overtorquing the kidney or renal pelvic lacerations and bleeding are also possible.[27]

The other issue to decide at the initial consultation with the referring urologist is whether the urologist should place a retrograde ureteral occlusion balloon prior to PCN. This balloon can be used to distend the renal pelvis and calyces, facilitating PCN manipulations in nonobstructed systems or collecting systems with a large stone burden. Of course, this step entails an additional procedure for the patient.

After the collecting system is accessed, a catheter should be manipulated down the ureter and into the bladder to ensure that access to the collecting system will not be lost during manipulations involving tract dilation, sheath, or endoscope insertion. Either a 5 Fr catheter that accepts a 0.038-inch guidewire can be placed into the bladder with an 8 Fr PCN left alongside it for drainage, or a nephroureteral stent can be inserted. If the radiologist performs the tract dilation, preferably with a balloon catheter rather than serial dilators, a 28 Fr Foley is left in the collecting system and the patient is transferred to the operating room. In some institutions, the entire procedure, including stone extraction, is performed in the interventional suite, although to do so is usually impractical because the second stage of the procedure ties up the suite for several hours and most interventional suites do not have the proper drainage systems to deal with the large amount of irrigation fluid used in nephrolithotomy procedures.

Access sites for various stones

Pelvic and posterior lower/midpole calculi are the simplest stones to access because the puncture is through a posterior or midpole calyx. For a pelvic stone, the puncture can be through any calyx that provides a good path to the stone. For a posterior or midpole calyx, direct puncture into the stone-bearing calyx should be performed.

The complex cases are those where staghorn calculi, upper pole calculi, anterior calculi, or multiple calculi are present. Staghorn calculi are difficult because there may be branches into multiple calyces, which are difficult for the urologist to access from one puncture site. The largest stone containing posterior lower pole calyx should be punctured. Residual fragments may require a second puncture or a "Y" tract from the first puncture.

Upper pole stones are likely to be located above the costal margin, increasing the chances of pneumothorax or liver or spleen puncture with a puncture above the 12th rib. If no infundibular stenosis is present and the stone is small, a posterior lower pole calyx can be punctured and a flexible endoscope can be directed upward into the calyx. If the stone is large or there is an infundibular stenosis, a direct puncture into the upper pole calyx will be necessary.

Anterior calyceal stones, multiple calculi, and other complex situations require careful analysis and will be challenging even to experienced operators. Puncture into a posterior upper pole calyx generally provides access into all calyceal stone sites. Many other approaches are possible, however, and the access site must be tailored to the individual situation. The reader is referred to an advanced text for additional reading on this subject.[28]

■ Troubleshooting

Most problems with nephrostomy tubes ultimately require a tube change in the department and cannot be resolved at the bedside or over the telephone. The most common problems are occlusion of the tube, which requires a tube change, and inadvertent removal or dislodgement of the tube, which requires that the tube be reinserted or repositioned. At the least, the tube needs to be evaluated by a contrast nephrostogram or "tube check." The following are commonly encountered problems.

- The PCN tube is not draining: The tube is either occluded or dislodged. The tubes are made of kink-resistant material; so external kinking of the tube occurs infrequently. The tube may not even be a PCN but is an NU tube that is draining the urine antegrade (see next item).
- The NU tube is not draining: The tube is either occluded or the urine is draining antegrade into the bladder. If the tube check demonstrates that the tube is patent and the patient is urinating without difficulty, then the external portion of the tube can be capped off because the external drainage bag is unnecessary.
- The NU tube is draining externally, but the patient is not urinating: Either the internal ureteral portion of the stent is occluded while the PCN external por-

tion is patent, or there is a bladder outlet obstruction with reflux or urine from the bladder up and out of the external portion of the tube. This situation could apply to a patient who has either one or two NU tubes. The tube also could be dislodged, but this is less likely to happen because long NU tubes are anchored more firmly than short PCN tubes.

- Urine is leaking around the tube: The tube is either occluded or dislodged, and urine is leaking alongside the tube through the tract to soak the dressing or clothing. The external portion of the tube also could be cracked or punctured. In this situation, the skin around the tube should be dry. Another possibility is that the pigtail retention suture on the Meditech tube was not cut short enough, thereby exiting the hub of the tube and getting caught in the Luer lock between the PCN tube and the connecting tube to the drainage bag, which will cause a urine leak.

- The tube is completely or partially dislodged: If the tube is partially dislodged, injecting the tube usually will opacify the tract and the collecting system. The tube should be removed carefully over a guidewire and replaced with a 5 Fr catheter. Further contrast injections should opacify the tract. Then the catheter can be advanced back into the collecting system over a floppy-tipped guidewire (Bentson) or a hydrophilic guidewire (Glidewire) and the tube replaced. If the tube has been removed completely, the chance of reinserting it through the same tract is best if urine is still leaking out of the tract. Local anesthesia should not be administered because to do so will cause the soft tissue to swell and compress the tract. The key to recannulating the tract is to opacify it with a contrast injection at the dermatotomy site through a vessel dilator, short directional catheter, or Christmas tree adapter, followed by advancement of the catheter over a guidewire back into the collecting system. Failure will necessitate a new puncture, which may convert an outpatient to an inpatient or at least require a longer period of observation before discharge.

- Bloody drainage is extremely common. Even a single-stick atraumatic nephrostomy procedure can cause pink urine, which usually clears within hours. Grossly bloody urine often is seen after procedures requiring multiple punctures. If blood pulses out of the tract while the tract is being dilated, a large catheter should be inserted to tamponade the tract. The blood generally clears in a few days, particularly with repeated flushing of the tube to ensure that it does not clot. If the urine fails to clear or the hematocrit drops, the tube should be exchanged for a larger tube to tamponade the tract. Larger tubes usually control the bleeding, although sometimes a segmental renal artery needs to be embolized.[29,30]

■ Outpatients

We routinely perform the following procedures on outpatients: PCN and NU tube changes and conversion of PCN to NU or double J stents. We also schedule initial PCN procedures on selected outpatients with the provision that the patient will be admitted if a complication occurs or if the patient is too drowsy to go home.[31]

Routine tube changes can be performed every 3 months. The patient should be encouraged to drink a lot of fluids to dilute the urine, which will help prevent tube occlusion by urine sediment. Most nephrostomy tubes do not need to be flushed routinely.

All outpatients should have the phone number and names of the physicians and nurses in the interventional radiology department where the tube was placed. They should be encouraged to call if they experience any signs of blockage of the tube or infection such as fever, chills, flank pain, or leakage around the tube. Patients with capped tubes should reattach them to external drainage bags until they arrive in the department for a tube change and possible antibiotic therapy.

Patients with skin infections around the tube also should contact the department. Many skin infections will resolve within 48 hr with increased home care. Those that do not resolve will need formal evaluation and possible antibiotic therapy.[32,33]

REFERENCES

1. Lang EK, Price ET. Redefinitions of indications for percutaneous nephrostomy. *Radiology* 1983;147:419–426.
2. Barbaric ZL. Percutaneous nephrostomy for urinary tract obstruction. *AJR, Am J Roentgenol* 1984;143:803–809.
3. Reznek RK, Talner LB. Percutaneous nephrostomy. *Radiol Clin North Am* 1984;22:393–406.
4. Keidan RD, Greenberg RE, Hoffman JP, et al. Is PCN for hydronephrosis appropriate in patients with advanced cancer? *Am J Surg* 1988;156:206–208.
5. Watkinson AF, A'Hern RP, Jones A, et al. Role of percutaneous nephrostomy in malignant urinary tract obstruction. *Clin Radiol* 1993;47:32–35.
6. Yoder IC, Lindfors KK, Pfister RC. Diagnosis and treatment of pyonephrosis. *Radiol Clin North Am* 1984;2:407–414.
7. Castaneda-Zuniga WR, Clayman R, Smith A, et al. Nephrostolithotomy: percutaneous technique for urinary calculus removal. *AJR Am J Roentgenol* 1982;139:721–726.
8. Matalon TAS, Thompson MJ, Patel SK, et al. Percutaneous treatment of urine leaks in renal transplantation patients. *Radiology* 1990;174:1049–1051.
9. Bell DA, Rose SC, Starr NK, et al. Percutaneous nephrostomy for nonoperative management of fungal urinary tract infections. *J Vasc Interv Radiol* 1993;4:311–315.
10. Whitaker RH, Chir M. The Whitaker test. *Urol Clin North Am* 1979;6:529–539.
11. Naidich JB, Rackson ME, Mossey RT, et al. Non-dilated obstructive uropathy: percutaneous nephrostomy performed for severe renal failure. *Radiology* 1986;160:653–657.

12. Lee WJ, Patel V, Patel S, et al. Emergency PCN: results and complications. *J Vasc Interv Radiol* 1994;5:135–139.
13. Babel SG, Winterkorn KG. Retrograde catheterization of the ureter without cystoscopic assistance. *Radiology* 1993;187:547–549.
14. Clayman RV. Nephrolithotomy (nephrostolithotomy): concepts and rationale. *Semin Intervent Radiol* 1984;1:75–78.
15. Dunnick NR, Carson CC III, Moore AV, et al. Percutaneous approach to nephrolithiasis. *AJR Am J Roentgenol* 1985;144:451–455.
16. Stables DP. Percutaneous nephrostomy: techniques, indications, and results. *Urol Clin North Am* 1982;9:15–29.
17. Papanicolaou N. Renal anatomy relevant to percutaneous interventions. *Semin Intervent Radiol* 1995;12:163–172.
18. Lang EK. Percutaneous management of ureteral strictures. *Semin Interv Radiol* 1987;4:79–89.
19. Cardella JF, Castaneda-Zuniga WR, Hunter DW. Long term ureteral stenting: techniques and effectiveness. *Radiology* 1986;161:313–318.
20. Salzman B. Ureteral stents: indications, variations and complications. *Urol Clin North Am* 1988;15:481–491.
21. Rackson ME, Mitty HA, Dan SJ, et al. Elevated bladder pressure: a cause of apparent ureteral stent failure. *AJR Am J Roentgenol* 1988;151:335–336.
22. de Baerre T, Denys A, Pappas P, et al. Ureteral stents: exchange under fluoroscopic control as an effective alternative to cystoscopy. *Radiology* 1994;190;887–889.
23. Mitty HA, Train JS, Dan SJ. Placement of ureteral stents by antegrade and retrograde techniques. *Radiol Clin North Am* 1986;24:587–600.
24. Lee WJ, Smith AD, Cubelli V, et al. Percutaneous nephrolithotomy: analysis of 500 consecutive cases. *Urol Radiol* 1986;8:61–66.
25. LeRoy AJ, May GR, Bender CE, et al. Percutaneous nephrostomy for stone removal. *Radiology* 1984;151:607–612.
26. Clayman RV, Surya V, Miller RP, et al. Percutaneous nephrolithotomy: extraction of renal and ureteral calculi from 100 patients. *J Urol* 1984;131:868–871.
27. Bjarnason H, Ferral H, Stackhouse DJ, et al. Complications related to percutaneous nephrolithotomy. *Semin Interv Radiol* 1994;11:213–225.
28. Castaneda-Zuniga WR, Tadavarthy SM, Hunter DW, et al. Interventional uroradiology. In: Castaneda-Zuniga WR, Tadavarthy SM, eds. *Interventional radiology*, 2nd ed, vol 2. Baltimore: Williams & Wilkins, 1992:777–989.
29. Ferral H, Stackhaus DJ, Bjarnason H, et al. Complications of percutaneous nephrostomy tube placement. *Semin Interv Radiol* 1994;11:198–206.
30. Cope C. Zeit RM. Pseudoaneurvsms after nephrostomy. *AJR Am J Roentgenol* 1982;139:255–261.
31. Cochran ST, Barbaric ZL, Lee JJ, et al. Percutaneous nephrostomy tube placement: an outpatient procedure? *Radiology* 1991:179:843–847.
32. Cronan JJ, Horn DL, Marcello A, et al. Antibiotics and nephrostomy tube care: preliminary observations. Part II. Bacteriuria. *Radiology* 1989;172:1043–1045.
33. *Nephrostomy catheter care.* Informational pamphlet for patients distributed by SCVIR, Fairfax, VA, 1992.

25

Pelvic and Obstetric Hemorrhage

ANDREW KERR

Life-threatening pelvic hemorrhage may result from blunt or penetrating trauma, pregnancy, malignancy, or arterial venous malformation. The pelvis is supplied by an extensive network of collateral vessels. Consequently, surgical ligation of the hypogastric artery origins has minimal effect on bleeding. Operative exposure and ligation of the bleeding distal hypogastric artery branches are a technical nightmare.[1] Dissection of the retroperitoneum to find the hypogastric artery origins at laparotomy often exacerbates bleeding by removing compression of the bleeding site provided by adjacent anatomic structures. Because of technical difficulties posed by the surgical approach, angiographic embolization is the treatment of choice for pelvic arterial hemorrhage. Embolic materials released into the internal iliac artery are carried by the bloodstream to occlude the artery beyond the larger collaterals. The arterial pressure at the bleeding site then decreases sufficiently to permit hemostasis.

■ Trauma

Approach to the patient with pelvic fractures and shock: Stop the bleeding!

The patient with life-threatening pelvic hemorrhage may be in florid shock or may not appear to be seriously injured at all when he or she is brought to the emergency department. Sometimes, flank and buttock hematomas are present. Displaced pelvic fractures may cause obvious leg-length discrepancies,[2] or no injuries may be visible. Blood pressure may be normal; baseline blood pressure varies from individual to individual. An adult can lose 30% of the blood volume acutely before systolic pressure begins to drop (although it then drops rapidly). Initially, the hematocrit is likely to be normal because it takes hours of equilibration with extravascular fluids before the serum hematocrit reflects an acute blood loss. Initially, the only abnormalities that may be observed are tachycardia (pulse > 100/min), tachypnea, coolness of the skin caused by peripheral vasoconstriction, a narrowed pulse pressure (actually an elevated diastolic pressure caused by catecholamine release), and low urine output. If the trauma patient has signs of shock after intravenous infusion of 2 L of fluid, it is most likely the consequence of active internal bleeding.[3] The overall mortality from pelvic fractures is 6 to 19%, and half of these deaths are from hemorrhage and the others from associated injuries. If tachycardia is attributed to pain from pelvic fractures, the diagnosis of shock may not be made until systolic blood pressure falls. The mortality rate rises to 50% when hypotension is present.[4] Hypotensive patients are treated with large volumes of intravenous crystalloid solution and packed red blood cells. If platelets and plasma are not infused as well, a dilutional coagulopathy develops. If the intravenous solutions are not warmed, the patient may become hypothermic. Hypothermia interferes with normal coagulation.[5] Consequently, fluid resuscitation for hypotension may worsen the bleeding. Patients who are hypotensive for prolonged periods often develop multiple organ-system failure and sepsis.[6] Therefore, it is essential to find the site of bleeding and to stop it before the patient's condition deteriorates.

The trauma patient with active hemorrhage usually

arrives in the emergency department with little clinical history but with many injuries. Complete evaluation of the patient requires numerous diagnostic tests. If the patient is to be saved, the sequence of tests must be prioritized so that potentially lethal injuries are addressed first and less dangerous (although frequently more obvious) injuries are evaluated later. The workup must proceed rapidly despite the fact that the patient may be hemodynamically unstable. Resuscitation and evaluation must take place simultaneously. Suspending the workup so that the patient can be "tuned-up" first will delay the time when a surgical or interventional procedure can be performed to stop the bleeding. Often, it is necessary to institute therapeutic procedures based on a probable diagnosis before a complete clinical picture is available.[7,8]

Diagnostic peritoneal lavage

The pelvic fracture patient with a patent airway in whom hemothorax, pneumothorax, cardiac contusion, and pericardial tamponade have been ruled out who shows signs of shock after vigorous intravenous fluid infusion is presumed to be actively bleeding. Supraumbilical diagnostic peritoneal lavage then is performed. If gross blood is found at lavage, it is likely that the bleeding emanates from a ruptured intraperitoneal organ (usually spleen or liver). The patient is taken for laparotomy. If the lavage does not reveal gross blood or if the patient remains unstable after laparotomy, ongoing retroperitoneal hemorrhage is probable. The patient then undergoes diagnostic pelvic angiography and possible embolization.[9]

Angiography and embolization

Hemorrhage from branches of the internal iliac artery requiring embolization occurs in 7 to 11% of patients with pelvic fractures.[10] The most commonly injured arteries are the superior gluteal, iliolumbar, and lateral sacral (associated with sacral fracture and sacroiliac joint disruption), and the internal pudendal and the obturator arteries (associated with pubic ramus and acetabular fractures) (Fig. 25-1).[11] Transcatheter embolization is successful in treating pelvic arterial hemorrhage in 85 to 90% of cases.[6,12,13] There is great potential for cross-pelvic collateralization via anterior and posterior division branches of the internal iliac arteries. Therefore, selective injections of both internal iliac arteries should be performed, and bilateral embolization is often necessary.

External fixation

Venous bleeding is common after pelvic fractures. An extensive venous plexus exists adjacent to the pelvic bones and is more fragile than the pelvic arteries (Fig. 25-2). The venous bed is a low-pressure, but high-capacity, structure. The pelvic veins are valveless and are therefore in open communication with the inferior vena cava, and they are also in open communication with the portal vein via the superior rectal vein. In dogs simultaneous ligation of the lumbar arteries, inferior mesenteric artery, medial sacral artery, right and left hypogastric, external iliac, and profunda femoral arteries had no effect on pelvic venous pressure.[14] Pelvic venous bleeding is stopped by the tamponade (compression) effect of surrounding structures. An unstable pelvic fracture (particularly of the open-book type) can greatly increase the potential volume of venous hemorrhage. A 3-cm diastasis of the pubic symphysis will increase the potential volume of the pelvis from the normal 4 L to 8 L.[15] Realigning the fractured and displaced bones by placement of external fixators is an orthopedic procedure performed to control venous bleeding. External fixation is helpful when there is a diastasis of the pubic symphysis. It decreases the potential space in which bleeding can take place and aids coagulation by preventing the fracture fragments from moving in relation to each other.[2] Angiographic embolization and external fixation treat different types of bleeding. External fixation controls osseous and venous bleeding but not arterial bleeding. Angiographic embolization controls arterial but not venous bleeding. At present, it is not possible to know initially whether a pelvic fracture patient is bleeding primarily from an arterial or a venous source; thus, which procedure should be performed first is a subject of controversy.

■ Indications for Other Radiographic Studies in the Pelvic Fracture Patient

Plain films

The only radiographs that an unstable blunt trauma patient should have are cervical spine, anteroposterior (AP) chest, and AP abdomen.[3] These studies will identify most of the potentially lethal injuries that can be visualized by plain films. The patient may well have obvious extremity fractures and facial lacerations. Evaluation and treatment of these must wait until life-threatening injuries have been treated or ruled out. Foley et al.[16] reported on four trauma patients who bled to death of ruptured spleens while plain films were being obtained in the emergency department.

Computed tomography scanning

Trauma patients with neurosurgical emergencies requiring immediate evacuation of intracranial hematomas usually present with one or more of the following: hy-

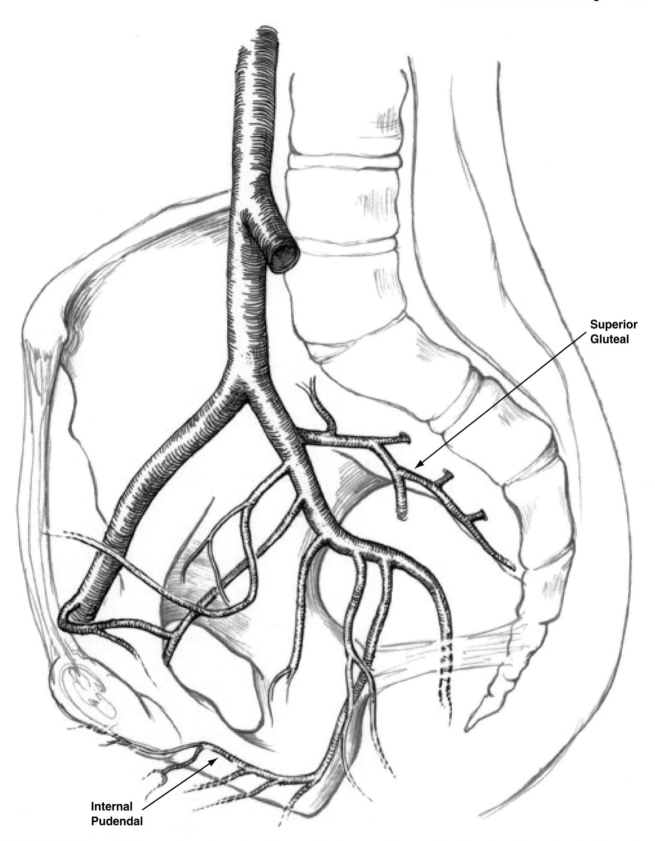

**Superior
Gluteal**

**Internal
Pudendal**

FIGURE 25-1. Internal iliac artery branches vulnerable to pelvic fractures. The superior gluteal and internal pudendal arteries are most commonly affected.

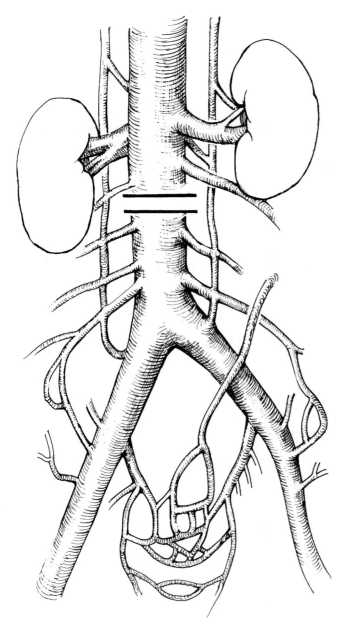

FIGURE 25-2. Pelvic venous plexus and collateral pathways.

pertension (not shock), bradycardia (not tachycardia), altered mental status (Glasgow coma scale of 8 or less), a dilated pupil on the side of the intracranial bleeding, and a peripheral neurological deficit on the side opposite the injury. For these patients, immediate computed tomography (CT) scan of the head is indicated.[3]

Chest and body CT scanning is appropriate for evaluation of the hemodynamically stable trauma patient but in general should not be performed on the patient in shock. Oral contrast should not be used when there is a possibility that angiography may follow CT scanning. In the unstable patient with pelvic fractures and when findings on the chest film suggest great vessel injury, both thoracic aortography and pelvic angiography should be performed.[10]

Uroradiographic studies

A patient in shock must have a catheter to drain the bladder and to measure urine output. Urethral injury in females is rare. If a male with pelvic trauma is unable to void, has blood at the meatus, has a prostate that is high riding or is not palpable, or has a scrotal hematoma, he may have sustained a urethral injury. To avoid converting a partial urethral tear to a complete transection, urethrography should be performed before a Foley catheter is placed.[17] A patient in shock should not undergo urethrography, cystography, or intravenous urography for two reasons: First, time is better spent stopping the bleeding than performing studies to evaluate injuries that are not life threatening; second, contrast that extravasates from an injured bladder may render pelvic angiography uninterpretable. Patients in shock who may have urethral injury and have an easily palpable bladder should have a suprapubic cystostomy placed at the bedside, which can be performed quickly and without contrast and is therapeutic. Many of these patients will require elective repair of urethral strictures after the urethral injury has healed.[18]

■ Obstetric Hemorrhage

Bleeding in excess of 1 L occurs in 1 to 2% of deliveries;[19] 11 to 13% of pregnancy-related maternal deaths in the United States are caused directly by hemorrhage, averaging 53 maternal deaths from bleeding each year.[20] The pregnant uterus is extremely vascular. It is perfused by the uterine branches of the internal iliac arteries as well as by the ovarian arteries, which in most cases originate from the abdominal aorta (Fig. 25-3). The ovarian arteries may arise from the renal, iliac, lumbar, or adrenal arteries.[21] The collateral blood supply to the uterus is excellent. Fatal obstetric hemorrhage can take place within minutes. Bilateral hypogastric artery ligation is successful in curtailing hemorrhage only 50% of the time. Bilateral uterine artery ligation is successful 95% of the time.[19] Packing the uterus with gauze when coagulopathy is present and even hysterectomy occasionally fails to stop uterine hemorrhage. When medical management fails, angiographic embolization in many cases can obviate laparotomy and may preserve fertility by making hysterectomy unnecessary.[22–26] When a patient is considered at high risk for postpartum bleeding, an angiographic catheter can be placed into the aorta through a left axillary approach while a lead apron shields the pelvis before the patient is taken to the operating room for cesarian section. Then intraoperative

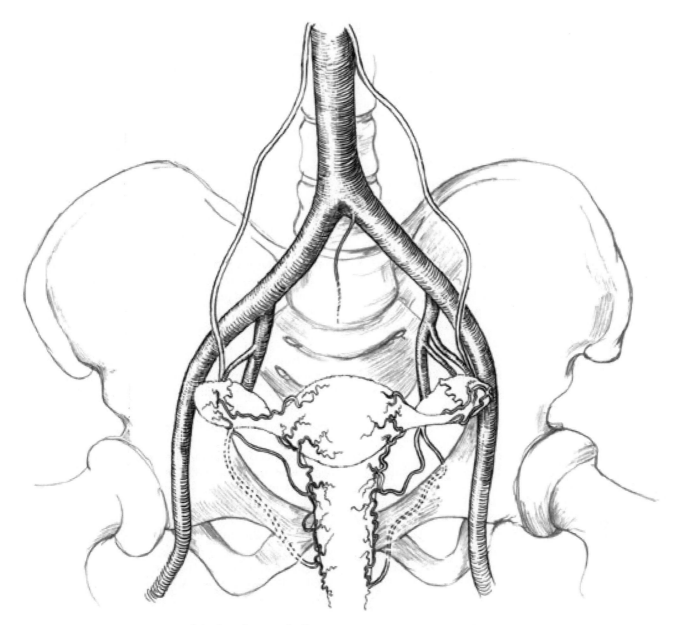

FIGURE 25-3. Arterial anatomy of the female reproductive organs.

embolization can be performed using C-arm fluoroscopy if hemorrhage is severe.[26,27] Because the placenta and the full-term uterus are extremely vascular structures, embolization to stop bleeding from a postpartum uterus or from an ectopic placenta frequently requires far larger quantities of Gelfoam than needed to control posttraumatic hemorrhage. Obstetric hemorrhage may be caused by bleeding from the placental implantation site, by trauma during delivery, or by the HELLP (hemolysis, elevated liver enzymes, and low platelet count) syndrome.

Bleeding from the site of placental implantation

The arterial flow to the placenta at term is approximately 600 mL/min.[20] When the placenta is expelled at delivery, the vessels connecting the uterus to the placenta are torn. Approximately 500 mL of blood is usually lost at this time. Contractions of the uterus occlude the disrupted vessels. If part of the placenta remains adherent to the uterus, bleeding will continue until the residual placenta is removed. If the uterus does not contract after delivery (*atonic uterus*), bleeding will persist. Atonic uterus usually responds to administration of oxytocin or, if this fails, to prostaglandin (15-methyl prostaglandin F_{2a}).[19] If the placenta attaches to the myometrium instead of to the endometrial decidua, it is called *placenta accreta;* if it invades deeply into the myometrium, *placenta increta;* and if it extends through the uterus and sometimes into adjacent organs, termed *placenta percreta.* Massive postpartum hemorrhage is probable in these situations because the abnormal placenta will not separate from the uterus at delivery. If the placenta separates from the uterus before labor begins (*placental abruption*), severe bleeding may occur and frequently is exacerbated by a coagulopathy caused by substances released by the placenta. Placental abruption associated with fetal distress or with continuing hemorrhage is treated by delivery of the fetus. If the placenta is near or covers the cervix (*placenta previa*), massive bleeding is likely to occur when labor begins. Placenta previa is detected by prenatal ultrasound. The patient is then delivered by cesarean section before labor begins.

In ectopic pregnancy, the placenta attaches and develops outside the uterus. Most commonly, the fetus develops in a fallopian tube (*tubal pregnancy*). Less commonly, the fetus may develop in the peritoneal cavity (*abdominal pregnancy*) or in the uterine cervix (*cervical pregnancy*). The ectopic gestation will establish blood vessels to nearby structures. These abnormal placental attachments may separate partially, causing massive hemorrhage. When an advanced abdominal or cervical pregnancy is removed at laparotomy, massive hemorrhage frequently occurs when the placenta is dissected from its abnormal insertion site. When preoperative embolization of the placenta is performed, operative blood loss is usually minimal. Gelfoam embolization should be performed less than 24 h before surgery because the vessels perfusing the ectopic gestation recanalize rapidly.[27,28]

Traumatic obstetric hemorrhage

Significant bleeding may occur from lacerations of the vagina caused by forceps delivery or by episiotomy. The uterus may bleed after spontaneous rupture during delivery or after cesarean section. The hemorrhage may be per the vagina, or it may be into the retroperitoneum and consequently not visible. Intractable bleeding usually is treated by hypogastric artery ligation, uterine artery ligation, or hysterectomy. Successful treatment of these injuries by angiographic embolization has been reported.[29]

Intraperitoneal hemorrhage associated with the HELLP syndrome

Preeclampsia, which occurs in 7% of pregnancies, is defined as hypertension associated with proteinuria developing during pregnancy. When seizures are also present, the condition is termed *eclampsia.* Approximately 10% of severely preeclamptic patients and 30 to 50% of eclamptic patients develop the HELLP syndrome. The cause of these disorders is unknown, but current research suggests that it may be an as yet unidentified toxic substance produced by the placenta. The placental toxin theory is supported by the fact that the disease resolves only after delivery of the fetus and placenta. Further, recovery has been more rapid in some patients treated with postpartum uterine curettage, plasma exchange, or steroids.[30] Patients with the HELLP syndrome develop disseminated intravascular coagulation (DIC). Liver infarction and intrahepatic hematoma formation are also common. After infarction, the affected portions of the liver sometimes rupture following minimal trauma or during labor. Liver rupture in the presence of coagulopathy is associated with massive intraperitoneal hemorrhage. If hepatic infarction or subcapsular hemorrhage is not associated with rupture of the liver capsule, the patient may be treated without surgery. Patients with intraperitoneal hemorrhage from liver rupture are treated with surgical packing at the rupture site and drainage of the intraperitoneal hemorrhage; this controls the bleeding in most cases. One study reported an 82% survival rate following this procedure.[31] Transcatheter hepatic artery embolization is an alternative to laparotomy for treatment of intraperitoneal hemorrhage from liver rupture in postpartum patients who have the HELLP syndrome. Arteriography usually demonstrates an avascular area with stretching of adjacent hepatic artery branches and small pseudoaneurysms.[32,33] Before hepatic artery embolization, arterial portography should be performed to show that there is adequate perfusion of the liver by the portal vein. Care must be taken during embolization to place the catheter distal to the cystic artery origin to avoid gallbladder infarction.

■ Pelvic Malignancy

Successful control of pelvic hemorrhage has been reported in patients with intractable bleeding from primary carcinoma of the cervix, uterus, and bladder as well as invasion of these organs by metastases. Bleeding from pelvic malignancy can be fatal; however, the rate of bleeding is often too slow to be demonstrated angiographically. The tumor usually can be well delineated angiographically, by CT scan, or magnetic resonance imaging. If continuing pelvic hemorrhage is clinically evident from a known pelvic tumor, angiographic demonstration of the bleeding site is not required before embolization.

Embolization of pelvic malignancy is a palliative procedure that does not eradicate the tumor. Bilateral embolization of the anterior divisions of the internal iliac arteries is necessary to minimize the risk of rebleeding. When an appropriate embolic agent is used, infarction of normal structures is unlikely because the collateral blood supply remains from the superior hemorrhoidal, iliac circumflex, gonadal, and profunda femoral arteries.

When embolization is performed for traumatic or obstetrical bleeding, a temporary occluding agent such as Gelfoam can be used because rapid healing is to be expected at the bleeding site. Unfortunately, pelvic malignancy will persist after embolization. Consequently, a permanent embolic agent must be used. Polyvinyl alcohol (PVA) 250-590 micron is the embolic agent of choice because it is permanent, it will occlude distal vessels, and yet it is not so small as to block the precapillary collateral plexus.[34,35]

■ Uterine Fibroids

Uterine fibroids are present in 20 to 40% of women older than 35 years of age. The standard treatment for sympto-matic patients (bleeding, pain) is hysterectomy or myomectomy. Since 1995 interventional radiologists have reported successful treatment of fibroid related symptoms by transcatheter embolization of the uterine arteries bilaterally (Fig. 25-4).[36] This causes infarction of fibroids but not of normal uterine tissue.

The procedure is performed using particulate polyvinyl alcohol, (500–710 microns). Technical success is achieved in over 95% of patients. Early and midterm follow up demonstrates that 80–94% of patients have moderate or marked improvement in symptoms, and over 90% of these patients have significant reduction in fibroid and uterine size.[37–39] Complication rates appear low. The effect on fertility is not yet known.

■ Pelvic Vascular Malformations

Vascular malformations are abnormal communications between arteries and veins. They are low-resistance pathways for arterial blood (high pressure) to enter the venous system (low pressure) without first perfusing nor-

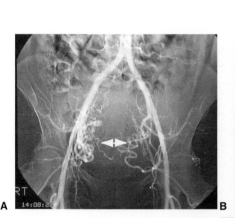

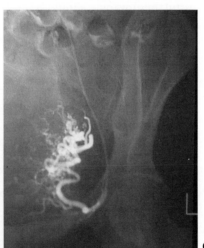

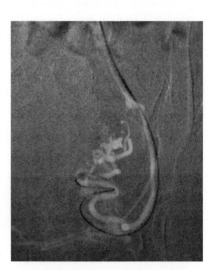

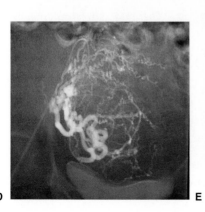

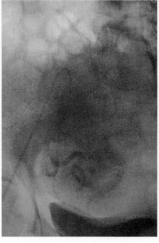

FIGURE 25-4. Bilateral uterine artery embolization. **A:** Pelvic arteriogram demonstrates bilateral large tortuous uterine arteries feeding hypervascular uterine fibroid. **B:** The left uterine artery has been selectively catheterized from the contralateral femoral approach. **C:** Superselective catheterization of the left uterine artery using a coaxial microcatheter system, prior to particulate PVA embolization. **D:** The right uterine artery has been catheterized. Note the marked hypervascularity of the uterine fibroid. **E:** Following embolization, there is marked decreased vascularity and marked arterial stasis.

mal structures. Consequently, blood will preferentially pass through this path of least resistance rather than go through the capillary bed of adjacent tissues. The size of vascular malformations tends to increase with time. Pelvic vascular malformations may cause a palpable mass, pain, bleeding, leg swelling, and, rarely, high output cardiac failure. The two types of vascular malformations are arterial venous malformations (AVM) and arteriovenous fistulas (AVF).

Arterial venous malformations are congenital. They result from incomplete differentiation of embryonic vascular tissue into arteries, capillaries, and veins. An arteriogram of a pelvic AVM usually shows a mass of innumerable vascular communications perfused by dilated arteries and drained by dilated early filling veins. Asymptomatic arterial venous malformations should be left alone. Complete obliteration of a pelvic AVM by embolization or surgical resection or both is successful about one third of the time.[40] In most cases after therapy, parts of the arterial venous malformation that have not been occluded or resected enlarge, causing reappearance of the mass. An arterial venous malformation is not a tumor. Its cells do not multiply or metastasize, but small, residual parts of the malformation can dilate enormously, leading to clinical relapse.[40,41] To date, no consistently successful therapy for this condition has been established (Fig. 25-5). One report describes successful embolization of 14 of 17 uterine

arterial venous malformations, with five subsequent pregnancies.[42] It seems that many of these cases were postsurgical arteriovenous fistulas and were not arterial venous malformations.

Arteriovenous fistula

A pelvic arteriovenous fistula is an acquired communication between a previously normal artery and vein (Fig. 25-6). Most are caused by penetrating trauma. Less commonly, an arteriovenous fistula can be caused by blunt trauma and, rarely, by rupture of an arterial aneurysm into a vein.[43] (An arteriovenous fistula is usually much easier to treat than is an AVM, because it consists of only a single arterial to venous connection. Occluding it cures the condition. Ideally, the AVF tract should be occluded by spring coils. Alternatively, the AVF can be treated by placing the coils in the feeding artery immediately proximal and distal to the AVF. This coil "sandwich" will prevent antegrade and retrograde filling of the AVF. The sandwich method, of course, will sacrifice at least a short segment of the feeding artery. Traumatic AVFs are often associated with a pseudoaneurysm at the fistula site.) If so, both the pseudoaneurysm and the feeding artery should be embolized with coils. Particulate agents such as Gelfoam or polyvinyl alcohol would be likely to pass through the fistula to become pulmonary emboli. Essen-

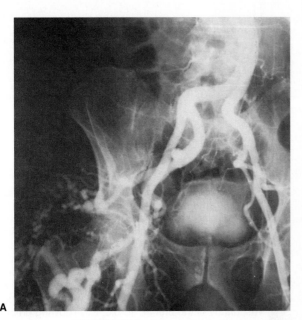
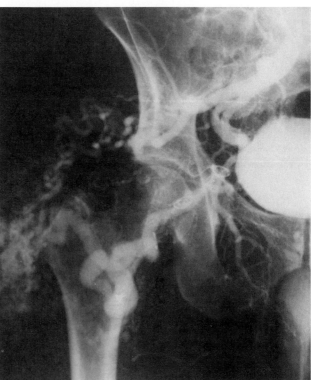

A   B

FIGURE 25-5. Congenital buttock arteriovenous malformation in a 47-year-old man. Note the numerous arteriovenous communications.

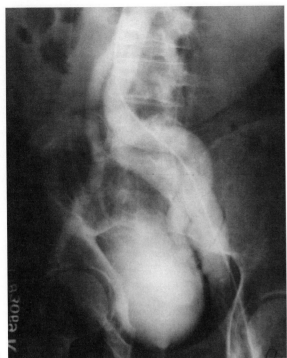
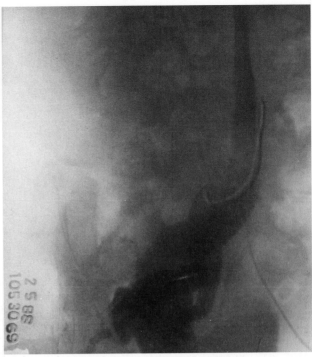

FIGURE 25-6. AP pelvic arteriogram (**A**) and oblique subtraction (**B**) review of selective internal iliac artery injection. Internal iliac arteriovenous fistula in a 33-year-old man who sustained pelvic fractures when he was hit by a bus at age 10. He came to the emergency department for treatment of gastroenteritis. A bruit was heard on auscultation of the abdomen. There is a single communication between the artery and vein. Also note the dilatation of the affected vessels caused by the long-standing fistula.

tial vessels such as the common and external iliac femoral, or subclavian arteries must remain patent while the internal iliac arteries and other branch vessels can usually be sacrificed. When major vessel patency is required open surgical repair or endovascular graft placement should be used.

■ Angiographic Technique for Diagnosis and Treatment of Pelvic Hemorrhage

Optimally, arterial catheterization should be performed from a femoral approach because it is usually easier and safer than an axillary artery puncture. If possible, the puncture should be made on the side of the patient opposite the suspected site of bleeding because it is easier to catheterize the internal iliac artery selectively on the side opposite the puncture site than to catheterize it on the same side. For example, if a trauma patient has left-sided pelvic fractures, angiography should be done from a right femoral artery approach. In several situations pelvic angiography for hemorrhage should be performed from a left axillary approach. The trauma patient may

have bilateral acetabular or pubic ramus fractures with extensive adjacent soft tissue hematomas obscuring the pulse and making manipulation painful. The patient may be in shock with inflated MAST pants (military antishock trousers) covering the femoral arteries. Alternatively, the patient may be a high-risk pregnancy patient in the angiography suite for prophylactic angiographic catheter placement before cesarean delivery. Radiation to the fetus must be minimized.

Intraarterial digital angiography can be done in less than half the time needed for cut-film angiography. Many pelvic hemorrhage patients are unable to cooperate fully. Consequently, it is necessary to study these patients by using unsubtracted digital angiography to avoid the motion artifacts that may occur using subtracted digital arteriography. With unsubtracted digital arteriography, the higher doses of contrast used for cut-film studies are necessary for good vessel opacification.

A nonselective pelvic flush study is done first using a 5 Fr pigtail catheter. The catheter tip is placed above the origin of the inferior mesenteric artery.[44] The superior hemorrhoidal branch of the inferior mesenteric artery perfuses the rectum. The rectum also is perfused by the

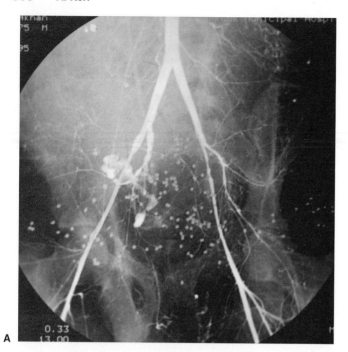
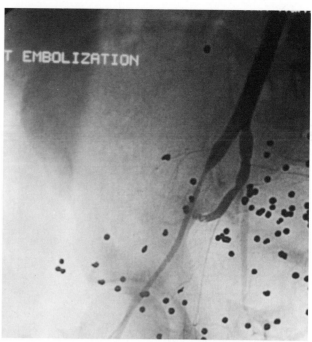

FIGURE 25-7. A: Active hemorrhage. Extravasation of contrast from the right superior gluteal artery demonstrated on the pelvic flush study. **B:** Following embolization with spring embolus coils and Gelfoam. Hemorrhage has been controlled. Mild persistent arterial spasm is present.

middle and inferior hemorrhoidal arteries, which originate from the obturator or internal pudendal branches of the internal iliac artery to form a collateral pathway so that bleeding from branches of the internal iliac artery may sometimes be demonstrated by inferior mesenteric artery injection and vice versa.

Next the pigtail catheter is exchanged for a cobra 2 catheter. If a bleeding site was demonstrated on the pelvic flush study, the bleeding vessel is selectively catheterized and embolized (Fig. 25-7). If no bleeding site was demonstrated on the pelvic flush study, selective right and left internal iliac artery injections are performed. First, the contralateral internal iliac artery is catheterized. Then the ipsilateral internal iliac artery is catheterized using the Waltman loop or other techniques (Fig. 25-8). If difficulty is experienced crossing the aortic bifurcation, the cobra 2 catheter should be exchanged for a hooked-shaped catheter such as a Rösch inferior mesenteric artery catheter or a SOS omni selective catheter or a Simmons catheter, which will allow easy placement of a guidewire across the aortic bifurcation. Once the guidewire tip is well seated within the contralateral iliac artery, the hooked-shaped catheter can be removed over the guidewire and then replaced by the cobra 2 catheter (Fig. 25-9A). If attempts to catheterize the ipsilateral internal iliac artery are unsuccessful using a cobra 2 cathe-

ter and the Waltman loop technique, a hooked-shaped catheter can be used instead (see Fig. 25-9B). In the internal iliac artery, 12 mm of contrast should be injected over 2 sec with filming obtained for 20 sec to identify extravasated contrast after intravascular contrast has cleared. The catheter tip must be in the proximal internal iliac artery to opacify the lateral sacral and the iliolumbar branches.

If a bleeding site or sites have been identified, transcatheter embolization is performed (Fig. 25-10). In most situations in which pelvic embolization is required, Gelfoam cubes are the agent of choice. Because this agent dissolves in several weeks, it is excellent for use in the treatment of traumatic and obstetric bleeding. Scatter embolization is the fastest way to stop the bleeding. The Gelfoam block should be cut into parallel strips 1 to 2 mm thick, leaving the bases of the strips attached like matches in a book. The block should then be turned 90° and a series of cuts made across the strips. This will produce 1 to 2 mm Gelfoam cubes. (This is more efficient than cutting each strip separately.) Several dozen cubes should be backloaded into a 10-mL syringe while the plunger is removed and then filled with contrast. The Gelfoam should be injected into the internal iliac artery under fluoroscopic guidance until flow is very slow, and embolization should be stopped before Gelfoam refluxes

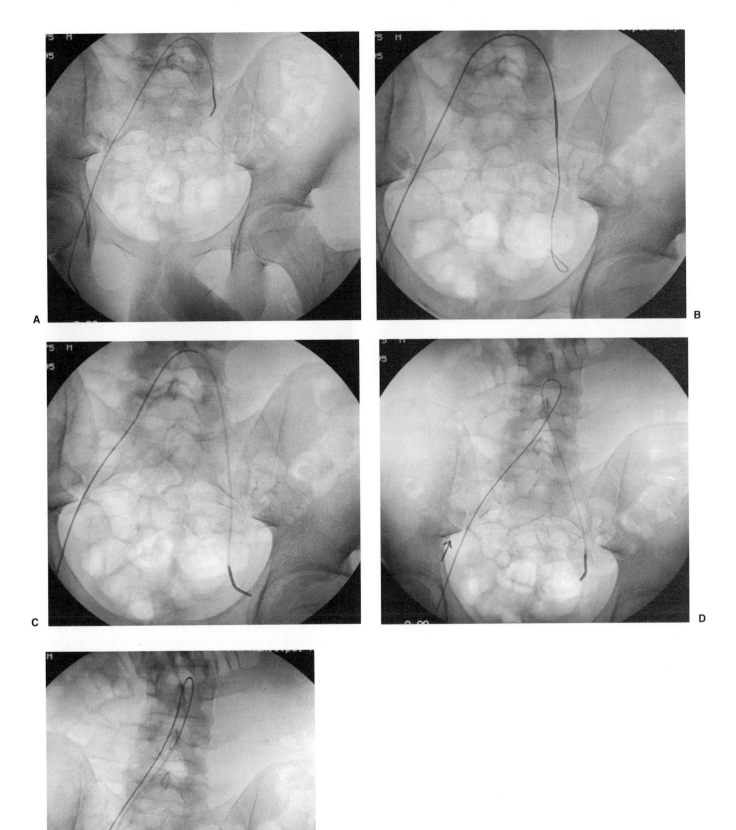

FIGURE 25-8. Waltman loop formed in the contralateral internal iliac artery. **A:** Cobra 2 catheter with distal tip in the contralateral internal iliac artery origin. **B:** The guidewire is advanced gently into a distal branch. **C:** The catheter is gently advanced as far as it will go. Then the guidewire is withdrawn to the aortic bifurcation. **D:** The catheter and guidewire are advanced as one unit and are turned 180 degrees clockwise, forming a loop. **E:** The catheter then is pushed up until the tip is in the abdominal aorta and then is pulled down into the ipsilateral internal iliac artery.

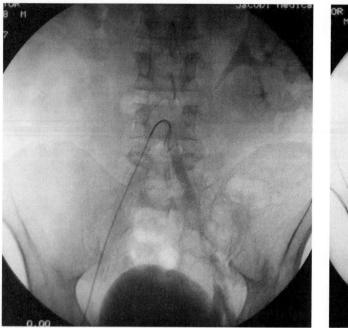 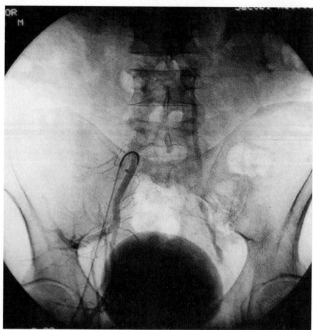

FIGURE 25-9. A: Rösch inferior mesenteric artery catheter crossing the aortic bifurcation. **B:** Rösch inferior mesenteric artery catheter in the ipsilateral internal iliac artery.

into the external iliac artery. After embolization is complete, pelvic flush arteriography should be performed to document that there is no further bleeding (Fig. 25-11).

If the patient is sufficiently stable, subselective embolization of the bleeding branch vessel or vessels can be performed instead of scatter embolization. If scatter embolization must be performed from the internal iliac artery trunk because expedient subselective catherization of the bleeding branch vessels is not possible, then protective spring coils can be placed into the origins of the superior and inferior gluteal arteries before scatter embolization. The coils will prevent Gelfoam from entering these internal iliac artery branches and will decrease the small risk of buttock ischemia and sciatic nerve injury. At this institution, "coil blockade" is not done frequently because patients who need scatter embolization are frequently unstable and placing the coils postpones the time when hemorrhage can be stopped. Most organs suffer irreversible injury within hours of acute arterial occlusion. Gelfoam's safety stems from its size, which is small enough to stop bleeding by causing occlusion distal to the larger collateral vessels and yet large enough to stop proximal to the precapillary network of collateral vessels, not from the fact that it dissolves in a few weeks. The bleeding site is therefore not deprived of all perfusion.

Other embolic agents

Gelfoam cubes are excellent for treating causes of bleeding that are temporary, such as traumatic or obstetric hemorrhage. Pelvic malignancies will persist and regenerate despite embolization, which is why a permanent agent such as polyvinyl alcohol (PVA) is more appropriate. Although the chemical formula of PVA is that of an alcohol, it is an inert solid. PVA is supplied by the manufacturer in several particle sizes. The term *absolute alcohol* refers to a solution of 99% ethyl alcohol. There is no role for absolute alcohol in pelvic embolization. It causes sclerosis of all arteries with which it comes in contact down to the capillary level, resulting in infarction of all tissues in the distribution of those vessels. Gelfoam powder can be purchased or made from a block of Gelfoam. Because of its small diameter, particles of Gelfoam powder occlude at the capillary level and is therefore likely to cause infarction. Like absolute alcohol, Gelfoam powder never should be used for treatment of pelvic hemorrhage.[45] Spring embolus coils are rarely used alone for treatment of pelvic bleeding. They usually occlude too proximally to stop bleeding from small collateral vessels. Coils are permanent. Therefore, it is not possible to recatheterize vessels in which they have been placed. They also create artifacts on magnetic resonance studies. Occasionally, a large proximal branch of the internal iliac artery is lacerated. Gelfoam cubes may be swept through the laceration into the extravascular space[46] and consequently have no effect on the bleeding. In these situations, spring embolus coils should be used. Optimally, coils are placed both distal and proximal to the bleeding site if the vessel has not been completely transsected. Distal embolization will prevent retrograde bleeding from collaterals beyond the

26

Pudendal Arteriography

SAMUEL I. WAHL, MICHAEL B. RUBIN, AND CURTIS W. BAKAL

Neurologic activity through the internal pudendal sensory nerves and the parasympathetic cavernosal motor nerves is responsible for developing and maintaining an erection. Arterial dilatation and a rapid increase in blood flow to the penis result from relaxation of the smooth muscles in the wall of the cavernosal arteries in response to parasympathetic stimulation. As distention increases, the small veins that drain the corpora are compressed against the tunica albuginea, preventing outflow of blood and maintaining penile erection.[1–3] Impotence is the inability to achieve and maintain an erection. In the patient with normal neurologic function and normal endocrine balance, impotence may be due to venous incompetence or arterial insufficiency. Duplex sonography and pulse-waved Doppler analysis have been widely used to evaluate penile arterial anatomy; pudendal arteriography remains the "gold standard" for penile arterial evaluation.[4–6] Arteriography has identified diffuse bilateral disease of the internal pudendal, common penile, and cavernosal arteries in impotent patients with atherosclerosis. Focal stenosis or occlusion involving the common penile or cavernosal artery is seen most often in young men who have a history of blunt perineal or pelvic trauma.[7]

Pudendal arteriography also can be useful in the evaluation and treatment of both low-flow (ischemic) and high-flow (nonischemic) priapism, a condition of persistent erection of the penis, often accompanied by pain and tenderness.

Traditionally, priapism has been classified as being either idiopathic or secondary. Hemodynamically and angiographically, it can be separated into two distinct types: more common low-flow (ischemic) priapism secondary to venous occlusion and less common high-flow (nonischemic) priapism caused by unregulated arterial flow.[8] The exact pathophysiology of high-flow priapism is unknown, but it is associated almost exclusively with direct penile trauma.[9–11]

■ Duplex Ultrasonography

Duplex ultrasonography is currently used as a screening modality to assess both function and anatomy.[12] A high-frequency linear transducer (7–10 MHz) is used to examine the penis in transverse axis both in a flaccid state and after intracavernosal injection of a vasoactive agent or prostaglandin E. Some authors advocate using the change in the cavernosal arterial diameter before and after injection as an indicator of arterial insufficiency.[3–5,13,14] Most authors agree that the most sensitive parameter for identifying a patient with arterial insufficiency is the mean peak systolic velocity.[5,13] Normal mean peak systolic velocity ranges from 35 to 60 cm per second. Peak systolic velocities of 25 to 35 cm per second indicate moderate arterial sufficiency, and velocities less than 25 cm per second correspond to severe arterial insufficiency, usually requiring surgical revascularization or prosthetic implantation.[7] Although the reported accuracy, noninvasiveness and relative expense of duplex sonography would appear to be advantageous compared with transcatheter arteriography, it is highly operator dependent. Arterial variability of the penis also may affect sonographic interpretation.[16–18] For example, in up to 30% of potent volunteers,[19] congenital anomalies such as either unilateral absence or hypoplasia of one dorsal artery may lead to frequent misinterpretation (Fig. 26-1). Other technical

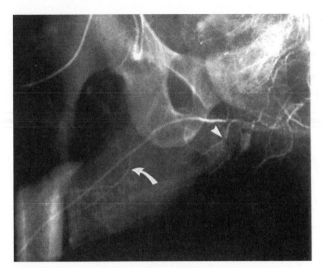

FIGURE 26-1. Aberrant origin of the left cavernosal artery (*curved arrow*). Sonographic evaluation at the base of the penis (*arrowhead*) may lead to misinterpretation.

limitations decrease the accuracy of ultrasound. Thus, ultrasound is used most frequently as a screening tool, and many urologic surgeons will proceed to pudendal arteriography to confirm the presence of arterial occlusive disease and plan intervention.

■ Pudendal Arteriography

Pudendal arteriography is an anatomic rather than a functional study, which we consider necessary in any potential candidate for penile arterial reconstruction. High-quality selective bilateral penile pharmacoarteriography is necessary to appreciate the type and frequency of anatomic variance, site of obstruction, and potential collateral routes in patients suspected of having arterial occlusions.

Impotence

We generally perform arteriography on an outpatient basis with the patient under mild conscious sedation. Multiplanar pelvic arteriography is performed to exclude the possibility of significant proximal lesions in the common and internal iliac arteries and to identify any anomalous origins of the penile arteries. This study usually is performed from the right common femoral artery with a 4- or 5-Fr pigtail catheter. We then proceed to selective left internal iliac artery catheterization with a 4- or 5-French Cobra 2 catheter. Superselective catheterization of the anterior division is often necessary to demonstrate the vascular anatomy adequately. The internal pudendal artery is identified by its characteristic course across the middle of the obturator foramen in the ipsilateral anterior oblique

position. We routinely use an intracavernosal injection of 60 mg of papaverine for optimal visualization of the penile vascular anatomy, especially if superselective catheterization of the internal pudendal artery is not possible. Some authors have found that vasodilatation with direct intrapudendal arterial injections of vasoactive drugs, such as nitroglycerin or papaverine, can overcome the vasoconstriction in the small or medium-sized arteries and consequent poor visualization of these vessels.[19] Others have found that intracavernosal papaverine–phentolamine combinations are helpful.[18] After completion of the left-sided study, it is usually possible to use the same cobra-shaped catheter to perform the ipsilateral, right-sided catheterization; in a few instances, a recurvant catheter, such as a Sos-1 catheter (Angiodynamics, Queensbury, NY), may be needed. We routinely use low osmolar contrast, filming in the ipsilateral anterior oblique projection. The penis is generally draped across the contralateral thigh in a profile position so that the cavernosal and dorsal arteries are not superimposed.

It is imperative that pudendal arteriography include visualization of both inferior epigastric arteries, because these arteries are the preferred donor vessels when planning penile revascularization surgery. There is no single type of revascularization surgery that fits every case; therefore, a pudendal arteriogram is also necessary for selection of the recipient vessel. Connecting the donor artery to a branch of the dorsal penile artery in an end-to-side fashion or, when possible, with an end-to-end anastomosis that allows the most efficient runoff is the preferred method of surgical revascularization. This method is possible if the dorsal penile artery has clearly demonstrated good branches to the cavernosal artery on the arteriogram. In the event that no such branches exist or no suitable dorsal arteries are available, revascularization of an isolated segment of deep dorsal vein with good communicators to the intracavernous tissue is the choice for the recipient vessel.[20,21]

The classic angiography pattern of penile anatomy demonstrates bilateral symmetry with a single pudendal artery on each side that gives rise to scrotal branches, where it becomes the common penile artery. The common penile artery divides into one dorsal penile artery, one cavernosal artery, and one bulbar artery (Fig. 26-2).[22,23] Generally, transverse root collaterals, a single spongiosal artery, and perforating arteries between the dorsal penile and cavernosal arteries also are seen. These vascular patterns are highly variable, and potent men may exhibit anatomy that differs from the classic pattern[24] which actually may be found only in a minority of patients. Occasionally, normal variance of penile anatomy may be confused with arterial occlusive disease when there is a unilateral origin of all cavernosal branches, unilateral hypoplasia of a dorsal penile artery, and aberrant origins of bulbar or cavernosal arteries (Table 26-1).

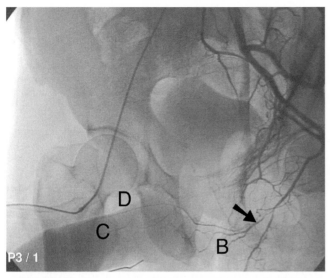

FIGURE 26-2. The classic penile arterial anatomy. The internal pudendal artery (*large arrow*) gives rise to a scrotal branch (*small arrow*), becoming the common penile artery (*arrowhead*). The common penile artery divides into the dorsal penile (*D*) and cavernosal artery (*C*) and the bulbar arteries (*B*).

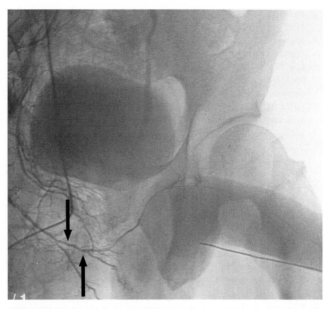

FIGURE 26-3. Right pudendal arteriogram demonstrating diffuse atherosclerotic changes (*arrows*).

In most patients who have arteriogenic impotence, the impaired penile perfusion is a component of generalized atherosclerosis (Fig. 26-3). Common risk factors associated with penile arterial insufficiency include hypertension, hyperlipidemia, diabetes mellitus, and cigarette smoking. Blunt perineal or pelvic trauma and pelvic irradiation are also well-known causes of insufficient penile blood flow.[7,25,26]

It is clinically important to be able to differentiate the cavernosal artery from the deep penile artery. Careful evaluation of the film and attention to technique usually will allow this differentiation.[17] Collateral roots that may assume functional impotence in patients with intrapenile occlusive disease include collateral communication from one side to another (for example, cavernosal artery to cavernosal artery through transverse communicators at the penile root) and communication between the dorsal and penile cavernosal arteries through perforating branches.

Priapism

On pudendal arteriography, only the dorsal penile and bulbar arteries are well visualized in low-flow priapism. Classically, the cavernosal arteries are not seen. Cavernosography will confirm the angiographic findings by demonstrating delayed venous drainage by as much as 15 minutes. In high-flow priapism resulting from trauma, abnormal rapid antegrade flow through the internal pudendal and penile arteries is seen, often with pooling of contrast in the corpus cavernosum from a ruptured cavernosal artery. Cavernosal artery to corpora cavernosal fistulae may be evident in an intense contrast blush at the base of the penis, frequently associated with rapid early filling of venous channels seen in the late arterial phase of filming.[8–11,27]

High-flow priapism often is treated effectively by using intracavernous vasoconstrictive agents or by surgical procedures designed to shunt blood away from the corpus cavernosum to the corpus spongiosum.[28] Surgical ligation of internal pudendal branch arteries also has been successful.[10] Successful superselective transcatheter embolization of the pudendal artery and its branches has been performed using autologous blood clot, absorbable gelatin sponge, and N-butyl-cyanoacrylate.[11,27–30] More recently, superselective embolization using platinum microcoils has been described.[31]

REFERENCES

1. Krane RJ. Sexual function and dysfunction. In: Walsh PC, Gittes RF, Perlmutter AD, Stanley TA, eds. *Campbell's urology.* Philadelphia: WB Saunders, 1986:700–735.

TABLE 26-1. *Penile Arterial Anatomic Variations*

Variant	Jarow et al. (5) (n = 42)	Bookstein and Lang (19) (n = 23)
Dorsal penile-cavernosal perforators	29%	91%
Accessory cavernosal branches	29%	57%
Bilateral cavernosals arising from one penile artery	41%	13%
Bilateral absence of cavernosals	2%	4%
Aberrant origin of cavernosal artery	12%	9%

2. Melman A. The evaluation of erectile dysfunction. *Urol Radiol* 1988;10:119–128.

3. Mueller SC, Lue TF. Evaluation of vasculogenic impotence. *Urol Clin North Am* 1988;15:65–76.

4. Lue TF, Hricek H, Marich KW, et al. Vasculogenic impotence evaluated by high-resolution, ultrasonography and pulsed Doppler analysis. *Radiology* 1987;59:777–781.

5. Jarow JP, Pugh VW, Routh WD, et al. Comparison of penile arterial anatomy affects interpretation of Doppler ultrasonography and pulsed Doppler spectrum analysis. *Invest Radiol* 1993;28:806–810.

6. Wahl SI, Rubin MB, Bakal CW. Radiologic evaluation of penile arterial anatomy in arteriogenic impotence. *Int J Impot Res* 1997;9:93–97.

7. Levine FJ, Greenfield AJ, Goldstein I. Arteriographically determined occlusive disease within the hypogastric-cavernous bed in impotent patients following blunt perineal and pelvic trauma. *J Urol* 1990;144:1147–1153.

8. Witt MA, Goldstein I, Saenz de Tejada I, et al. Traumatic laceration of intracavernosal arteries: the pathophysiology of nonischemic, high flow, arterial priapism. *J Urol* 1990;143:129–132.

9. Hauri D, Spycher M, Bruhlmann W. Erection and priapism: a new physiologic concept. *Urol Int* 1983;38:138.

10. Ricciardi R Jr, Bhatt GM, Cynamon J, et al. Delayed high flow priapism: pathophysiology and management. *J Urol* 1993;149:119–121.

11. Walker TG, Grant PW, Goldstein I, et al. "High-flow" priapism: treatment with superselective transcatheter embolization. *Radiology* 1990;174:1053–1057.

12. Lue TF, Hricek H, Marich KW, et al. Vasculogenic impotence evaluated by high-resolution ultrasonography and pulsed Doppler analysis. *Radiology* 1985;155:777.

13. Benson CB, Vickers MA. Sexual impotence caused by vascular disease: diagnosis by using duplex sonography. *AJR Am J Roentgenol* 1989;153:1149–1153.

14. Collins JP, Lewandowski BJ. Experience with intracorporal injection of papaverine and duplex ultrasound scanning for assessment of arteriogenic impotence. *Br J Urol* 1987;59:84–88.

15. Mellinger BC, Fried JT, Vaughn ED. Papaverine-induced penile blood flow acceleration in impotent men measured by duplex scanning. *J Urol* 1990;144:827.

16. Rajfer J, Canan V, Dorey FJ, et al. Correlation between penile angiography and duplex scanning of cavernous arteries in impotent men. *J Urol* 1990;143:1128.

17. Quam JP, King BF, James EM, et al. Duplex and color Doppler sonographic evaluation of vasculogenic impotence. *AJR Am J Roentgenol* 1989;153:1141–1147.

18. Chiang PH, Chiang CP, Wu CC, et al. Colour duplex sonography in the assessment of impotence. *Br J Urol* 1991;68:181–186.

19. Bahren W, Gall H, Scherb C, et al. Arterial anatomy and arteriographic diagnosis of arteriogenic impotence. *Cardiovasc Intervt Radiol* 1988;11:195–210.

20. Hatzichristou D, Goldstein I. Penile microvascular and arterial bypass surgery. *Urol Clin North Am* 1993;1:39–60.

21. Hawatmeh IS, Houttuin E, Gregory JG, et al. Vascular surgery for the treatment of the impotent male. In: Krane RJ, Siroky MB, Goldstein I, eds. *Male sexual dysfunction.* Boston: Little, Brown, 1983:683–690.

22. Ferner H, Straubesand J, eds. *Sobotta atlas of human anatomy,* vol 2, 10th ed. Baltimore: Urban & Schwartzberg, 1983:200–201.

23. Kadir S. *Atlas of normal and variant angiographic anatomy.* Philadelphia: WB Saunders, 1991:227–293.

24. Bookstein JJ, Lang EV. Penile magnification pharmacoarteriography: details of intrapenile arterial anatomy. *AJR Am J Roentgenol* 1987;146:883–888.

25. Goldstein I, Feldman MI, Deckers PJ, et al. Radiation-associated impotence: a clinical study of its mechanism. *JAMA* 1984;251:259–266.

26. Rosen MP, Greenfield AJ, Walker TG, et al. Arteriogenic impotence: findings in 195 impotent men examined with selective internal pudendal angiography. *Radiology* 1990;151:80–90.

27. Steers WD, Selby JB. Use of methylene blue and selective embolization of the pudendal artery for high flow priapism refractory to medical and surgical treatments. *J Urol* 1991;146:1361–1363.

28. Bertram RA, Webster GD, Carson CC III. Priapism: etiology, treatment, and results in series of 35 presentations. *Urology* 1985;26:229–235.

29. Alvarez Gonzalez E, Pamplona M, et al. High flow priapism after blunt perineal trauma: resolution with bucrylate embolization. *J Urol* 1994;151:426–428.

30. Numan F, Cakirer S, Islak C, et al. Post-traumatic high-flow priapism treated by N-butyl-cyanoacrylate embolization. *Cardiovasc Intervent Radiol* 1996;19:278–280.

31. Kerlan RK, Gordon RL, LaBerge J, et al. Superselective microcoil embolization in the management of high-flow priapism. *J Vasc Interv Radiol* 1998;9:85–89.

27

Varicocele and Female Infertility

MELVIN ROSENBLATT and KEVIN W. DICKEY

Since the beginning of recorded history, humans have placed an emphasis on fertility. In many cultures, childlessness is viewed as a deficiency on the part of both male and female partners. Even in today's modern society, procreation is considered a basic human right, and infertile couples must cope with difficult psychological and social problems. Unfortunately, the incidence of infertility in newly married couples is on the rise. In industrialized countries, the incidence of infertility has increased from 7 to 8% in 1960 up to 20 to 35% today.[1] In response to the growing problem, new medical therapies have been advanced both to diagnose and to treat the wide variety of disorders that can cause infertility. Over the past two decades, advances in fluoroscopically guided catheter techniques have helped to treat some of these disorders. This chapter reviews these techniques as they pertain to the treatment of varicoceles, fallopian tube occlusions, and cervical stenosis.

■ Varicoceles

Varicocele, defined as abnormal distention of veins in the pampiniform plexus, has long been recognized to be associated with testicular dysfunction (Fig. 27-1). As early as the first century AD, Celsus described the association between swollen veins over the testes and testicular atrophy.[2] The realization that varicocele ablation can restore testicular function was made in the late 1800s when Barwell described the restoration of testicular function with subsequent conception after varicocele occlusion.[3] Although the association with testicular dysfunction was recognized, treatment was primarily directed toward the relief of painful symptoms. The procedure was not used to repair varicoceles in infertile males. It was not until 1952, when Tuloch reported the restoration of fertility in an azospermic male, that varicocele ligation as a treatment for infertility gained widespread acceptance.[4] Since then, varicocelectomy has become the most common operation performed for male infertility.[5]

The importance of the varicocele and its role in infertility lies in its common occurrence in the general population. Among young men, the reported incidence of varicoceles in the literature ranges from 5 to 26% with a mean incidence of approximately 15%.[6-11] The incidence among infertile men is much higher, occurring in approximately 40% of patients.[12,13]

Treatment for this disorder has focused on the ligation of the spermatic vein, and various surgical techniques have been described in the literature.[14-17] In 1977, Iaccarino described a percutaneous technique for radiologically sclerosing the spermatic vein.[18] Since its introduction, technical enhancement and the development of newer embolic agents has made this a safe, effective, and relatively simple procedure.

Anatomy

The veins of the spermatic cord emerge from the mediastinum of the testicle to form the pampiniform plexus, which consists of three groups of freely anastomosing veins: the anterior, middle, and posterior. The external spermatic vein and the cremasteric veins constitute the posterior group. These veins course posterior to the spermatic cord and drain into the inferior epigastric veins at the level of the external inguinal ring. The middle group

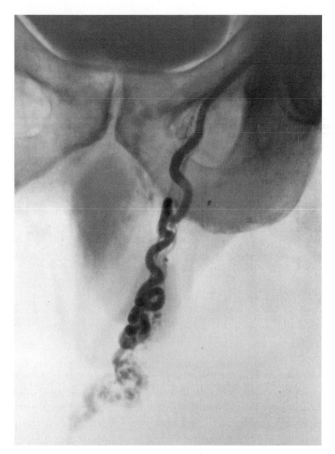

FIGURE 27-1. Internal spermatic vein (ISV) venogram demonstrating the reflux of contrast material into the dilated veins of a left varicocele. This image normally should not be obtained because the scrotum should be shielded from radiation exposure during venography.

courses medially along the vas deferens and drains into the internal iliac veins. The anterior group, or the internal spermatic vein (ISV), accompanies the spermatic artery as it courses through the retroperitonium. On the left side, the ISV drains into the left renal vein. On the right, the ISV usually enters the inferior vena cava (IVC) just below the origin of the right renal vein (Fig. 27-2). Drainage of the right ISV into the right renal vein has been noted in 10% of cases.[19] In most instances, the ISV contains valves that are normally located within one centimeter of the vein opening.[20]

The anatomy of the ISV is highly variable, and multiple collateral pathways exist. Knowledge of these pathways offers insight into the pathogenesis of varicoceles and is important in providing effective treatment.[21,22] Several collateral pathways anastomose with the upper portion of the ISV. These pathways include hilar, capsular, intrarenal, retroperitoneal and colonic communications (see Fig. 27-2). Hilar collaterals, which emanate from the hilar portion of the renal vein and anastomose with the

ISV, are present in 14% of patients (Fig. 27-3).[23] Capsular collaterals arise from intrarenal or capsular veins and pursue a tortuous course before joining the ISV. Retroperitoneal collaterals, which are present in 40% of patients, provide communications between the upper ISV and lumbar veins (Fig. 27-4).[24] Communications occur frequently between the colic veins, the inferior mesenteric vein on the left, and the superior mesenteric vein on the right.[24] These vessels usually contain valves and join with the ISV at the level of the iliac crest. Bridging collaterals, draining directly into the IVC, also occur but involve the right ISV far more often than the left.[24] All these collateral pathways, when present, can permit venous reflux by bypassing competent ISV valves.

Collaterals that anastomose with the lower portion of the ISV include parallel channels and venous communications to the internal iliac and inferior epigastric veins. Parallel channels are fine, multiple, threadlike veins that originate and terminate in the ISV (Fig. 27-5). If left unoccluded, these seemingly insignificant vessels can, in time, enlarge and reconstitute the ISV. Collaterals to the internal iliac and inferior epigastric veins are infrequent; for example, internal iliac vein anastomoses were found to be present in only 2% of cases.[24]

Etiology

Varicoceles can be primary or secondary. Secondary varicoceles usually occur in older patients and result from spermatic or renal vein obstruction by tumor or massive hydronephrosis.[25,26] Primary varicocele, by far the more common type, is most prevalent in adolescent males and occurs on the left side in approximately 90% of cases.[27] It is bilateral in 8 to 9% and is right-sided in 1 to 2%.[28] Several hypotheses have been advanced to explain this asymmetric presentation. Incomplete or absent valves, which occur more frequently on the left side, have been cited as one possible explanation (Fig. 27-6). Ahlberg et al. found absent valves in 40% of left spermatic veins examined at autopsy compared with 23% on the right.[19] Unfortunately, the frequent occurrence of valvular abnormalities is inconsistent with the relatively low 15% incidence of varicoceles in the general population. Additionally, several investigators have noted varicoceles in patients with competent ISV valves.[29] Other hypotheses, such as the vertical course and perpendicular insertion of the left spermatic vein[30] and the nutcracker phenomenon, have been proposed. The *nutcracker phenomenon* is compression of the left renal vein between the aorta and the superior mesenteric artery in the upright position.[31–33] The physiologic obstruction of the renal vein leads to increased hydrostatic pressure in the left ISV and formation of the varicocele. More recently, a developmental etiology has been advanced. The embryogenesis of the left venous system is more complex than the right,

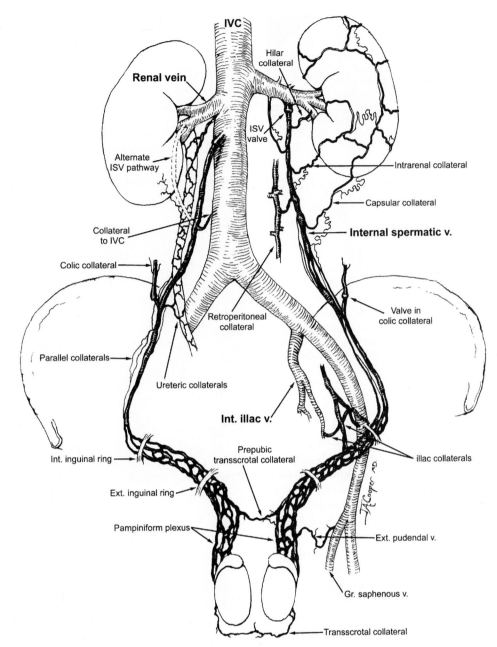

FIGURE 27-2. Venous anatomy of the internal spermatic veins.

and developmental anomalies are common. Disordered involution of the cardinal veins during development results in persistent intercardinal vein anastomoses. These collaterals permit retrograde flow in the ISV and varicocele formation.[29]

Pathophysiology

There is great debate about whether and how varicoceles effect spermatogenesis. Some investigators claim that the relationship, if any, is coincidental.[34] Others have dem-

onstrated significant alterations in sperm density motility and morphology in association with varicoceles.[35, 36] How the varicocele, which is predominantly a unilateral process, causes bilateral testicular dysfunction is obscure. Several hypotheses, including scrotal hyperthermia,[37] retrograde flow of toxic metabolite such as prostaglandin's E_2 and $F_2\alpha$[38,39] and hypoxia due to venous stasis, have been advanced.[40] It is possible that many of these factors act in conjunction to cause impaired spermatogenesis. This damage, once begun, progresses over time and results in testicular atrophy and irreversible cellular damage.

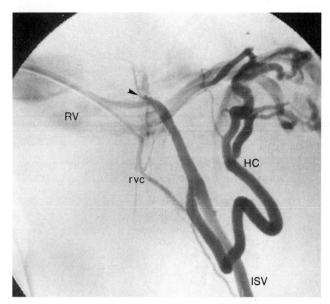

FIGURE 27-3. Left internal spermatic vein (ISV) venogram demonstrating an atypical origin of the ISV from the superior aspect of the left renal vein (*arrowhead*) as well as a large hilar and smaller renal vein (RV) collateral. RVC, renal vein collateral; HC, hilar collateral.

Diagnosis

Varicoceles are diagnosed most often on clinical examination and are described by their size. A grade 1 varicocele is small and can be palpated only while the patient performs a valsalva maneuver. Grade 2 varicoceles are easily palpable but are not visible, whereas grade 3 varicoceles can be detected by visual scrutiny alone.[41] Varicoceles that cannot be detected by careful clinical examination have been termed *subclinical varicoceles,* which are defined as reflux in the ISV without palpable distention of the pampiniform plexus.[42] The significance of the subclinical varicocele, as it relates to infertility, is a subject of ongoing debate. A recent review by Marshman et al. discovered that most investigators believe this type of varicocele can cause infertility and they argue in the favor of treatment.[43] These arguments are based on observed improvement in fertility after subclinical varicocelectomy[44] and the lack of correlation between varicocele size and degree of infertility.[45,46]

Several noninvasive diagnostic modalities are used to detect subclinical varicoceles; including thermography,[47] Doppler ultrasound,[48] radionuclide imaging,[49] and real-time ultrasound,[46] which have varying degrees of sensitivity and specificity.[50,51] At present, real-time scrotal ultrasound is the preferred noninvasive imaging modality used to detect subclinical venous dilatation and reflux. The presence of a varicocele is confirmed by the visualization of two to three dilated venous channels with diameters larger than 3 mm that increase in size in the erect position or with a valsalva maneuver.[46] Using these criteria, Hamm

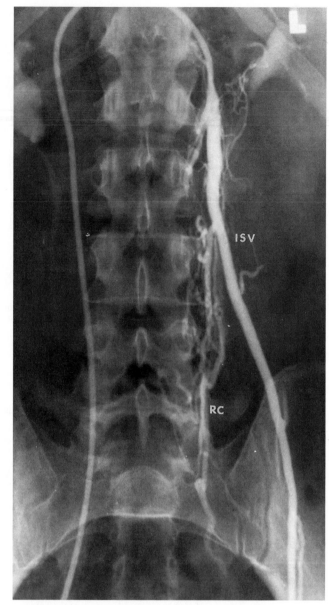

FIGURE 27-4. Left internal spermatic vein (ISV) venogram demonstrating multiple retroperitoneal collaterals (RC).

et al. reported a sensitivity of 92.2% and a specificity of 100%.[52]

Spermatic venography was considered the most accurate means by which venous reflux could be demonstrated.[19] Recently, the value of venography has been questioned. Netto et al. demonstrated reflux in normal subjects and showed no correlation between the presence of reflux and alteration in spermatogenesis.[53] A criticism of this study is that the venograms were performed with the catheter tip in the spermatic vein orifice, which can bypass a proximal valve and artificially demonstrates reflux. Considering the controversial value of venography and its invasive nature, this procedure should be reserved

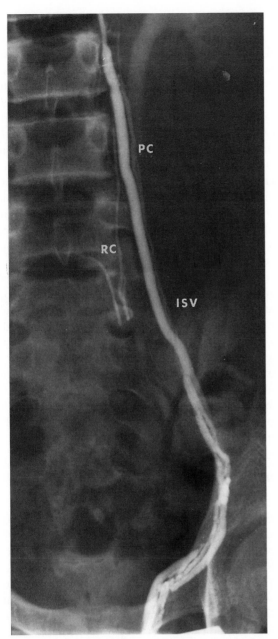

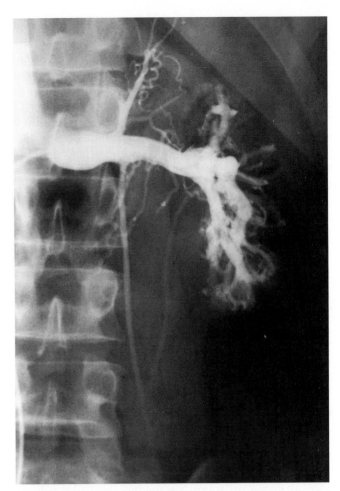

FIGURE 27-6. Left renal venogram demonstrating an incompetent proximal internal spermatic vein (ISV) valve with retrograde filling of the ISV. RV, renal vein.

FIGURE 27-5. Left spermatic venogram demonstrating multiple threadlike parallel veins as well as a small retroperitoneal collateral (RC). IVC, internal spermatic vein; PC, parallel collaterals.

for the determination of venous anatomy just prior to percutaneous occlusion.

Treatment

Indications

Indications for therapeutic varicocele occlusion include pain, disfigurement, male-factor infertility, and, in the adolescent, early evidence of testicular dysfunction. Although discomfort and disfigurement are straightforward

indications for treatment, infertility is not. In the infertile couple, the presence of a varicocele in the male partner, although known to cause progressive deterioration in spermatogenesis, is not indicative of oligospermia. In fact, a majority of patients with varicoceles have sperm counts well above the accepted lower limits of normal. These limits, established by the World Health Organization (WHO), are 20 million sperm per milliliter, with a progressive motility of 40 to 60%.[54] Hargreave reported a 20% incidence of varicoceles among the men seen in his infertility clinic: however, only 6.4% had a varicocele associated with sperm densities lower than 20 million per milliliter.[2] To confuse the issue further, many men with oligospermia have been able to father children. In 1993 Hargreave et al. reported that in the absence of other factors, the future chances of pregnancy decrease only when the motile sperm concentration (percent motility × sperm density) falls below 2 million per milliliter, which is well below the WHO lower limits of normal.[2] In this same study, an inverse relationship was shown to exist between the duration of involuntary infertility and the likelihood of future pregnancy. Thus, the longer a couple has been trying, the less likely they are to conceive without therapeutic intervention. Taking these issues into consideration, our current indication for therapeutic varicocele occlusion as a treatment for male infertility is the lack of conception after 12 months of unprotected intercourse in association with a sperm motile density below WHO lower limits.

In the adolescent, an asymptomatic varicocele is cause for concern because of potential future deleterious effects on fertility. The progressive, time-dependent, spermatotoxic effects of varicoceles have been demonstrated in both animal and human studies.[35,55,56] There is a large difference in the incidence of palpable varicoceles between men of couples who have never been able to produce children (*primary infertility*) and men of couples who have produced children in the past but are currently infertile (*secondary infertility*).[57] This difference, 35% versus 81%, respectively, strongly suggests that infertility is acquired from the presence of a long-standing varicocele. Cheval and Purcell demonstrated a time-dependent decline in sperm density and motility in a group of men with varicoceles who initially had normal semen parameters.[58] The difficulty is that not all varicoceles will cause clinically relevant future testicular damage. Therapy based on the presence of a varicocele alone could result in substantial overtreatment. Therefore, specific features need to be identified that will indicate which patients are at higher risk for future infertility. The most commonly used indicators are based on sperm parameters, testicular volume measurements, and endocrine assessment.

In the older teenager, semen samples are often not difficult to obtain. An abnormal result in a teenager with a varicocele is an indication for treatment. In an adolescent in whom it is not possible to obtain a semen specimen, loss of testicular volume ipsilateral to the varicocele indicating testicular growth arrest is considered to be the primary indication for treatment.[59,60] Testicular volume can be measured by careful physical examination[61] or by ultrasonography.[60] Typically, there should be no more than a 2-mL difference between testes. When the volume difference exceeds 3 mL, varicocele occlusion should be performed.[56] In the absence of discernible testicular volume loss, the gonadotropin releasing hormone stimulation test (Gn/RH) can help to identify men who show early evidence of testicular injury. A supranormal leuteinizing hormone and follicle stimulating hormone response to intravenous Gn/RH indicates Leydig's cell and seminiferous tubule dysfunction.[56,59] This type of response, if noted in an adolescent with a varicocele, is an indication for therapy.

Surgical treatment

The surgical approach to the treatment of varicoceles can be low (inguinal) or high (retroperitoneal) ligation of the ISVs. The inguinal approach, or *modified Ivanissevich procedure*, involves making a small incision over the inguinal canal to expose the spermatic and cremasteric veins. These veins are dissected free of the surrounding structures (vas deferens and testicular artery) and ligated.[16] The retroperitoneal approach, or modified *Palomo procedure*, exposes the ISV within the retroperitoneum after it exits the inguinal canal[17] To accomplish this, a small abdominal incision is made at the level of the internal inguinal ring. The fibers of the external oblique faschia and internal oblique muscle are divided to expose the dilated ISVs. Once identified, the veins are ligated and divided. Recently, laparoscopic ligation of the ISVs has become popular. This technique requires three intraperitoneal entry points for placement of the laparoscope and operative instruments.[62] With the laparoscope, the inner surface of the abdominal wall can be visualized, revealing either the right or left ISV coursing through the retroperitoneum just above the internal inguinal ring. To access these veins, the parietal peritoneum is incised and the veins are isolated and ligated. Proponents of this technique have demonstrated its safety and efficacy.[63,64] Critics argue that the laparoscopic approach transforms a simple extraperitoneal procedure performed through a single incision with local anesthesia into an intraabdominal procedure requiring three separate incisions and general anesthesia.[65,66]

Percutaneous occlusion

Approach

A method for selectively catheterizing the ISV from a femoral vein approach was first described in 1976;[67] just one year later, this approach was used to occlude a refluxing ISV percutaneous.[18,68] Today, femoral vein catheterization is the most commonly used approach for embolization of spermatic veins.[69,70] From the right common femoral vein, the left ISV can be catheterized with a 7.3 Fr Hopkins curved catheter (Cordis Corp., Miami, FL) (Fig. 27-7). This catheter is placed in the distal left renal vein and is gently pulled back to engage the orifice of the left ISV (Fig. 27-8A). The right ISV, arising from IVC, can be catheterized with a 6 or 7 Fr Simmons-shaped catheter (Fig. 27-8B). The acute angle at which the right ISV arises from the IVC makes catheterization from the femoral route more difficult. Great care must be taken to avoid inadvertent dissection of the vein orifice with the catheter tip. After engaging the ISV orifice, subselective catheterization is often required to deliver the embolic agent, which can be difficult from a femoral approach because the direction of catheter tip travel is opposite the direction of applied force. The use of a 7 or 8 Fr Hopkins curved guiding catheter permits coaxial catheterization of the ISV and remedies this problem.[71]

The difficulties associated with the catheterization of

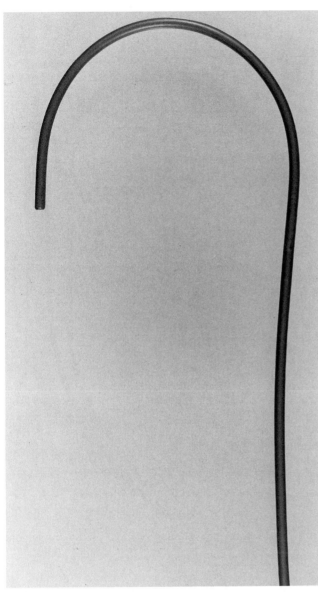

FIGURE 27-7. A 7.3 Fr Hopkins curved catheter (Cook, Bloomington, IN).

the ISV from the femoral vein prompted other investigators to advocate an internal jugular or basilic vein approach.[72–75] From the internal jugular vein, a modified 7 Fr headhunter catheter can be used to select the origin of the right or left ISV.[73,74] From this route, catheter travel and applied force are in alignment, thus facilitating deep catheterization of the vein. Additionally, the recovery period required after catheterization of the internal jugular vein is somewhat shorter than the recovery period required after femoral vein catheterization.

Venography

Irrespective of the route used, once the origin of the ISV is catheterized, a venogram must be performed. This is accomplished by vigorously injecting 10 to 20 mL of contrast material into the vein orifice while the patient performs a valsalva maneuver. Alternatively, if a tilt table is available, the contrast can be injected with the patient in reverse Trendelenberg position. The resulting images can be recorded digitally or on a series of cut-film radiographs. The purpose of the venogram is to confirm the presence of venous reflux and to delineate the highly variable anatomy of the ISV. The anatomic information helps determine which embolic agent will best provide effective occlusion. On occasion, even with a clinically obvious varicocele, a competent ISV valve is present and no reflux can be demonstrated. In this setting, anastomosing bypass channels to the distal renal vein, capsular veins, or retroperitoneal veins must be present.[23,76,77] A renal venogram sometimes can help to identify these collaterals. Unfortunately, the collateral branches are often small and tortuous and will not fill from an injection into the main renal vein. Furthermore, many of the collateral branches responsible for retrograde flow in the ISV do not drain into the renal vein. To demonstrate these collaterals more reliably, a venogram should be performed after catheterizing across the competent valve. This approach not only better defines the anatomy of the ISV it also allows an embolic agent to be deposited below the insertion of these collaterals, thus permanently preventing reflux into the veins of the pampiniform plexus (Fig. 27-9).[78]

Embolotherapy

The goal of percutaneous therapy is to eliminate congestion in the veins of the pampiniform plexus by occluding the refluxing ISV and all its collateral tributaries. Sclerosing agents, tissue adhesives (histoacryl), stainless steel coils, and detachable balloons all have been used to accomplish this task. Of these, no single agent has proved to be clearly superior. Each agent possesses its unique advantages and disadvantages.

Sclerotherapy

Several different sclerosing agents are used for the treatment of varicoceles. Aethoxysklerol (polidocanol),[79] Sotradecol (sodium, tetradecyl, sulfate),[80] Varicocid (sodium, morrhuate, benzyl alcohol),[81] ethanol,[82] and boiling contrast[83] all have proved effective. Aethoxysklerol and Varicocid are not approved by the U.S. Food and Drug Administration (FDA) and therefore not available in the United States. Sclerosants are easily delivered by directly injecting them into the proximal ISV. Effectiveness depends on the amount injected and the length of time the sclerosant remains in contact with the veins. Ideally, the entire ISV and all its parallel collaterals should be filled with sclerosant medium for several minutes. For this reason, relative stasis in the ISV should be

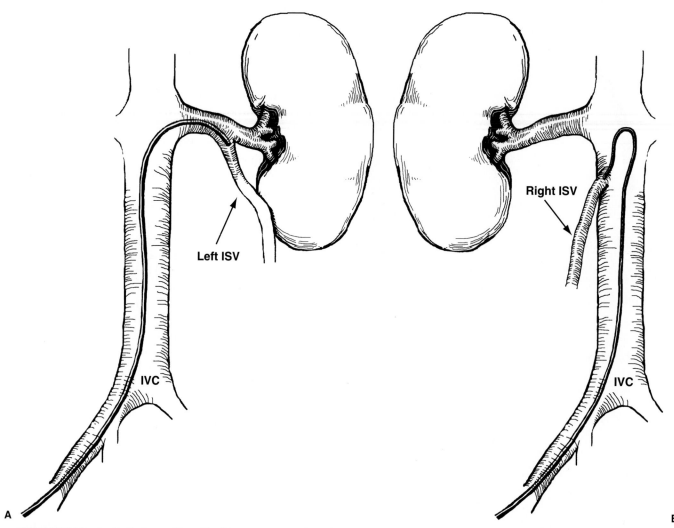

FIGURE 27-8. A: Catheters with a Hopkins curve permit catheterization of left internal spermatic vein (ISV) from the femoral vein. **B:** From the femoral vein, Simmons-shaped catheters can be used to select the origin of the right ISV when it arises from the inferior vena cava (IVC).

present. Often, just catheterization of the vein orifice can cause significant stasis. With larger ISVs, stasis can be achieved by placing a proximal occlusion balloon.[84] Once flow in the ISV has been halted, the sclerosant can be injected. The sclerosant, if not radiopaque, should be mixed with contrast so that its venous distribution can be monitored with fluoroscopy. The total amount injected depends on the capacitance of the ISV. An occlusion rate of 100% was accomplished when the ratio of the injected sclerosant to the calculated ISV volume was greater than 40%. To do so, an average of 24 mL of boiling contrast was used.[83] With other sclerosants, such as Varicocid, only 3 to 5 mL is injected.[81,85] It is important, however, to avoid overinjection and reflux of sclerosant into critical vascular beds. Proximal reflux can cause renal vein thrombosis. Distal reflux into the pampiniform plexus can result in severe thrombophlebitis, testicular atrophy, and aspermia[83] this can be prevented by externally compressing

the ISV against the superior pubis ramus. Compression, which can be applied with a specially designed device,[86] always should be used when a sclerosant is used. Some investigators have mixed the sclerosant medium with Gelfoam particles (Upjohn, Kalamazoo, MI) or air in an effort to slow its flow in the ISV.[87] This approach reduces the likelihood of reflux and increases the time the agent remains in contact with the veins.

The advantages of sclerotherapy are several. For one, because the sclerosant is a fluid, it can enter and obliterate all the numerous collateral channels, thus reducing the likelihood of recurrence. Recurrence rates after sclerotherapy have been reported to range from 2 to 19%;[85] however, most studies report a recurrence rate of only 2 to 3%. Another advantage is the ability to deliver the agent through small vessels that are difficult to catheterize and still effect distal occlusion. Lastly, these agents are inexpensive compared with other types of embolic agents.

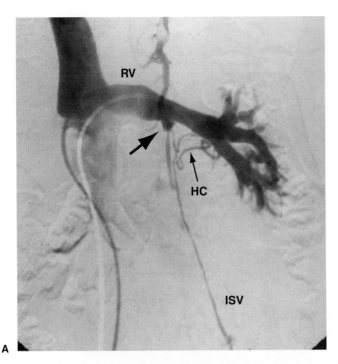

A

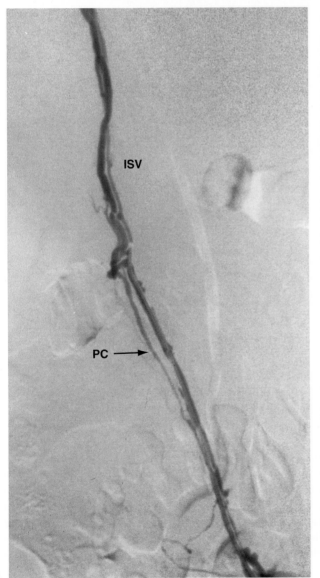

B

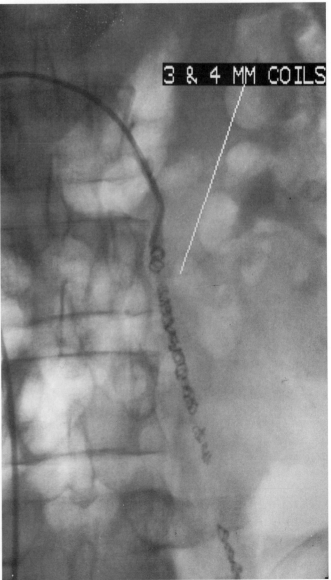

C

FIGURE 27-9. **A:** Left renal vein venogram demonstrating a competent internal spermatic vein (ISV) valve (*solid arrow*) with partial opacification of the ISV through hilar collaterals (HC). **B:** A venogram performed after selective catheterization across the proximal valve better demonstrates the venous anatomy of the ISV. Parallel collateral (PC) is noted. **C:** Catheterization across the valve permits distal embolization of the ISV. The entire ISV is filled with 3- and 4-mm coils to occlude all parallel collaterals and to prevent recurrence.

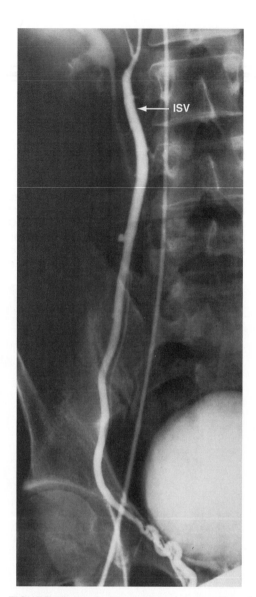

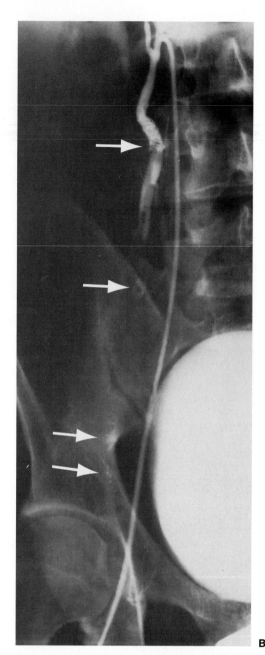

FIGURE 27-10. A: Right internal spermatic vein (ISV) venogram demonstrating reflux. **B:** Coils are deposited at various levels to occlude the ISV and all collaterals (*solid arrows*).

Disadvantages of sclerotherapy are severe pain on injection, pampiniform thrombophlebitis, and renal vein thrombosis. Injection discomfort is noted with all these agents but is most pronounced with the injection of hot contrast.[83] The discomfort is short-lived, lasting from several seconds to a few minutes. Pampiniform plexitis from the sclerosant has a reported incidence of 0.5 to 1.5%.[69,87–89] Renal vein thrombosis rarely occurs but has been reported.[83] Both complications can be prevented by balloon occlusion to prevent proximal reflux, adequate external compression to prevent distal reflux, and careful fluoroscopic monitoring.

Tissue Adhesive

In 1979 Kunnen described the technique of varicocele occlusion with tissue adhesive.[90] Histoacryl (N-butyl cyanoacrylate), which is currently not FDA approved and therefore unavailable in the United States, polymerizes on contact with blood to form an occluding cast of the vessel injected. The material must be delivered inferior to the lowest anastomosis between the ISV and perirenal venous plexus, which requires subselective coaxial catheterization with a mirocatheter. Although a complete description of this technique is beyond the scope of this chapter, several technical points are important. Because the material polymerizes on contact with any ionic solution, steps must be taken to avoid this from occurring prematurely by mixing the material with an oil-based contrast material (Ethiodol, Savage Laboratories, Melville, NY) in a ratio of approximately 1 to 3 parts contrast to 1 part tissue adhesive. Thus, the agent is opacified and its polymerization is slowed. The resulting mixture can be delivered to the site of embolization only by flushing it through the microcatheter with a nonionic glucose solution (D5W). The delivery catheter, which should be used only once, must be flushed thoroughly with the glucose solution before the agent is introduced. After delivering the agent, the catheter must be retracted immediately to avoid inadvertent adherence of the catheter to the vein wall.

The merits of tissue adhesive are its ability to penetrate and rapidly occlude the multiple collateral channels of the ISV without extending into critical vascular beds. Unfortunately, this technique has numerous drawbacks. Preparation and use of this material require extensive experience. If the material is not mixed or delivered properly, several complications can occur. Slow delivery or rapid polymerization can result in inadvertent permanent adherence of the catheter tip to the vein wall.[91] Rapid delivery or slow polymerization can result in reflux and embolization to the pampiniform plexus, renal vein, or lung.

Coils

Stainless steel coils, developed in 1975 for vascular occlusion, first were used by Thelen to treat varicoceles in 1979.[92] These devices, which come in sizes ranging from 3 to 15 mm, can be extruded from the tip of a catheter to fill and occlude a vessel. Today, commonly used coils are constructed from wire ranging in thickness from 0.018 to 0.038 inch. The 0.018-inch coils can be delivered through 3 Fr microcatheters and usually are constructed from platinum wire to increase their radiopacity. The 0.038-inch coils are relatively inexpensive and are the most commonly used type. These coils can be delivered through 5 Fr or larger catheters. To occlude the varicocele effectively using this device, subselective catheterization of the ISV is necessary. Ideally, the distal nest of coils should be placed below the inferior-most collateral entering the ISV, usually at the level of the internal inguinal ring. After placing the distal-most coils, the catheter is retracted and the ISV is occluded at various levels adjacent to the takeoff of parallel channels. The last series of coils is placed near the origin of the ISV (Fig. 27-10). Great care must be taken to avoid prolapse of the coils into the renal vein or IVC. On occasion, subselective catheterization can be difficult particularly from a femoral vein approach. Jugular access eases deep catheterization of the ISV, and several investigators favor this approach.[72,74] The use of a coaxial microcatheter through a larger guiding catheter also permits deep catheterization

of the ISV.[93] Unfortunately, only the more expensive microcoils can be delivered through these small catheters. Even with these limitations, the success rates for this technique have been reported to range from 80 to 100% for the left ISV and 73 to 90% for the right.[74,92–96]

Availability, reduced cost, and ease of use are the main advantages of coil embolization. The disadvantages are those associated with the difficulty in subselective catheterization and precise placement of a foreign body. Complications related to use of coils in the ISV include severe venous spasm,[74] coil extension into the renal vein or IVC, and transient groin and flank pain in 17% of patients.[97] Rarely, this discomfort is persistent. Hargreave reported a single case in which coils had to be surgically removed after six months because the patient experienced persistent pain.[2]

Detachable balloons

In 1981 White et al. reported their initial experience with varicocele occlusion using a detachable balloon occlusion device known as the Silicone Mini Balloon (Becton-Dickinson, Rutherford, NJ).[98] This device gained FDA approval in 1982 and was used extensively for treatment of this and other disorders. In 1990, the manufacturer withdrew this device from the market for financial reasons. At that time, two other detachable balloons existed. The detachable latex balloon, developed by Debrun (Nycomed-Ingenor, Paris, France), was approved for use in Canada, Europe, and the Far East. Its availability in the United States, however, was limited because it was never submitted for FDA evaluation. The ITC-DSB detachable silicone balloon, developed by Hieshima (ITC-DSB: Interventional Therapeutics, Fremont, CA), was used in the United States for ISV occlusion during a multiinstitutional trial that ended in 1993. Since completion of this trial, the device has not been available for use in the treatment of varicoceles. Currently, this device, now manufactured by Target Therapeutics (Fremont, CA), has recently become commercially available.

The technique for varicocele occlusion by a detachable balloon involves the use of an 8 Fr guided catheter, placed at the origin of the ISV. After a venogram is performed, the appropriately sized balloon is mounted on a 3 Fr catheter and advanced into the ISV through the guide catheter. The first balloon is positioned just above the internal inguinal ring and inflated with isoosmotic contrast to occlude the vessel. Before detachment, contrast is injected through the guide catheter to assess for bypass channels. If bypass channels are present, the balloon can be deflated and repositioned to achieve the most effective occlusion. Once a satisfactory position is obtained, the balloon is detached. A second balloon then is positioned proximally, near the origin of the internal spermatic vein. Before the balloon is inflated, a sclerosant, such as 70% glucose mixed with contrast, is injected while the patient

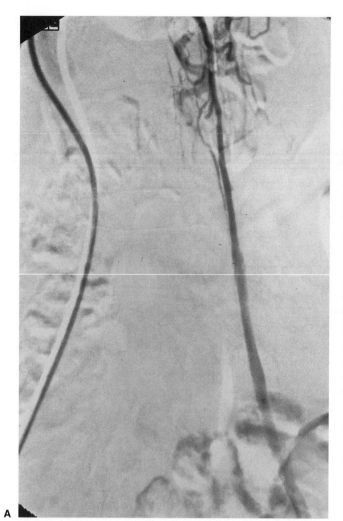

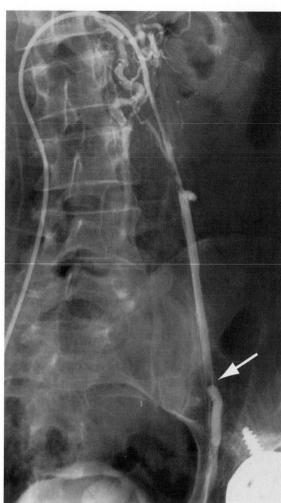

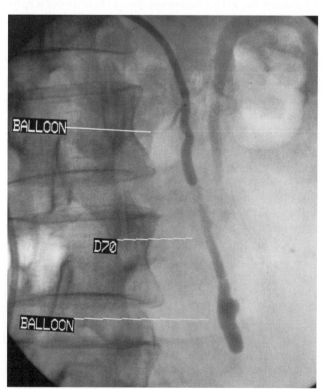

FIGURE 27-11. **A:** Left internal spermatic vein (ISV) veno-gram demonstrating reflux. **B:** A detachable balloon is placed to occlude the distal ISV (solid arrow). Postplacement veno-gram demonstrating multiple bypass channels reconstituting the ISV. **C:** A second balloon is placed at the origin of a large parallel collateral, and a third balloon is placed near the origin of the ISV. Before inflating this balloon, a 70% dextrose (D70) sclerosing solution is injected and trapped in the ISV between the two balloons.

performs a valsalva maneuver. The proximal balloon then is rapidly inflated, trapping the sclerosant in the ISV. This maneuver has been described as the *sandwich technique* (Fig. 27-11).[99] Technical success rates of 89 to 100% have been reported.[98,100–102]

The advantages of the detachable balloons are similar to those of mechanical occluding agents. One important advantage of this device over the other embolic agents is its ability to be repositioned as needed before detachment. This feature ensures optimal occlusion of the ISV. Additionally, the ability to trap a sclerosant in the ISV between two balloons enhances the effectiveness of the sclerosant. At the same time, this technique reduces the risk of sclerosant reflux and injury to other vessels. Disadvantages of the detachable balloon include a lack of availability, higher cost, and complexity of use. Significant experience with proper use of this device is needed to avoid premature detachment and inadvertent embolization to the lung.

Complications

The incidence and type of complications encountered after percutaneous varicocele occlusion are related to the properties of the embolic agents. Liquid sclerosants can reflux out of the ISV during delivery and injure nearby structures, which can result in pampiniform thrombophlebitis, testicular atrophy, renal vein thrombosis, and inguinal or scrotal pain.[68,79,81,83,85] Pain is the most commonly encountered complication, and its severity is related to the caustic nature of the sclerosant. With boiling contrast, a 46% incidence of mild and a 13% incidence of severe scrotal and inguinal pain lasting up to 4 weeks have been reported.[83] Additionally, a 13% incidence of numbness or paresthesia over the anterior aspect of the thigh was reported which took 3 to 6 months to resolve. What caused this is unclear. It is likely that penetration of the severely caustic sclerosant into other vascular beds, causing tissue damage, is to blame. Other less caustic agents do not cause such a high incidence of discomfort or tissue injury. Particulate agents differ from liquid sclerosants in that they can be precisely positioned in the ISV, thus avoiding extention into small vessels and tissue injury. On occasion, these devices can dislodge and embolize to the lung.[98,103] This complication, while seemingly harmful, rarely if ever causes any symptoms.[104]

The overall complication rate for percutaneous varicocele occlusion is approximately 10%.[79,81,83,91,95,100,105] Most of these complications are transient and require no intervention. The incidence of major complications is less than 2% and includes renal vein thrombosis (0.6%), testicular atrophy from pampiniform plexus thrombophlebitis (0.6%), and pulmonary embolization (2%). In contrast, the complication rate for surgical ligation of the ISV is much higher. In a comparative study by Lenk et al., the incidence of complications for an open operation

was 23% versus 16% for laparoscopic varicocele treatment and 6% for percutaneous therapy.[79] Additionally, some complications noted in the surgical groups were quite severe. With open surgical ISV ligation, hydrocele was common, occurring in 19% of treated patients. In the laparoscopic group, intraabdominal bleeding occurred. Other severe complications, such as wound infections and genital femoral nerve injury also have been reported with laparoscopic techniques.[64,106]

Treatment outcome

Infertility is the most common indication for varicocele treatment and, hence, pregnancy is the most important outcome measure. The literature is replete with studies documenting pregnancy rates after interruption of the ISV. The results of these studies vary widely. Pregnancy rates of 0 to 63% have been reported.[107,108] The largest series involved 986 patients treated over a 12-year period and reported a pregnancy rate of 55% after surgical ligation of the ISV.[109] A recent review and metaanalysis of the postvaricocele treatment pregnancy rates reported in 65 studies involving 6,983 patients from 1954 to 1992 revealed a posttreatment pregnancy rate of approximately 37%.[110] The results of this review speak more to the pregnancy rate expected after surgical ligation of the ISV because only 5 of the studies reviewed involved transcatheter occlusion. However, two randomized studies demonstrated no difference in pregnancy rates between surgical ligation and embolization.[111,112] Furthermore, an additional study reported a pregnancy rate of 57% in the long-term follow-up of varicocele patients who were treated with detachable balloons and coils.[100] Thus, pregnancy rates of at least 35 to 40% can be expected after transcatheter occlusion of the ISV.

Recently, doubts about the efficacy of varicocele occlusion by any technique have been expressed. These doubts were fueled by the wide variation in pregnancy rates reported in multiple nonrandomized retrospective studies and have been substantiated by the results of randomized control trials that have found no difference between treatment and observation. One recent well-designed prospective randomized trial of 95 patients comparing treatment to observation alone, found no difference in pregnancy rates.[113] In sharp contrast to these findings are the results reported as part of an ongoing WHO-sponsored large-scale multicenter prospective trial; a 60% pregnancy rate was found in the treatment group versus 10% in the control group.[114] Thus, the debate about the efficacy of varicocele treatment continues. Only additional well-designed prospective studies will resolve this question definitively. At present, the preponderance of studies attests to the benefits of varicocele occlusion on both sperm parameters and pregnancy.[94,100,115] We therefore advocate varicocele treatment for infertile males.

■ Female Infertility

Infertility in women can have multiple causative factors, from hormonal to mechanical. In many cases, patients present with coexistent factors leading to inability to conceive. Interventional techniques in the female reproductive tract, those focusing on obstruction of the fallopian tubes, uterus, and cervix, are relatively new options for treatment of these mechanical problems, although the concept was initially described in the nineteenth century by Smith. He also theorized that proximal obstruction of the fallopian tubes may be due to cellular debris, and if dislodgement of that debris could be performed, fecundity could be increased.[116] It was not until the 1970s and 1980s that selective salpingography and nonsurgical techniques for treating proximal fallopian tube obstruction were described using fluoroscopic guidance.[117, 118]

Proximal fallopian tube obstruction

Tubal obstruction contributes to female infertility in as many as 30 to 50% of cases; ampullary (distal) obstruction is the most common site.[119] Obstruction at or near the uterotubal junction (proximal tube) is present in as many as 20 to 25% of patients who have tubal abnormalities on hysterosalpingography (HSG).[119–121] Tubal obstruction may be due to one or a combination of factors, including tubal spasm, cellular debris, polyps, peritubal adhesions, previous pelvic surgery (including tubal ligation), tumors, tubal pregnancy, synechiae from Asherman syndrome, or pelvic inflammatory disease (PID) (Fig. 27-12A). Although controversial, it has been postulated that the most common cause of proximal (cornual) fallopian tube obstruction is a "plug" of cellular debris and mucus.[119–121] Routine HSG has been reported to increase fertility, possibly by washing away the plugs of debris.[122–125]

Selective salpingography and fallopian tube recanalization

In our institution, selective salpingography is the next step in the workup of patients with proximal tubal obstruction demonstrated by HSG. Often, selective salpingography is all that is required to restore tubal patency. Fallopian tube recanalization (FTR), or transcervical salpingoplasty, is most effective in the treatment of proximal tubal obstruction. The technique involves the use of a guidewire–catheter system to engage the tubal orifice

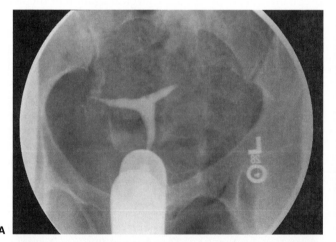

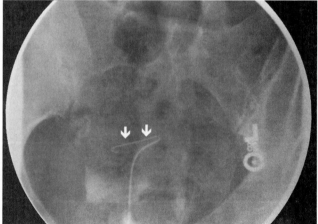

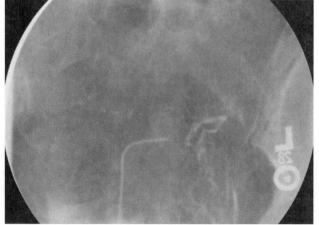

FIGURE 27-12. Hysterosalpingogram (HSG) and selective salpingography. **A:** HSG in a patient with infertility showing nonfilling of the left fallopian tube. The spherical filling defect in the uterine cavity is an air bubble. **B:** A 0.035-inch guidewire is buckled within the uterine cavity and a 6 Fr catheter (*arrows*) is advanced coaxially into the left tubal ostium. **C:** Selective injection (salpingogram) of the left tube reveals the tube to be patent after injection alone. No further intervention was performed.

under fluoroscopic guidance and "dilate" the proximal tube with a tapered catheter, small angioplasty balloon, or the guidewire alone.[126-131] Before the advent of FTR, patients with proximal tubal obstruction could be treated only with open or laparoscopic surgical resection of the uterine horn and microsurgical anastomosis of the affected tube. With current techniques, patients with distal isthmic or ampullary tubal obstruction are not candidates for FTR.

Technique

In our institution, a modification of the protocol described by Thurmond and colleagues for selective tubal catheterization and FTR is used.[126,127] This technique uses a coaxial catheter and guidewire system. Except for the occasional case performed in the operating room, FTR can be performed in a standard fluoroscopic room on a table fitted with stirrups. After the procedure is discussed with the patient and informed consent is obtained, the patient is placed on the fluoroscopic table in the dorsal lithotomy position, and the perineum is prepared and draped. An antibiotic (doxycycline) is given intravenously during the procedure. A speculum is inserted, and the exocervix is directly visualized. A cervical cannula then is inserted to perform HSG and to serve as a working channel into the uterine cavity. A number of instruments and techniques are available for this purpose. An example is the Thurmond-Rosch Hysterocath (Cook, Bloomington, IN), which uses an acorn cannula to engage the cervical os and a suction device to secure the cannula. Cervical catheters fitted with a distal balloon as a securing device such as the one manufactured by Conceptus (San Carlos, CA), are also available. This cannula has a 14 Fr outer diameter, is stiff, and will allow traction on the uterus for easier passage of catheters and wires through the cervical canal. The cervical catheter usually is placed under direct visualization through the speculum. When the cervical catheter is in place, an initial HSG is performed. In patients who have cervical stenosis, a diagnostic HSG cannot be performed because of inadequate filling of the uterine cavity and fallopian tubes. The patient then may require cervical dilation, which is described later in this chapter. If, during an adequate HSG, a tube fills throughout its length and contrast spills out the fimbriated end of the tube into the peritoneum, there is no need for selective tubal injection or FTR of that tube. If proximal tubal obstruction is demonstrated, an effort should be made to select the tubal orifice. Under fluoroscopic guidance, an 0.035-inch J-wire is advanced through the cervical cannula and coiled or "buckled" in the uterine cavity (Fig. 27-12B). This buckling technique is a reliable way to direct the catheter toward the fallopian tubal orifice. This maneuver should be done gently, because certain patients can experience discomfort with instrumentation in the re-

gion of the uterine fundus. In most cases, a curved 6 Fr catheter (Soft Torque, Conceptus, Inc.) will readily engage the ostia of the fallopian tubes after placement over a wire. As the catheter tip approaches the tubal ostium, the guidewire is removed and the catheter is advanced to engage the ostium. Contrast medium then is injected through the catheter to determine its relationship to the tubal orifice. If the catheter tip is close to the ostium, a straight 0.035-inch guidewire is advanced through it to direct the catheter accurately toward the fallopian tube, and the catheter is pushed to a wedged position. If the catheter is not wedged correctly in the tubal ostium, selection of the fallopian tube with a microcatheter and wire can be difficult. Contrast medium is injected for a selective salpingogram. Quite often, this contrast injection demonstrates a patent tube, although the initial HSG does not (Fig. 27-12C). This phenomenon suggests that the tube may have been blocked by a plug of cellular debris that was washed away merely by the contrast injection, or the tube was in spasm at the time of the initial HSG.

If the tube remains obstructed after selective contrast injection (Fig. 27-13A), FTR is performed. An 0.018-inch flexible-tip (Mandrel) guidewire (Cook) is fitted through a microcatheter that tapers to 2.4 Fr at the tip (VS Catheter, Conceptus). This combination is advanced coaxially through the lumen of the 6 Fr catheter. The guidewire is manipulated carefully into the fallopian tube and advanced through the obstruction (Fig. 27-13B). If this maneuver fails, a 0.018-inch wire with a hydrophilic coating (Glidewire, Medi-tech, Watertown, MA) can be used. We make a point not to advance the wire or catheter beyond the first turn in the isthmic portion of the tube so as to guard against perforation (Fig. 27-13C). After the wire is advanced beyond the site of obstruction, the microcatheter is advanced over the wire to dilate the lumen. The microcatheter is the dilation tool; that is, no devices such as balloon catheters are used. Confirmation of recanalization of the fallopian tube then is documented by selective injection, done through the microcatheter both distal to the dilated area to detect any concomitant tubal disease and proximal to confirm obliteration of the obstruction (Fig. 27-13D). The procedure is terminated and the instruments are removed. The patient is allowed to recover and is monitored by the nursing staff for 30 min to 1 hr. The patient then is given a prescription for oral antibiotics to be given for 3 to 5 days after the procedure (doxycycline 100 mg, taken orally twice a day). The patient and her partner are instructed not to have sexual intercourse for 48 hr postprocedure as a precaution against infection.

Outcome

The technical success rate, defined as successful tubal cannulation and visualization of distal tubal anatomy ranges between 76 and 95%.[128,129,132-135] Pregnancy rates after

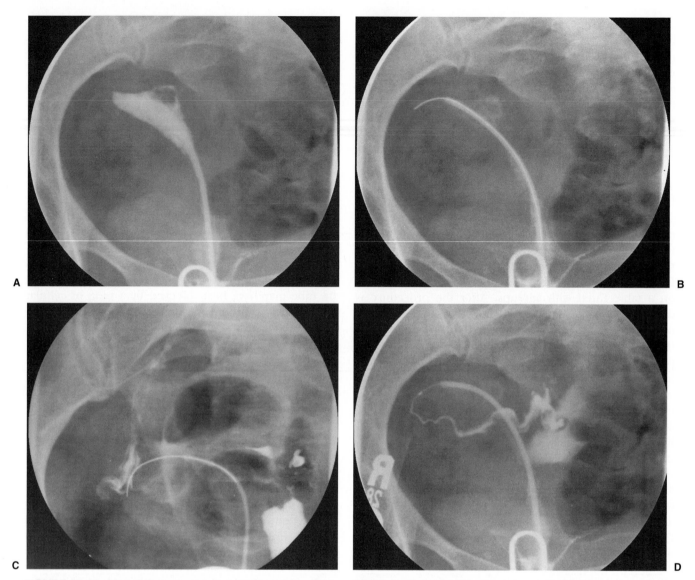

FIGURE 27-13. The technique of fallopian tube recanalization (FTR). **A:** Selective injection of a right fallopian tube reveals obstruction of the cornual portion. **B:** An 0.018-inch curved guidewire is used to cross the area of obstruction. Over this wire, a 2.4 Fr microcatheter will be advanced past the obstruction. **C:** FTR in another patient demonstrates the maximum advancement of the wire for a proximal (cornual) tubal obstruction. **D:** Selective injection of the same tube in (**A**) and (**B**) showing patency and spillage of contrast into the peritoneum. Note the radiopaque marker at the tip of the microcatheter and that the injection is made slightly proximal to the area dilated to document obliteration of the obstruction.

recanalization range from 17 to 58% with as long as 12 months' follow-up. In one group of 37 patients, with total obstruction and significant concomitant tubal disease (adhesions, salpingitis, isthmica nodosa, hydrosalpinx), treatment with FTR achieved technical success in 45 of 63 tubes treated (71%). FTR resulted in 14 (33%) conceptions, 11 intrauterine and 3 ectopic. Of the intrauterine pregnancies, seven occurred in women with diseased tubes. There were five full-term deliveries.[136] One series in which FTR was performed in patients who had previously undergone tubal surgery, FTR failed in all patients with tubal fistulae,[4] but was highly successful in patients with stenoses/stric-

tures (13 of 15 patients, 87%).[137] There is histologic evidence that failure of FTR may be due to severe intrinsic tubal disease [obliterative fibrosis (61%), chronic salpingitis (57%), and salpingitis isthmica nodosa (42%)] and not to technical error.[119]

The complication rate for FTR ranges from 3 to 11%; fallopian tube perforation is the most commonly reported complication, and hemorrhage or infection is rare. The most common site for perforation is in midisthmic occlusions. If a fallopian tube is perforated by a guidewire, the patient usually does not experience pain and suffers no known sequellae.[138] Concern about radiation dose to the ovaries has been raised; the average absorbed dose to the ovaries has been reported to be 8.5 mGy ± 5.6 (0.85 rad ± 0.56), which is comparable to the uterine dose during an excretory urogram (8 mGy) and less than that received during a barium enema (35 mGy).[139] The use of ultrasound guidance for fallopian tube catheterization has been reported to cannulate the tube 43% of the time. Although the patient is spared ionizing radiation, the technique has severe limitations, such as the inability to image small catheters in the uterus and tubes.[140] The incidence of ectopic pregnancy in patients after FTR has ranged from 4 to 7%, which is less than the 10% ectopic pregnancy rate quoted after surgical tubocornual reanastomosis.[118,136,138] Other devices for the dilation of the proximal fallopian tube have been reported, including the use of balloon catheters much like those used for small vessel angioplasty. In studies using a balloon catheter for FTR, technical success rates have been reported to range from 82 to 92%, and pregnancy rates have approached 34 to 35%, although small numbers of ectopic pregnancies and spontaneous losses occurred.[130,141]

Cervical stenosis and false passages

Stenosis of the exocervical os, cervical canal, or endocervical os has been described in patients with infertility.[142,143] The etiology of cervical stenosis includes congenital anomalies, previous cone biopsy, trauma, or idiopathic disease. Stenoses may be so severe as to cause oligomennorhea or even amennorhea. The routine procedure used by gynecologists for access to the uterine canal is to probe the cervical canal with sequentially enlarging sounds and then to introduce the instrument needed for a certain task, such as endometrial biopsy device or curette. If the cervical canal is narrow or the uterus is markedly anteverted, causing an acute bend in the endocervix, it is possible to create false passages within the canal by using rigid instruments. In patients undergoing workup for infertility, which in our institution requires an HSG and endometrial biopsy, access to the uterine cavity without imaging guidance may be difficult, especially in the presence of cervical stenosis or false passages resulting from previous instrumentation. In this type of patient, the technique of cervical dilation may be helpful for both the treatment of cervical stenosis and to help facilitate an infertility workup.[144]

Technique

The procedure uses both routine angiographic materials and techniques. No specific contraindications to this procedure have been identified. After informed consent is obtained, doxycycline 100 mg is administered intravenously 30 min to 1 hr before the procedure. Most procedures are performed in the radiology department in a standard radiography/fluoroscopy unit using conscious sedation. The patient is placed in the dorsal lithotomy position, and the perineum is prepared and draped. A metal speculum is passed into the vagina, and the exocervical os is identified. Under direct visualization, the cervical os is cannulated with a 5 to 8 Fr, 23-cm vascular sheath (Cordis Corporation, Miami, FL) or a Thurmond-Rosch hysterocath (Cook). Water-soluble contrast material is injected into the cervical canal (Fig. 27-14A). If a cervical stenosis or false channel is seen, attempts are made to traverse the true cervical canal using a guidewire–catheter combination. The wires used most often for this purpose are an 0.035-inch, 3-mm J-wire (Cook), or an 0.035-inch Bentson wire (Cook). A 5 Fr catheter with a distal curve such as a Berenstein curve (Medi-tech) has proved useful. Once a wire has been passed across the stenosis, the catheter is placed in the uterine canal and the wire is exchanged for a stiffer 0.035-inch wire (Amplatz Super-Stiff, Medi-tech). Over this wire the narrowing is dilated with an angioplasty balloon measuring 6–8 mm in diameter (Medi-tech) (Fig. 27-14B). The cervix is dilated until the "waist" of the balloon obliterates or a postdilation contrast injection reveals a patent canal. The minimum balloon diameter chosen in each case is 6 mm, which is the normal adult diameter of the cervical canal. In each case, a postdilation contrast injection is performed to assess the dilation result (Fig. 27-14C). If the injection opacified the uterine canal and proximal tube obstruction is diagnosed, attempts are made to recanalize the tubes. After the procedure patients are given a prescription for a 3-day course of antibiotics and are monitored closely. Following dilation, patients can undergo procedures that require uterine access, such as endometrial biopsy, in vitro fertilization for embryo transfer (IVF-ET), or artificial insemination.

Outcome

In a series reported at our institution, 17 cervical dilation procedures were performed in 15 patients. Technical success was achieved in 14 of 15 patients (93.3%). No evidence of infection was noted. No patient experienced pain or bleeding for more than 48 hr. All patients underwent endometrial biopsy without difficulty 2 weeks to 7 months postdilation. Of the 15 patients in this preliminary study, four have become pregnant (pregnancy rate, 26.7%). Of those four, one underwent IVF and one had artificial insemination. Two became pregnant spontaneously. Of these four, three have delivered healthy infants and one had a spontaneous abortion at 8 weeks' gestational age.

One theoretic concern for this technique is the potential to cause cervical incompetence. Of the patients who conceived and delivered, none showed signs of cervical incompetence. In our patient whose fetus aborted, the fetal loss occurred at too early a gestational age to suspect cervical incompetence. Cervical dilation may provide op-

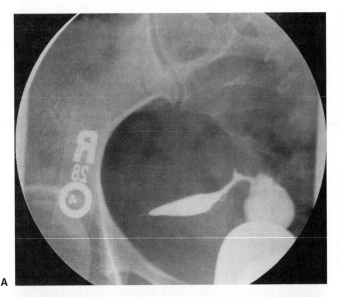

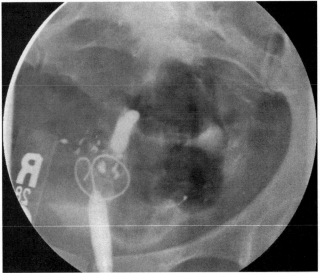

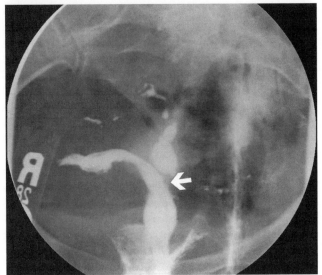

FIGURE 27-14. The technique of cervical dilation in a patient who has previously had multiple unsuccessful attempts at hysterosalpingogram (HSG) and endometrial biopsy. **A:** HSG via a balloon catheter in the lower cervix reveals the uterus to be markedly anteverted. Note also that there is nonfilling of the right fallopian tube. **B:** An 8-mm × 2-cm angioplasty balloon is inflated over a wire within the true cervical canal in the region of cervical stenosis and false passage. **C:** HSG after cervical dilation shows the cervical canal to be patent (*arrows*), and the false passages do not fill.

tions for treatment that otherwise would not be available to a select number of infertile patients who have intractable cervical stenosis or false passage.[144]

■ Conclusion

Treatment of the infertile couple can be complex, and many widely varying therapies are advocated. Catheter-directed therapy offers a nonsurgical alternative for the treatment of infertility. In women, advancements in catheter-directed techniques have offered noninvasive solutions for mechanical obstruction of the reproductive tract. In men, these techniques permit nonsurgical occlusion of varicoceles. Catheter-directed techniques are effective and safe and have exceptionally low complication rates. Recovery is rapid, and most patients usually can return to normal activities within 24 hr of treatment.

These techniques have distinct advantages over surgical alternatives. The use of radiographic imaging often can identify pathology that would be unrecognized at surgery. Examples include the inability to identify complex venous collaterals during surgical ligation, thus resulting in varicocele recurrence, and the creation of false passages in the cervix when treating women with cervical stenoses. In addition to the imaging advantage, catheter-directed therapy is often more cost effective than the myriad of surgical alternatives.[145–147] Thus, we recommend that these treatment methods be considered instead of surgical methods in most cases.

REFERENCES

1. Page H. Estimation of the prevalence and incidence of infertility in a population: a pilot study. *Fertil Steril* 1989;51:571–577.

2. Hargreave TB. Varicocele—a clinical enigma. *Br J Urol* 1993;72: 401–408.

3. Barwell R. One hundred cases of varicocele treated by the subcutaneous wire loop. *Lancet* 1885;1:978.

4. Tulloch WS. A consideration of sterility factors in the light of subsequent pregnancies. II. Subfertility in the male. *Trans Edinb Obstet Soc* 1952;59:29–34.

5. McClure RD, Hricak H. Scrotal ultrasound in the infertile man: detection of subclinical unilateral and bilateral varicoceles. *J Urol* 1986;135:711–715.

6. Steeno O, Knops J, Declerck L, Adimoelja A, van de Voorde H. Prevention of fertility disorders by detection and treatment of varicocele at school and college age. *Andrologia* 1976;8:47–53.

7. Pyror JL, Howards SS. Varicocele. *Urol Clin North Am* 1987;14: 499–513.

8. Lund L, Rasmussen HH, Ernst E. Asymptomatic varicocele testis. *Scand J Urol Nephrol* 1993;27:395–398.

9. Meacham RB, Townsend RR, Rademacher D, Drose JA. The incidence of varicoceles in the general population when evaluated by physical examination, gray scale sonography and color Doppler sonography. *J Urol* 1994;151:1535–1538.

10. Risser WL, Lipshultz LI. Frequency of varicocele in black adolescents. *J Adolesc Health Care* 1984;5:28–29.

11. de Castro MP, Mastrorocco DA. Reproductive history and semen analysis in prevasectomy fertile men with and without varicocele. *J Androl* 1984;5:17–20.

12. Jarow JP, Coburn M, Sigman M. Incidence of varicoceles in men with primary and secondary infertility. *Urology* 1996;47:73–76.

13. Marks JL, McMahon R, Lipshultz LI. Predictive parameters of successful varicocele repair. *J Urol* 1986;136:609–612.

14. Musella M, Imbimbo C, Palmieri A, Mirone V, Musella S. Laparoscopic surgery in varicocele: description of the technique and preliminary data. *Ann Ital Chir* 1995;66:537–542.

15. Pauwels RP, Festen C, Janknegt RA, Moonen WA. Varicocele and subfertility. Results of Ivanissevich's operation. *Ned Tijdschr Geneeskd* 1970;114:1565–1572.

16. Ivanissevich O. Left varicocele due to reflux: experience with 4,470 operative cases in forty-two years. *Intl Coll Surg* 1960;34: 742–755.

17. Palomo A. Radical cure of varicocele by a new technique: preliminary report. *Urology* 1949;61:604–607.

18. Iaccarino V. Trattamento conservatio del varicoseles: flebografia selettiva o scleroterapia delle vene gonadiche. *Riv Radiol* 1977;17: 107–117.

19. Ahlberg NE, Bartley O, Chidekel N, Fritjofsson A. Phlebography in varicocele scroti. *Acta Radiol Diagn* (Stockh) 1966;4:517–528.

20. Nadel SN, Hutchins GM, Albertsen PC, White RI, Jr. Valves of the internal spermatic vein: potential for misdiagnosis of varicocele by venography. *Fertil Steril* 1984;41:479–481.

21. Hill JT, Hirsh AV, Pryor JP, Kellett MJ. Changes in the appearance of venography after ligation of a varicocele. *J Anat* 1982;135(Part 1):47–52.

22. Lenz M, Hof N, Kersting-Sommerhoff B, Bautz W. Anatomic variants of the spermatic vein: importance for percutaneous sclerotherapy of idiopathic varicocele. *Radiology* 1996;198:425–431.

23. Comhaire F, Kunnen M, Nahoum C. Radiological anatomy of the internal spermatic vein(s) in 200 retrograde venograms. *Int J Androl* 1981;4:379–387.

24. Bigot JM, Chatel A. The value of retrograde spermatic phlebography in varicocele. *Eur Urol* 1980;6:301–306.

25. Hanna GB, Byrne D, Townell N. Right-sided varicocele as a presentation of right renal tumours. *Br J Urol* 1995;75:798–799.

26. White S. Acute varicocele due to the pressure of a greatly distended left kidney (non-malignant). *BMJ* 1914;2:177.

27. Slot B, Meijenhorst GC. Venography of the left internal spermatic vein in patients with fertility problems. *Diagn Imaging* 1982; 51:214–223.

28. Tjia TT, Rumping WJ, Landman GH, Cobben JJ. Phlebography of the internal spermatic vein (and the ovarian vein). *Diagn Imaging* 1982;51:8–18.

29. Braedel HU, Steffens J, Ziegler M, et al. A possible ontogenic etiology for idiopathic left varicocele. *J Urol* 1994;151: 62–66.

30. Saypol DC. Varicocele. *J Androl* 1981;2:61.

31. Barnes RW, Fleisher HLD, Redman JF, et al. Mesoaortic compression of the left renal vein (the so-called nutcracker syndrome): repair by a new stenting procedure. *J Vasc Surg* 1988;8:415–421.

32. Stassen CM, Weil EH, Janevski BK. Left renal vein compression syndrome ("nutcracker phenomenon"). *Rofo Fortschr Geb Rontgenstr Neuen Bildgeb Verfahr* 1989;150:708–710.

33. Takihara H, Sakatoku J, Cockett AT. The pathophysiology of varicocele in male infertility. *Fertil Steril* 1991;55:861–868.

34. Nilsson S, Edvinsson A, Nilsson B. Improvement of semen and pregnancy rate after ligation and division of the internal spermatic vein: fact or fiction? *Br J Urol* 1979;51:591–596.

35. Nagao RR, Plymate SR, Berger RE, et al. Comparison of gonadal function between fertile and infertile men with varicoceles. *Fertil Steril* 1986;46:930–933.

36. Takihara H, Ishizu K, Ueno T, et al. Pathogenesis of varicocele: experimental study using flow cytometric DNA analysis. *Andrologia* 1990;22:137–143.

37. Zorgniotti AW. Testis temperature, infertility, and the varicocele paradox. *Urology* 1980;16:7–10.

38. Ito H, Fuse H, Minagawa H, et al. Internal spermatic vein prostaglandins in varicocele patients. *Fertil Steril* 1982;37:218–222.

39. Schlegel W, Rotermund S, Farber G, Nieschlag E. The influence of prostaglandins on sperm motility. *Prostaglandins* 1981;21:87–99.

40. Chakraborty J, Hikim AP, Jhunjhunwala JS. Stagnation of blood in the microcirculatory vessels in the testes of men with varicocele. *J Androl* 1985;6:117–126.

41. Dubin L, Amelar RD. Varicocele size and results of varicocelectomy in selected subfertile men with varicocele. *Fertil Steril* 1970; 21:606–609.

42. Comhaire F, Monteyne R, Kunnen M. The value of scrotal thermography as compared with selective retrograde venography of the internal spermatic vein for the diagnosis of "subclinical" varicocele. *Fertil Steril* 1976;27:694–698.

43. Marsman JW, Schats R. The subclinical varicocele debate. *Hum Reprod* 1994;9:1–8.

44. Marsman JW. Clinical versus subclinical varicocele: venographic findings and improvement of fertility after embolization. *Radiology* 1985;155:635–638.

45. Wheatley JK, Bergman WA, Green B, Walther MM. Transvenous occlusion of clinical and subclinical varicoceles. *Urology* 1991;37: 362–365.

46. Demas BE, Hricak H, McClure RD. Varicoceles: radiologic diagnosis and treatment. *Radiol Clin North Am* 1991;29:619–627.

47. Comhaire F. Scrotal thermography in varicocele. *Adv Exp Med Biol* 1991;286:267–270.

48. Greenberg SH, Lipshultz LI, Wein AJ. A preliminary report of "subclinical varicocele": diagnosis by Doppler ultrasonic stethoscope: examination and initial results of surgical therapy. *J Reprod Med* 1979;22:77–81.

49. Prenen JA, Van Dis P, Feijen HL. Varicocele scintigraphy: a simplified screening method for the detection of spermatic vein reflux. *Clin Nucl Med* 1996;21:921–927.

50. Geatti O, Gasparini D, Shapiro B. A comparison of scintigraphy, thermography, ultrasound and phlebography in grading of clinical varicocele. *J Nucl Med* 1991;32:2092–2097.

51. Trum JW, Gubler FM, Laan R, van der Veen F. The value of palpation, varicoscreen contact thermography and colour Doppler ultrasound in the diagnosis of varicocele. *Hum Reprod* 1996; 11:1232–1235.

52. Hamm B, Fobbe F, Sorensen R, Felsenberg D. Varicoceles: com-

bined sonography and thermography in diagnosis and postthera-peutic evaluation. *Radiology* 1986;160:419–424.

53. Netto Junior NR, Lerner JS, Paolini RM, de Goes GM. Varicocele: the value of reflux in the spermatic vein. *Int J Fertil* 1980;25:71–74.

54. World Health Organization. *Laboratory Manual for the Examination of Human Semen and Semen-cervical Mucus Interaction,* 2nd ed. New York: Cambridge University Press, 1987.

55. Harrison RM, Lewis RW, Roberts JA. Pathophysiology of varicocele in nonhuman primates: long-term seminal and testicular changes. *Fertil Steril* 1986;46:500–510.

56. Witt MA, Lipshultz LI. Varicocele: a progressive or static lesion? *Urology* 1993;42:541–543.

57. Gorelick JI, Goldstein M. Loss of fertility in men with varicocele. *Fertil Steril* 1993;59:613–616.

58. Cheval MJ, Purcell MH. Deterioration of semen parameters over time in men with untreated varicocele: evidence of progressive testicular damage. *Fertil Steril* 1992;57:174–177.

59. Podesta ML, Gottlieb S, Medel R Jr, et al. Hormonal parameters and testicular volume in children and adolescents with unilateral varicocele: preoperative and postoperative findings. *J Urol* 1994;152(2 Part 2):794–797.

60. Costabile RA, Skoog S, Radowich M. Testicular volume assessment in the adolescent with a varicocele. *J Urol* 1992;147:1348–1350.

61. Nasu T, Takihara H, Hirayama A. A new apparatus for the measur-ment of testicular volume. *Jpn J Fertil Steril* 1979;24:12.

62. Aaberg RA, Vancaillie TG, Schuessler WW. Laparoscopic varico-cele ligation: a new technique. *Fertil Steril* 1991;56:776–777.

63. Wuernschimmel E, Lipsky H, Noest G. Laparoscopic varicocele ligation: a recommendable standard procedure with good long-term results. *Eur Urol* 1995;27:18–22.

64. Tan SM, Ng FC, Ravintharan T, et al. Laparoscopic varicocelec-tomy: technique and results [see comments]. *Br J Urol* 1995; 75:523–528.

65. Mandressi A, Buizza C, Antonelli D, Chisena S. Is laparoscopy a worthy method to treat varicocele? Comparison between 160 cases of two-port laparoscopic and 120 cases of open inguinal spermatic vein ligation. *J Endourol* 1996;10:435–441.

66. Enquist E, Stein BS, Sigman M. Laparoscopic versus subinguinal varicocelectomy: a comparative study. *Fertil Steril* 1994;61:1092–1096.

67. Comhaire F, Kunnen M. Selective retrograde venography of the internal spermatic vein: a conclusive approach to the diagnosis of varicocele. *Andrologia* 1976;8:11–24.

68. Lima SS, Castro MP, Costa OF. A new method for the treatment of varicocele. *Andrologia* 1978;10:103–106.

69. Seyferth W, Jecht E, Zeitler E. Percutaneous sclerotherapy of vari-cocele. *Radiology* 1981;139:335–340.

70. Riedl P, Lunglmayr G, Stackl W. A new method of transfemoral testicular vein obliteration for varicocele using a balloon catheter. *Radiology* 1981;139:323–325.

71. Trerotola SO, Venbrux AC, Savader SJ, et al. Guiding catheter for varicocele embolization. *J Vasc Interv Radiol* 1993;4:433–434.

72. Morag B, Rubinstein ZJ, Goldwasser B, Yerushalmi A, Lunnenfeld B. Percutaneous venography and occlusion in the management of spermatic varicoceles. *AJR Am J Roentgenol* 1984;143:635–640.

73. Smith TP, Hunter DW, Craff AH, et al. Spermatic vein emboliza-tion with hot contrast material: fertility results. *Radiology* 1988; 168:137–139.

74. Formanek A, Rusnak B, Zollikofer C, et al. Embolization of the spermatic vein for treatment of infertility: a new approach. *Radiol-ogy* 1981;139:315–321.

75. Kuroiwa T, Hasuo K, Yasumori K, et al. Transcatheter embolization of testicular vein for varicocele testis. *Acta Radiol* 1991;32:311–314.

76. Coolsaet BL. The varicocele syndrome: venography determining the optimal level for surgical management. *J Urol* 1980;124:833–839.

77. Vajda J, Bohm K, Horvath L, Molnar Z. Retrograde phlebography of the internal spermatic vein in varicocele. *Int Urol Nephrol* 1981;13:175–184.

78. Rooney MS, Gray RR. Varicocele embolization through competent internal spermatic veins. *Can Assoc Radiol J* 1992;43:431–435.

79. Lenk S, Fahlenkamp D, Gliech V, Lindeke A. Comparison of different methods of treating varicocele. *J Androl* 1994;15(Suppl): 34S–37S.

80. Trombetta C, Salisci E, Deriu M, et al. Echo-flowmetric control 6 years after percutaneous treatment of varicocele. *Arch Ital Urol Androl* 1993;65:363–7.

81. Braedel HU, Steffens J, Ziegler M, Polsky MS. Out-patient sclero-therapy of idiopathic left-sided varicocele in children and adults. *Br J Urol* 1990;65:536–540.

82. Usuki N, Nakamura K, Takashima S, et al. Embolization of varico-cele with ethanol. *Nippon Igaku Hoshasen Gakkai Zasshi* 1994; 54:870–875.

83. Hunter DW, King NJD, Aeppli DM, et al. Spermatic vein occlusion with hot contrast material: angiographic results. *J Vasc Interv Radiol* 1991;2:507–515.

84. Fuochi C, Moser E, dalla Palma F, et al. Value of percutaneous sclerotherapy in the treatment of varicocele. Technic and results. *Ann Urol* (Paris) 1986;20:252–256.

85. Fobbe F, Hamm B, Sorensen R, Felsenberg D. Percutaneous trans-luminal treatment of varicoceles: where to occlude the internal spermatic vein. *AJR Am J Roentgenol* 1987;149:983–987.

86. Hunter DW, Bildsoe MC, Amplatz K. Aid for safer sclerotherapy of the internal spermatic vein. *Radiology* 1989;173:282.

87. Sigmund G, Bahren W, Gall H, Lenz M, Thon W. Idiopathic varicoceles: feasibility of percutaneous sclerotherapy. *Radiology* 1987;164:161–168.

88. Bigot JM. Percutaneous sclerotherapy of varicocele. *Ann Radiol* (Paris) 1986;29:173–177.

89. Riedl P, Kumpan W, Hajek PC, Salomonowitz E. Left spermatic vein sclerotherapy. A seven-year retrospective analysis. *Ann Radiol* (Paris) 1986;29:165–168.

90. Kunnen M. New techniques for embolization of the internal sper-matic vein: intravenous tissue adhesive (author's transl). *ROFO Fortschr Geb Rontgenstr Neuen Bildgeb Verfahr* 1980;133:625–629.

91. Kunnen M, Comhaire F. Nonsurgical cure of varicocele by tran-scatheter embolization of the internal spermatic vein(s) with a tissue adhesive (Bucrylate). In: Castaneda-Zuniga WR, Tadavarthy SM, eds. *Interventional Radiology.* Baltimore: Williams & Wilkins, 1988:128–153.

92. Weissbach L, Thelen M, Adolphs HD. Treatment of idiopathic varicoceles by transfemoral testicular vein occlusion. *J Urol* 1981; 126:354–356.

93. Berkman WA, Price RB, Wheatley JK, et al. Varicoceles: a coaxial coil occlusion system. *Radiology* 1984;151:73–77.

94. Punekar SV, Prem AR, Ridhorkar VR, et al. Post-surgical recurrent varicocele: efficacy of internal spermatic venography and steel-coil embolization. *Br J Urol* 1996;77:124–128.

95. Ferguson JM, Gillespie IN, Chalmers N, et al. Percutaneous varico-cele embolization in the treatment of infertility. *Br J Radiol* 1995;68:700–730.

96. Gonzalez R, Narayan P, Formanek A, Amplatz K. Transvenous embolization of internal spermatic veins: nonoperative approach to treatment of varicocele. *Urology* 1981;17:246–248.

97. Thelen M, Weissbach L, Franken T. Die bernandlung der idiopa-thischen varikozele durch transfemorale spiralokklusion der ven testicularis sinistra. *Fortschr Rontgenstrahlen* 1979;131:24–29.

98. White RI, Jr., Kaufman SL, Barth KH, et al. Occlusion of varicoce-les wih detachable balloons. *Radiology* 1981;139:327–334.

99. Halden W, White RI, Jr. Outpatient embolotherapy of varicocele. *Urol Clin North Am* 1987;14:137–144.

100. Zuckerman AM, Mitchell SE, Venbrux AC, et al. Percutaneous

varicocele occlusion: long-term follow-up. *J Vasc Interv Radiol* 1994;5:315–319.

101. Reyes BL, Trerotola SO, Venbrux AC, et al. Percutaneous embolotherapy of adolescent varicocele: results and long-term follow-up. *J Vasc Interv Radiol* 1994;5:131–134.

102. Shuman L, White RI Jr, Mitchell SE, et al. Right-sided varicocele: technique and clinical results of balloon embolotherapy from the femoral approach. *Radiology* 1986;158: 787–791.

103. Matthews RD, Roberts J, Walker WA, Sands JP. Migration of intravascular balloon after percutaneous embolotherapy of varicocele. *Urology* 1992;39:373–375.

104. Nemcek A Jr. Varicocele embolization. *J Vasc Interv Radiol* 1996;7: 541–542.

105. Rivilla F, Casillas JG, Gallego J, Lezana AH. Percutaneous venography and embolization of the internal spermatic vein by spring coil for treatment of the left varicocele in children. *J Pediatr Surg* 1995;30:523–527.

106. Jarow JP, Assimos DG, Pittaway DE. Effectiveness of laparoscopic varicocelectomy. *Urology* 1993;42:544–547.

107. Palti Z, Kedar S, Polishuk WZ. Oligospermia treatment. *Fertil Steril* 1968;19:631.

108. Davidson HA. Testicular temperature and varicoceles. *Practitioner* 1954;173:703.

109. Dubin L, Amelar RD. Varicocelectomy: 986 cases in a twelve-year study. *Urology* 1977;10:446–449.

110. Schlesinger MH, Wilets IF, Nagler HM. Treatment outcome after varicocelectomy. A critical analysis. *Urol Clin North Am* 1994;21: 517–529.

111. Sayfan J, Soffer Y, Orda R. Varicocele treatment: prospective randomized trial of 3 methods. *J Urol* 1992;148:1447–1449.

112. Nieschlag E, Behre HM, Schlingheider A, et al. Surgical ligation vs. angiographic embolization of the vena spermatica: a prospective randomized study for the treatment of varicocele-related infertility. *Andrologia* 1993;25:233– 237.

113. Nieschlag E, Hertle L, Fischedick A, Behre HM. Treatment of varicocele: counseling as effective as occlusion of the vena spermatica. *Hum Reprod* 1995;10:347–353.

114. Madgar I, Weissenberg R, Lunenfeld B, et al. Controlled trial of high spermatic vein ligation for varicocele in infertile men. *Fertil Steril* 1995;63:120–124.

115. Hirokawa M, Matsushita K, Iwamoto T, et al. Assessment of Palomo's operative method for infertile varicocele. *Andrologia* 1993;25:47–51.

116. Smith TW. New method of treating sterility by the removal of obstructions of the fallopian tube. *Lancet* 1849;1:603–605.

117. Rouanet JP CJ. An application of selective catheterization: salpingography: preliminary note (letter). *Nouv Presse Medi* 1977;6: 2785.

118. Platia MP KA. Transcervical fluoroscopic recanalization of a proximally occluded oviduct. *Fertil Steril* 1985;44:704–706.

119. Letterie GS SE. Histology of proximal tubal obstruction in cases of unsuccessful tubal canalization. *Fertil Steril* 1991;56:831–835.

120. Sulak PJ LG, Coddington, et. al. Histology of proximal tubal occlusion. *Fertil Steril* 1987;48:437–440.

121. Wadin K LM, Rasmussen C, et. al. Frequency of proximal tubal obstruction in patients undergoing infertility evaluation. *Acta Radiol* 1994;35:357–360.

122. Gillespie HW. The therapeutic aspect of hysterosalpingography. *Br J Radiol* 1965;38:301.

123. Horbach JG M, van Hall EV. Factors influencing the pregnancy rate following hysterosalpinography and their prognostic significance. *Fertil Steril* 1973;24:15–18.

124. DeCherney AH KH, Barney JB, et. al. Increased pregnancy rate with oil-soluble hysterosalpingography dye. *Fertil Steril* 1980;33: 407–410.

125. Mackey RA, Glass RH, Olson LE, Vaidya R. Pregnancy following hysterosalpingography with oil and water soluble dye. *Fertil Steril* 1971;22:504–507.

126. Thurmond AS NM, Uchida BT, Rosch J. Fallopian tube obstruction: selective salpingography and recanalization. Work in progress. *Radiology* 1987;163:511–514.

127. Thurmond AS RJ, Patton PE, et al. Fluoroscopic transcervical fallopian tube catheterization for diagnosis and treatment of female infertility caused by tubal obstruction. *Radiographics* 1988;8: 621–640.

128. Thurmond AS RJ. Nonsurgical fallopian tube recanalization for treatment of infertility. *Radiology* 1990;174:371–374.

129. Thurmond AS. Selective salpinography and fallopian tube recanalization. *AJR Am J Roentgenol* 1991;156:33–38.

130. Confino E T-KI, DeCherney A, et. al. Transcervical balloon tuboplasty: multicenter study. *JAMA* 1990;264:2079–2082.

131. Millward SF CP, Leader A, et. al. Technical report: Fallopian tube recanalization: a simplified technique. *Clin Radiol* 1994;49:496– 497.

132. Lang EK DH, Roniger WE. Selective osteal salpingography and transvaginal catheter dilitation in the diagnosis and treatment of fallopian tube obstruction. *AJR Am J Roentgenol* 1990;154:735– 740.

133. Kumpe DA ZS, Rothbarth LJ, et. al. Proximal fallopian tube occlusion: diagnosis and treatment with transcervical fallopian tube catheterization. *Radiology* 1990;177:183–187.

134. Winfield AC MD, Segars J, et. al. Selective fallopian tube canalization. *AJR Am J Roentgenol* 1990;154:195.(abst)

135. Amendola MA BM, Pollack HM, et. al. Preliminary experience with fluoroscopic transcervical fallopian tube recanalization. *AJR Am J Roentgenol* 1990;154:196.(abst)

136. Hovsepian DM BJ, Eschelman DJ, et. al. Fallopian tube recanalization in an unrestricted patient population. *Radiology* 1994;190: 137–140.

137. Lang EK DH. Transcervical recanalization of strictures in the postoperative fallopian tube. *Radiology* 1994;191:507–512

138. Darcy MD MB, Picus D, et. al. Transcervical salpingoplasty: current techniques and results. *Urol Radiol* 1991;13:74–79.

139. Hedgpeth PL, Thurmond AS, Fry R, et al. Radiographic fallopian tube recanalization: absorbed ovarian radiation dose. *Radiology* 1991;180:121–122.

140. Thurmond AS PP, Hector DM, et. al. US-guided fallopian tube catheterization. *Radiology* 1991;180:571–572.

141. Gleicher N CE, Corfman R, et. al. The multicenter transcervical tuboplasty study: conclusions and comparison to alternative technologies. *Hum Repro* 1993;8:1264–1271.

142. Baggish MS BP. Carbon dioxide laser treatment of cervical stenosis. *Fertil Steril* 1987;48:24–28.

143. Luesley DM RC, Buxton EJ, et. al. Prevention of post-cone biopsy cervical stenosis using a temporary cervical stent. *Br J Obstet Gynecol* 1990;97:334–337.

144. Dickey KW ZT, Hsia HC, et. al. Transvaginal fluoroscopically-guided uterine cervical dilation: preliminary results in patients with infertility. *Radiology* 1996.

145. Dewire DM, Thomas AJ Jr, Falk RM, et al. Clinical outcome and cost comparison of percutaneous embolization and surgical ligation of varicocele. *J Androl* 1994;15:(Suppl): 38S–42S.

146. Belgrano E, Puppo P, Quattrini S, et al. The role of venography and sclerotherapy in the management of varicocele. *Eur Urol* 1984;10:124–129.

147. Comhaire F, Zalata A, Mahmoud A. Critical evaluation of the effectiveness of different modes of treatment of male infertility. *Andrologia* 1996;28(Suppl 1):31–35.

28

Anatomy of the Gastrointestinal Tract, Liver, and Biliary System

JAMES E. SILBERZWEIG

Familiarity with the normal and variant anatomy of the gastrointestinal (GI) tract, liver, and biliary system is essential for the interventional radiologist. Pathologic conditions may distort normal anatomy and make therapeutic interventions difficult or impossible. An understanding of variant vascular and ductal anatomy, as well as of the presence and location of collateral pathways is essential to both diagnosis and therapy.

■ Arterial Anatomy

The arterial supply to the GI tract is by the three main ventral branches of the abdominal aorta (Fig. 28-1): the celiac artery, the superior mesenteric artery (SMA), and the inferior mesenteric artery (IMA). There is considerable variation in the branching pattern from these three main vessels. Furthermore, there are copious collateral pathways between the vascular territories.

Celiac artery

The celiac artery arises from the aorta at the level of the T12 vertebral body.[1] Its branches supply the liver, gallbladder, stomach, proximal duodenum, pancreas, and spleen. The three major branches of the celiac artery are the left gastric artery (LGA), splenic artery, and common hepatic artery (Figs. 28-2 through 28-4).

Left gastric artery
The LGA is a branch of the celiac artery in 90% of all persons. It arises from the superior margin of the proximal celiac artery and courses vertically toward the lesser curvature of the stomach. The origin and orientation of the LGA sometimes make selective catheterization of the LGA difficult. Accessory LGA branches may arise from the left hepatic artery. The LGA arises directly from the aorta in 1 to 5% of all persons[2-4] and supplies the lower esophagus, cardia, fundus, and body of the stomach.

Splenic artery
The splenic artery is the largest branch of the celiac artery and is tortuous in adults. It courses superior and anterior to the splenic vein and may arise directly from the aorta in 2% of persons.[3] The splenic artery supplies the spleen, the pancreas, and the stomach.

Branches of the splenic artery include the posterior gastric artery, short gastric arteries, left gastroepiploic artery, and the superior and inferior terminal branches supplying the spleen. The splenic artery gives rise to three pancreatic branches: the dorsal pancreatic artery supplies the neck and body of the pancreas; the great pancreatic artery (arteria pancreatica magna) supplies the body of the pancreas; and the caudal pancreatic artery supplies the tail of the pancreas. The transverse pancreatic artery runs within the pancreas and originates from the left branch of the dorsal pancreatic artery. The transverse pancreatic artery anastomoses with the other pancreatic branches from the splenic artery.[5]

Common hepatic artery
The main branch of the common hepatic artery is the gastroduodenal artery (GDA). The superior pancreaticoduodenal artery arises from the GDA, which continues as the right gastroepiploic artery along the greater curvature of the stomach. The right gastroepiploic artery then

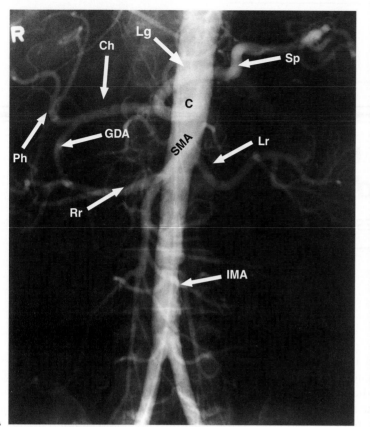
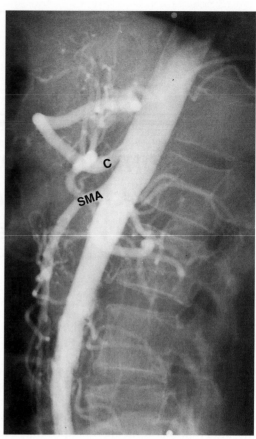

FIGURE 28-1. Abdominal aortogram. Frontal (**A**) and lateral (**B**) projections. C, celiac artery; SMA, superior mesenteric artery; IMA, inferior mesenteric artery; Sp, splenic artery; Ch, common hepatic artery; GDA, gastroduodenal artery; Ph, proper hepatic artery; Rr, right renal artery; Lr, left renal artery; Lg, left gastric artery.

forms an anastomosis with the left gastroepiploic artery. The left gastroepiploic artery arises from the distal splenic artery.

The common hepatic artery courses to the right and becomes the proper hepatic artery after giving rise to the GDA. The right and left hepatic arteries arise from the proper hepatic artery, and the middle hepatic artery arises from either the left or right hepatic artery and supplies the medial segment of the left lobe of the liver.[6]

Cystic artery

The cystic artery is usually a branch of the right hepatic artery, but it may arise from the left or common hepatic artery (Fig. 28-5).[3] This artery is inconsistently visualized on arteriography.

Right gastric artery

This small vessel arises from the proper hepatic or left hepatic artery in 80% of persons. In the remaining 20%, the right gastric artery arises from the GDA or from the right or middle hepatic artery.[3] The right gastric artery forms an anastomosis with the left gastric artery along the

lesser curvature of the stomach. This vessel usually is not visualized on arteriography.

Hepatic Arterial Variants

There is considerable anatomic variation in the arterial supply to the liver.[3,6] The most common variations include the following:

1. The *left hepatic artery* arises from the LGA (10–30%) and also may be referred to as the *aberrant left hepatic branch.*
2. The *accessory left hepatic artery* arises from the LGA (8%).
3. The *replaced right hepatic artery* arises from the SMA (14–20%) and also may be referred to as the *aberrant right hepatic branch.* It runs behind the pancreas and the portal vein.
4. The *accessory right hepatic* artery (partial replacement) arises from the SMA (6%).
5. The *replaced common hepatic artery* (Fig. 28-6), arises from the SMA with no hepatic artery branches originating from the celiac artery (2.5%).[7]

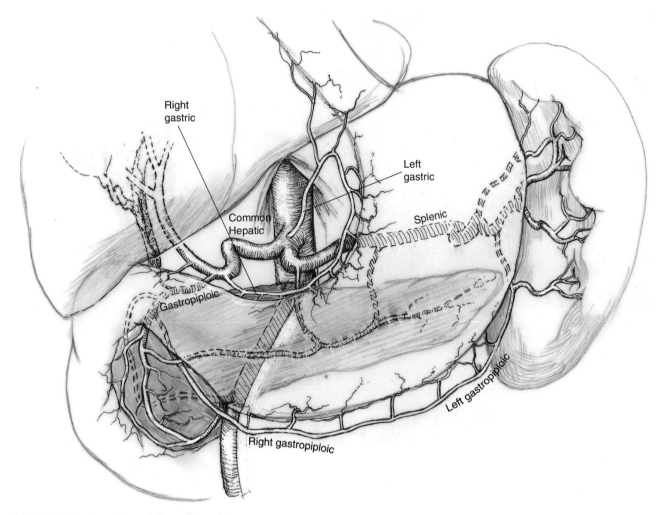

FIGURE 28-2. Branches of the celiac artery.

The presence of a replaced hepatic artery branch is an important variant that may affect arterial anastomoses during liver transplant surgery, dissection during liver resection, portocaval shunt surgery, or pancreaticoduodenectomy (*Whipple procedure*). Variant anatomy, such as an LGA branch arising from the left hepatic artery or a replaced hepatic artery branch, must be recognized in cases of percutaneous transarterial tumor chemoembolization. Failure to recognize these variants may result in inadequate embolization or unintentional embolization of the vessels supplying the bowel. During papaverine infusion into the SMA in a patient with a replaced hepatic

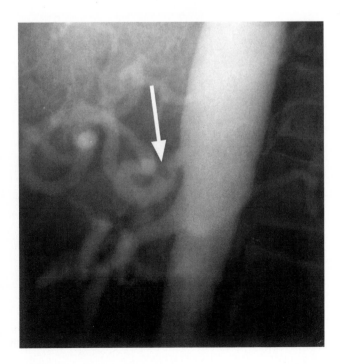

FIGURE 28-3. Celiac axis compression. Lateral abdominal aortogram shows a smooth narrowing of the superior aspect of the celiac artery that resulted from crural fibers of the diaphragm (median arcuate ligament).[16] This finding is common and should not be considered a pathologic condition in asymptomatic persons. It remains unresolved whether compression of the celiac axis by the median arcuate ligament, as an isolated finding, can result in clinically significant mesenteric ischemia.[17]

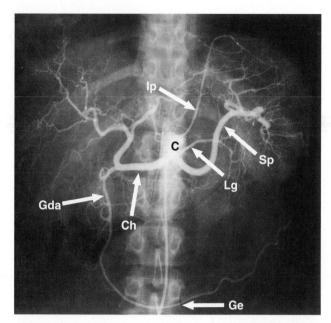

FIGURE 28-4. Celiac arteriogram. C, celiac trunk; Sp, splenic artery; Lg, left gastric artery; Ch, common hepatic. Gda, gastroduodenal artery; Ge, gastroepiploic artery; Ip, inferior phrenic artery.

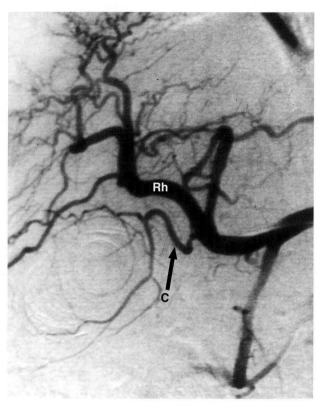

FIGURE 28-5. The cystic artery, (C) typically arises from the right hepatic (RH) artery.

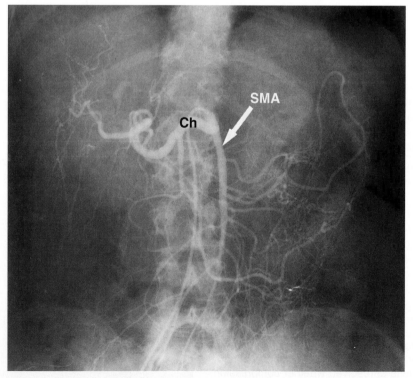

FIGURE 28-6. Replaced common hepatic artery. Superior mesenteric artery (SMA) injection shows the common hepatic artery origin from the proximal SMA. Ch, common hepatic artery.

artery branch, the catheter tip must be positioned distal to the replaced hepatic artery branch for an effective infusion.

Inferior phrenic artery

The inferior phrenic artery can arise from the celiac artery in 35% to 65% of persons or directly from the aorta. The right and left inferior phrenic arteries may have a common or separate origins. Before entering the diaphragm, the left inferior phrenic artery may give off a small gastroesophageal branch. The inferior phrenic arteries may not be well opacified on celiac arteriography, because they arise from the most proximal aspect of this vessel.[8,9]

Superior mesenteric artery

The SMA arises from the aorta approximately 1 to 2 cm inferior to the origin of the celiac artery at the level of L1 vertebral body[1] (Figs. 28-7 and 28-8). The celiac artery and the SMA from the aorta (celiacomesenteric trunk) have a common origin in 0.4% of persons (Fig. 28-9).[3] Branches of the SMA include the inferior pancreatico-duodenal artery, the jejunal and ileal arteries, the middle colic artery, right colic artery, and ileocolic artery. Branches of the SMA supply the head of the pancreas, duodenum, jejunum, ileum, cecum, ascending colon, and proximal half of the transverse colon.

Inferior pancreaticoduodenal artery (IPDA)

The first branch of the SMA, the IPDA occasionally may have a common origin with a jejunal artery. It divides into anterior and posterior branches, which anastomose with the corresponding branches of the superior pancreaticoduodenal arteries from the GDA to form the pancreaticoduodenal arcades. The IPDA may arise as a single artery or as one anterior branch and one posterior branch with separate origins.[3,6]

Jejunal and ileal arteries

Ten to 14 of these arteries arise from the left lateral border of the SMA. The *ileal arteries* are the branches that arise from the SMA beyond the origin of the ileocolic artery. Multiple arcade-like anastomoses exist between these branches. The arcades closest to the small intestine (*marginal artery of Dwight*) give off the vasa recta.[10]

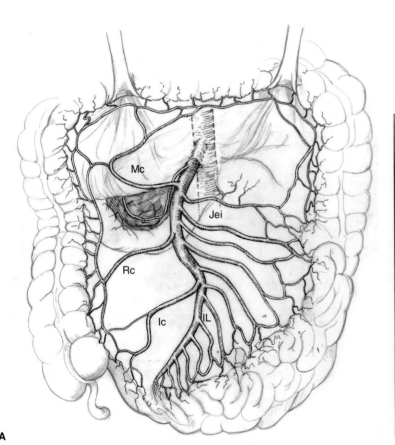

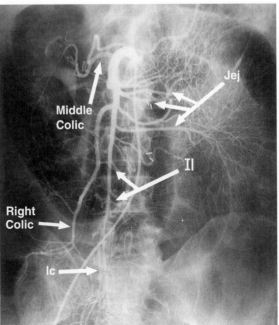

A   B

FIGURE 28-7. A: The superior mesenteric artery. **B:** Superior mesenteric arteriogram. Jej, jejunal branches; Il, ileal branches; Mc, middle colic artery; Rc, right colic artery; Ic, ileocolic artery.

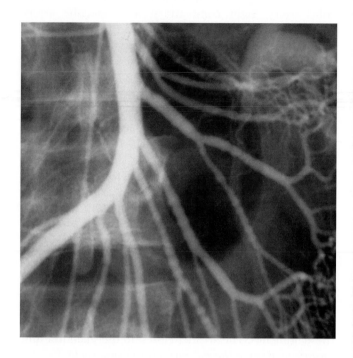

FIGURE 28-8. Standing wave phenomenon. Uniform wave-like changes in arterial contour of superior mesenteric (SMA) branches are seen in this normal vessel. These changes may be seen after one injection and may not be present on subsequent injection of the same vessel. This phenomenon is not associated with any known pathologic process within the vessel.[18]

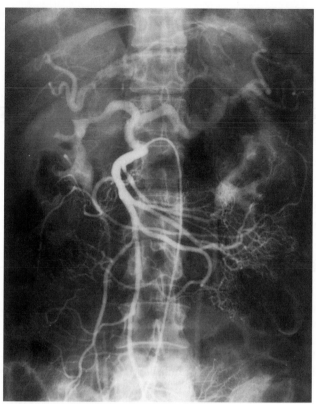

FIGURE 28-9. Common origin of celiac artery and superior mesenteric artery (SMA).

Middle colic artery

This vessel arises from the proximal SMA at the level of the first jejunal artery. The middle colic artery divides into left and right branches: The left branch anastomoses with the ascending branch of the left colic artery, and the right branch of the middle colic artery anastomoses with the ascending branch of the right colic artery. The middle colic artery supply occasionally originates from the celiac artery or one of its branches (0.5%).[3] The left branch of the middle colic artery may have an accessory branch that arises from the dorsal pancreatic artery (3%).[3]

Right colic artery

The right colic artery may arise from the SMA, middle colic artery, or ileocolic artery. The right colic artery typically is described to originate from the SMA but is found in only 13% of cases.[6] The right colic artery divides into an *ascending branch,* which anastomoses with the right branch of the middle colic artery, and a *descending branch,* which anastomoses with the ascending branch of

the ileocolic artery. The right colic artery supplies the ascending colon and hepatic flexure.

Ileocolic artery

The last major branch of the SMA, the ileocolic artery is the only constant branch of the SMA and it has a characteristic course downward and to the right, is the only constant branch of SMA, and therefore serves as an important angiographic landmark. It distributes branches to the terminal ileum, cecum, appendix, and the lower third of the ascending colon.[10]

Inferior mesenteric artery

The inferior mesenteric artery (Fig. 28-10) arises at the level of the left pedicle of L3, descends to the left, and divides into the left colic artery, sigmoid arteries, and superior hemorrhoidal artery. The inferior mesenteric artery supplies the distal half of the transverse colon, the descending colon, sigmoid colon, and rectum.

Left colic artery

The ascending branch of the left colic artery anastomoses with the left branch of the middle colic artery to form the

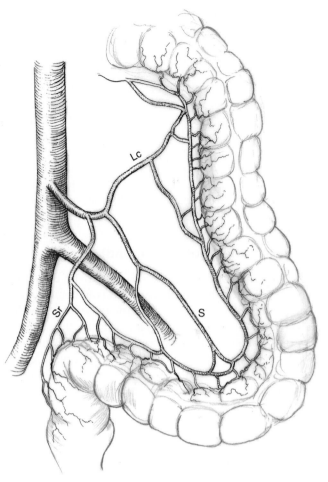

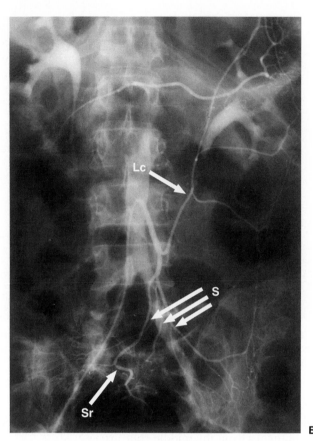

FIGURE 28-10. A: Inferior mesenteric artery. **B:** Inferior mesenteric arteriogram, Lc, left colic artery; S, sigmoid branches; Sr, superior rectal artery.

marginal artery (of Drummond). This vessel divides into ascending and descending branches. The ascending branch anastomoses with the left branch of the middle colic artery, and the descending branch anastomoses with branches of the sigmoid arteries.

Sigmoid arteries
Usually two to three of these arteries are present.

Superior hemorrhoidal artery
The branches of the superior hemorrhoidal artery anastomose with the middle and inferior hemorrhoidal arteries, which are branches from the anterior division of the internal iliac artery. This anastomosis can act as a collateral pathway to the lower extremity in cases of common iliac artery occlusion. An internal iliac artery angiogram should be considered in cases of lower GI bleeding in which the SMA and IMA injections demonstrate no abnormality.

■ Anastomotic Arteries

Arc of Riolan

This inconstant anastomotic artery joins the proximal portion of the middle colic artery and the ascending branch of the left colic artery. It is located near the root of the colonic mesentery.[6,10]

Arc of Buehler

This represents a persistent congenital anastomosis between the celiac artery and the SMA (Fig. 28-11).

Arc of Barkow (greater omental arcade)

The omental arteries act as potential collaterals between hepatic, splenic, and superior mesenteric arteries. The arc of Barkow receives anterior epiploic arteries from the right and left gastroepiploic arteries and posterior epi-

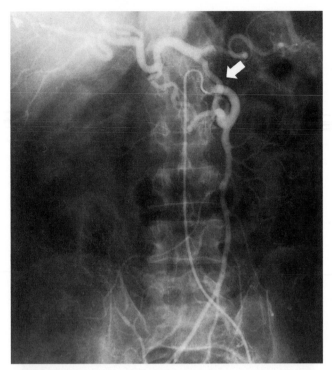

FIGURE 28-11. Arc of Buehler. Superior mesenteric artery (SMA) injection shows congenital connection between the SMA and celiac artery (*arrow*).

ploic arteries from the transverse pancreatic artery as well as branches from the middle colic artery.[10]

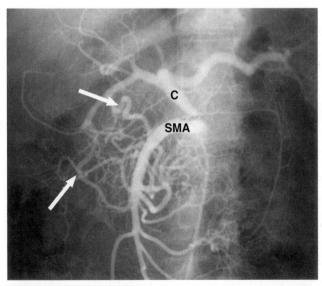

FIGURE 28-12. Pancreaticoduodenal arcades. Superior mesenteric artery (SMA) injection shows prominent pancreaticoduodenal arcades acting as a collateral pathway in this case of celiac artery origin stenosis. C, celiac trunk.

Pancreaticoduodenal arcades

The superior and inferior pancreaticoduodenal arteries (Fig. 28-12) supply the pancreatic head and proximal portion of the duodenum. The anterior and posterior branches of the superior pancreaticoduodenal artery form anastomoses with the anterior and posterior branches of the inferior pancreaticoduodenal artery, a branch of the proximal SMA. The pancreaticoduodenal arcades can act as an important collateral pathway in cases of celiac artery or SMA origin occlusion. The presence of this dual arterial supply to the duodenum can make bleeding duodenal ulcers difficult to treat by transarterial embolization.

Marginal artery (of Drummond)

The marginal artery is a vessel formed by the vascular arcades of the right, middle, and left colic arteries. It runs within the mesentery parallel to the mesenteric border of the colon and gives off the vasa recta to the colon. The marginal artery can act as a collateral pathway in cases of occlusion of the SMA or IMA. The marginal artery is usually not complete because the vasa recta of the transverse colon often will arise directly from the middle colic artery.[10]

Griffith's point

Located at the splenic flexure, Griffith's point is a watershed area between the SMA and IMA circulations. It is vulnerable to ischemia because the marginal artery is often incomplete at the splenic flexure and has no anastomotic arcades linking the left branch of the middle colic artery with the ascending branch of the left colic artery.[10]

Central anastomotic artery

The central anastomotic artery represents a direct anastomosis of the middle colic and left colic arteries. It is located within the colonic mesentery between the marginal artery and the arc of Riolan.[10]

Meandering artery

This artery (Fig. 28-13) may be identified angiographically when either the superior or the inferior mesenteric artery is occluded. The meandering artery is a dilated central anastomotic artery or a dilated arc of Riolan. The direction of the blood flow in the meandering artery is from the patent to the occluded main artery. The medical literature contains great variety concerning the definitions and the angiographic appearance of the central anastomotic artery and the meandering artery.[10,11]

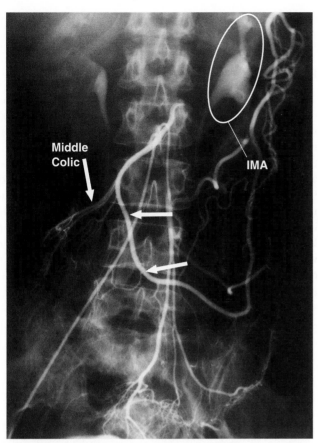

FIGURE 28-13. Meandering mesenteric artery. A large collateral vessel arising from the inferior mesenteric artery (IMA) with flow toward the middle colic artery (*arrows*) in this case of superior mesenteric artery (SMA) origin occlusion.

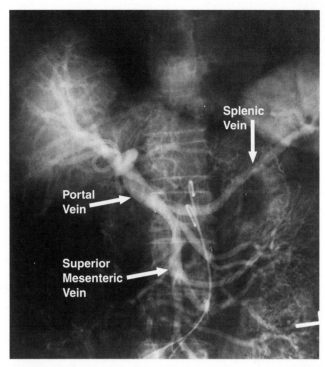

FIGURE 28-14. Portal venous anatomy. Venous phase of simultaneous injection of celiac artery and superior mesenteric artery (SMA).

■ Venous Anatomy

Portal venous system

The portal venous system drains blood from the small intestine, stomach, spleen, pancreas, gallbladder, and colon (except the lower part of the rectum). The superior mesenteric vein (SMV) and the splenic vein join to form the portal vein posterior to the head of pancreas (Fig. 28-14).

The splenic vein arises at the splenic hilus and receives the pancreatic veins; the short gastric veins, which drain the fundus and the left part of the greater curvature of the stomach; the left gastroepiploic veins; and the inferior mesenteric vein (IMV) (Fig. 28-15). The IMV is formed by the left colic vein, sigmoid veins, and superior hemorrhoidal vein and usually drains into the splenic

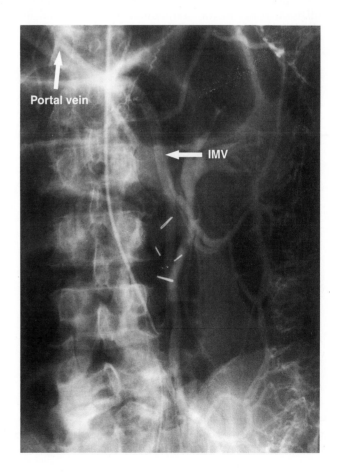

FIGURE 28-15. Inferior mesenteric vein (IMV) opacification following inferior mesenteric artery injection.

vein proximal to the confluence of the splenic vein and the SMV. In 10% of cases, the portal vein is formed by the confluence of the SMV, IMV, and splenic vein.[3] The right gastric and left gastric (coronary) veins drain into the splenic vein or directly into the portal vein. The SMV receives the jejunal, ileal, ileocolic, right colic, and middle colic veins as well as the right gastroepiploic and the pancreaticoduodenal veins.

The portal vein enters the liver and divides into right and left portal vein branches. The portal vein branches divide into smaller branches that run with the hepatic artery branches and biliary ducts, terminating in the sinusoids. The sinusoids represent the point of origin of the hepatic venules, which eventually drain into the inferior vena cava by the hepatic veins.

The paraumbilical veins are small vessels that establish an anastomosis between the anterior abdominal wall, the portal vein, and internal iliac veins. The paraumbilical veins extend along the ligamentum teres.[5] In cases of portal hypertension, the paraumbilical veins can become enlarged, especially in the event of portal vein thrombosis. The *umbilical vein* (Fig. 28-16) originates at the umbilicus and courses dorsally and upward, between the layers of the falciform ligament along the surface or within the ligamentum teres, and ends in the left branch of the portal vein. The umbilical vein can act as a major collateral vessel to the abdominal wall or internal iliac

veins in the presence of portal hypertension (*Cruveilhier-Baumgarten syndrome*).

Hepatic veins

The hepatic veins (Figs. 28-17 and 28-18) provide venous return from the liver to the systemic circulation. The right, middle, and left hepatic veins converge at the posterior surface of the liver and drain into the inferior vena cava near its termination at the right atrium. The middle and left hepatic veins often have a common trunk, and the right hepatic vein joins the inferior vena cava separately.[3] Often a right inferior hepatic vein drains directly into the inferior vena cava. The caudate lobe of the liver has a separate venous drainage directly into the inferior vena cava.[6] The location, angulation, and large diameter of the right hepatic vein makes it the vein most commonly used for creation of a transjugular portosystemic shunt (TIPS).

Pressure measurements obtained from a catheter

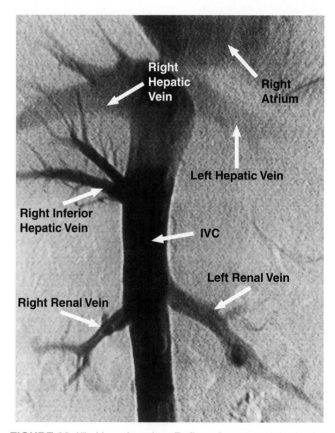

FIGURE 28-17. Hepatic veins. Reflux of contrast into the hepatic veins is demonstrated during inferior vena cava (IVC) contrast injection. Reflux into the hepatic veins during IVC injection is often seen in patients with an elevated right heart pressure or during Valsalva maneuver. The middle hepatic vein is superimposed over the inferior vena cava.

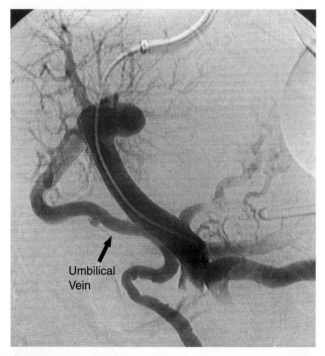

FIGURE 28-16. Umbilical vein. Portal vein injection during transjugular portosystemic shunt (TIPS) procedure. Hepatofugal flow is demonstrated in a patent umbilical vein.

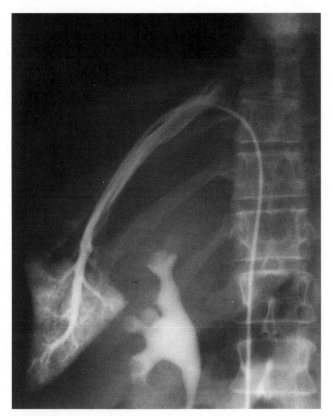

FIGURE 28-18. Right hepatic vein. Selective right hepatic venogram shows normal intrahepatic branching pattern and parenchymal stain.

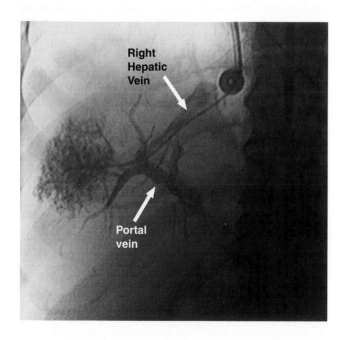

FIGURE 28-19. Wedged hepatic venogram. Injection of contrast into the right hepatic vein with the catheter wedged into a venule results in reflux of contrast into portal vein branches. This injection was performed during a transjugular portosystemic shunt (TIPS) procedure.

wedged in a hepatic venule can act as a reflection of portal venous pressure. A wedged hepatic venogram opacifies the portal venous system by reflux of contrast through the hepatic sinusoids into the portal vein (Fig. 28-19) and most often is performed for localization of the portal vein during a TIPS procedure.

Portosystemic anastomoses

Multiple communications exist between the portal and systemic venous systems and serve as collateral pathways to decompress the portal venous system in patients with portal hypertension. These collaterals may be identified at portography as enlarged and tortuous vessels with hepatofugal flow. The most common collateral pathways encountered at portography include the following:

1. Esophageal (coronary) → azygous vein
2. Gastric/splenic → azygous and/or left renal vein
3. Mesenteric → left renal, gonadal, or retroperitoneal veins
4. Intrahepatic portal veins → paraumbilical veins or umbilical vein
5. Inferior mesenteric vein → hemorrhoidal veins[12]

■ Liver Anatomy

The liver has a dual blood supply. The hepatic blood supply comprises 75% by the portal vein and 25% by the hepatic artery. The right and left lobes of the liver are divided by the middle hepatic vein. The right lobe is divided into an anterior and posterior segment by the right hepatic vein, and the left lobe is divided into medial and lateral segment by the left hepatic vein. The caudate lobe has an independent venous drainage directly into the IVC. The Couinaud and Bismuth numbering systems of segmental anatomy divides the liver into eight segments based on the distribution of the three hepatic veins and the right and left main portal trunks (Fig. 28-20).[13] The segmental numbering system provides a means for detailed description of the location, extent, and relation to the venous structures of a liver lesion. This functional division of the liver is used to determine the surgical approach for liver tumor resection and for reduced-size orthotopic liver transplantation.[14]

■ Biliary System Anatomy

The hepatic ducts have a lobar and a segmental distribution (Fig. 28-21). The right hepatic duct is formed by the anterior and posterior segmental ducts. The left hepatic duct is formed by the medial and lateral segmental ducts.

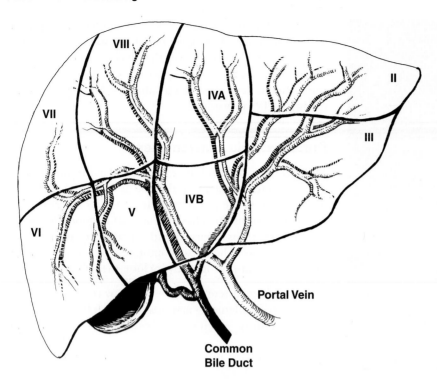

FIGURE 28-20. Segmental anatomy of the liver.

Bile ducts from the caudate lobe drain into either the left or the right hepatic ducts. The main left duct is usually longer than the main right duct.

The common hepatic duct (CHD) forms at the porta hepatis by the junction of the left and right hepatic ducts. The distal 1 to 2 cm of the right and left hepatic ducts lies outside the liver parenchyma. The CHD is closely related to the hepatic artery and portal vein. The hepatic artery lies to the left of the CHD, and the portal vein runs posterior and to the left of the CHD. Insertion of the cystic duct into the CHD defines the origin of the common bile duct (CBD), which is joined by the pancreatic duct at the ampulla. The ampulla drains into the second portion of the duodenum at the papilla of Vater.[15]

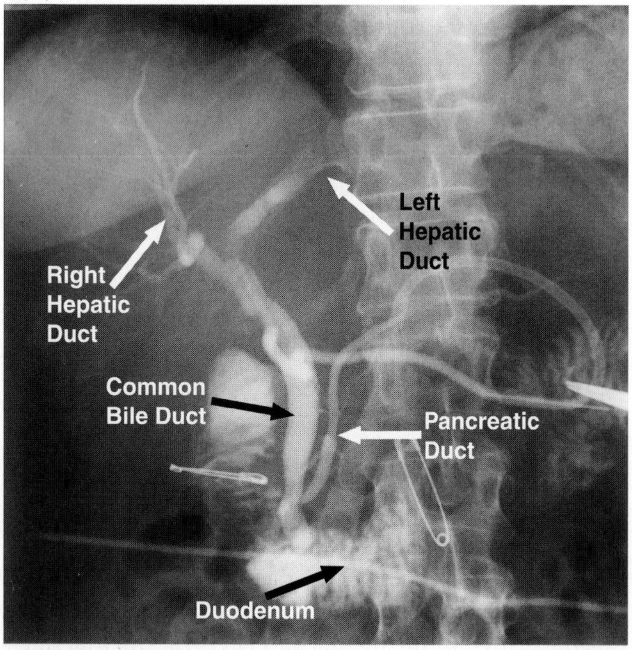

REFERENCES

1. Kao GD, Whittington R, Coia L. Anatomy of the celiac axis and superior mesenteric artery and its significance in radiation therapy. *Int J Radiat Oncol Biol Phys* 1992;25:131–134.
2. Nebesar RA, Kornblith PL, Pollard JJ, et al. *Celiac and Superior Mesenteric Arteries: A Correlation of Angiograms and Dissections.* Boston: Little, Brown and Company; 1969.
3. Michels NA. *Blood Supply and Anatomy of the Upper Abdominal Organs, with a Descriptive Atlas.* Philadelphia: JB Lippincott; 1955.
4. Naidich JB, Naidich TP, Sprayregen S, et al. The origin of the left gastric artery. *Radiology* 1978;126:623–626.
5. Clemente CD. *Gray's Anatomy.* 30th American ed. Philadelphia: Lea and Febiger; 1985.
6. VanDamme JPJ. Behavioral anatomy of the abdominal arteries. *Surg Clin North Am* 1993;73:699–725.
7. Kadir S. *Atlas of Normal and Variant Angiographic Anatomy.* Philadelphia: WB Saunders; 1991.
8. Swigart LL, Siekert RG, Hambley WC, et al. The esophageal arteries: an anatomic study of 150 specimens. *Surg Gynecol Obstet* 1950; 90:234–243.
9. Kahn PC. Selective angiography of the inferior phrenic arteries. *Radiology* 1967;88:1–8.
10. Kornblith PL, Boley SJ, Whitehouse BS. Anatomy of the splanchnic circulation. *Surg Clin North Am* 1992;72:1–30.
11. Moskowitz M, Zimmerman H, Felson B. The meandering mesenteric artery of the colon. *AJR Am J Roentgenol* 1964;92:1088.

FIGURE 28-21. T-tube cholangiogram.

12. Johnsrude IS, Jackson DC, Dunnick NR. *A Practical Approach to Angiography.* 2nd ed. Boston: Little, Brown and Company; 1987.

13. Dodd GD. An American's guide to Couinaud's numbering system. *Am J Roentgenol* 1993;161:574–575.

14. Dodson TF. Surgical anatomy of hepatic transplantation. *Surg Clin North Am* 1993;73:645–659.

15. Kadir S. *Diagnostic Angiography.* Philadelphia: WB Saunders Company, 1986.

16. Szilagi DE, Rian RL, Elliot JP, Smith RP. The celiac artery compression syndrome: does it exist? *Surgery* 1972;72:849–863.

17. Bech F, Loesberg A, Rosenblum J, et al. Median arcuate ligament compression syndrome in monozygotic twins. *J Vasc Surg* 1994;19: 934–938.

18. Lehrer H. The physiology of angiographic arterial waves. *Radiology* 1967;89:11–19.

29

Interventional Management of Gastrointestinal Strictures

MICHAEL J. HALLISEY AND STEVEN G. MERANZE

Strictures of the gastrointestinal (GI) tract have many causes, including malignant, congenital, benign, and postsurgical lesions. Although these strictures can be difficult to manage, surgery has been the standard method of treatment; however, endoscopic and interventional radiologic treatments are rapidly proving to be effective methods in caring for these patients. In the upper GI tract, esophageal stenoses are the most common lesions, followed by gastric and duodenal lesions; newer techniques now allow interventional management of colonic strictures. All these lesions are amenable to stricture dilation.

■ Esophageal Strictures

Strictures of the esophagus may be secondary to primary congenital anomaly, caustic ingestion, malignant disorders, esophageal surgery, or esophagitis. Malignant strictures arise directly from a primary esophageal carcinoma or from an adjacent lung or mediastinal malignancy invading the esophagus. In the midesophagus, 90% of the primary esophageal malignancies are due to squamous cell carcinoma. In the distal third of the esophagus, the most common malignancy is gastric adenocarcinoma. Treatment of these malignant disorders has included surgical bypass, stent placement, or primary repair. Although 50% of esophageal tumors are deemed resectable, the 5-year survival rate of these patients is only 10%, regardless of the treatment.[1,2] The most commonly encountered benign etiology for strictures in adults is reflux esophagitis. Other causes include achalasia, caustic ingestion, postradiation changes, and iatrogenic trauma. Traditional treatment of these benign strictures is repetitive dilation with mercury bougies.

Transluminal dilation with angioplasty balloons has added yet another effective tool to the treatment armamentarium of these stenotic lesions. When used with fluoroscopic and standard guidewire techniques, these balloons have proved safe and effective. The recent availability of expandable metallic stents has added to the interventional radiologists ability to assist in the treatment of these patients, particularly those with malignant disease.

Surgical and endoscopic treatments

Traditional surgical methods for the treatment of esophageal strictures include patching the esophagus in the region of the stricture or bypassing the stricture with colon or jejunum. Although the former method may result in excellent relief of dysphagia and reflux symptoms, about one half of patients undergoing patching may require dilation at a later date. Intestinal interposition operations are effective but also are associated with significant morbidity and mortality and constitute a major surgical procedure. For malignant disease, radiation therapy and chemotherapy have short-lived effects, and although laser treatment is used for exophytic tumors, it must be repeated frequently.

Bougienage has been performed for centuries and involves the use of an instrument with a straight or rounded olive-shaped tip inserted through the stricture, progressively stretching the narrowed segment to achieve the desired lumen. In the past, these instruments could be passed repeatedly by the patient using bougies (such as

353

the Hurst or Maloney dilators); however, the use of endoscopic techniques has encouraged the development of types of bougies that pass over guidewires, reducing the likelihood of perforation. The most popular of these models are the Celestine and Eder-Puestow devices.

Although effective, these devices have one major disadvantage: They provide a significant radial force on the stricture but also exert longitudinal force on the adjacent, normal esophagus. This additional stress can lead to perforation or mucosal tears.[3] Angioplasty balloons passed over a wire and placed directly across the lesion may overcome the shortcomings of bougienage. These balloons can be introduced on a small catheter that then can be inflated to a large outer diameter, thus maximizing the radial force on the lesion while reducing the longitudinal force on the adjacent esophagus.

General intubation techniques

Before esophageal dilation, an esophagram is required to help delineate the anatomy of the stricture. Stricture dilation generally does not require analgesics, and sedation with intravenous midazolam hydrochloride (Versed) is usually adequate. Atropine may be helpful if the patient develops signs of increased vagal tone (e.g., bradycardia) or if secretions are copious. The use of topical analgesia such as anesthetic gels or oral sprays are recommended to avoid patient discomfort and to reduce the gag reflex.

A soft nasogastric tube is passed transorally and placed just above the level of the stricture. The transoral intubation approach usually is employed for esophageal stricture dilation. This transoral route is easier and better tolerated, and it will permit passage of catheters larger than those used in the transnasal approach. Moreover, this route must be used for the placement of stents. The transnasal approach is preferred if a feeding tube is to be placed over the same guidewire. By enlarging the side hole in the nasogastric tube, the rounded tip of the tube can be maintained while still allowing guidewires to be inserted through the tube. After the tube is in position, a small amount of contrast is injected to define the proximal aspect of the stricture. In patients at risk for aspiration, dilute barium or oily contrast may be used.

A flexible-tipped standard 0.035-inch guidewire then is passed through either the endhole or sidehole of the nasogastric tube, which then is exchanged for a 5 Fr selective angiographic catheter. Although the stricture often can be traversed using a flexible guidewire, a torque-control guidewire or hydrophilic guidewire may be used to cross the lesion if the stricture is particularly tight or irregular. Great care must be exercised to minimize the risk of esophageal perforation, particularly in patients who have malignant strictures. Once the guidewire and catheter are through the lesion, the guidewire is removed and

replaced with a long exchange wire (> 180 cm), which is advanced well into the stomach or small bowel. At this point, the catheter can be exchanged for the balloon dilating catheter, which is placed across the stricture.

A diameter of 20 mm in the esophagus is recommended to permit normal oral intake. With extremely tight strictures (i.e., ≤ 3 mm) a 6- to 8-mm predilating balloon is used and then exchanged for larger-diameter sizes as needed. If no "waist" persists with the small balloon, it is exchanged for one with a larger diameter (i.e., 12, 15, or 20 mm) until the 20-mm diameter is achieved. Whereas most patients experience some discomfort, a significant degree of discomfort during dilation should signal the interventional radiologist to limit the increase in balloon size, at least for the current session. In patients with achalasia, overdistention of the esophagus may be desired, and multiple balloons may be used to achieve the desired lumen diameter. In patients who have strictures resulting from caustic ingestion, great care must be taken to avoid perforation.

An esophagram should be performed after the dilation procedure to evaluate for possible esophageal tears. The appearance of the lesion at this point is not predictive of clinical success, however. A postprocedural success rate of 90 to 95% in the esophageal lesions, with approximately 70% of benign lesions remaining asymptomatic 2 years following dilation, should be expected.[4]

Although long-term relief is unlikely, dilation of malignant lesions can be used to assist in the placement of enteric feeding tubes, and some degree of palliation can occur, if only for a short time. The use of stents has greatly changed the ability to palliate these patients.

Stents

Plastic stents have largely been replaced by metallic stents because of problems with food impaction and perforation. In one review, the complication rate was 36% the dislodgment rate 20%, and the morbidity rate 16% during endoscopic placement of these plastic stents.[5] As in other locations, the use of metallic stents in the esophagus is intended to maintain a stable lumen diameter, with a small and well-tolerated introducing system. Currently, three metallic stents are available that have been approved for use in the esophagus. The Cook Gianturco (Cook Inc., Bloomington, IN) stent and the Schneider Wallstent (Schneider USA, Minneapolis MN) are covered. The third, the Ultraflex nitinol stent (Medi-tech, Boston Scientific, Watertown, MA), is a tightly woven metal mesh. All three stents were designed to provide a large-lumen diameter while preventing ingrowth of tumor at the ends or through the body of the stent.

The procedure for placing these stents is similar to performing a balloon dilation (Fig. 29-1). It is necessary

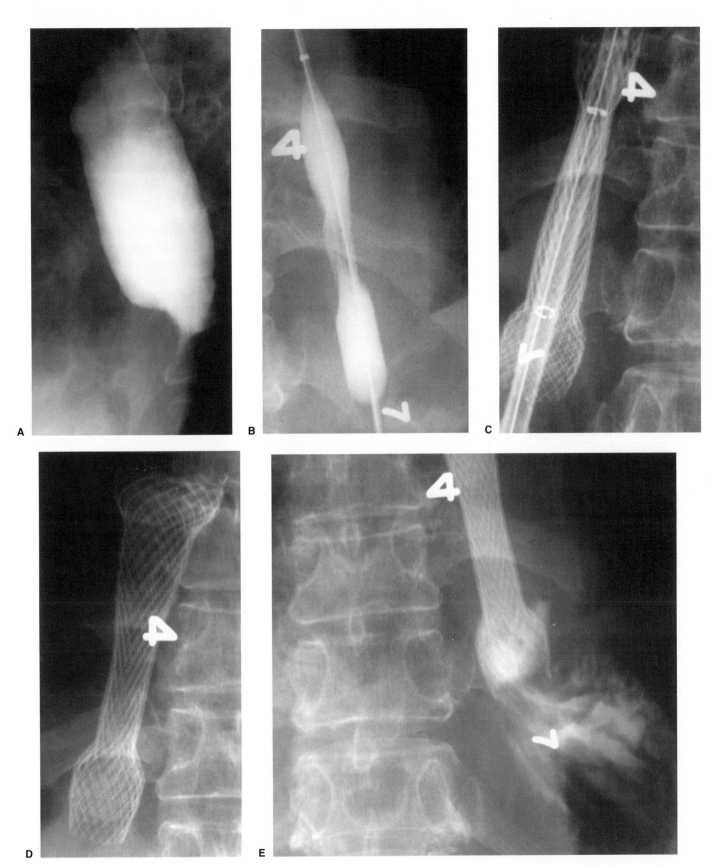

FIGURE 29-1. Transluminal stent placement for the relief of esophageal obstruction. **A:** A 55-year-old man with esophageal carcinoma originating just above the gastroesophageal junction. Note the "bird's beak" appearance of the stenotic segment and the proximal esophageal dilation. **B:** The stenotic area was dilated with a 15-mm balloon before the stent was placed. **C:** An 18-mm diameter by 6 cm Wallstent is deployed under fluoroscopic guidance across the stenotic segment by releasing the constraining membrane. **D:** The stent fully expands after balloon dilation, which provides the patient with a large enough lumen for passage of the food bolus. **E:** After stent placement, contrast empties from the esophagus into the stomach. The stent terminates just above the gastroesophageal junction in an attempt to avoid reflux.

to extend the neck fully to insert these stents because of size and rigidity of introducer device. It is important to predilate the lesions to at least 12 to 14 mm to allow the device to be inserted and withdrawn without difficulty.

The results obtained with these stents have been encouraging. In most series, with properly selected patients, no problem with initial insertion has been encountered. Most patients have had prompt relief of dysphagia (within 24 hr). Complications can include migration, perforation, tumor overgrowth (all types), and tumor ingrowth (uncovered stents). Erosion with hemorrhage (some fatal) has occurred, particularly in patients who have previously undergone radiation therapy. Tracheoesophageal fistulas that occur as a consequence of malignancy[6] or infection[7] also have been treated by placing covered stents.

Because of their short life expectancy, long-term follow-up is a relative concept in these patients. Complications or tumor overgrowth have been treated either by redilating or repeat stenting. In cases of tumor ingrowth, laser cauterization or restenting is usually adequate to reestablish patency. Treatment of benign stenoses with stents is still controversial. Long-term sequelae from these stents may be esophageal erosion or intense tissue hyperplasia.[8]

■ Gastric and Duodenal Strictures

Strictures of the antral and pyloric regions as well as the body of the stomach and duodenum also may be dilated. Balloons larger than 20 mm may be required. If balloons larger than 20 mm are not readily available, multiple balloons are necessary to achieve a diameter this large. The use of two balloons will result in an oblong-shaped dilation surface. Therefore, three balloons are recommended to create a shape more closely approximating a round dilation surface.[9]

Compared with the esophagus, the stenotic antrum, pylorus, or duodenum may require more skill in intubation. The stomach may be fluid filled and distended, making the use of standard angiographic techniques difficult. In these patients, stiffer tubes such as those used for duodenal intubation or cooperation with the endoscopist may be necessary during the initial stricture passage. Although the endoscope may not pass through the stricture, it can be used to support the angiographic catheters and to assist in the direction of the guidewire. Once the lesion has been traversed, the techniques are similar to those used in the esophagus, with exchanges made over a stiff exchange-length guidewire. A final lumen size of approximately 12 mm is ideal. In our series, long-term follow-up has demonstrated that approximately 75% of patients developed some degree of relief following dilation.[4]

■ Postoperative and Anastomotic Strictures

Postoperative and anastomotic strictures also can be treated with balloon dilation, particularly if the patients are poor surgical candidates. Moreover, conventional endoscopic techniques can be difficult in these patients.

The techniques for dilating anastomotic strictures are similar to those in other areas; however, the challenge with anastomotic strictures is due more to difficulties in the intubation technique than that of the dilation procedure itself. Endoscopic assistance can be used to access and treat these strictures, using the endoscope to assist in finding the lumen. Balloons of 12 to 15 mm are generally adequate. To our knowledge, balloon rupture of an esophagogastric anastomosis has not occurred.

Postoperative pyloric stenosis can develop following vagotomy and pyloroplasty. The stenosis can be secondary to pylorospasm (in the immediate postoperative period related to an incomplete pyloromyotomy) or surrounding fibrosis (which can occur many years after surgery). Recently, Denys et al.[10] advocated overdilation of the pyloric channel with a 30-mm balloon as the initial treatment procedure to reduce the likelihood of repeat dilation. Because the pylorus has a relatively smaller normal diameter than the esophagus or stomach, many interventional radiologists previously had approached these stenoses with a 10-mm or smaller diameter angioplasty balloon, but when balloons this size are used to treat these pyloric stenoses, multiple repeat dilations may become necessary because of recurrence of the stenosis.

■ Colonic Strictures

Large, expandable metallic stents are now available for the palliative treatment of colonic obstruction. They have not been approved for the treatment of benign strictures. Interventional management of malignant strictures has several advantages: (a) prompt relief of obstructive symptoms, (b) elimination of the need for emergent colostomy in the presence of unprepped bowel, (c) a less invasive procedure compared with surgery, and (d) in some cases, an outpatient procedure. The stents reach a maximum diameter of 22 mm and a maximum length of 9 cm.[11]

The treatment procedure (Fig. 29-2) is similar to stent placement in other locations within the GI tract. The lesion is localized and measured using standard barium techniques. A small catheter is used to cross the lesion. A stiff wire is placed across the lesion. The stent is placed across the lesion under fluoroscopic guidance and expanded by withdrawing the constraining membrane. Decompression of the obstructed segment is immediate, but

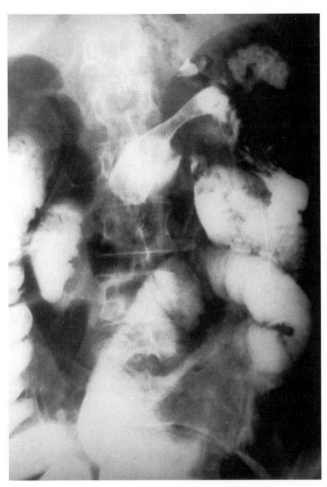

FIGURE 29-2. A 60-year-old patient presenting with colonic obstruction secondary to a malignancy. Following stent placement across the transverse colon, the large bowel obstruction is relieved.

luminal size can be increased by balloon dilation of the stent.

Although these larger-diameter stents are now available for the palliative decompression of colonic obstruction, there are emerging indications for which the stents are proving beneficial. These indications include (a) poor

surgical or medical risk, (b) no potential cure of a malignancy with resection, (c) repeat dilation of recurrent stenoses, and (d) postoperative strictures. More research in these newer areas will be necessary before widespread use and clinical approval are achieved.

■ Summary

Gastrointestinal strictures are amenable to transluminal balloon dilation and stent placement. Newer catheters, wires, and stent materials are now making these procedures easier to perform by interventional radiologists.

REFERENCES

1. Sons Hu, Borchard F. Cancer of the distal esophagus and cardia: incidence, tumorous infiltration and metastatic spread. *Ann Surg* 1986;203:188–195.
2. Muller JM, Erasmi H, Stelzner M, et al. Surgical therapy of oesophagel carcinoma. *Br J Surg* 1990;77:845–857.
3. McLean GK, LeVeen RF. Shear stress in the performance of esophageal dilation: comparison of balloon dilation and bougienage. *Radiology* 1989;172:983–986.
4. McLean GK, Cooper GS, Hartz WH, et al. Radiologically guided balloon dilation of gastrointestinal strictures. *Radiology* 1987;165:35–43.
5. Fugger R, Niederle B, Jantsch H, et al. Endoscopic tube implantation for the palliation of malignant esophageal stenosis. *Endoscopy* 1990;22:101–104.
6. Song H-Y, Young-Soo D, Young-Min H, et al. Covered, expandable esophageal metallic stent tubes: experiences in 119 patients. *Radiology* 1994;193:689–695.
7. Nelson DB, Silvis SE, Ansel HJ. Management of a tracheoesophageal fistula with a silicone-covered self-expanding metal stent. *Gastrointest Endosc* 1994;40:497–499.
8. Cwikiel W, Willen R, Stridbeck H, et al. Self-expanding stent in the treatment of benign esophageal strictures: experimental study in pigs and presentation of clinical cases. *Radiology* 1993;187:667–671.
9. Gaylord GM, Pritchard WF, Chuang VP, et al. The geometry of triple-balloon dilation. *Radiology* 1988;166:541–555.
10. Denys A, De Baere T, Lasser P, et al. Single-step balloon dilation of postoperative pyloric stenosis: benefit of large-balloon technique. *J Vasc Interv Radiology* 1994;5:781–782.
11. Mainar A, Tejero E, Maynar M, et al: Colorectal obstruction: treatment with metallic stents. *Radiology* 1996;198:761–764.

30

Nonvariceal Upper GI Bleeding

SEYMOUR SPRAYREGEN

Upper gastrointestinal (UGI) bleeding refers to a bleeding site proximal to the ligament of Treitz and accounts for 80% of all gastrointestinal bleeding.[1] From its onset, this entity must be recognized as potentially lethal, so diagnosis, resuscitation, and definitive treatment should be undertaken concomitantly. The mortality from acute nonvariceal UGI bleeding is approximately 10% and has remained fairly constant over the past 50 years;[2] it has been postulated that, despite advances in pharmacologic and endoscopic therapy, the mortality rate has remained the same because older, sicker patients have made up an increasing proportion of patients with gastrointestinal bleeding.[3] On the other hand, in one article suggesting that there is some evidence of a decline in mortality over the past 10 years, endoscopic advances and the wider availability and increased effectiveness of treatment in intensive care units are credited with the improved survival.[4]

The epidemiology of UGI bleeding is not static. The number of hospitalizations for gastric ulcers increased by 20% and the frequency of bleeding gastric ulcers increased by 100% between 1980 and 1985; during the same period, however, hospital admissions for nonbleeding duodenal ulcers decreased dramatically.[5] The increase in bleeding gastric ulcers has been attributed to the frequent use of nonsteroidal antiinflammatory drugs (NSAIDs), and the lower incidence of duodenal ulcers has been attributed to the availability of histamine 2-receptor antagonists (H_2RAs).[6]

UGI bleeding from a wide variety of sources stops spontaneously in approximately 80% of patients. Recurrent bleeding, however, occurs in as many as 25% of cases. In patients who have continued bleeding or rebleeding, mortality rates may be as high as 30 to 40%.[7] Patients must receive prompt, effective treatment to preclude the onset of hemorrhagic shock and coagulopathy. Even when bleeding rapidly ceases spontaneously, identifying the source of the hemorrhage will facilitate rapid treatment if rebleeding occurs.

■ Clinical Approach to UGI Bleeding

History and physical examination

A careful history and physical examination often will direct the physician to the cause of the bleeding and yield information regarding coexisting diseases and medications that may impact diagnosis and treatment. A history of pain preceding presentation or a history of peptic ulcer disease suggests peptic ulcer disease. The use of aspirin or other NSAIDs should raise the suspicion of peptic ulcer. A history of retching or vomiting before bleeding is classic for a Mallory-Weiss tear. Alcohol use or a history of blood transfusions increases the likelihood of liver disease with congestive gastropathy or varices. A previous history of pancreatitis should lead the physician to consider hemorrhage resulting from a pseudoaneurysm or pancreatic pseudocyst. Renal disease often is associated with GI bleeding.[8] Approximately 50% of patients with acute renal failure have GI bleeding, often from peptic ulcer disease. Aortoduodenal fistula must be the primary consideration in patients with an aortic graft for aneurysm or occlusive disease, but it may occur with abdominal aortic aneurysms without previous surgery. A history of epistaxis, especially with skin telangiectasias, should raise the possibility of Osler-Weber-Rendu disease.

Physical evaluation should include evaluating for stigmata of cirrhosis, abdominal tenderness, and a rectal examination. Inspection of nasogastric and rectal contents may provide information regarding the prediction of mortality; with bleeding from peptic ulcers, mortality rates of 30% when there was a red nasogastric aspirate and red stool and 9% when the nasogastric aspirate and stool were black have been reported.[9] Hematemesis generally indicates a more severe bleeding episode than melena.

Orthostatic hypotension (an increase in pulse rate by more than 20 beats per minute, a decrease in systolic blood pressure by more than 20 mm, and a decrease in diastolic blood pressure by more than 10 mm) may be the only physical finding and this usually occurs when there is a loss of 20% of intravascular volume or 1500 mL. Frank shock with supine hypotension and tachycardia indicates a volume loss approaching 40% or 2500 mL. Hypotension may result in transient hemostasis, and bleeding may recur when the blood pressure is restored to normal levels.

Resuscitation and management

An algorithm for the management of UGI bleeding is shown in Figure 30-1.

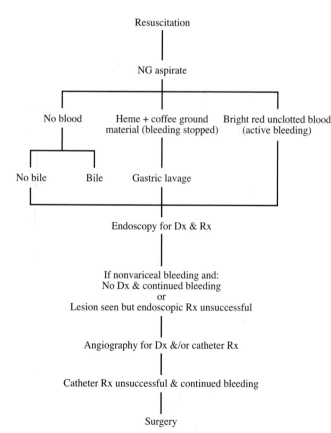

FIGURE 30-1. Algorithm for management of upper gastrointestinal bleeding.

Nasogastric tube and gastric lavage

A nasogastric tube should be passed. Black coffee-ground material (due to gastric acid acting on hemoglobin to form acid hematin) that tests positive for blood is indicative of recent hemorrhage, and bright red unclotted blood suggests continued rapid bleeding. If the nasogastric aspirate does not show evidence of blood, it is important to note the presence or absence of bile; if bile is present, it is likely that the bleeding is from the lower GI tract or that a UGI source has stopped. If neither blood nor bile is present, the bleeding may still be from a duodenal ulcer with no reflux of duodenal contents into the stomach (one large survey showed that 12% of patients with no blood on nasogastric aspirate demonstrated active UGI bleeding on endoscopy).[10] This same study showed a higher correlation between nasogastric return and endoscopy with gastric lavage and more prolonged nasogastric monitoring. Although melena (black tarlike stool) typically is seen with UGI or small bowel bleeding, it occasionally is seen with colonic bleeding. Frankly bloody bowel movements also can be due to bleeding from the stomach or duodenum and in these latter cases indicates rapid loss of more than 500 mL of blood.[10] The airway should be protected in patients with a reduced level of consciousness or repeated episodes of vomiting.

Gastric lavage has been used since the late 1950s, when Wangensteen and colleagues introduced the principle of gastric hypothermia for control of UGI bleeding.[11] Subsequent studies showed that lavage with saline at room temperature works as well as with ice solutions; indeed, cold-fluid lavage may impair coagulation, which occurs optimally at room temperature. Gastric lavage with a large-bore tube, regardless of the temperature and type of solution (saline, water, epinephrine), is a mainstay of treatment of UGI bleeding in most centers. Decreased gastric distension results in decreased gastrin release (and therefore decreased acid secretion). Although hemoglobin in the stomach helps to buffer acid, the fibrinolytic activity of retained blood outweighs the acid neutralizing action of blood.

Venous access lines

Large-bore (at least 16 gauge) peripheral or central venous access lines and (often) a urinary catheter should be placed. A Swan-Ganz catheter should be placed in patients who have underlying cardiac or renal disease or in patients in shock. Blood should be analyzed for type and cross-match for packed red blood cells. Blood should be drawn for hemoglobin, hematocrit, platelet count, prothrombin time, partial thromboplastin time, blood urea nitrogen (BUN), creatinine, calcium, and glucose. The hematocrit and hemoglobin do not change for the first few hours after hemorrhage because proportional amounts of plasma and red blood cells are lost; only as extracellular fluid enters the vascular space do these values fall, and this equilibration process may take from 24 to 72 hours. An elevated BUN with normal creatinine suggests a UGI source of bleeding. Oxygen should be administered because oxygen-carrying capacity is lost due to the loss of red blood cells (RBCs). The patient must receive appropriate blood and fluid replacement to maintain adequate intravascular volume and red cell mass, and coagulation defects must be corrected (usually with vitamin K or fresh frozen plasma). A hematocrit of 30% is a reasonable goal for most patients and provides a buffer should bleeding recur.

Histamine 2-receptor antagonists (H₂RAs)

H₂RAs reduce gastric acid secretion and are useful for ulcer healing, but they have not been shown to stop active bleeding or to definitely prevent rebleeding.[12] H₂RAs are extremely effective in preventing the formation of, and bleeding from, stress ulcers;[13,14] their use in intensive care unit (ICU) patients accounts for the marked reduction in stress ulcers seen in ICU patients in recent years.

Endoscopy

Emergency endoscopy should be the first diagnostic test in patients with continued bleeding or if esophageal varices are suspected to be the source of bleeding. It should be noted that 20 to 30% of bleeding patients with varices will be bleeding from a source other than varices.[15,16] Endoscopy should be performed as soon as all melenic material and clots have been evacuated by lavage. Endoscopy should be performed when bleeding persists after lavage, because endoscopy usually will be successful even in the presence of persistent bleeding. It is likely that hemorrhage from lesions bleeding so rapidly as to preclude endoscopic diagnosis most likely will not be stopped by further lavage.

The accuracy of endoscopy in identifying the cause of UGI bleeding ranges from 74 to 96%.[17] It is important that endoscopy be performed as close to the bleeding episode as possible, because the longer the delay between cessation of bleeding and endoscopy, the less revealing will endoscopy be. In one study, the diagnostic accuracy decreased from 90% when endoscopy was performed within 48 hr of a bleeding episode to 33% when endoscopy was performed more than 48 hr from the cessation of the bleeding episode.[18] The complication rate for emergency endoscopy has been reported to range from 0.1 to 8%, which contrasts with a complication rate of only 0.01% when elective endoscopy is used.[19] All patients who do not undergo endoscopy emergently should have elective endoscopy within 24 hr

of the initial bleed. This timing is important because (a) endoscopic signs (especially seeing pulsatile arterial blood) can be used to predict the risk for continued or recurrent hemorrhage with peptic ulcer,[20] (b) multiple lesions are present in about 25% of cases and early endoscopy can identify the lesion actually responsible for the bleeding, (c) superficial lesions can heal in a short time, and (d) identification of the lesion responsible for bleeding makes it possible to direct therapy appropriately.

■ Causes of UGI Bleeding

Endoscopic surveys[10,21] show that acid peptic diseases account for up to 75% of cases of UGI bleeding, with equal numbers caused by gastritis, gastric ulcer, and duodenal ulcer; varices, esophagitis, duodenitis, and Mallory-Weiss tears account for most of the remaining cases. The following is a brief description of some of the major causes of nonvariceal UGI bleeding.

Peptic ulcer disease (PUD)

Whereas the number of hospitalizations, operations, and deaths from PUD have decreased in recent years, hospitalizations for bleeding ulcers have not decreased.[22] PUD is particularly a problem of the elderly: the incidence of PUD increases with age. Of patients hospitalized for PUD complications, 70% are 60 years of age or older, approximately 80% of ulcer deaths occur in patients over 65 years, and the average mortality from complicated PUD in the elderly is 30%.[22] Overall mortality from bleeding PUD is approximately 6%. Clinical risk factors that are correlated with an adverse outcome from bleeding PUD are hematemesis, red nasogastric aspirate that does not clear, clinical shock, age greater than 60 years, and associated illnesses. Endoscopic features associated with a poor outcome are location (high gastric ulcer, posterior duodenal ulcer), large size, and endoscopic stigmata of recent hemorrhage.[20]

Gastric ulcers penetrate the muscularis mucosa, which distinguishes them from superficial erosions. Although ulcers can occur anywhere in the stomach, the most frequent location is on the lesser curvature near the angularis.[23] In 2 to 8% of cases, ulcers are multiple.[24] Gastric ulcers are one fourth as common as duodenal ulcers.

There are many theories regarding the pathogenesis of gastric ulcers.[25] Of patients who take NSAIDs, 25% develop gastric ulcers, and the risk of bleeding is twice that of gastric ulcers in patients who do not take NSAIDs.[9] NSAID-induced duodenal ulcers occur slightly less frequently.[26] The use of aspirin is associated with acute mucosal lesions and chronic ulcers.[25,27] Smoking also has been associated with gastric ulcers.[25]

Helicobacter pylori is a gram-negative bacterium that was first isolated in 1982 and is believed to have a dominant causal role in chronic superficial gastritis.[28] Because only a small percentage of patients with *H. pylori* develop ulcerations and because of the lack of strong evidence from animal models, it has been difficult to prove that *H. pylori* directly causes PUD; however, it is believed that infection with the organism may be a prerequisite for the occurrence of almost all duodenal ulcers in the absence of other specific precipitating factors.[28] As mentioned, the prevalence of *H. pylori* is much higher than the incidence of peptic ulcers; however, almost all patients with duodenal ulcer and a somewhat smaller percentage of patients with gastric ulcer have *H. pylori* colonization of the stomach.[29] Additional strong evidence that *H. pylori* causes peptic ulcers is the marked decrease in the recurrence rate of ulcers following eradication of the organism.[28] It is not clear whether *H. pylori* and NSAIDs act synergistically to cause ulcers.

Acute hemorrhagic gastritis

This term describes superficial gastric mucosal lesions (which do not penetrate the muscularis mucosa) that result in bleeding. The erosions are found primarily in the body and fundus of the stomach. Hemorrhagic gastritis is associated with physiologic stress (related to trauma, surgery, burns, or severe medical problems), NSAIDs, alcohol abuse, and portal hypertension. Less frequent causes are gastric irradiation, ingestion of caustic substances, bile reflux, and long-distance running. In only 20% of cases is a predisposing cause absent.[30] Duodenal erosions and gastric or duodenal ulcers may coexist with hemorrhagic gastritis.

Stress-related mucosal disease (SRMD)

This is a common cause of acute hemorrhagic gastritis and also a cause of duodenal mucosal bleeding. The formation of stress ulcers is multifactorial; factors that have been implicated are coagulopathy, reduced mucosal blood flow, inhibition of prostaglandin synthesis, bile reflux, reduced secretion of mucus and bicarbonate, and possibly increased gastric acidity.[12,31,32] Following a major physiologic stress, nearly all patients show evidence of acute mucosal injury. Although SRMD occurs in most critically ill patients, it is particularly common with major trauma, severe burns, sepsis, and respiratory, renal, and hepatic failure. Endoscopic studies have shown that the incidence of gastroduodenal damage within 18 to 24 hours of admission to an ICU is between 52 and 100%.[30] Before the use of H$_2$RAs, clinically significant bleeding occurred in 5 to 20% of patients who had experienced a major physiologic stress, with a mortality rate approaching 50%.[31,33]

Mallory-Weiss tear

The Mallory-Weiss syndrome, a mucosal tear at the esophagogastric junction, was first described in 1929.[34] Approximately two thirds of patients have an antecedent history of retching or vomiting, and 70% of patients are men.[35] Alcohol ingestion traditionally is associated with Mallory-Weiss tears and is present in 40 to 75% of patients. Recent use of aspirin or NSAIDs (30%), blunt trauma, straining at stool, coughing, seizures, heavy lifting, primal scream therapy, cardiopulmonary resuscitation, increased intracranial pressure, pregnancy, and endoscopy are also associated with this lesion.[36,37] 80 to 90% of tears are on the gastric side of the esophagogastric junction, and the remaining 10 to 20% are in the esophagus.[38] Other authors state that although tears may extend to the esophagus, they usually do not involve the esophagus alone.[37] Hematemesis occurs in 85% of cases; 10% of patients present only with melena. Abdominal pain is rare. The diagnosis is made at endoscopy with visualization of a single linear mucosal tear in 80 to 90% of cases, with two or three tears seen in the remainder. Transfusions are required in only 40% of patients, and bleeding stops spontaneously in more than 90% of cases. Management is usually supportive. When intervention is necessary, electrocoagulation, compression with the gastric balloon of a Sengstaken-Blakemore or Minnesota tube, vasopressin (systemic or into the celiac or left gastric artery), and left gastric artery embolization all have been effective.[37,39]

Esophageal causes of UGI bleeding

Hemorrhage is an infrequent complication of peptic esophagitis and is more likely related to an inflamed hiatus hernia or Barrett's esophagus. Hemorrhage in these cases may be the presenting symptom or may be superimposed on other symptoms of esophagitis. Hemorrhage usually is associated endoscopically with a discrete esophageal ulcer and less frequently by diffuse ulcerative esophagitis.[40] Other esophageal diseases that may cause melena and hematemesis are fungal and viral infections and aortoesophageal fistula (as a result of foreign bodies, lung and esophageal cancer, aortic aneurysm, or perforation of an esophageal ulcer).[41] Bleeding is usually fatal with aortoenteric fistulas.

Gastric tumors

Overt bleeding, more frequently melena than hematemesis, infrequently may be the presenting symptom of gastric cancer,[42] or it may occur in patients with known tumors.[43] Bleeding also can be the presenting symptom with gastric polyps, carcinoid, leiomyoma and leiomyosarcoma, lipoma, and liposarcoma. Bleeding also occurs with lymphoma, metastatic disease to the stomach, and pancreatic rests.

Dieulafoy's disease

Dieulafoy's disease is bleeding that occurs from a defect in an unusually large but histologically normal submucosal artery, through a minute mucosal erosion, usually in the proximal stomach; 75 to 95% of lesions occur within 6 cm of the gastroesophageal junction.[44] Lesions also have been described in the gastric antrum, duodenum, jejunum, colon, and rectum.[44] Whereas Dieulafoy's disease is uncommon, it has been reported to account for 1.7 to 5.8% of cases of nonvariceal UGI bleeding.[44,45] Although alcohol, aspirin, NSAIDs, and PUD have been reported to be associated with Dieulafoy's,[45] these associations remain controversial.[37]

It is not known why the enlarged submucosal artery is present or what causes the mucosal erosion or defect over the artery. The two main theories are that a normal artery becomes elongated with aging, and that a large submucosal artery is congenitally abnormally close to the mucosa. In either case, the tortuous artery may cause pressure on the mucosa, leading to mucosal ischemia and erosion, which are followed by arterial rupture.[44] Dieulafoy's disease can cause massive bleeding and can be difficult to see endoscopically because of the small mucosal defect. The Dieulafoy lesion is identified endoscopically in 82% of cases (49% were identified on initial endoscopy, 33% during a second examination, and 18% were seen only at surgery).[46] The typical presentation is a middleaged or elderly man (the male-to-female ratio is 2:1) with sudden massive hematemesis, melena, and hemodynamic instability. Angiography can identify extravasation when bleeding is active, but Dieulafoy's lesions have no specific angiographic signs.[47] A review of endoscopic treatment of Dieulafoy's disease in 1991 showed that permanent hemostasis was achieved in 85% of cases and that 15% rebled, requiring a second therapeutic endoscopic procedure.[46]

Aneurysms and pseudoaneurysms

Chronic pancreatitis causes pseudoaneurysms by enzymes eroding arterial walls and by pseudocysts eroding into arteries (variceal bleeding resulting from splenic vein occlusion also may occur). These problems are unusual but life-threatening complications of chronic pancreatitis. Pseudoaneurysms of pancreatitis rupture and bleed more frequently than true splenic artery aneurysms. Hemorrhage from these pseudoaneurysms tends to be intermittent, repetitive, and sometimes massive. Pseudoaneurysms can bleed into the pancreatic parenchyma or the GI tract through the pancreatic duct; presentation usually is associated with bleeding into the lumen of the GI tract, but patients may present with pain resulting from pancreatitis or the pseudocyst. The splenic, gastroduodenal, and pancreaticoduodenal arteries most frequently are involved, but pseudoaneurysms can originate from any branch of the celiac or superior mesenteric arteries. Ten percent of patients with chronic pancreatitis will demonstrate pseudoaneurysms on arteriography.[48] Of pseudocysts, 2 to 10% have been reported to hemorrhage with a mortality rate of 40 to 80%.[49]

Hemobilia

Hemobilia refers to bleeding originating in the liver, biliary tree, or pancreas and passing through the ampulla of Vater. Trauma, both iatrogenic (40%) or accidental (20%), is the most common cause; less frequent causes are hepatic artery aneurysms, gallstones eroding the cystic artery, metastatic disease to the liver, and invasion of the biliary or pancreatic ducts by tumor or parasitic infection, particularly with ascaris.[37]

Percutaneous biliary drainage (PBD) is a commonly performed procedure; the incidence of vascular complications requiring therapy is 4 to 6.6%.[50–52] Hemorrhage may come from a communication of a side hole of the catheter with the vascular system of the liver or from vascular trauma.[53] If bleeding is not related to a side hole of the catheter communicating with hepatic vessels, selective hepatic arteriography is performed.[53] If no lesion is identified on the arteriogram, selective hepatic venography has been advocated.[53] to detect the rate fistula between a hepatic vein and the biliary tract. Hemobilia has been reported to occur from 1 day to 1 year following PBD.[51] Asymptomatic hemobilia occurs in 8% of patients and usually responds to either repositioning the catheter or catheter upsizing.[51] A mortality rate of 22% has been reported;[54] thus, diagnosis and treatment should be aggressive. The classic triad of biliary colic, jaundice, and GI bleeding is present in approximately 40% of cases. Endoscopy shows blood or clots at the ampulla in 40% of cases; it has been suggested that clots favor hepatic hemobilia (because blood remains in the biliary system for longer periods), and oozing blood favors a pancreatic origin.[55] Confirmation of hemobilia requires celiac or hepatic arteriography; isolated case reports of diagnosis by computed tomography (CT) scanning[56] and by technetium-99m scintigraphy[57] have been reported. Transcatheter embolization with particles of Gelfoam or ivalon or with coils is the treatment of choice and is usually effective.[58] See Chapter 31 for details regarding diagnosis and treatment of hemobilia.

Aortoenteric fistula

Aortoenteric fistula is an infrequent (0.4–2.4%) but life-threatening late complication of aortic vascular grafting[59] and must be considered in any patient with UGI bleeding who has had previous aortic surgery; a fistula may occur even more rarely with a mycotic or noninfected aortic aneurysm without previous surgery, erosion of a tumor, or a pancreatic pseudocyst into the aorta or as a sequela of radiation therapy. Aortoduodenal fistulas account for 80% of all aortoenteric fistulas. The postsurgical mechanisms include direct fistulous communication between the graft lumen (due to disruption of the suture line) and bowel (duodenum), pseudoaneurysm at the suture line with erosion into the bowel lumen, and erosion of the graft body into the bowel lumen remote from a vascular suture line.[59] GI bleeding occurs in nearly all patients with these conditions. Characteristically, the initial bleed, whether hematemesis, melena, hematochezia, or a combination of these, is brief and self-limited and followed from several hours to days by massive GI bleeding; rarely, there is massive initial GI bleeding without a sentinel bleed. Lesser degrees of chronic bleeding occur when the graft erodes into the duodenum; these patients may also present with septicemia. The third and fourth portions of the duodenum most commonly are involved, with the small bowel or colon involved in 10 to 20% of cases. Endoscopy is the diagnostic procedure of choice, but because the fistulas are usually in the third or fourth portion of the duodenum, they may not be seen endoscopically. Any bleeding or erosion distal to the second portion of the duodenum should arouse the suspicion of an aortoduodenal fistula. CT may show an aneurysm, and the diagnosis is confirmed if extraluminal gas is detected at the site of previous surgery. Angiography may show extravasation, an aneurysm, or pseudoaneurysm, but it also may be normal. All diagnostic studies may be normal; when the possibility of an aortoenteric fistula is considered, surgery must be performed because up to one third of patients die within 6 to 12 hours of the sentinel bleeding.

Vascular lesions

Two infrequent vascular lesions that cause UGI bleeding, usually in patients aged 60 to 80 years, are gastric antral vascular ectasia (*watermelon stomach*) and gastroduodenal arteriovenous malformations (AVMs).[37] Watermelon stomach is much more common in women than men; there is no sex predilection in AVMs. Both can present with occult bleeding or melena. Diagnosis usually is made by characteristic endoscopic findings, and patients can be treated by endoscopic techniques. Angiography may show a feeding artery, nidus, and early draining vein in AVMs.[60]

■ Endoscopic Therapy

Many lesions causing UGI bleeding, including 85% of bleeding ulcers, can be treated effectively by endoscopy.[20,61] Therapeutic modalities currently used in conjunction with endoscopy are the heat probe, electrocoagulation, injection (with ethanol, epinephrine, or hypertonic saline), combinations of these modalities, and laser therapy. There is no conclusive evidence that one modality is more effective or safer than the others. Lesions that have been treated successfully by endoscopy include gastric and duodenal ulcers, Mallory-Weiss tears, angiodysplasias, and Dieulafoy's lesions. Erosive gastritis is usually not amenable to endoscopic treatment because of the diffuse nature of the lesion. Gastric ulcers high on the lesser curvature and ulcers in the posteroinferior aspect of the duodenal bulb are at high risk for bleeding during endoscopic therapy (as well as for catastrophic rebleeding) as a result of their close relationship to the left gastric artery and the gastroduodenal artery, respectively; therefore, most endoscopists do not treat these lesions endoscopically.[20] Complications of endoscopic hemostatic therapy include ulceration, bleeding, and perforation.[20,61] In only 1 to 2% of cases is induced bleeding not controlled with further therapy. Ulceration is self-limited and does not appear to prolong ulcer healing rates. The rate of perforations is usually 1% or less but may be as high as 3%.

■ Diagnostic Arteriography

Diagnostic arteriography for acute UGI bleeding is indicated when continued bleeding and unsuccessful or indeterminate endoscopy occur. The arteriogram should be directed toward the suspected site of bleeding as determined clinically and endoscopically. The angiographic sign of bleeding is contrast extravasation (Figs. 30-2A, 30-3, and 30-4), which may be tubular and simulate a vein (Fig. 30-3), but differentiation from a vein is possible because contrast does not drain into more central veins and remains in its original position. This angiographic sign of bleeding (which also applies to bleeding in other areas) was first described in the upper GI tract and is referred to as the *pseudovein sign*.[62] It has been shown experimentally that a bleeding rate as low as 0.5 mL/min can be demonstrated angiographically.[63] On the other hand, even massive bleeding may not be demonstrated if the angiogram is not performed at the exact instant that bleeding is occurring, because bleed-

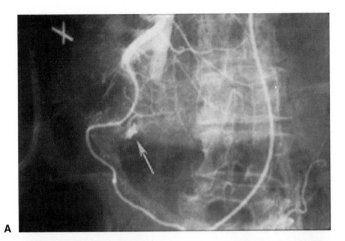

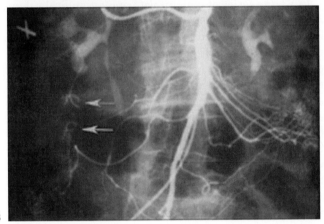

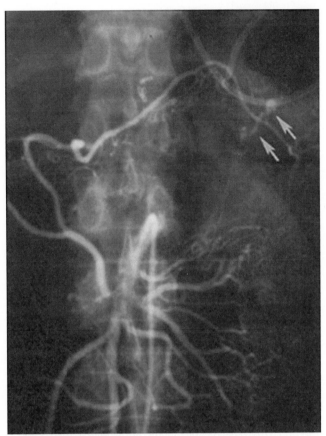

FIGURE 30-2. Bleeding duodenal ulcer: angiographic demonstration and embolization. **A:** Gastroduodenal artery injection shows extravasation (*arrow*). Coils then were placed in the gastroduodenal artery, obstructing it. **B:** Superior mesenteric arteriogram shows no extravasation in the duodenum. Note the coils (*arrows*) in gastroduodenal artery.

FIGURE 30-3. Bleeding marginal ulcer with pseudovein sign. Extravasation in the left upper quadrant (*arrows*) fed by a jejunal artery. The patient had a Billroth II operation.

ing is frequently intermittent.[64] For a reasonable chance at demonstrating extravasation, blood loss should be in the order of at least two to three units per day.[65] Extravasation on angiography with UGI bleeding is more frequent than with lower GI bleeding.[66–68] Extravasation has been demonstrated in up to 97% of patients[67] with UGI bleeding; the highest reported rate with lower GI bleeding is 72%.[68] Arteriography can show only arterial and capillary bleeding but will not show venous bleeding (as in bleeding esophageal varices).

The arteriogram usually is performed from the femoral artery and far less frequently from the left axillary or brachial artery. Aortography is not performed unless an aortoduodenal fistula is suspected. Aortography may show a nipple at the site of the fistula,[65] or it may show no evidence of the fistula. One report emphasizes the value of a prone lateral view to visualize an aortoenteric fistula.[69]

Although many different catheters can be used for selective studies, we favor the 5 F Sos Omni catheter (Angio-

Dynamics, Queensbury, NY) because it can be used for superior mesenteric, celiac, and left gastric catheterizations. If the Sos Omni catheter is not successful in catheterizing the left gastric artery, a Rosch left gastric catheter (Cook Incorporated, Bloomington, IN) or the Waltman loop technique may be used with a cobra catheter; this latter technique is said to be successful in catheterizing 90% of left gastric arteries.[70] Using cut-film or nonsubtracted digital acquisition, celiac and superior mesenteric arteries are injected with 50 mL of contrast (approximately half the amount of contrast is used with digital subtraction technique) and filmed at a rate of 1 film/sec for 10 sec followed by 1 film/every other second for 20 sec. For left gastric arteriography, approximately 15 mL at 3 mL/sec is injected with filming at 1/sec for 15 sec. The angiographer should be aware that a normal adrenal stain (Fig. 30-5), hyperemic or compressed mucosa, or staining caused by injection with the catheter wedged all may produce stains that can be mistaken for contrast extravasation.[71]

Aortography is rarely indicated, except, as mentioned, when there is clinical suspicion of an aortoenteric fistula or occasionally for a distal esophageal lesion, which may

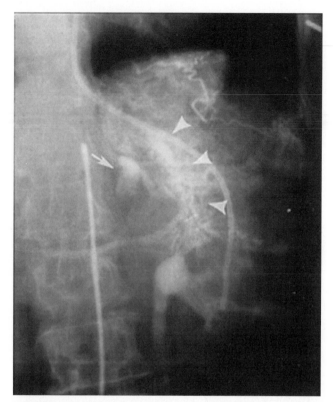

FIGURE 30-4. Erosive gastritis. Late capillary/venous phase of left gastric arteriogram shows extravasation of contrast (*arrow*) and hyperemic gastric fundus (*arrowheads*). Also noted is filling of left inferior phrenic artery branches.

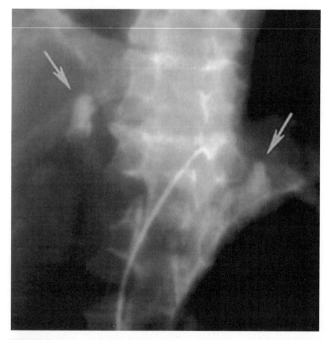

FIGURE 30-5. Normal adrenal stain. Capillary phase of celiac arteriogram shows bilateral adrenal stains. (Courtesy of Jonathan Trambert, M.D.)

be fed directly by small aortic branches. If endoscopy demonstrates bleeding from the distal esophagus or stomach, the first injection should be into the left gastric artery. For duodenal bleeding, a common hepatic or gastroduodenal arteriogram should be obtained first. If no abnormality is seen, the superior mesenteric artery should be studied; it is even more desirable with duodenal bleeding to perform a selective inferior pancreaticoduodenal arteriogram (the inferior pancreaticoduodenal artery arises from the first jejunal artery in 50% of cases). If endoscopy cannot be performed or does not reveal a bleeding site, celiac and superior mesenteric arteriograms should be obtained; all the arterial branches that could supply a UGI bleeding lesion must be well visualized.

In a large series of patients with angiographically demonstrated gastric bleeding,[72] extravasation was from a branch of the left gastric artery in 85% of cases, the right gastric and the short gastric arteries each in 5%, the gastroepiploic artery in 3%, and the gastroduodenal and the left inferior phrenic artery each in 1%. Bleeding was at the gastroesophageal junction in 11%, in the fundus and proximal two thirds of the body in 81%, and in the distal third of the body and antrum in 8%. Most cases were stress mucosal bleeding, which in 95% of these cases was in the proximal stomach. The authors pointed out that there was a 33% correlation between endoscopy and angiography in localizing bleeding sites, but they also showed that despite endoscopic findings of diffuse oozing or bleeding from multiple sites, angiography revealed more than one bleeding site in only two of the 103 patients with extravasation. Figure 30-4 demonstrates extravasation from the left gastric artery resulting from erosive gastritis. Other authors have reported that often gastric stress bleeding does not demonstrate extravasation but rather demonstrates diffuse hypervascularity, mucosal hyperemia, and prominent draining veins (Fig. 30-6).[73]

It is usually difficult to state with certainty based on the angiographic extravasation whether the bleeding is from a stress erosion, Dieulafoy's lesion, or Mallory-Weiss tear because all these bleeding sites are in the proximal stomach; gastric ulcers also may occur in the proximal stomach. Not infrequently, a left adrenal blush is produced from injection of the left inferior phrenic artery, which can originate from or near the left gastric artery and should not be mistaken for a gastric bleed.

Clinically significant bleeding occurs in up to 5% of patients following endoscopic sphincterotomy[74] and usually is identified endoscopically immediately after sphincterotomy. Angiography identified the bleeding site in four of five patients in one report,[75] and the usual source is a branch of the gastroduodenal artery. Hemobilia due to PBD can be diagnosed and managed via the angiographic catheter as discussed in Chapter 31.

TABLE 30-1. *Results of Embolotherapy for Pyloroduodenal Bleeding*

Artery embolized	No. of patients	Initial control of bleeding	Long-term control of bleeding	Duodenal stenosis with obstruction
Pancreaticoduodenal	28	27	15	5
Gastroduodenal	29	25	8	2

From Lang EK. Transcatheter embolization in management of hemorrhage from duodenal ulcer: long-term results and complications. *Radiology* 1992;1882:703–707.

pressin infusion mentioned previously in regard to gastric bleeding also pertain to pyloroduodenal bleeding. The largest series on embolotherapy for pyloroduodenal bleeding was reported by Lang,[92] who described the results of embolotherapy for bleeding duodenal ulcer in 57 patients. The results are shown in Table 30-1. In summary, selective embolization of a pancreaticoduodenal artery supplying the bleeding site offers better initial and long-term control of bleeding than gastroduodenal occlusion. The main complication of embolotherapy, duodenal stenosis with obstruction, occurs more than twice as frequently with pancreaticoduodenal than gastroduodenal embolization.

It is perhaps somewhat surprising that only a few cases of infarction after embolotherapy or vasopressin infusions have been reported. Duodenal infarction requiring surgery has been reported in only two cases of somewhat more than 100 cases of pyloroduodenal bleeding in the literature treated by catheter-directed techniques;[93,94] in one additional case of embolization of both the gastroduodenal and pancreaticoduodenal arteries, postmortem examination revealed pancreatitis.[95] Thus, in all three cases, further ischemic insult in addition to embolization (gastroduodenal surgery and vasopressin infusion) was found.

Should the angiographer embolize when endoscopy shows a bleeding site but the angiogram does not demonstrate extravasation? Reports in the literature have conflicting conclusions. Lang et al.[96] reported that approximately 20% of patients with endoscopically confirmed UGI bleeding had normal findings at angiography; additionally, two thirds of the lesions that were not treated during angiography had massive rebleeding, and lesions supplied by the left gastric artery that were prophylactically embolized did not rebleed. On the other hand, Dempsey et al.[97] retrospectively studied patients with nonvariceal massive UGI bleeding. Embolization, mostly of the left gastric artery, was performed based on clinical, endoscopic, and angiographic findings in patients who did not show extravasation. Subsequent surgery to control bleeding was necessary in approximately 30% of both embolized and nonembolized patients. It is

our policy to embolize the appropriate artery when a bleeding site is demonstrated endoscopically but not angiographically. We are less certain regarding embolization if a nonbleeding lesion (such as an ulcer) is endoscopically demonstrated; in view of the low morbidity of embolization, we lean toward embolotherapy in these cases.

Duodenal bleeding following endoscopic sphincterotomy often cannot be controlled endoscopically. As stated, bleeding is usually from a branch of the gastroduodenal artery. Bleeding usually can be successfully treated by embolization; in the four cases (of the five studied) with extravasation, Saeed et al.[75] successfully treated three patients by Gelfoam pledget embolization of the bleeding branch (in the fourth, celiac stenosis precluded selective catheterization). The author's treatment plan for catheter-directed therapy of endoscopically demonstrated pyloroduodenal bleeding is shown in Figure 30-8.

In the largest series dealing with embolotherapy of pancreatic pseudoaneurysms,[98] the authors successfully occluded 15 of 19 (79%) peripancreatic aneurysms and pseudoaneurysms (13 were due to pancreatitis). The article did not specify precisely what embolic materials were used, but in the single case described, the splenic artery was occluded with coils and Gelfoam. Two patients died of sepsis, and four additional patients required ancillary surgery, including "drainage of pseudocyst and intraabdominal sepsis." Most other articles also describe coils as the most appropriate agent for arterial occlusion, although Gelfoam often has been used for small arteries leading to pseudoaneurysms. Two principles of embolotherapy of pseudoaneurysms to ensure optimal treatment and to prevent recurrence must be emphasized: (a) if possible, the artery distal and proximal to the pseudoaneurysm should be occluded (also, coils should be deposited directly into the pseudoaneurysm), and (b) angiography of potential collaterals should be performed, because it is not unusual for these pseudoaneurysms to be fed by more than one artery. Success and follow-up can be monitored by duplex sonography.[99] Figure 30-9 shows a pseudoaneurysm of a pancreaticoduodenal artery before and after coil embolization.

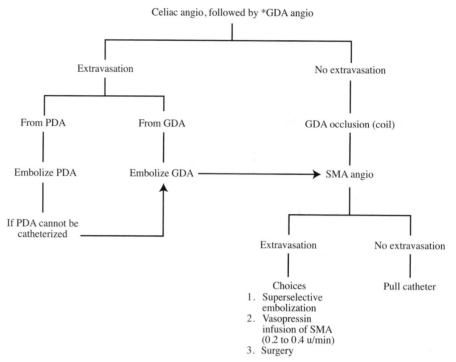

Celiac angio, followed by *GDA angio

Extravasation

No extravasation

From PDA

From GDA

GDA occlusion (coil)

Embolize PDA

Embolize GDA ⟶ SMA angio

If PDA cannot be
catheterized

Extravasation

No extravasation

Choices
1. Superselective
   embolization
2. Vasopressin
   infusion of SMA
   (0.2 to 0.4 u/min)
3. Surgery

Pull catheter

FIGURE 30-8. Algorithm for catheter-directed therapy of endoscopically demonstrated polyro-duodenal bleeding. If it is not possible to catheterize the gastroduodenal artery (GDA) vasopres-sen can be infused into the celiac artery, following the algorithm in Figure 30-7.[2] Following pancreaticoduodenal artery (PDA) embolization, GDA angiography should be performed to make certain that there is no additional bleeding from PDA or GDA; † then do superior mesenteric artery (SMA) angiography and follow flow chart for SMA angiography. Danger of infarction from embolization is heightened with pre-embolization or gastroduodenal surgery (see text).‡

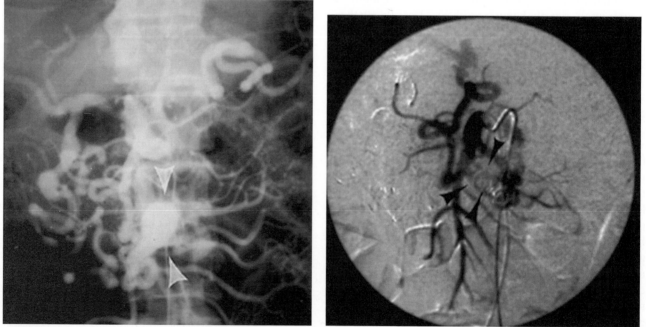

FIGURE 30-9. Pseudoaneurysm of pancreaticoduodenal artery. **A:** Before treatment (*arrowheads*). **B:** After coil embolization. Coils in aneurysm, with aneurysm no longer opacified (*arrowheads*).

REFERENCES

1. Forde KA: Lower gastrointestinal bleeding: the magnitude of the problem. In: Sugawa C, Schuman BM, Lucas CE, eds. *Gastrointestinal bleeding.* New York: Iqaku-Shoin, 1992:13–25.
2. Pitcher JL. Therapeutic endoscopy and bleeding ulcers: historical overview. *Gastrointest Endosc* 1990;36(Suppl 5):S2–S7.
3. Pimpl W, Boeckl O, Waclawiczek HW, et al. Estimation of the mortality rate of patients with severe gastroduodenal hemorrhage with the aid of a new scoring system. *Endoscopy* 1987;19:101–106
4. Walt RP, Langman MJS. Acute bleeding peptic ulcer. In: Bouchier IAD, Allan RN, Hodgson HJF, eds. *Gastroenterology clinical science and practice,* 2nd ed. London: WB Saunders, 1993:309.
5. Kurata JH, Corboy ED, Current peptic ulcer time trends: an epidemiological profile. *J Clin Gastroenterol* 1988;10:259–268.
6. Greene FL, Williams RB, Pettigrew FC. Upper gastrointestinal bleeding: the magnitude of the problem. In: Sugawa C, Schuman BM, Lucas CE, eds. *Gastrointestinal bleeding.* New York: Iqaku-Shoin, 1992:3–12.
7. Fleischer D. Etiology and prevalence of severe persistent upper gastrointestinal bleeding. *Gastroenterology* 1983;84:538–543.
8. Kankaria AG, Fleischer DE. The critical care management of nonvariceal upper gastrointestinal bleeding. *Crit Care Clin* 1995;11: 347–368.
9. Hawkey G. NSAIDS and peptic ulcers. *BMJ* 1990;300:278–281.
10. Silverstein FE, Gilbert DA, Tedesco FJ, et al. The National ASGE Survey on upper gastrointestinal bleeding. *Gastrointest Endosc* 1981;27:80–93.
11. Wangensteen OH, Root HD, Salmon PA, et al. Depressant action of local gastric hypothermia on gastric digestion. *JAMA* 1959;169: 1601–1604.
12. Feldman M, Burton ME. Histamine 2-receptor antagonists: standard therapy for acid peptic diseases (Part 11). *N Engl J Med* 1990; 323:1749–1755.
13. Puera DA, Johnson L. Cimetidine for prevention and treatment of gastroduodenal mucosal lesions in patients in an intensive care unit. *Ann Intern Med* 1985;103:173–177.
14. Lacroix J, Infante-Rivard C, Jenicek M, et al. Prophylaxis of upper gastrointestinal bleeding in intensive care units: a metaanalysis. *Crit Care Med* 1989;17:862–869.
15. Sutton FM. Upper gastrointestinal bleeding in patients with esophageal varices. *Am J Med* 1987;83:273–275.
16. Tabibian N, Graham DY. Source of upper gastrointestinal bleeding in patients with esophageal varices seen at endoscopy. *J Clin Gastroenterol* 1987;9:279–282.
17. Birkett DH. Gastrointestinal bleeding: common dilemmas in management. *Surg Clin North Am* 1991;71:1259–1269.
18. Allen HM, Block MA, Schuman BM. Gastroduodenal endoscopy: management of acute upper gastrointestinal hemorrhage. *Arch Surg* 1973;106:450–455.
19. Gogel HK, Tandberg D. Emergency management of upper gastrointestinal hemorrhage. *Am J Emerg Med* 1986;4:150–162.
20. Fleischer DE. Endoscopic control of upper gastrointestinal bleeding. *J Clin Gastroenterol* 1990;12(Suppl 2):S41–S47.
21. Gilbert DA. Epidemiology of upper gastrointestinal bleeding. *Gastrointest Endosc* 1990;(Suppl 5): S9–S13.
22. Peterson WL. Bleeding peptic ulcer: epidemiology and nonsurgical management. *Gastroenterol Clin North Am* 1990;19:155–170.
23. Gelfand DW, Dale WJ, Ott DJ. The location and size of gastric ulcers: radiologic and endoscopic evaluation. *AJR Am J Roentgenol* 1984;143:755–758.
24. Boyle JD. Multiple gastric ulcers. *Gastroenterology* 1971;61:628–631.
25. Richardson CT. Gastric ulcer. In: Sleisenger MH, Fordtran JS, eds. *Gastrointestinal Disease,* 4th ed. Philadelphia: WB Saunders, 1989: 879–909.
26. Graham DY. The relationship between nonsteroidal anti-inflammatory drug use and peptic ulcer disease. *Gastroenterol Clin North Am* 1990;19:171–182.
27. Aspirin Myocardial Infarction Study Research Group of National Heart, Lung and Blood Institute. A randomized, controlled trial of aspirin in persons recovered from myocardial infarction. *JAMA* 1980;243:661–669.
28. NIH Consensus Conference. *Helicobacter pylori* in peptic ulcer disease. NIH Consensus Development Panel on *Helicobacter pylori* in Peptic Ulcer Disease. *JAMA* 1994;272:65–69.
29. Tytgat GNJ, Rauws EAJ. *Campylobacter pylori* and its role in peptic ulcer disease. *Gastroenterol Clin North Am* 1990;19:183–196.
30. Chamberlain CE. Acute hemorrhagic gastritis. *Gastroenterol Clin North Am* 1993;22:843–873.
31. Shuman RB, Schuster DP, Zuckerman GR. Prophylactic therapy for stress ulcer bleeding: a reappraisal. *Ann Intern Med* 1987;106: 562–567.
32. Cannon LA, Heiselman D, Gardner W, et al. Prophylaxis of upper gastrointestinal tract bleeding in mechanically ventilated patients: a randomized study comparing the efficacy of sucralfate, cimetidine and antacids. *Arch Intern Med* 1987;147:2101–2106.
33. Robert A, Kauffman GJ. Stress ulcers, erosions and gastric mucosal injury. In: Sleisenger MH, Fordtran JH, eds. *Gastrointestinal disease,* 4th ed. Philadelphia; WB Saunders, 1989:772–792.
34. Mallory GK, Weiss S. Hemorrhages from lacerations of the cardiac orifice of the stomach due to vomiting. *Am J Med Sci* 1929;178: 506–515.
35. Graham DY, Schwartz JT. The spectrum of Mallory-Weiss tear. *Medicine* 1978;57:307–318.
36. Gupta PK, Fleischer DE. Nonvariceal upper gastrointestinal bleeding. *Med Clin North Am* 1993;77:973–992.
37. Katz PO, Salas L. Less frequent causes of upper gastrointestinal bleeding. *Gastroenterol Clin North Am* 1993;22:875–889.
38. Sugawa C, Benishek D, Walt A.J. Mallory-Weiss syndrome: a study of 224 patients. *Am J Surg* 1983;145:30–33.
39. Carsen GMS, Casarella WJ, Spiegel RM. Transcatheter embolization for treatment of Mallory-Weiss tears of the esophagogastric junction. *Radiology* 1978;128:309–313.
40. Hogan WJ, Dodds WJ. Gastroesophageal reflux disease (reflux esophagitis). In: Sleisenger MH, Fordtran JS, eds. *Gastrointestinal disease,* 4th ed. Philadelphia: WB Saunders, 1989:594–619.
41. McDonald GB. Esophageal diseases caused by infection, systemic illness and trauma. In: Sleisenger MH, Fordtran JS, eds. *Gastrointestinal disease,* 4th ed. Philadelphia: WB Saunders 1989:640–656.
42. Davis GR. Neoplasms of the stomach. In: Sleisenger MH, Fordtran JS, eds. *Gastrointestinal disease,* 4th ed. Philadelphia: WB Saunders, 1989: 45–772.
43. Goldstein HM, Medellin H, Ben-Menachem Y, et al. Transcatheter arterial embolization in the management of bleeding in the cancer patient. *Radiology* 1975;115:603–608.
44. Stark ME, Gostout CJ, Balm RK. Clinical features and endoscopic management of Dieulafoy disease. *Gastrointest Endosc* 1992;38: 545–550.
45. Baettig B, Haecki W, Lammer F, et al. Dieulafoy's disease: endoscopic treatment and follow up. *Gut* 1993;34:1418–1421.
46. Reilly HF, Al-Kawas FH. Dieulafoy's lesion: diagnosis and management. *Dig Dis Sci* 1991;36:1702–1707.
47. Durham JD, Kumpe DA, Rothbarth LJ, et al. Dieulafoy's disease: arteriographic findings and treatment. *Radiology* 1991;174:937–941.
48. White AF, Baum S, Buranasari S. Aneurysms secondary to pancreatitis. *AJR Am J Roentgenol* 1976;127:393–396
49. Kane MG, Kreis GJ. Pancreatic pseudocyst. *Adv Intern Med* 1984; 29:271–300.
50. Hoevels J, Nillson U. Intrahepatic vascular lesions following percutaneous transhepatic bile duct intubation. *Gastrointest Radiol* 1980; 5:127–135.

51. Savader SJ, Trerotota SO, Merine DS. Hemobilia after percutaneous transhepatic biliary drainage: treatment with transcatheter embolotherapy. *J Vasc Intervent Radiol* 1992;3:345–352.

52. Mitchell SE, Shuman LS, Kaufman SL, et al. Biliary catheter drainage complicated by hemobilia: treatment by balloon embolotherapy. *Radiology* 1985;157:645–652

53. Rosch J, Putnam JS, Keller FS. Diagnosis and management of hemobilia. *Semin Intervent Radiat* 1988;5:49–60

54. Yoshida J, Donahue PE, Nyhus LM. Hemobilia: review of recent experience with a worldwide problem. *Am J Gastroenterol* 1987;82:448–453.

55. Blackstone MO. *Endoscopic interpretation.* New York: Raven Press, 1984:392–393.

56. Lutter DR, Berger ML. Diagnosis of nontraumatic hematobilia by computerized tomography of the abdomen. *Am J Gastroenterol* 1988;83:329–330.

57. Jackson DE, Floyd JL, Levesque PH. Hemobilia associated with hepatic artery aneurysms: scintigraphic detection with technetium-99m-labeled red blood cells. *J Nucl Med* 1986;27:491–494.

58. Uflacker R, Moourao GS, Piske RL, et al. Hemobilia: transcatheter occlusive therapy and long term follow up. *Cardiovasc Intervent* Radiol 1989;12:136–141.

59. Bernhard VM. Aortoenteric fistula. In: Bernhard VM, Towne JB, eds. *Complications in vascular surgery,* 2nd ed. Orlando: Grune & Stratton, 1985:513.

60. Roberts LK, Gold RE, Routt WE. Gastric angiodysplasia. *Radiology* 1981;139:355–359.

61. Standards of Practice Committee. The role of endoscopy in the management of non-variceal acute upper gastrointestinal bleeding. *Gastrointest Endosc* 1992;38:760–764.

62. Ring WJ, Athanasoulis CA, Waltman AC, et al. The pseudovein: an angiographic appearance of arterial hemorrhage. *J Can Assoc Radiol* 1973;24:242–244.

63. Baum S, Athanasoulis CA, Waltman AC, et al. Gastrointestinal hemorrhage: angiographic diagnosis and control. *Adv Surg* 1973;7:149–198.

64. Sos TA, Lee JG, Wixson D, et al. Intermittent bleeding from minute to minute in acute massive gastrointestinal hemorrhage: arteriographic demonstration. *AJR Am J Roentgenol* 1978;131:1015–1017.

65. Dorfman GS, McKusick KA, Waltman AC. Gastrointestinal hemorrhage: Radiologic diagnosis and treatment. In: Taveras JM, Ferrucci JT, eds. *Radiology: diagnosis-imaging-intervention.* Philadelphia: JB Lippincott, 1984:1–22.

66. Rahn NH, Tishler JM, Han SY, et al. Diagnostic and interventional angiography in acute gastrointestinal hemorrhage. *Radiology* 1982;143:361–366.

67. Eckstein MR, Kelemouridis V, Athanasoulis CA, et al. Gastric bleeding: therapy with intraarterial vasopressin and transcatheter embolization. *Radiology* 1984;152:643–646.

68. Browder W, Cerise EJ, Litwin MS. Impact of emergency angiography in massive lower gastrointestinal bleeding. *Ann Surg* 1986;204:530–536.

69. Pingoud EG, Cerise EJ, Litwin MS. Usefulness of the prone position for aortography of aortic graft-intestinal fistulae. *AJR Am J Roentgenol* 1979;132:836–838.

70. Waltman AC, Courey WR, Athanasoulis CA, et al. Techniques for left gastric artery catheterization. *Radiology* 1973;109:732–734.

71. Baum S. Arteriographic diagnosis and treatment of gastrointestinal bleeding. In: Abrams H, ed. *Abrams angiography: vascular and interventional radiology,* 3rd ed. Vol 2. Boston: Little, Brown, 1983:1669–1700.

72. Kelemouridis V, Athanasoulis CA, Waltman AC. Gastric bleeding sites: an angiographic study. Radiology 1983;149:643–648.

73. Hilleren DJ. Treatment of gastric bleeding. In: Kadir S, ed. *Current practice of interventional radiology.* Philadelphia: B.C. Decker 1991:414–418.

74. Goodall RJR. Bleeding after endoscopic sphincterotomy. *Ann R Coll Surg Engl* 1985;67:87–88.

75. Saeed M, Kadir S, Kaufman S, et al. Bleeding following endoscopic sphincterotomy: angiographic management by transcatheter embolization. *Gastrointest Endosc* 1989;35:300–303.

76. Rosch J, Gray RK, Grollman JH Jr, et al. Selective arterial drug infusions in the treatment of acute gastrointestinal bleeding: a preliminary report. *Gastroenterology* 1970;59:341–349.

77. Rosch J, Dotter CT, Antonovic R. Selective vasoconstrictor infusion in the management of arterio-capillary gastrointestinal hemorrhage. *AJR Am J Roentgenol* 1972;116:279–288.

78. Athanasoulis CA, Baum S, Waltman AC, et al. Control of acute gastric mucosal hemorrhage: intra-arterial infusion of posterior pituitary extract. *N Engl J Med* 1974;290:597–603.

79. Athanasoulis CA, Simmons JT, Sheehan B, et al. Gastric blood flow alterations during intraarterial and systemic infusions of vasopressin. *Invest Radiol* 1976;11:369(abst).

80. Gomes AS, Lois JF, McCoy RD. Angiographic treatment of gastrointestinal hemorrhage: comparison of vasopressin infusion and embolization. *AJR Am J Roentgenol* 1986;146:1031–1037.

81. Rosenbaum A, Siegelman SS, Sprayregen S. The bleeding marginal ulcer: catheterization diagnosis and therapy. *AJR Am J Roentgenol* 1975;125:812–815.

82. Brown JR, Derr JW. Arterial blood supply of human stomach. *Arch Surg* 1952;64:616–621.

83. Prochaska JM, Flye MW, Johnsrude IS. Left gastric artery embolization for control of gastric bleeding: a complication. *Radiology* 1973;107:521–522.

84. Goldman ML, Land WC, Bradley EL III, et al. Transcatheter therapeutic embolization in the management of massive upper gastrointestinal bleeding. *Radiology* 1976;120:513–521.

85. Rosch J, Keller FS, Kozak B, et al. Gelfoam powder embolization of the left gastric artery in treatment of massive small-vessel gastric bleeding. *Radiology* 1984;151:365–370.

86. Michal JA III, Brody WR, Walter J, et al. Transcatheter embolization of an esophageal artery for treatment of a bleeding esophageal ulcer. *Radiology* 1980;134:246.

87. Encarnacion CE, Kadir S, Beam CA, et al. Gastrointestinal bleeding: treatment with gastrointestinal arterial embolization. *Radiology* 1992;183:505–508.

88. Waltman AC, Greenfield AJ, Novelline RA, et al. Pyloroduodenal bleeding and intraarterial vasopressin: clinical results. *AJR Am J Roentgenol* 1979;133:643–646.

89. Ring EJ, Oleaga JA, Ereiman D, et al. Pitfalls in the angiographic management of hemorrhage: hemodynamic considerations. *AJR Am J Roentgenol* 1977;129:1007–1013.

90. Baum S, Nusbaum M. The control of gastrointestinal hemorrhage by selective mesenteric arterial infusion of vasopressin. *Radiology* 1971;98:497–505.

91. Rosch J, Dotter CT, Brown MJ. Selective arterial embolization: a new method for control of acute gastrointestinal bleeding. *Radiology* 1972;102:303–306.

92. Lang EV. Transcatheter embolization in management of hemorrhage from duodenal ulcer: long-term results and complications. *Radiology* 1992;182:703–707.

93. Miller RE, Baer JW, Nizin JS, et al. Hemorrhagic pancreatitis: a complication of transcatheter embolization treated successfully by total pancreatectomy. *Am J Surg* 1985;149:802–808.

94. Shapiro N, Brandt L, Sprayregen S, et al. Duodenal infarction after Gelfoam embolization of a bleeding duodenal ulcer. *Gastroenterology* 1981;80:176–180.

95. Bell SD, Lau KY, Sniderman KW. Synchronous embolization of the gastroduodenal artery and the inferior pancreaticoduodenal artery in patients with massive duodenal hemorrhage. *J Vasc Intervent Radiol* 1995;6:531–536.

96. Lang EV, Picus D, Marx MV, et al. Massive upper gastrointestinal

hemorrhage with normal findings on arteriography: value of prophylactic embolization of the left gastric artery. *AJR Am J Roentgenol* 1992;158:547–549.

97. Dempsey DT, Burke DR, Reilly RS, et al. Angiography in poor-risk patients with massive nonvariceal upper gastrointestinal bleeding. *Am J Surg* 1990;159:282–286.

98. Mandel SR, Jaques PF, Mauro MA, et al. Nonoperative management of peripancreatic arterial aneurysms: a 10-year experience. *Ann Surg* 1987;2:126–128.

99. Lim SM, Jeffrey RB Jr, Tolentino CS. Pancreatic pseudoaneurysm: monitoring success of transcatheter embolization with duplex sonography. *J Ultrasound Med* 1989;8:643–646.

31

Liver and Spleen

JAMES E. SILBERZWEIG

The use of angiography and venography for the diagnosis and staging of liver and splenic lesions has been nearly eliminated in recent years as a result of the advent of sonography, computed tomography (CT), and magnetic resonance imaging (MRI); however, interventional radiology procedures are being used more frequently for the treatment of these disorders. Advances in catheter, guidewire, stent, and embolization technology resulted in the development of innovative percutaneous procedures for the management of tumors, trauma, and portal hypertension.

■ Liver

Liver tumors

The two most frequent types of primary malignant liver tumors are hepatocellular carcinoma and cholangiocarcinoma. Metastases are the most common malignant neoplasms affecting the liver. Most patients with multiple liver metastases are not candidates for surgical resection and have a poor prognosis. Patients with metastases from neuroendocrine tumors have a better prognosis but may experience severe symptoms related to excessive hormone production.

Hepatocellular carcinoma

Hepatocellular carcinoma (HCC, or hepatoma) is the most common primary liver malignancy, with most cases occurring in Asia and southern Africa.[1] More than one million patients die of HCC per year worldwide. The prognosis of HCC without treatment is poor, with a me-

dian survival of 1.6 months reported in the Asian population.[2] The development of HCC is associated with a history of hepatitis B or hepatitis C infection and cirrhosis. Seventy-five percent of hepatomas occur in cirrhotic livers. Ninety percent of patients with hepatomas are hepatitis B or C virus antigen carriers.[1]

Frequently, HCC is discovered as an incidental finding in patients with cirrhosis and portal hypertension. Symptoms include hepatomegaly, abdominal pain, fever, weight loss, ascites, and jaundice. HCC produces alpha-fetoprotein, which is elevated in the serum of about 70% of patients.[3] Alpha-fetoprotein level can be used for diagnosis as well as a measure of response to therapy.

Sonography, CT, and MRI are commonly used imaging modalities for the screening, diagnosis, and staging of HCC.[4] HCC may be solitary, multicentric, or diffuse. Angiographic features that may be found in HCC include enlarged feeding arteries, neovascularity, irregular tumor stain, arteriovenous (AV) shunting, and portal vein invasion (Fig. 31-1). Hepatic vein invasion may be identified during the parenchymal phase of a hepatic arteriogram or an inferior venacavogram. The arteriographic findings of hypervascular metastases or hemangiomas may appear similar on arteriography. Therefore, arteriography frequently lacks specificity for the diagnosis of HCC.

Portal hypertension that is newly diagnosed or worsening may be the first clinical sign of HCC. HCC may invade the portal venous system and lead to portal hypertension. During angiography, invasion of the portal vein by HCC may be identified as a filling defect within the portal vein or thrombosis of the portal vein (Fig. 31-2). The tumor thrombus may contain vascular "threads and streaks."[5] The portal vein normally is not opacified on hepatic artery

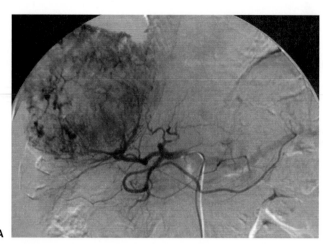

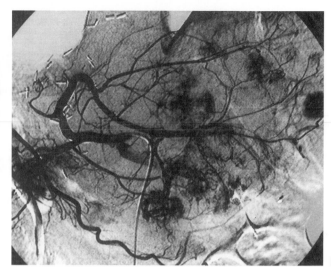

FIGURE 31-1. A: Solitary. **B:** Multicentric hepatocellular carcinomas.

injection; however, arteriovenous shunting is often present in cases of HCC. This high-output communication between the hepatic artery and the portal vein may cause reversal of portal venous flow and portal hypertension.

Surgical resection and liver transplantation are the treatment methods most likely to result in cure; however, they are not options in patients with diffuse disease. At initial diagnosis, many patients already have satellite nodules, extrahepatic metastases, or vascular invasion that

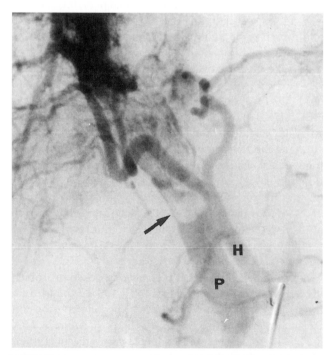

FIGURE 31-2. Hepatocellular carcinoma. Hepatic artery injection demonstrates arteriovenous shunting and invasion of the portal vein (*arrow*). H, hepatic artery; P, portal vein.

may preclude surgical therapy. The median survival is 4 to 6 months for patients with unresectable tumors. Systemic chemotherapy has not been shown to be effective.[6]

Several percutaneous techniques have been described for the treatment of HCC and unresectable metastatic liver disease. These include percutaneous injection of ethanol, acetic acid, or hot saline into the tumor and thermal ablation with radiofrequency, laser, microwaves, or freezing (*cryoablation*). Therapy can be delivered through a catheter into the hepatic artery, including chemotherapy infusion, hepatic artery embolization, or hepatic artery chemoembolization.[7–13] The rationale for therapy via the hepatic artery is that the blood supply to hepatic tumors is typically from the hepatic artery, not from the portal vein.

Chemoembolization is a combination of intraarterial infusion of a chemotherapeutic agent and the introduction of an embolizing agent for occlusion of the tumor vascular supply. Chemoembolization decreases blood flow to the tumor, resulting in ischemia and extending the time of contact of the chemotherapeutic drug with the tumor.[14] Embolization materials such as polyvinyl alcohol (PVA), gelfoam, and iodized oil (Ethiodol) have been used in combination with chemotherapeutic agents.[15] One study described the use of hepatic artery embolization with PVA particles without any chemotherapeutic agent.[1] No treatment method has proven to be superior.

Chemoembolization can be technically challenging, with a great potential for complications. Preembolization arteriography of the celiac, superior mesenteric, and hepatic arteries is performed to define the blood supply of the tumors, to identify variant arterial anatomy, and to assess the patency of portal vein and the direction of portal venous flow. The presence of portal vein occlusion is a poor prognostic factor that increases the risk of liver necrosis following chemoembolization. Other contraindications to chemoembolization are severe liver failure, tumor involvement of greater than 70% of the liver, and biliary obstruction.[6]

Complications of chemoembolization include liver failure, liver abscess, liver infarction, biloma, cholecystitis, and unintentional embolization to extrahepatic organs.[16] Prophylactic intravenous antibiotics are routinely used. Coil embolization of the gastroduodenal artery may be required to prevent inadvertent chemoembolization of the pancreas and duodenum. A postembolization syndrome may occur that may include fever, nausea, and pain for several days following the procedure.

Cholangiocarcinoma

Cholangiocarcinoma is the only primary liver tumor that commonly causes vascular encasement and arterial occlusion.[17] Encasement of the hepatic artery and splenic artery is seen frequently in cases of pancreatic carcinoma (Fig. 31-3).

Metastases

Hepatic metastases arise from hypervascular or hypovascular primary tumors and usually reflect the vascularity of the primary lesion. Unlike HCC, metastases typically are not associated with arteriovenous shunting or portal venous occlusion. The most frequent tumors that metastasize to the liver arise from the gastrointestinal tract (Fig. 31-4). Currently, hepatic resection is the only potentially curative therapy for patients with colorectal cancer metastases.[18] The use of hepatic arterial chemotherapy infu-

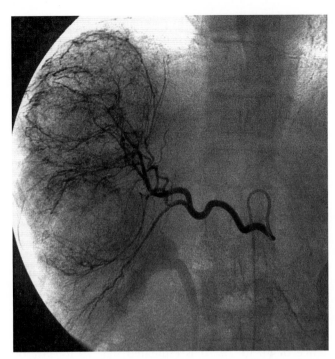

FIGURE 31-4. Metastasis to liver from colon carcinoma.

sion and chemoembolization for colorectal metastases is being investigated.[19–21]

Resection of hepatic metastases has been associated with prolonged survival, particularly for metastases from colorectal primaries.[22] Patients with more than four hepatic metastases, involvement of both hepatic lobes, or an estimated remaining liver that is less than 30% of the initial liver volume are not considered good candidates for resection.[23]

Computed tomography arterial portography and MRI are the imaging studies used to determine the extent of hepatic metastases. CT arterial portography is based on portal enhancement of the liver by infusion of contrast material through the superior mesenteric artery or splenic artery. Because all the injected contrast medium is delivered to the liver from the portal vein, the enhancement of the disease-free liver is high. Hepatic tumors generally do not have a portal venous blood supply, and they are detected as areas of low attenuation compared with the normal enhanced liver.

Neuroendocrine tumors

The two most common neuroendocrine tumors that metastasize to the liver are carcinoid and islet cell tumors. These are slow-growing neoplasms that frequently produce hormonal substances. The appendix is the most common site or origin of carcinoid tumors. Islet cell tumors typically arise from the pancreas. Patients with hepatic metastases from neuroendocrine tumors may remain relatively free of symptoms until the tumor replaces

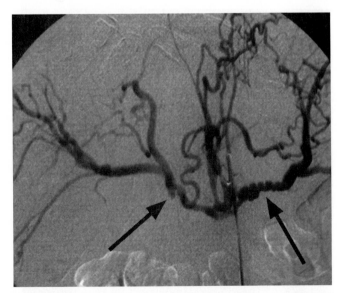

FIGURE 31-3. Hepatic artery and splenic artery encasement by pancreatic carcinoma. Irregular "sawtooth" narrowing of the hepatic and splenic arteries (*arrows*) is caused by tumor encroachment on the arterial walls.

a significant volume of liver parenchyma. Symptoms are caused by production of hormones or mass effect. Surgical resection of neuroendocrine tumors is not a therapeutic option because these tumors are often metastatic at presentation. Hepatic artery embolization or chemoembolization is a recognized method of controlling hormonal symptoms and tumor bulk.[24–26] Patients with carcinoid tumor refractory to other therapy can experience considerable relief of symptoms by such treatment. In addition, somatostatin is used during and after chemoembolization to prevent a carcinoid crises in hormonally active tumors. Somatostatin also can be used intravenously in the event of a carcinoid crisis.

Cavernous hemangioma

Cavernous hemangiomas are benign hepatic tumors that consist of thin-walled, endothelium-lined, septated vascular spaces. Cavernous hemangiomas frequently are identified incidentally during imaging. Hemangiomas are the most common benign tumors in the liver with an incidence of up to 7%. It is estimated that 70 to 95% of hemangiomas occur in women. Multiple hemangiomas have been identified in 10% of cases.[27] Rarely, a large hemangioma (>4 cm) may cause symptoms from mass effect or bleeding.[28]

Hemangiomas may be seen on ultrasound as hyperechoic masses. On dynamic contrast-enhanced CT, hemangiomas initially appear hypodense and then show peripheral areas of focal enhancement, followed by diffuse hyperdensity at 2 minutes, and finally isodense on delayed scans. Red cell radionuclide scanning also can be used to make a reliable diagnosis. Hemangiomas produce intense signal on T2-weighted MR images.[29] Rare cavernous hemangiomas may not exhibit conventional features and require needle biopsy for diagnosis.

Angiographic features of cavernous hemangiomas include a well-marginated tumor arising in the late arterial or capillary phase and persisting into the venous phase with early peripheral opacification. Cavernous hemangiomas have a normal-sized feeding artery with no neovascularity or arteriovenous shunting (Fig. 31-5).

Focal nodular hyperplasia

Focal nodular hyperplasia (FNH) is a benign tumor that contains liver elements, including hepatocytes, Kupffer cells, and bile ducts. FNH occurs in young women, is asymptomatic, and is not associated with oral contraceptive use; nor is it associated with malignant degeneration or spontaneous hemorrhage. An enhancing central scar is sometimes seen on CT or MR, but findings in FNH are typically nonspecific.[30] The angiographic features include a well-marginated hypervascular tumor with feeding vessels entering from the periphery and a dense parenchymal stain (Fig. 31-6). There is no neovascularity or arteriovenous shunting present. There may be a central scar resulting in a "spoke-wheel" appearance.

Hepatic adenoma

Hepatic adenoma is a neoplasm that is associated with hemorrhage caused by spontaneous necrosis. There ex-

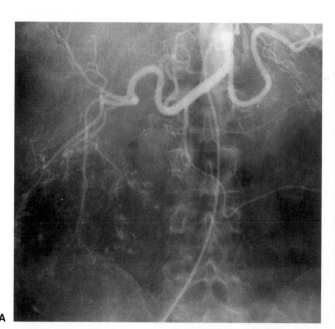
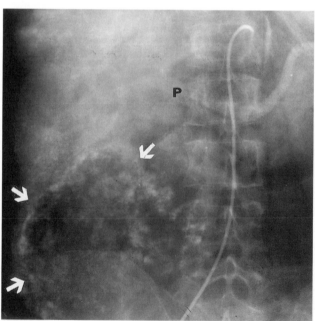

A   B

FIGURE 31-5. Giant cavernous hemangioma. **A:** Arterial Phase. **B:** Venous phase of a celiac trunk injection shows progressive opacification of the tumor periphery (*arrows*). P, portal vein. The feeding hepatic artery branches are of normal size with no hypervascularity or arteriovenous shunting.

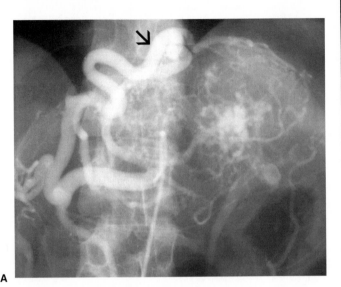
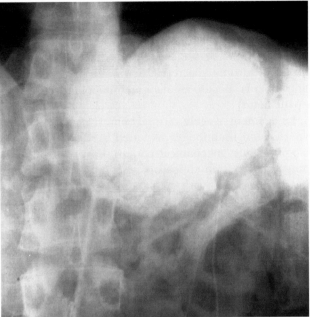

A   B

FIGURE 31-6. Focal nodular hyperplasia. (A). Large feeding artery (*arrow*) at the periphery of the lesion. (B). Dense parenchymal stain.

ists a small potential for malignant degeneration. Most hepatic adenomas arise in young women, and there is a strong association with the use of oral contraceptives.[31] Because of hemorrhage and necrosis, most adenomas are symptomatic when discovered. The CT and angiographic appearances of hepatic adenomas are nonspecific.

Portal hypertension

Cirrhosis is characterized by hepatic necrosis, regeneration, and fibrosis. In early cirrhosis, fibrosis develops around the sinusoidal spaces and obstructs central veins while preserving portal venules. Portal venous hypertension results from an increase in the vascular resistance within the liver. The portal venous system is decompressed through enlarged portosystemic collateral channels.

Several hemodynamic changes in the portal venous system occur as cirrhosis progresses. The most important is the enlargement of portosystemic collateral vessels. The direction of flow in the portal vein also changes as portal hypertension worsens. With mild cirrhosis, portal vein flow is hepatopetal. As resistance increases, bidirectional flow in the portal vein may develop, and the portal vein may not fill at all. With severe portal hypertension, the portal vein becomes an outflow conduit for the liver, and flow is hepatofugal. In patients with advanced cirrhosis, the hepatic arteries may have a corkscrew appearance because of increased arterial flow and liver shrinkage. As hepatic fibrosis worsens and portal flow decreases, cirrhotic patients become increasingly dependent on arterial perfusion of the liver.

The most common complication of portal hypertension is bleeding from gastroesophageal varices (Fig. 31-7). Normally, the portosystemic gradient is less than 5 mm Hg. Portal hypertension is defined as a portosystemic gradient of 6 mm Hg or greater. The risk of bleeding from gastroesophageal varices becomes significant when

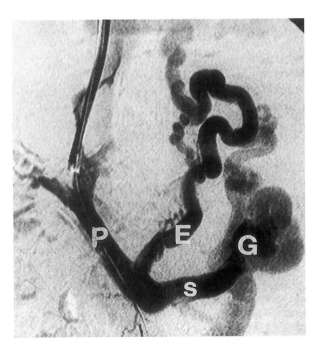

FIGURE 31-7. Gastroesophageal varices. Portal venogram during a TIPS procedure. P, portal vein; S, splenic vein; E, esophageal varices; G, gastric varices.

the gradient is 12 mm Hg or greater.[32,33] Between 40 and 70% of patients die of the first episode of variceal bleeding. Other complications of cirrhosis and portal hypertension include ascites, hepatic encephalopathy, hepatorenal syndrome, bacterial peritonitis, splenomegaly, pancytopenia, hepatocellular carcinoma, and fulminant hepatic failure.

Management of acute variceal hemorrhage from portal hypertension traditionally included the use of pharmacologic agents, mechanical compression with tamponading balloons, and endoscopic techniques that include sclerotherapy and variceal banding. Intravenous infusions of medications—including vasopressin, nitroglycerin, propranolol, and octreotide—have been used for temporary control of variceal bleeding. Systemic infusion is as effective as intraarterial administration. Endoscopic banding and sclerotherapy are effective techniques for the initial management of variceal hemorrhage in most patients; however, sclerotherapy and banding do not correct portal hypertension.

Surgical treatments for portal hypertension include ligation and portosystemic shunt creation. Surgical shunt procedures provide long-term prevention of variceal hemorrhage by reducing portal venous pressure; however, surgical mortality of operative shunts has been reported to be as high as 20%.[34] Liver transplantation is the definitive treatment for relieving portal hypertension from chronic liver disease.

Transjugular intrahepatic portosystemic shunts

The transjugular intrahepatic portosystemic shunt (TIPS) procedure was developed to relieve portal hypertension without the mortality and morbidity of an open surgical procedure. In this percutaneous procedure, an expandable metallic stent is placed in the liver to create a channel between the portal vein and hepatic vein (Fig. 31-8).

The most common indications for the TIPS procedure include acute or recurrent variceal bleeding unresponsive to medical therapy, including endoscopic banding and sclerotherapy. Preliminary endoscopic examination is mandatory because bleeding actually may arise from nonvariceal causes such as peptic ulcer disease, alcoholic gastritis, esophageal ulcer, and Mallory–Weiss tear. TIPS has been performed to treat intractable ascites and to treat portal hypertension from Budd–Chiari syndrome.

Contraindications for the TIPS procedure include severe hepatic failure, severe right-sided heart failures, severe hepatic encephalopathy, primary or metastatic liver tumor, polycystic liver disease, portal vein thrombosis, and severe active infection.

TIPS procedure

Duplex sonography is performed before the procedure to establish portal and splenic vein patency and flow direction, to determine the status of the hepatic veins, to

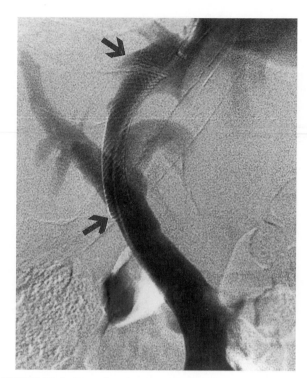

FIGURE 31-8. Transjugular intrahepatic portosystemic shunt. Wallstent extends from the portal vein to the hepatic vein (*arrows*).

assess liver size, and to exclude the presence of a liver tumor or polycystic liver disease.

Access for the TIPS procedure usually is gained through the right internal jugular vein. A vascular sheath is passed into the right hepatic vein. The portal vein catheter–needle access system then is inserted through the sheath and passed from the hepatic vein through liver parenchyma into a branch of the intrahepatic portal vein. Several methods are used to select a site for puncture from the hepatic vein toward the portal vein. The most commonly used techniques are the use of bony landmarks and wedged injection of iodinated contrast material or carbon dioxide, which usually fills the central portal venous system.[35–37]

The needle access system then is exchanged over a guidewire for a diagnostic catheter. Portal venography and pressure measurements then are obtained. The parenchymal tract from the hepatic vein to the portal vein then is dilated with an 8-mm angioplasty balloon. A 10- or 12-mm diameter self-expandable Wallstent is deployed across the parenchymal tract. The stent then is dilated with a 10- or 12-mm balloon. Additional stents may be required to cover the entire tract from the hepatic vein to the portal vein.

The procedural complication rate for TIPS is less than 10%. Major complications of TIPS procedure include bleeding, liver dysfunction, sepsis, and stent malposition or migration. Between 5 and 35% of patients experience new or worsened hepatic encephalopathy.[38,39] Rarely, needle passes may result in gallbladder perforation, hepatic artery pseudoaneurysms, and arteriovenous fistula formation.[40] Massive hemorrhage from extracapsular, inferior vena cava, or portal vein perforation is rare.

The immediate procedure-related mortality rate is less than 2%. Early death is usually the result of bleeding related to extracapsular liver perforation or hepatic artery injury, hepatic artery thrombosis with fulminant hepatic failure, extrahepatic portal vein puncture, or acute right heart failure.[38,39]

The TIPS procedure is technically successfully in more than 95% of cases.[38] In patients treated for variceal hemorrhage, rebleeding within 6 months occurs in up to 15% of patients; however, late rebleeding may occur in up to 30% of cases. Most patients treated for intractable ascites have partial or complete resolution within 1 month of placement.[41]

Despite the excellent short-term results of the TIPS procedure, most shunts require secondary interventions such as angioplasty of the shunt or additional stent insertion to maintain patency. Late post-TIPS stenoses may develop within the stent, portal vein, or most commonly the draining hepatic vein. TIPS stenosis or occlusions occur in 25 to 37% of patients within 6 months.[42–44]

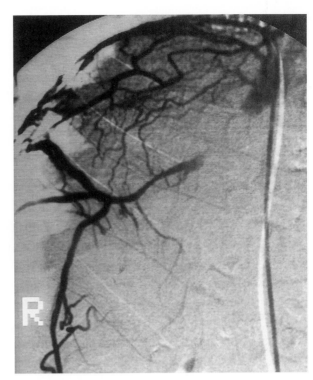

FIGURE 31-9. Budd–Chiari syndrome. Right hepatic venogram shows occlusion (arrow) with spider web–like collaterals.

Budd–Chiari syndrome

Budd-Chiari syndrome (BCS) is caused by occlusion of hepatic venous outflow resulting in hepatic congestion, hepatic necrosis, and ultimately cirrhosis and portal hypertension. The onset of BCS may be acute, with rapidly progressive liver failure or chronic. BCS has been associated with congenital webs of the inferior vena cava, neoplasms, myeloproliferative disorders, hypercoagulable states, paroxysmal nocturnal hemoglobinuria, and oral contraceptive use.[45] No definite cause can be identified in most cases.[46] Typical initial symptoms include abdominal pain, hepatomegaly, and ascites.

Budd–Chiari syndrome is diagnosed by liver biopsy and imaging studies. BCS can be definitively diagnosed by inferior cavography and hepatic venography. An inferior vena cavogram may show narrowing of the inferior vena cava as a result of compression from an enlarged caudate lobe or occlusion from thrombosis or venous webs. Catheterization of the hepatic veins may not be possible if the veins are occluded at their origins. Injection of contrast in a wedged position may show a spider web–like system of collaterals from the hepatic veins to other venous channels (Fig. 31-9). Contrast-enhanced CT demonstrates hepatomegaly with a diffuse mottled pattern of enhancement throughout the liver.

Surgical treatment of BCS consists of portosystemic shunt placement and liver transplantation.[47] Several percutaneous interventions have emerged as treatment options to recanalize the hepatic vein, including thrombolysis, percutaneous transluminal angioplasty, and stent implantation.[48] Transjugular intrahepatic portosystemic shunt insertion has been used to treat portal hypertension caused by BCS.[46,49]

Hepatic artery aneurysms

About 15% of visceral artery aneurysms occur in the hepatic artery. Hepatic artery aneurysms are the second most common visceral aneurysm after splenic artery aneurysms. Hepatic artery aneurysms are usually extrahepatic, solitary, and atherosclerotic (Fig. 31-10). Multiple aneurysms of small hepatic artery branches are seen in polyarteritis nodosa. Intrahepatic artery pseudoaneurysms are usually posttraumatic. The most common iatrogenic causes of traumatic hepatic artery pseudoaneurysms include percutaneous liver biopsy and percutaneous biliary drainage (Fig. 31-11).

Bleeding into the bile ducts (*hemobilia*) may occur when the aneurysm is intrahepatic and intraperitoneal bleeding may occur when the aneurysm is extrahepatic. The treatment of choice for hemobilia caused by a hepatic artery pseudoaneurysm is superselective embolization of the hepatic artery branch supplying the lesion. All hepatic artery aneurysms should be treated because of

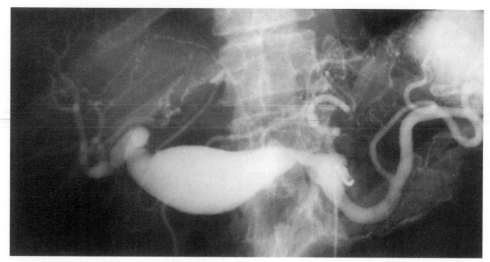

FIGURE 31-10. Hepatic artery aneurysm.

the high risk of rupture. Most extrahepatic aneurysms are treated with surgical resection and bypass grafting.

Liver transplantation

Indications

Orthotopic liver transplantation (OLT) in adults is indicated for irreversible liver diseases, including acute fulminant hepatic necrosis, congenital or acquired end-stage cirrhosis, sclerosing cholangitis, metabolic disorders resulting in liver failure, BCS, and primary hepatocellular malignancy.

Liver-transplant techniques

The orthotopic liver-transplant surgical procedure typically consists of four end-to-end vascular anastomoses and

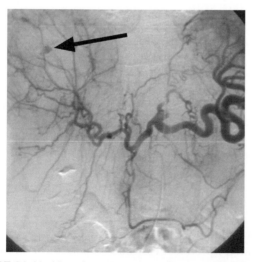

FIGURE 31-11. Hepatic artery pseudoaneurysm. Pseudoaneurysm (*arrow*) following percutaneous liver biopsy.

a biliary anastomosis. The donor hepatic artery anastomotic site is at the branch point of the common hepatic and splenic arteries or at the celiac axis with an aortic Carrel patch (aortic patch containing the origin of the celiac axis). The recipient hepatic artery anastomotic site is at the bifurcation of the right and left hepatic arteries or at the branch point of the gastroduodenal and proper hepatic arteries. Sometimes a donor iliac artery interposition graft is anastomosed directly to the supraceliac or infrarenal aorta if adequate inflow from the native celiac artery cannot be ensured, as in extremely small vessels or in severe celiac artery stenosis.

During removal of the diseased liver, the inferior vena cava is transected superior and inferior to the intrahepatic segment. End-to-end suprahepatic and infrahepatic inferior vena cava anastomoses then are made with the donor intrahepatic inferior vena cava.

An end-to-end anastomosis is made between the donor and recipient portal veins. A venous jump graft from the donor portal vein to the recipient superior mesenteric vein may be used in cases of portal vein thrombosis.

The biliary anastomosis is usually made between the donor and recipient common ducts. A T-tube may be left in place to stent the anastomosis and facilitate cholangiography. If the recipient common hepatic duct is diseased, too short, or too narrow, a choledochojejunostomy is performed. A cholecystectomy is routinely performed.

Complications

The most common transplant complications include vascular thrombosis or stenosis, biliary obstruction or leakage, hepatic infarction, hemorrhage, posttransplantation neoplasms, and rejection. Factors that affect OLT outcome include the extent of pretransplantation liver disease, complexity of the transplantation surgical procedure, and the use of immunosuppressive drugs.[50] Sonography is frequently the initial diagnostic modality used to evaluate for complications. Arteriography and venography are used as confirmatory examinations or during percutaneous interventions.

Vascular complications

After transplantation, the donor bile duct is entirely dependent on the hepatic arterial blood supply. Occlusion of the hepatic artery leads to bile duct ischemia and necrosis. Clinical presentations of hepatic artery thrombosis (HAT) include massive hepatic necrosis, delayed biliary leak/biloma, and intermittent episodes of sepsis without an obvious source (Fig. 31-12). Causes of HAT include faulty surgical technique, clamp injury, intimal trauma caused by perfusion catheters, disrupted vasa vasorum leading to ischemia of the arterial ends, and rejection. HAT has been reported to occur in 4 to 25% of liver transplants.[51–53] Sonographic evaluation demonstrates the absence of proper hepatic and intrahepatic arterial flow. Abrupt hepatic artery cutoff is identified during arteriography. In adult patients with HAT, collateral vessels to the transplanted liver do not form. The treatment for acute HAT consists of surgical thrombectomy or retransplantation.

Hepatic artery stenosis occurs in up to 11% of cases, with most stenoses occurring at the anastomosis (Fig. 31-13). Nonanastomotic stenoses are usually the result of rejection. Sonographic features of hepatic artery stenosis include focal accelerated velocity of greater than 200 to 300 cm per second, with turbulence present at or distal to the stenosis.[54] Treatment for hepatic artery stenosis is surgical anastomotic revision, retransplantation, or balloon angioplasty.[55,56] Frequently, chronic irreversible changes are present within the liver parenchyma by the time a hepatic artery stenosis is diagnosed.

Hepatic artery pseudoaneurysm is an uncommon but potentially fatal complication. Pseudoaneurysms typically

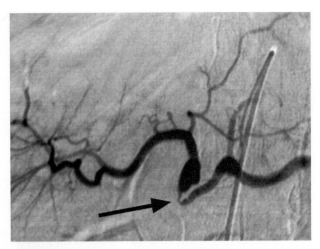

FIGURE 31-13. Hepatic artery stenosis following liver transplantation. Tortuous hepatic artery with stenosis (*arrow*) at the surgical anastomosis.

occur at vascular anastomoses; however, intrahepatic pseudoaneurysms may occur following percutaneous needle biopsy, biliary procedure, or focal infection.

Inferior vena cava stenosis or thrombosis is a rare complication of liver transplantation. Sonography shows echogenic thrombus or obvious narrowing, with a substantially increased flow velocity through the stenosis or reversal of flow in the hepatic veins.[57,58] Venography demonstrates the stenosis at the surgical anastomosis (Fig. 31-14). Successful balloon angioplasty and stent placement in the treatment of inferior vena cava stenosis have been reported.[59] Care must be taken that a potential size discrepancy between donor and recipient inferior vena cavae not be mistaken for a stenosis.

Portal vein thrombosis or anastomotic stenosis occurs in fewer than 3% of liver-transplant recipients. The clinical presentation includes symptoms of portal hypertension, hepatic failure, massive ascites, or edema.[60]

Biliary complications

Biliary complications occur in 13 to 25% of cases after liver transplantation. Most biliary complications present within the first 3 months after transplantation. Biliary stricture is the most common cause of biliary obstruction after transplantation. Nonanastomotic bile leaks and strictures usually are caused by bile duct ischemia resulting in bile duct necrosis. Causes of bile duct ischemia include hepatic artery thrombosis, prolonged cold ischemia time of the donor liver, ABO blood-type incompatibility, and chronic rejection.[61,62]

Biliary stricture may occur anywhere in the liver. Ischemic strictures often start at the liver hilus and progress to involve the intrahepatic bile ducts. Anastomotic strictures are usually secondary to scar formation or ischemia. Anastomotic strictures are treated with balloon dilatation

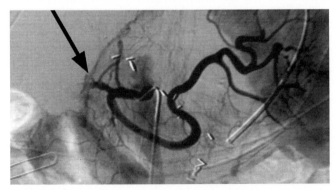

FIGURE 31-12. Hepatic artery thrombosis following liver transplantation. Celiac trunk injection demonstrating abrupt cutoff of the hepatic artery (*arrow*).

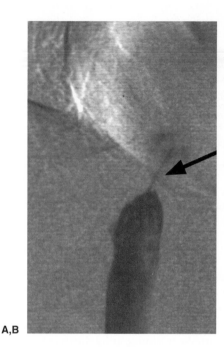
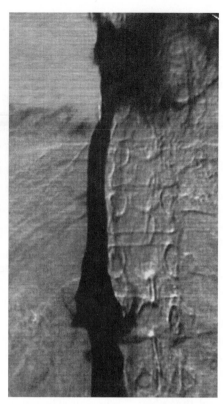

A,B

FIGURE 31-14. Inferior vena cava stenosis following liver transplantation. (**A**). Marked focal stenosis at the upper inferior vena cava anastomosis (*arrow*). (**B**). The stenosis was treated with percutaneous balloon angioplasty.

or surgical anastomotic revision. Most nonanastomotic strictures are due to bile duct ischemia. Percutaneous stents and dilation can be used in the management of nonanastomotic strictures that develop within 3 months after transplantation in the absence of pretransplantation primary sclerosing cholangitis, ductopenic rejection, cytomegalovirus infection, or hepatic artery thrombosis.[63–65]

Nonanastomotic biliary leaks that are not at the T-tube site are associated with hepatic artery thrombosis in 89% of cases.[66] These leaks are usually hilar or intrahepatic. Bile leaks can be treated with percutaneous biliary decompression and drainage. If hepatic artery thrombosis is present, the outcome is poor despite drainage. In some liver-transplant recipients, biloma drainage can prevent the need for retransplantation or prolong graft survival until a donor liver becomes available.

Acute transplant rejection
Acute transplant rejection cannot be reliably detected by radiologic methods. Biopsy of the graft with histologic examination remains the standard for detecting hepatic graft rejection.[50]

Posttransplant malignancy
Transplant recipients undergoing immunosuppressive therapy are at increased risk of developing malig-

nancy. The estimated prevalence of malignancy in OLT patients is increased 100-fold compared with that of age-matched populations. Most of these malignancies are non-Hodgkin's lymphoma or squamous cell skin cancer.[67]

■ Spleen

The spleen contributes to the removal of cellular elements from the circulating blood. Abnormal and aged erythrocytes, abnormal granulocytes, normal and abnormal platelets, and cellular debris are cleared by the spleen. The spleen also has an immunologic function. Patients who have had a splenectomy are at increased risk for overwhelming bacterial infection.[68,69]

Pathologic conditions that may be evaluated and treated with splenic arteriography and embolization include splenic trauma, splenic artery aneurysms, and hypersplenism. Splenic artery embolization may be performed before elective open or laparoscopic splenectomy to minimize operative blood loss.

Trauma

The spleen is the most frequently injured abdominal organ in patients with blunt abdominal trauma.[70] Splenic injury may manifest immediately after trauma or become apparent several days or weeks later. Conventional operative treatment of splenic injury consists of splenectomy. Partial splenectomy and splenorrhaphy have been successful in preserving splenic tissue and function.[71] Nonoperative management of blunt splenic trauma that includes observation and bed rest has been used as an alternative to laparotomy. The rationale for this treatment method is that many splenic injuries are not actively bleeding at the time of laparotomy; however, a failure of nonoperative management carries the risk of hemodynamic instability necessitating blood transfusion and urgent laparotomy. Reports demonstrated a 31 to 48% failure rate of nonoperative management.[72,73]

The aggressive use of arteriography and splenic artery embolization in cases of splenic injury has improved significantly the rate of splenic salvage with nonoperative management.[74,75] In most trauma centers, abdominal CT is used for the initial identification of splenic injury in hemodynamically stable patients. CT also is used for follow-up evaluation of splenic injury in patients who undergo nonoperative management. Findings indicative of splenic injury by CT include intraparenchymal hematomas, subcapsular hematomas, an irregular splenic outline, and hemoperitoneum. Indications for splenic arteriography vary by trauma center. At some trauma centers,

arteriography is performed in all cases of splenic injury identified by CT, whereas at other centers arteriography is performed only in cases in which there is the presence of an intraparenchymal contrast collection hyperdense with respect to the surrounding parenchyma.

The angiographic findings in splenic trauma may be subtle and vary with the severity of injury. Splenic arteriography often may show a mottled parenchymal blush, which should not be confused with contusion or laceration. Cases of extremely fine punctate extravasations (*Seurat spleen*) do not represent a significant sign of bleeding and therefore do not require embolization.[74]

The presence of splenic hematomas may result in an inhomogeneous parenchymal phase with splaying of smaller splenic artery branches. Overall spleen size may appear normal or enlarged. Extravasations resulting from splenic injury often are coarse, irregular, blotchy swirls of contrast material that may not appear to originate from a specific arterial branch. This finding has been called the "starry night" appearance and may involve a portion of or the entire spleen (Fig. 31-15). This appearance has been attributed to pooling and leaking of blood from the fragmented sinusoids.[76] Other angiographic findings include well-defined arterial pseudoaneurysms, arterial extravasation, arterial or venous branch occlusion, and arteriovenous shunting (Fig. 31-16).

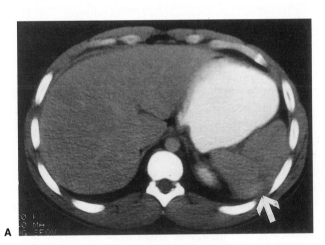

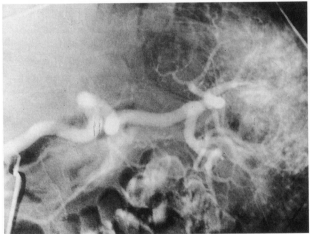

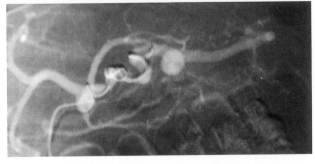

FIGURE 31-15. Splenic trauma. (**A**). Abdominal computed tomography image shows splenic injury (*arrow*) following a motor-vehicle accident. (**B**). Splenic arteriogram shows a "starry night" pattern. (**C**) Coil embolization of the splenic artery was performed. (Courtesy of S. Sclafani)

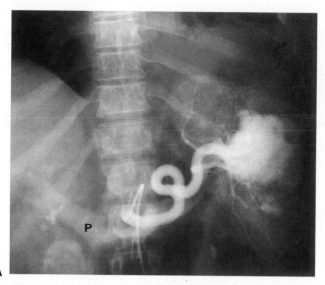
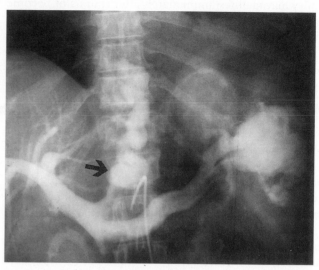

FIGURE 31-16. Splenic injury with arteriovenous shunting. This patient was involved in a motor-vehicle accident 6 months before the arteriogram was taken. (**A**) Arterial phase shows the splenic injury with arteriovenous shunting. P, portal vein. The massive shunting resulted in portal hypertension. (**B**). Venous phase of the splenic arterial injection shows opacification of esophageal varices (*arrow*).

Discrete pseudoaneurysms arising from intrasplenic or other smaller branches can be treated with selective coil embolization. An alternative to selective splenic artery branch embolization is main splenic artery embolization. If extravasation of contrast material is seen within or extended beyond the spleen, the proximal splenic artery just distal to the dorsal pancreatic artery is occluded with coils. Embolization is performed in the proximal splenic artery between the origin of the dorsal pancreatic branch and the next most distal pancreatic branch. Several coils can be packed into the splenic artery to accelerate occlusion. Occlusion of the splenic artery with coils lowers the distal perfusion pressure without causing ischemia and tissue infarction.

Splenic artery aneurysms

Although visceral artery aneurysms are rare, nearly half of all visceral artery aneurysms occur in the splenic artery. The incidence of splenic artery aneurysms is less than 1 in 1000 in the general population. Splenic artery aneurysms occur twice as frequently in women as in men. Most splenic artery aneurysms are present in the main trunk of the splenic artery (Fig. 31-17). Splenic artery aneurysms frequently are multiple. The etiology of splenic artery aneurysms is medial degeneration with superimposed atherosclerosis. Predisposing conditions include atherosclerosis, pregnancy, and portal hypertension.[77,78] Specific symptoms related to the presence of a splenic artery aneurysm are usually absent, but patients may present with pain in the left upper quadrant. Calcifi-

cation in the aneurysm wall is reported in as many as two thirds of patients. Causes of pseudoaneurysms of the splenic artery include pancreatitis (Fig. 31-18), infection, surgery, and trauma.

Splenic artery aneurysms may rupture, embolize, or thrombose. The most frequent complication is aneurysm rupture, which occurs in about 10% of patients.[77–79] There is an increased risk of splenic artery aneurysm rupture in pregnant women or women of childbearing age.[79] Calcified aneurysms also rupture, although less frequently. Splenic artery aneurysms typically rupture into the peritoneal cavity or rarely into the gastrointestinal tract, spleen, or pancreas.[80]

Because of the high mortality from rupture, all symptomatic splenic artery aneurysms should be resected. Asymptomatic aneurysms exceeding 2.5 cm in diameter should be treated.[81] The conventional treatment has been surgical ligation or excision of the aneurysm with or without splenectomy. Patients at increased surgical risk can be treated with percutaneous transarterial embolization.[82,83] If the aneurysm arises from the main splenic artery, the "sandwich" embolization technique is used. A nest of embolization coils is placed distal and proximal to the aneurysm with the purpose of excluding it from the circulation.

Hypersplenism

Hypersplenism refers to overactivity of splenic function leading to accelerated removal of any or all of the circulating cellular elements of the blood. Typical features of

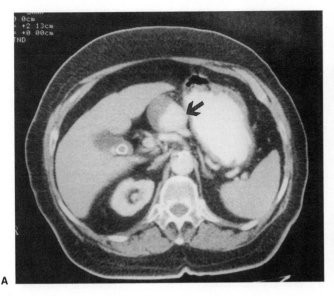

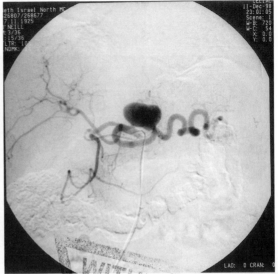

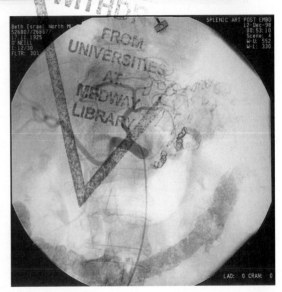

FIGURE 31-17. Splenic artery aneurysm. (**A**). Abdominal computed tomogram shows a large aneurysm (*arrow*) of the splenic artery containing mural thrombus. (**B**). Arteriography. (**C**). Coil embolization of the splenic artery proximal and distal to the aneurysm was performed. (Courtesy of B. Kanner)

hypersplenism include splenomegaly, anemia, leukopenia, and thrombocytopenia.[84] Surgical splenectomy is the traditional therapy for hypersplenism; however, partial splenic embolization is an accepted alternative to surgical splenectomy.[85]

Several diseases have been treated by partial splenic embolization as an alternative to splenectomy. Partial splenic embolization has been useful in the treatment of hypersplenism related to idiopathic thrombocytopenic purpura, portal hypertension, and thalassemia. Partial splenic embolization has been used for the treatment of hypersplenism in children.[84]

Embolization is performed with the catheter positioned in the distal splenic artery beyond the pancreatic and gastric branches. Gelfoam pledgets or polyvinyl alcohol particles may be used. The goal is to reduce splenic

perfusion by 70 to 80%. The procedure often is performed in a staged manner over several weeks to reduce the risk of complication from excessive infarction of splenic tissue. Patients are given broad-spectrum antibiotics before the procedure. Postembolization pain, fever, and leukocytosis are expected to be present for several days after the procedure. The spleen shrinks markedly over 3 to 4 months after the embolization procedure, with improvement in platelet and leukocyte count. The results of partial splenic embolization are long lasting in most patients. Repeat embolization may be necessary if less than 50% of the splenic volume is embolized initially.

Complications of partial splenic artery embolization include splenic rupture, pancreatitis, pneumonia, splenic abscess formation, and overwhelming sepsis. These major complications can occur with excessive

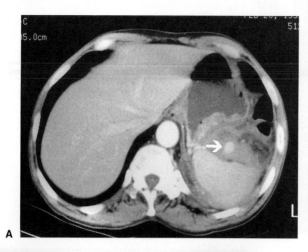

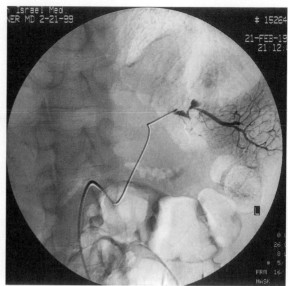

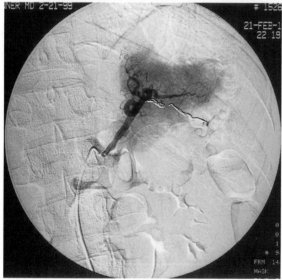

FIGURE 31-18. Splenic artery pseudoaneurysm. (**A**). Abdominal computed tomogram demonstrates a splenic artery aneurysm (*arrow*) in a patient with acute pancreatitis. (**B**). Selective catheterization and embolization of the affected splenic artery branch were performed. (**C**). Completion arteriogram shows no opacification of the pseudoaneurysm and preservation of most of the splenic parenchyma. (Courtesy of B. Kanner)

splenic devascularization. Inadvertent nontarget embolization to the liver, stomach, or pancreas can occur. Transient respiratory complications, such as pleural effusion and atelectasis, commonly occur and are related to the extent of embolization and the size of the spleen.

REFERENCES

1. Brown KT, Nevins AB, Getrajdman GI, et al. Particle embolization for hepatocellular carcinoma. *J Vasc Interv Radiol* 1998;9:822–828.
2. Okuda K, Ohtsuki T, Obata H, et al. Natural history of hepatocellular carcinoma and prognosis in relation to treatment. *Cancer* 1985; 56:918–928.
3. Colombo M. Hepatocellular carcinoma. *J Hepatol* 1992 15:225–236.
4. Itoh K, Nishimura K, Togashi K, et al. Hepatocellular carcinoma: MR imaging. *Radiology* 1987;164:21–25.
5. Okuda K, Musha H, Yoshida T, et al. Demonstration of growing casts of hepatocellular carcinoma in the portal vein by celiac angiography: the thread and streaks sign. *Radiology* 1975;117:303–309.
6. Gates J, Hartnell GG, Stuart KE, et al. Chemoembolization of hepatic neoplasms: safety, complications, and when to worry. *Radiographics* 1999;19:399–414.
7. Livraghi TL, Giorgio A, Mario G, et al. Hepatocellular carcinoma and cirrhosis in 746 patients: long term results of percutaneous ethanol injection. *Radiology* 1995;197:101–108.
8. Honda N, Guo Q, Uchida H, et al. Percutaneous hot saline injection therapy for hepatic tumors: an alternative to percutaneous ethanol injection therapy. *Radiology* 1994;190:53–57.
9. Murakami R, Yoshimatsu S, Yamashita Y, et al. Treatment of hepatocellular carcinoma: value of percutaneous microwave coagulation. *AJR Am J Roentgenol* 1995;164:1159–1164.
10. Livraghi T, Goldberg SN, Lazzaroni S, et al. Hepatocellular carcinoma: radio-frequency ablation of medium and large lesions. *Radiology* 2000;214:761–768.
11. Ngan H, Lai C, Fan S, et al. Transcatheter arterial chemoembolization in inoperable hepatocellular carcinoma: four-year follow-up. *J Vasc Interv Radiol* 1996;7:419–425.

12. Park JH, Han JK, Chung JW, et al. Superselective transcatheter arterial embolization with ethanol and iodized oil for hepatocellular carcinoma. *J Vasc Interv Radiol* 1993;4:333–339.

13. Dodd GD III, Soulen MC, Kane RA, et al. Minimally invasive treatment of malignant hepatic tumors: at the threshold of a major breakthrough. *Radiographics* 2000;9–27.

14. Nakamura H, Hashimoto T, Oi H, et al. Transcatheter oily chemoembolization of hepatocellular carcinoma. *Radiology* 1989;170:783–786.

15. Bronwicki JP, Vetter D, Dumas F, et al. Transcatheter oily chemoembolization for hepatocellular carcinoma. *Cancer* 1994;74:16–24.

16. Soulen MC. Chemoembolization of hepatic malignancies. *Oncology* 1994;8:77–84.

17. Reuter SR, Redman HC, Bookstein JJ. Angiography in carcinoma of the biliary tract. *Br J Radiol* 1971;44:636–641.

18. Butler J, Attiyeh FF, Daly JM. Hepatic resection for metastases of the colon and rectum. *Surg Gynecol Obstet* 1986;162:109–113.

19. Martinelli DJ, Wadler S, Bakal CW, et al. Utility of embolization or chemoembolization as second-line treatment in patients with advanced or recurrent colorectal carcinoma. *Cancer* 1994;74:1706–1712.

20. Kemeny N, Huang Y, Cohen AM, et al. Hepatic arterial infusion of chemotherapy after resection of hepatic metastases from colorectal cancer. *N Engl J Med* 1999;341:2039–2048.

21. Patt YZ, Peters RE, Chuang VP, et al. Effective retreatment of patients with colorectal cancer and liver metastases. *Am J Med* 1983;75:237–240.

22. Sugarbaker PH. Surgical decision making for large bowel cancer metastatic to the liver. *Radiology* 1990;174:621–626.

23. Soyer P, Bluemke DA, Fishman EK. CT during arterial portography for the preoperative evaluation of hepatic tumors: how, when, and why? *AJR Am J Roentgenol* 1994;163:1325–1331.

24. Mitty HA, Warner RP, Newman LH, Train JS, Parnes IH. Control of carcinoid syndrome with hepatic artery embolization. *Radiology* 1985;155:623–626.

25. Brown KT, Koh BY, Brody LA, et al. Particle embolization of hepatic neuroendocrine metastases for control of pain and hormonal symptoms. *J Vasc Interv Radiol* 1999;10:397–403.

26. Carrasco CH, Charnsangavej C, Ajani J, et al. The carcinoid syndrome: palliation by hepatic artery embolization. *Am J Roentgenol* 1986;147:149–154.

27. Abrams RM, Bernbaum ER, Santos JS, et al. Angiographic features of cavernous hemangioma of the liver. *Radiology* 1969;92:308–312.

28. Adam YG, Huvos AG, Fortner JG. Giant hemangiomas of the liver. *Ann Surg* 1970;172:230–245.

29. Nelson RC, Chezmar JL. Diagnostic approach to hepatic hemangiomas. *Radiology* 1990;176:11–13.

30. Powers C, Ros PR, Stoupis C, et al. Primary liver neoplasms: MR imaging with pathologic correlation. *Radiographics* 1994;14:459–482.

31. Baum JK, Bookstein JJ, Holtz F, et al. Possible association between benign hepatomas and oral contraceptives. *Lancet* 1973;2:926–929.

32. Cavaluzzi JA, Sheff R, Harrington DP, et al. Hepatic venography and wedge hepatic vein pressure measurements in diffuse liver disease. *AJR Am J Roentgenol* 1977;129:441–446.

33. Garcia-Tsao G, Groszmann RJ, Fisher RL, et al. Portal pressure, presence of gastroesophageal varices and variceal bleeding. *Hepatology* 1985;5:419–424.

34. Orloff MJ, Orloff MS, Orloff SL, et al. Three decades of experience with emergency portocaval shunt for acutely bleeding esophageal varices in 400 unselected patients with cirrhosis of the liver. *J Am Coll Surg* 1995;180:257–272.

35. Rees CR, Niblett RL, Lee SP, et al. Use of carbon dioxide as a contrast medium for transjugular intrahepatic portosystemic shunt procedures. *J Vasc Interv Radiol* 1994;5:383–386.

36. Uflacker R, Reichert P, D'Albuquerque LC, et al. Liver anatomy applied to the placement of transjugular intrahepatic portosystemic shunts. *Radiology* 1994;191:705–712.

37. Zemel G, Becker GJ, Bancroft JW, et al. Technical advances in transjugular intrahepatic portosystemic shunts. *Radiographics* 1992;12:615–622.

38. LaBerge JM, Ring EJ, Gordon RL, et al. Creation of transjugular intrahepatic portosystemic shunts with the Wallstent endoprosthesis: results in 100 patients. *Radiology* 1993;187:413–420.

39. Freedman AM, Sanyal AH, Tisnado J, et al. Complications of the transjugular intrahepatic portosystemic shunt: a comprehensive review. *Radiographics* 1993;13:1185–1210.

40. Haskal ZJ, Cope C, Shlansky-Goldberg RD, et al. Transjugular intrahepatic portosystemic shunt-related arterial injuries: prospective comparison of large- and small-gauge needle systems. *J Vasc Interv Radiol* 1995;6:911–915.

41. Nazarian GK, Bjarnason H, Dietz CA, et al. Refractory ascites: midterm results of treatment with a transjugular intrahepatic portosystemic shunt. *Radiology* 1997;205:173–180.

42. Sterling KM, Darcy MD. Stenosis of transjugular intrahepatic portosystemic shunts: presentation and management. *AJR Am J Roentgenol* 1997;168:239–244.

43. Nazarian GK, Ferral H, Castaneda-Zuniga WR, et al. Development of stenosis in transjugular intrahepatic portosystemic shunts. *Radiology* 1994;192:231–234.

44. Haskal ZJ, Pentecost MJ, Soulen MC, et al. Transjugular intrahepatic portosystemic shunt stenosis and revision: early and midterm results. *AJR Am J Roentgenol* 1994;163:439–444.

45. Mitchell MC, Boitnott JK, Kaufman S, et al. Budd–Chiari syndrome: etiology, diagnosis and management. *Medicine* 1982;61:199–218.

46. Blum U, Rossle M, Haag K, et al. Budd–Chiari syndrome: technical, hemodynamic, and clinical results of treatment with transjugular intrahepatic portosystemic shunt. *Radiology* 1995;197:805–811.

47. Bismuth H, Sherlock DJ. Portosystemic shunting versus liver transplantation for the Budd–Chiari syndrome. *Ann Surg* 1991;214:581–589.

48. Ishiguchi T, Fukatsu H, Itoh S, et al. Budd–Chiari syndrome with long segmental inferior venal cava obstruction: treatment with thrombolysis, angioplasty, and intravascular stents. *J Vasc Interv Radiol* 1992;3:421–425.

49. Peltzer MY, Ring EJ, LaBerge JM, et al. Treatment of Budd–Chiari syndrome with a transjugular intrahepatic portosystemic shunt. *J Vasc Interv Radiol* 1993;4:263–267.

50. Nghiem HV, Tran K, Winter TC, et al. Imaging of complications in liver transplantation. *Radiographics* 1996;16:825–840.

51. Sanchez-Urdazpal L, Sterioff S, Janes C, et al. Increased bile duct complications in ABO incompatible liver transplant recipients. *Transplant Proc* 1991;23:1440–1441.

52. Tzakis A, Bordon R, Shaw B Jr, et al. Clinical presentation of hepatic artery thrombosis after liver transplantation in the cyclosporine era. *Transplantation* 1985;40:667–671.

53. Flint E, Sumkin J, Zajko A, et al. Duplex sonography of hepatic artery thrombosis after liver transplantation. *AJR Am J Roentgenol* 1988;151:481–483.

54. Dodd GD III, Memel D, Zajko A, et al. Hepatic artery stenosis and thrombosis in transplant recipients: Doppler diagnosis with resistive index and systolic acceleration time. *Radiology* 1994;192:657–661.

55. Raby N, Karani J, Thomas S, et al. Stenoses of vascular anastomoses after hepatic transplantation: treatment with balloon angioplasty. *AJR Am J Roentgenol* 1991;157:167–171.

56. Orons PD, Zajko AB, Bron KM, et al. Hepatic artery angioplasty after liver transplantation: experience in 21 allografts. *J Vasc Interv Radiol* 1995;6:52–55.

57. Skolnick ML, Dodd GD III. Doppler sonography in liver transplan-

tation: pre- and posttransplant evaluation. In: Thrall JH, ed. *Current Practice in Radiology*. Philadelphia: Dekker; 1993;161–172.

58. Rossi A, Pozniak M, Zarvan N. Upper inferior vena caval anastomotic stenosis in liver transplant recipients: Doppler US diagnosis. *Radiology* 1993;187:387–389.

59. Orons PD, Zajko AB. Angiography and interventional procedures in liver transplantation. *Radiol Clin North Am* 1995;33:541–558.

60. Godoy MA, Camunez F, Echenagusia A, et al. Percutaneous treatment of benign portal vein stenosis after liver transplantation. *J Vasc Interv Radiol* 1996;7:273–276.

61. Stratta R, Wood R, Langans A, et al. Diagnosis and treatment of biliary tract complications after orthotopic liver transplantation. *Surgery* 1989;106:675–684.

62. Lerut J, Gordon R, Iwatsuki S, et al. Biliary tract complications in human orthotopic liver transplantation. *Transplantation* 1987;43:47–51.

63. Ward E, Kiely M, Maus T, et al. Hilar biliary strictures after liver transplantation: cholangiography and percutaneous treatment. *Radiology* 1990;177:259–263.

64. Campbell WL, Sheng R, Zajko AB, et al. Intrahepatic biliary strictures after liver transplantation. *Radiology* 1994;191:735–740.

65. Sheng R, Campbell WL, Zajko AB, et al. Cholangiographic features of biliary strictures after liver transplantation for primary sclerosing cholangitis: evidence of recurrent disease. *AJR Am J Roentgenol* 1996;166:1109–1113.

66. Kaplan S, Zajko A, Koneru B. Hepatic bilomas due to hepatic artery thrombosis in liver transplant recipients: percutaneous drainage and clinical outcome. *Radiology* 1990;174:1031–1035.

67. Holbert BL, Campbell WL, Skolnick ML. Evaluation of the transplanted liver and postoperative complications. *Radiol Clin North Am* 1995;33:521–540.

68. Green JB, Shackford SR, Sise MJ, et al. Late septic complications in adults following splenectomy for trauma: a prospective analysis in 144 patients. *J Trauma* 1986;26:999–1004.

69. Chaudry IH, Tabata Y, Schleck S, et al. Effect of splenectomy on reticuloendothelial function and survival following sepsis. *J Trauma* 1980;20:649–656.

70. Roberts JL, Dalen K, Bosanko CM, et al. CT in abdominal and pelvic trauma. *Radiographics* 1993;13:735–752.

71. Hebeler RF, Ward RE, Miller PW, et al. The management of splenic injury. *J Trauma* 1982;22:492–495.

72. Shackford SR, Molin M. Management of splenic injuries. *Surg Clin North Am* 1990;70:595–620.

73. Godley CD, Warren RL, Sheridan RL, et al. Nonoperative management of blunt splenic injury in adults: age over 55 years as a powerful indicator for failure. *J Am Coll Surg* 1996;183:133–139.

74. Sclafani SJA, Weisberg A, Scalea TM, et al. Blunt splenic injuries: nonsurgical treatment with CT, arteriography, and transcatheter arterial embolization of the splenic artery. *Radiology* 1991;181:189–196.

75. Davis KA, Fabian TC, Croce MA, et al. Improved success in nonoperative management of blunt splenic injuries: embolization of splenic artery pseudoaneurysms. *J Trauma* 1998;44:1008–1013.

76. Scatliff JH, Fisher ON, Guilford WB, et al. The "starry night" splenic angiogram. *AJR Am J Roentgenol Radium Ther Nucl Med* 1975;125:91–98.

77. Busuttil RW, Brin BJ. The diagnosis and management of visceral artery aneurysms. *Surgery* 1980;88:619–624.

78. Graham JM, McCollum CH, DeBakey ME. Aneurysms of the splanchnic arteries. *Am J Surg* 1980;140:797–810.

79. Stanley JC, Thompson NW, Fry WJ. Splanchnic artery aneurysms. *Arch Surg* 1970;101:689–697.

80. Bishop NL. Splenic artery aneurysm rupture into the colon diagnosed by angiography. *Br J Radiol* 1984;57:1149–1150.

81. Mattar SG, Lumsden AB. The management of splenic artery aneurysm: experience with 23 cases. *Am J Surg* 1995;169:580–584.

82. Baker KS, Tisnado J, Cho S, et al. Splanchnic artery aneurysms and pseudoaneurysms: transcatheter embolization. *Radiology* 1987;163:135–139.

83. Carr SC, Pearce WH, Vogelzang RL, et al. Current management of visceral artery aneurysms. *Surgery* 1996;120:627–633.

84. Harned RK, Thompson HR, Kumpe DA, et al. Partial splenic embolization in five children with hypersplenism: effects of reduced-volume embolization efficacy and morbidity. *Radiology* 1998;209:803–806.

85. Miyazaki M, Itoh H, Kaiho T, et al. Partial splenic embolization for the treatment of chronic idiopathic thrombocytopenic purpura. *AJR Am J Roentgenol* 1994;163:123–126.

32

The Biliary Tree and Pancreas

JONATHAN J. TRAMBERT

Radiological evaluation and percutaneous transcatheter intervention in the pancreas and biliary tree constitute a substantial subset of gastrointestinal radiology and intervention. The anatomic proximity of the pancreas and biliary tree and the fact that disease in one area often has a profound effect on the other make it logical to consider both in the same chapter.

■ Biliary Tree

Percutaneous radiological evaluation and intervention are usually sought in a patient with suspected obstructive jaundice. Before percutaneous procedures are undertaken in the bile duct, as much information as possible should be obtained from the clinical history and physical examination. Noninvasive studies should be obtained to confirm the presence of an obstruction and to evaluate for any related findings that could significantly affect the safety and feasibility of the percutaneous intervention.

Workup

The clinical background can yield much useful information. For example, the onset of jaundice associated with pain usually is due to an acute mechanical obstruction such as acute choledocholithiasis or acute pancreatitis. Painless jaundice usually is associated with malignant obstruction.

Imaging studies

If obstructive jaundice is clinically suspected, ultrasound should be one of the initial imaging studies. It is nonin-

vasive, it is excellent for detecting bile duct distentsion (Fig. 32-1), and it can yield information about the state of the liver parenchyma. At times, in addition to the intrahepatic bile ducts, the pancreas and distal bile ducts can be evaluated. Ultrasound also can yield information about the presence of ascites, which is extremely relevant when planning percutaneous interventions, as will be discussed later.

Computerized tomography (CT) is also valuable, especially if it is performed with intravenous contrast (Fig. 32-2). Although slightly less sensitive to intrahepatic bile duct dilation than ultrasound, CT yields additional important information that is often difficult to obtain with ultrasound (e.g., the cause of distal bile duct obstruction, the presence of liver metastases or primary tumors elsewhere in the body that may be metastatic to the liver). CT is also less operator dependent than ultrasound, although it is more expensive and the use of intravenous contrast makes it slightly more invasive.

Cholescintigraphy with hepatic 2,6-dimethyliminodeacetic acid (HIDA) and related agents is sometimes useful for assessing biliary tract functional status. A mechanical obstruction usually is associated with the absence of radionuclide activity in the bowel even on delayed images.

Magnetic resonance (MR) imaging and MR cholangiography hold promise for the noninvasive evaluation of the biliary tree. With MR cholangiography, computer manipulation and reconstruction of stacked cross-sectional images can yield three-dimensional maximum intensity projection (MIP) reconstructions, which can be rotated in different directions to provide views of the bile ducts from different angles. Various MR techniques are available for

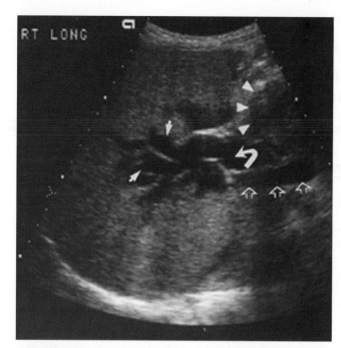

FIGURE 32-1. Ultrasound of the liver demonstrating dilated intrahepatic ducts (*solid white arrows*) and extrahepatic duct (*curved arrow*) resulting from metastatic gastric carcinoma to peripancreatic lymph nodes (*white arrowheads*). Portal vein (*open white arrows*) lies posterior to the common hepatic duct.

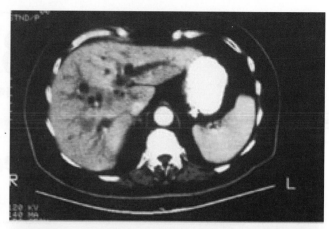

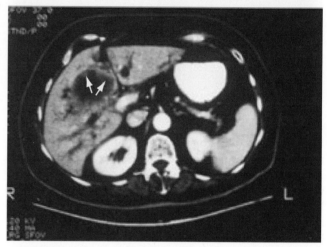

FIGURE 32-2. Computed tomography (CT) with intravenous contrast in a patient with gallbladder carcinoma and biliary obstruction. **A:** Dilated intrahepatic ducts are seen as circular and tubular hypodense structures. **B:** Thickened irregular gallbladder wall *(arrows)* is seen in a more caudal image.

suppressing surrounding tissues and enhancing the cholangiographic quality of the acquired image.[1]

Contrast cholangiography can be performed either by direct retrograde catheterization of the bile ducts through an endoscope (endoscopic retrograde cholangiography or ERC) (Fig. 32-3) or by percutaneous transhepatic cholangiogram (PTC) using a skinny needle (21 or 22 gauge). The endoscopic approach has the advantage of studying the biliary tract without some of the risks associated with the percutaneous transhepatic needle route. It also affords the possibility of studying the pancreatic duct as well as the common bile duct (endoscopic retrograde cholangiopancreatography, or ERCP). In addition, if desired, definitive therapy for a biliary stricture may be instituted in the form of transendoscopic papillotomy or placement of an internal stent.

ERCP does have potential complications, including a 1% incidence of pancreatitis and 0.8% incidence of septic cholangitis in experienced hands. The rate of complications is approximately four times higher in less experienced hands.[2]

ERCP is technically infeasible in certain situations, such as previous Roux-en-Y hepaticojejunostomies and high proximal biliary strictures refractory to contrast opacification of the peripheral intrahepatic bile ducts. In such situations as well as in centers that do not have skilled endoscopists, contrast cholangiography can be obtained

only through the percutaneous transhepatic route. In percutaneous transhepatic cholangiography, a 21- or 22-gauge needle is passed through an anesthetized area on the overlying skin, through the liver parenchyma, to a biliary radicle, allowing direct contrast opacification of the bile duct.

Specific cholangiographic findings

Contrast cholangiography yields definitive information about the morphology and location of the stricture or obstruction. The morphology of the stricture can often give an indication as to its etiology (Fig. 32-4). The location of the stricture provides additional clues to its etiology (Table 32-1).[3]

Stricture etiology

Nonmalignant etiologies

Nonmalignant etiologies of bile duct strictures, or "benign" bile duct strictures, include postoperative strictures,

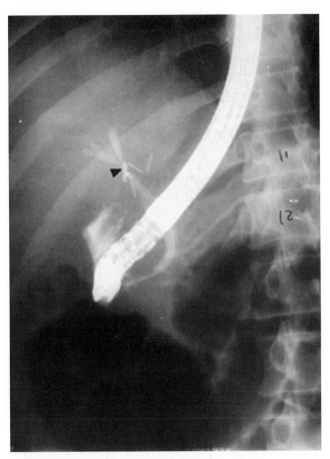

FIGURE 32-3. Endoscopic retrograde cholangiopancreatography (ERCP) showing proximal common hepatic duct stricture *(arrowhead)* that resulted from inadvertent duct injury during cholecystectomy (see also Fig. 32-14).

calculi, inflammatory strictures related to chronic cholecystitis (Mirizzi syndrome), chronic pancreatitis, and sclerosing cholangitis. Postoperative strictures can occur at the site of previous duct injury or repair (see Fig. 32-3) or at a site unassociated with the previous duct anastomosis. Strictures that occur after duct transsection and reanastomosis are often due to scar formation at the anastomosis site. Strictures that occur somewhat remote to the original site of ductal manipulation are presumed to be ischemic in etiology, perhaps related to pressure injury or thermal injury.

Purely inflammatory strictures of the common hepatic duct (CHD) or common bile duct (CBD) are usually the result of chronic cholecystitis or chronic pancreatitis. In chronic cholecystitis, inflammation of the gallbladder and cystic duct can cause them to thicken to the extent that they extrinsically compress and obstruct the adjacent CHD or CBD (Mirizzi syndrome) (Fig. 32-5). Chronic pancreatitis also can result in more distal extrinsic narrowing or stricturing of the CBD (Fig. 32-6).

Sclerosing cholangitis is a disease of unknown etiology characterized by diffuse periductal fibrosis. Intrahepatic or extrahepatic ducts or both can be involved. The incidence of ulcerative colitis and Crohn's disease is increased in patients with sclerosing cholangitis, although the exact relationship between inflammatory bowel disease and sclerosing cholangitis is unknown. The typical cholangiographic finding in sclerosing cholangitis is diffuse multifocal strictures of the intrahepatic or extrahepatic bile ducts, which gives them a "beaded" appearance. Diffuse intrahepatic and extrahepatic bile duct disease, identical cholangiographically to sclerosing cholangitis, can be seen after liver transplantation as a result of transplant ischemia and in patients with the acquired immunodeficiency syndrome (AIDS). Diffuse cholangiocarcinoma and diffuse liver metastases encasing the bile ducts are sometimes cholangiographically indistinguishable from sclerosing cholangitis (Fig. 32-7) (see the discussion of malignant biliary strictures following).

Malignant etiologies

Malignant bile duct strictures comprise both primary hepatobiliary tract neoplasms and extrinsic bile duct involvement by metastatic lesions (Table 32-1). Primary hepatobiliary tumors include bile duct epithelial adenocarcinomas (referred to as *cholangiocarcinoma* when they involve the intrahepatic or most proximal extrahepatic ducts) and hepatocellular carcinoma (hepatoma). Cholangiocarcinoma frequently involves the confluence of the right and left hepatic ducts and proximal common hepatic duct (Fig. 32-8). Pancreatic carcinoma displays the prototypical appearance of extrinsic malignant duct encasement, often with a "rat tail"-like luminal termination (Fig. 32-9). Metastatic disease to extrahepatic periductal lymph nodes can produce abrupt obstruction or irregular encasement of the CHD or CBD (Figs. 32-10 and 32-11).

Unfortunately, much overlap may exist between the cholangiographic appearance of benign and malignant strictures. Sclerosing cholangitis can be mimicked by diffuse liver metastases and cholangiocarcinoma. Postoperative or inflammatory strictures or obstructions occasionally are indistinguishable from those of malignant etiology. The clinical and surgical history might be helpful in differentiating malignant from nonmalignant causes. A brush biopsy by endoscope or percutaneous transhepatic tract can be used to help make a diagnosis, as can percutaneous needle biopsy of periductal tissue using a previously placed biliary stent for fluoroscopic guidance to the lesion. Occasionally, the definitive diagnosis is not known until surgery.

Biliary tract intervention

The best possible therapeutic option for a patient with obstructive jaundice is a surgical resection of the offen-

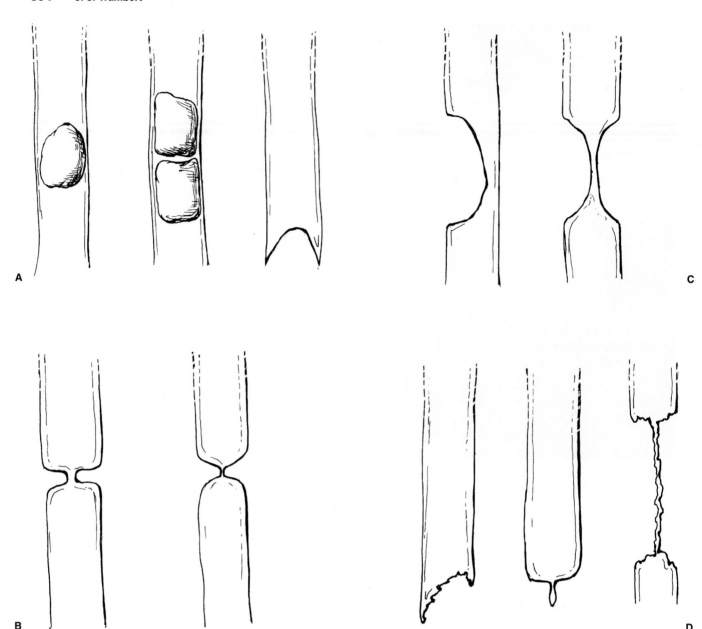

FIGURE 32-4. Cholangiographic appearances of bile duct pathologies. **A–C:** Nonmalignant diseases. Calculi typically produce intraluminal rounded filling defects or meniscus-shaped lumen termination (**A**). Extrinsic inflammatory disease (chronic cholecystitis, pancreatitis) usually produces a rounded compression of the adjacent bile duct (**B**). Postoperative fibrotic strictures usually appear as a short, focal stricture or short segmental duct occlusion (**C**). Malignant diseases (**D**). Suggestive cholangiographic features include ragged lumen termination (e.g., ampullary carcinoma, polypoid primary bile duct carcinoma), "rat tail"-shaped lumen termination (e.g., encasement by pancreatic carcinoma) and long irregular strictures (e.g., primary bile duct carcinoma, duct encasement by extrinsic tumor).

ding lesion and revision of the bile duct, which has the potential for long-term cure and is feasible in patients with nonmalignant strictures in such anatomic locations that complete resection of the stricture still allows for tension-free anastomoses. In many medical centers, this category is limited to lesions in the extrahepatic duct (CHD or CBD). Occasionally, malignant strictures can be curatively resected and bypassed. Sclerosing cholangitis involving only the extrahepatic duct (unusual) is also amenable to surgical bypass. One study noted an 88% five-year sympton-free outcome in patients who underwent surgical correction of benign postoperative strictures.[4] In patients in whom surgery is not a viable option, percutaneous biliary intervention should be considered.

TABLE 32-1. Biliary Strictures—Location versus Etiology

Intrahepatic bile duct strictures
    Cholangiocarcinoma
    Encasement by liver metastases or hepatoma
    Sclerosing cholangitis
Hepatic duct confluence, common hepatic duct
    Cholangiocarcinoma
    Gallbladder carcinoma
    Metastatic porta hepatis lymphadenopathy
    Postoperative strictures
Common hepatic duct, Common bile duct
    Bile duct carcinoma
    Pancreatic carcinoma
    Lymphoma, or other metastatic hepato-duodenal ligament
      lymphadenopathy
    Chronic pancreatitis
    Postoperative stricture
Distal common bile duct, Ampulla
    Pancreatic carcinoma
    Ampullary carcinoma

Percutaneous biliary interventions include biliary drainage catheter placement, antegrade placement of internal bile duct stents, bile duct stricture balloon dilatation, percutaneous cholecystostomy, and gallstone extraction.

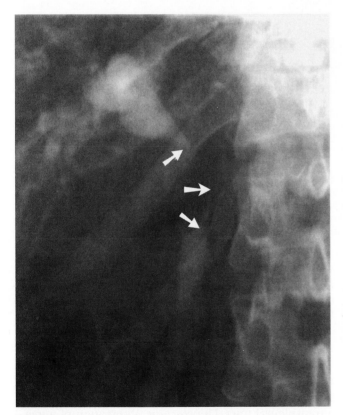

FIGURE 32-5. Percutaneous transhepatic cholangiogram (PTC) demonstrating smooth extrinsic compression of common hepatic duct (CHD) and common bile duct (CBD) (*arrows*) secondary to chronic cholecystitis (Mirizzi syndrome).

Percutaneous biliary drainage

Indications

The main indications for percutaneous biliary drainage (PBD) are the relief of jaundice resulting from inoperable obstruction or relief of septic cholangitis. Many patients who present with obstructive jaundice are unfit for surgery because their disease is too advanced (i.e., short life expectancy), they are poor medical risks for the required major surgery that the biliary reconstruction requires, or the offending lesions are in anatomic positions that are not amenable to durable surgical bypass (e.g., the intrahepatic ducts or hepatic duct confluence.) Such patients are committed to transcatheter prosthesis palliation. Such a prosthesis can be placed either by retrograde endoscopic approach or by percutaneous transhepatic access. Patients with obstructive jaundice who are surgical candidates but who have septic cholangitis should undergo external biliary drainage to allow resolution of the cholangitis before surgery. The value of preoperative percutaneous biliary drainage in patients who are not septic is controversial because there is no published evidence to suggest that preoperative reduction of the bilirubin level has any beneficial effect on subsequent surgical morbidity or mortality.[5,6] Despite this lack of published proof, many surgeons believe that preoperative drainage is of some benefit and

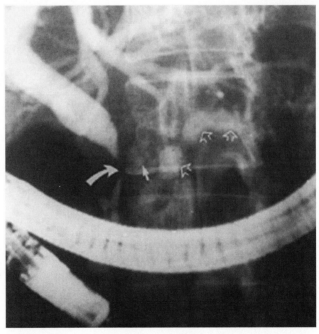

FIGURE 32-6. Endoscopic retrograde cholangiopancreatography (ERCP) revealing a smoothly tapered common bile duct (CBD) stricture due to chronic pancreatitis (*curved white arrow*). Corroborating this diagnosis are the faintly visible adjacent pancreatic head calcifications (*solid white arrow*). Also note contrast in the distened irregular pancreatic duct (*hollow white arrows*).

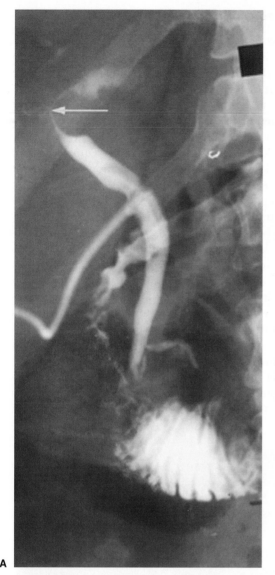

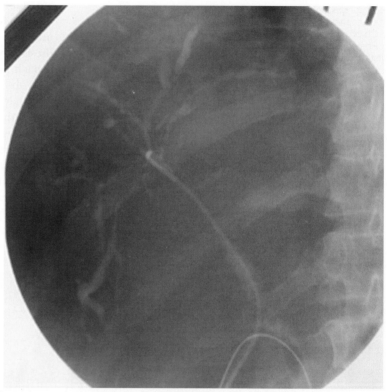

A   B

FIGURE 32-7. Metastatic adenocarcinoma to liver and porta hepatis nodes. **A:** T-tube cholangiogram showing stricture involving main hepatic duct (HD) confluence and proximal common hepatic duct (CHD) caused by encasement by porta hepatis lymphadenopathy (*arrow*). **B:** Retrograde selective right cholangiogram via T-tube tract demonstrating diffuse intrahepatic duct encasement by the liver parenchymal metastases. The resultant multifocal strictures and beadlike appearance of virtually all the opacified ducts shown here are cholangiographically similar to primary sclerosing cholangitis and diffuse cholangiocarcinoma.

continue to refer patients. Furthermore, many surgeons prefer mapping by PTC before bile duct revision, and if this study discloses biliary obstruction, decompression is mandated.

Method

If present, coagulopathies need to be corrected before percutaneous biliary intervention. Preprocedure and periprocedure antibiotics are mandatory to minimize the risk of sepsis from biliary duct manipulation. Antibiotic prophylaxis usually consists of intravenous (IV) cefazolin or cefoxitin 1 g before the procedure and 1 g every 8 hr for 48 hr. A common alternative would be ampicillin 2 g

IV, prior to the procedure, and 1 g every 6 hr for 48 hr in addition to gentamicin 1.5 mg/kg IV, preprocedure followed by 1.5 mg/kg IV, every 8 hr for 48 hr.

A suitable skin entry site is chosen in the region of the right mid to anterior axillary line over the right upper quadrant of the abdomen. The exact location is guided by fluoroscopic observation of the liver and diaphragm, taking care to choose an approach with minimum risk of a transpleural tract. Fluoroscopic observation of a metal marker at the planned entry site while the patient takes a deep breath is usually enough to accomplish this step. The tract, by necessity, is almost always intercostal. Entry should be over the lower rib rather than under the upper

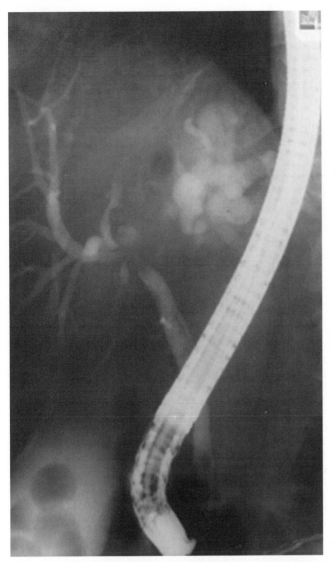

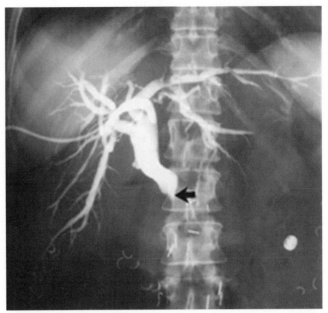

FIGURE 32-9. Percutaneous transhepatic external biliary drainage catheter. Transcatheter cholangiogram shows typical "rat tail" rapid taper common bile duct (CBD) obstruction caused by pancreatic carcinoma (*arrow*).

FIGURE 32-8. Endoscopic retrograde cholangiography (ERC) demonstrating a cholangiocarcinoma involving the confluence of the right and left hepatic ducts and proximal common hepatic duct. Left hepatic ducts are totally obstructed. This type of lesion is sometimes referred to as a *Klatzkin tumor*.

rib of the intercostal space to minimize risk of trauma to the intercostal artery and irritation of the intercostal nerve that might render the drainage catheter more painful.

Adequate conscious sedation is needed because percutaneous biliary manipulation can be quite painful, especially in patients with fibrotic livers resistant to catheter advancement. Lidocaine anesthesia is given along the tract from the skin to the peritoneum. Then a percutaneous transhepatic cholangiogram is performed by advancing a 21- or 22-gauge needle into the liver. Dilute contrast is infused gently into the needle as it is slowly retracted under fluoroscopic observation until the characteristic pattern of bile duct filling is identified. This is manifested by filling of tubular lumina with contrast that does not wash away (Fig. 32-10A). In attempting to opacify the biliary tree, the needle tip may traverse or lodge in a portal vein, hepatic vein, hepatic artery, or lymphatic. Each of these nonbiliary lumina has a characteristic orientation and appearance that differentiate it from a bile duct, and contrast invariably will wash out of the lumen in all of these nonbiliary structures.

Once a biliary radicle is entered, contrast is injected slowly and gently. Care should be exercised to avoid overdistension of the obstructed biliary tree, which could increase the chance of sepsis. A few milliliters of contrast are injected, followed by aspiration of an equal number of milliliters through the same needle to progressively exchange bile for contrast to visualize as much of the biliary tree as possible. Because iodinated water soluble contrast flows into the most dependent locations, tilting the patient semiupright can be helpful in allowing opacification of the central bile ducts with less overall volume of injected contrast. When sufficient anatomy is apparent, diagnostic images are obtained. The definitive drainage procedure is completed by the originally entered duct, if it is suitable in location and vector or by advancing another needle into a more suitable duct under fluoroscopic guidance (see Fig 32-10B). A rotating C-arm fluoroscopy unit is most helpful for delineating the three-dimensional array of the biliary system in planning definitive access. Coaxial micropuncture access systems are used most often to achieve definitive drainage, either by the initial PTC site or by a different duct (see Fig. 32-10).

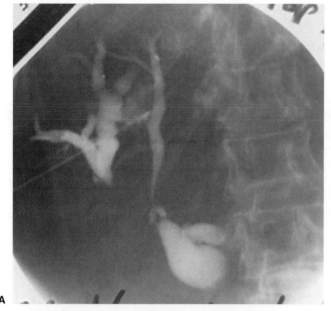

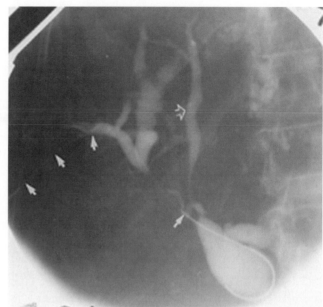

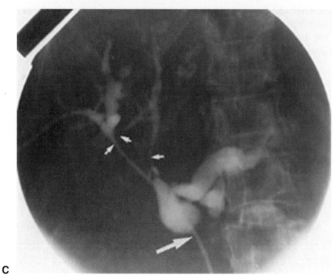

FIGURE 32-10. Procedure for performing percutaneous transhepatic biliary drainage in a patient with adenocarcinoma metastatic to liver and porta hepatis nodes: sequential steps. **A:** Thin-needle percutaneous transhepatic cholangiogram (PTC). The particular duct entered is not suitable for definitive catheterization because of the unfavorable direction of entry, which would direct subsequent wires and catheters peripherally. **B:** After opacification of bile ducts by skinny-needle PTC, more favorably oriented peripheral right hepatic duct tributary then was entered with the skinny needle and 0.018-inch diameter wire (*solid white arrows*) advanced centrally. The site of initial duct puncture for PTC (*open arrow*). **C:**. After coaxial dilation over 0.018-inch diameter wire, a working catheter was used to cross more distal strictures for internal-external drainage catheter placement. Intrahepatic duct strictures (*small arrows*) caused by duct encasement by liver metastases. Common hepatic duct stricture (*large arrow*) caused by lymphadenopathy in porta hepatis and hepaticoduodenal ligament.

External biliary drainage usually is completed by positioning an 8 Fr pigtail catheter proximal to the obstruction and connecting it to a drainage bag. If internal stenting is desired, the stricture or obstruction must be crossed. Crossing the stricture or obstruction is accomplished by a torque catheter, such as a cobra or Levin shape (Cook) and a soft tip Bentson guidewire (Cook) or hydrophilic glide wire (Terumo) to facilitate atraumatic passage through the blockage to the bowel. If the lesion cannot be crossed easily on the first day, then an external drainage catheter is temporarily left in place upstream of the obstruction, and another attempt to cross the lesion is made a few days later. External bile decompression allows for a decrease in the inflammation and edema, thereby making it easier to cross the obstruction at a later date. Furthermore, external bile decompression will less-

en the risk of procedure-related sepsis if multiple manipulations are needed to cross a lesion. It is rare that an obstruction cannot be traversed on either the first or second attempt.

Complications
Pain control can be difficult, especially when advancing catheters through severely fibrotic livers. This problem is compounded by the presence of a history of chronic alcohol or narcotic abuse with consequent tolerance to analgesic drugs.

Despite prophylactic antibiotics, blood-borne infection still occurs in 2 to 12% of patients treated.[5,7,8] A pneumothorax and a biliary pleural fistula are additional risks, given the proximity of the working area to the diaphragm and pleural space. One or both of these complications

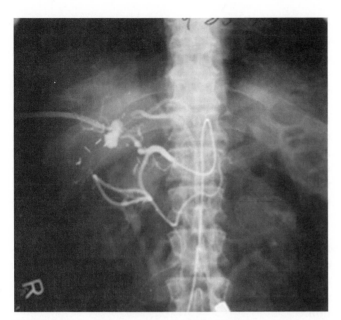

FIGURE 32-11. Hepatic artery branch pseudoaneurysm complicating chronic biliary catheter drainage that was successfully treated by superselective transcatheter embolotherapy.

were noted in approximately 8% of percutaneous biliary drainage procedures.[8]

Clinically significant bleeding is encountered in 4 to 15% of percutaneous biliary drainage procedures.[5,9] Fortunately, hepatic artery extravasation or pseudoaneurysms complicating PTC and biliary drainage (Fig. 32-11) are amenable to percutaneous transcatheter embolotherapy. Ascites increases the risk of complications, particularly that of intraperitoneal hemorrhage. Without ascites, the close apposition of the hepatic capsule to the parietal peritoneum provides a tamponade effect. This advantage is lost when the punctured or lacerated hepatic capsule is surrounded by fluid. In addition, the presence of ascites between the abdominal wall and the liver renders percutaneous biliary drainage or stent placement more difficult. Guidewires and catheters are more likely to buckle and coil in that space when attempts are made to advance them through the liver parenchyma; use of a sheath can be helpful in this situation. These difficulties are often circumvented by performing PBD left biliary drainage from the anterior approach (usually because of gravity there is less ascites anterior) or removing some of the ascites by paracentesis prior to biliary drainage. An internal stent can also be placed via a transjugular, transhepatic approach, thereby avoiding the peritoneal cavity.[10]

Biliary drainage options

There are three biliary drainage options. The first is external drainage (see Fig. 32-9). The disadvantage of this arrangement is that the patient is committed to wear-

ing a leg bag. External drainage is also nonphysiologic; the fluid and electrolytes in the excreted bile are lost and careful fluid replacement may become necessary. For this reason, external biliary drainage is not an acceptable long-term option when it is possible to traverse the obstruction.

The second arrangement is "internal-external" biliary drainage (see Fig. 32-12). Advantages of this arrangement are that bile drains back into the patient eliminating the fluid and electrolyte loss, and the catheter can be exchanged easily over a guidewire. The disadvantages include annoyance to the patient of a prosthesis protruding from the skin, which can affect the patient's lifestyle and self-image as well as the small but finite risk of introducing an infection.

A third option is placement of an indwelling stent. The advantage of this option is that no catheters protrude from the skin; therefore, patients are not burdened by an externally protruding prosthesis. The disadvantage of totally internal stents is that they do obstruct eventually, and then they must be exchanged or revised either transendoscopically or by a new percutaneous transhepatic biliary access procedure.

Endoscopic or percutaneous stent placement

Most biliary stents are placed transendoscopically at many institutions, including ours. Percutaneous stent placement is preferred in the following situations: (a) in high biliary strictures or obstructions where it is technically more successful than endoscopic stenting or (b) unfavorable anatomy such as gastric outlet obstruction or presence of a Roux-en-Y hepaticojejunostomy. Percutaneous

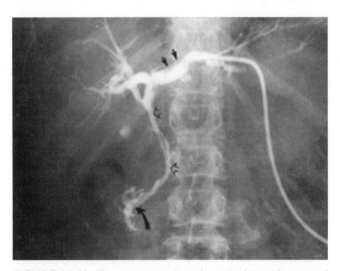

FIGURE 32-12. Percutaneous transhepatic internal–external biliary drainage catheter. Patient with encasement of virtually entire common hepatic duct–common bile duct (CHD–CBD) by metastatic breast carcinoma (*open arrows*). Some of the catheter sideholes proximal to obstruction are faintly visible (*solid black arrows*). Catheter pigtail is in duodenum (*curved arrow*).

stent placement may often succeed when strictures are refractory to endoscopic retrograde advancement of the stent.

Plastic stents

Probably the most common plastic stent that has been in use by interventional radiologists is the Carey Coons stent (Medi-Tech Inc.), a straight plastic tube with side holes along its length and a nylon string attached to its proximal end that can be used to retract the stent if it is initially advanced too far. The string then is connected to a Silastic button, which is embedded in subcutaneous tissue via a small 1.5-cm incision. The nylon string thus prevents stent dislodgement and migration. It is sometimes possible to regain entry into the bile duct containing the proximal end of the stent by reexposing the silastic button, mobilizing the nylon string, tying a suture to the string, and then advancing a small catheter over this suture-nylon string guidewire into the bile duct, allowing a possible stent exchange or replacement.[11] Stent exchange can be accomplished by engaging the old occluded stent coaxially with an angioplasty balloon, pushing it into the duodenum or jejunum, and placing a new stent over the guidewire. The old stent almost invariably passes through the bowel by peristalsis and out with the stool.

Internal plastic stents have an average life expectancy of 3 to 4 months.[12] Frequently, patients treated with stents for malignant obstructions die before their stents occlude. Sometimes, however, patients can survive for 1 or 2 years following the palliative stent bypass. This is particularly true of slow growing, indolent malignancies such as some cholangiocarcinomas or rarely in the case of slow growing pancreatic carcinomas.

A patient with nonmalignant strictures may require stenting, perhaps because the stricture has failed more than one attempt at operative repair, has an anatomically unfavorable location for operative repair (such as intrahepatic strictures or multiple strictures), or has failed balloon dilatation treatment. Patients with refractory nonmalignant strictures may have a normal lifespan if their bile flow and hepatic integrity are maintained either by stenting or in selected situations by liver transplantation. Such patients will outlive their stents, therefore, long-term stent maintenance and possible replacement must be considered at the time of stent placement.

When internal–external stenting is used, the stent may be exchanged easily over a guidewire, a simple outpatient procedure, usually done prophylactically every 3 months, treating the patient with one dose of antibiotics (like those administered for percutaneous biliary drainage) before the exchange. Unfortunately, an exchange is more complicated for patients who have internal stents. Exchange of internal stents, if not possible endoscopically, requires a new percutaneous transhepatic bile duct access, with its associated discomfort and potential complications.

One of the major disadvantages of placing large plastic stents from the percutaneous approach is the need for a transhepatic tract at minimum the size of the stent caliber (usually 12–14Fr). Thus, the risks of bleeding and pain from stent advancement, particularly through a fibrotic or cirrhotic liver, are increased. In the past, this problem was ameliorated by the combined percutaneous–endoscopic team approach to stent placement. Because lower profile metallic stent for malignant etiologies have replaced plastic stents in many institutions, this potential problem is encountered much less frequently.

Percutaneous transhepatic stent placement   The percutaneous placement of an internal biliary stent involves the advancement of the stent transhepatically over a guidewire and carefully positioning it across the obstruction.

Plastic stents are advanced over the guidewire using a "pusher catheter," which is retracted after the stent is in position. Expandable metal stents are positioned on their delivery device and then deployed either by retraction of a containment membrane or sheath (Wallstent and Gianturco-Rosch Z-stent, respectively) or by balloon expansion (Palmaz stent). Expandable metal stents are discussed in greater detail later. When the internal stent is in position, an external catheter usually is temporarily positioned upstream of the stent. The external catheter is removed when adequate internal stent function has been confirmed clinically and cholangiographically and external drainage or transhepatic access is no longer needed.

Percutaneous–endoscopic team approach   The combined antegrade–retrograde team approach involves creation of a catheter tract from the skin through the biliary obstruction to the bowel. A transhepatic entry into the biliary tree is made, and the interventional radiologist advances a guidewire across the obstruction and out into the bowel; the wire is then grasped by the endoscopist and retracted out through the oral cavity. Retrograde transoral stent placement is then made possible because the guidewire can be held taut at both ends.

When the stent is safely in position, the guidewire is removed, which allows the advancement of a 12 Fr stent while only needing a 4 or 5 Fr tract in the skin and liver parenchyma, resulting in a significant decrease in pain and morbidity.[13]

Expandable metal stents

The advantage of the expandable metal stent is that it can be introduced through a small transhepatic tract, and it then expands, either by inherent spring tension or balloon dilatation to a much larger caliber than the introducer itself. The stents available in the United States

The Biliary Tree and Pancreas

that are approved by the Food and Drug Administration (FDA) for use in the biliary system include the Wallstent (Schneider Incorporated), the Gianturco-Rosch Z-stent (Cook Incorporated), and the Palmaz stent (Johnson and Johnson). The Wallstent and Gianturco-Rosch Z-stent are self-expanding (Fig. 32-13). The Palmaz stent requires balloon expansion. In Europe, the Strecker stent is also available, but this stent is not yet approved for use in the United States.

The most popular stents for use in the bile ducts are the Wallstent and the Gianturco-Rosch Z-stent. At my institution, the Wallstent is used most frequently. The Wallstent introducer is only 7 Fr, and some interventionalists place them without using a sheath (7 Fr ID, 8.5 Fr OD). This means the maximum size transhepatic tract needed is only 7-8.5Fr compared to the 12–14 Fr tract needed to place a Carey-Coons type plastic stent. Unlike the plastic stents with lumina of only 4 mm or smaller, the Wallstent and Gianturco-Rosch Z-stent can expand to 10 mm or larger.

It would seem that a 10 mm diameter lumen would remain patent longer than a 4 mm plastic stent lumen. Initially, this impression was not corroborated by experience; however, one recent double-blind trial comparing plastic stents and Wallstents shows an approximately two-fold patency duration advantage for Wallstents compared with plastic stents1.[14] This, in addition to the decreased pain and morbidity involved in the transhepatic placement of expandable metal stents, offsets the disadvantage of their relatively high price (the cost of a single metal stent is approximately 20 times higher than that of a plastic stent).

Self-expanding metal stents, despite their larger maximum lumen, do occlude. Occlusion occurs either by tumor overgrowth at the ends of the stent, bile inspissation, or, less commonly, tumor ingrowth through the wire mesh of the stent. Tumor overgrowth at stent ends can be forestalled by careful positioning of the stent and by selection of a stent at least 1 cm longer than the stricture at either end. Not much can be done to prevent bile sludge inspissation occlusion, and patients differ in their propensity for this problem. Some interventional radiologists believe that the Gianturco-Rosch Z-stent is more susceptible to tumor ingrowth through the stent interstices than the Wallstent, which possesses a much tighter wire mesh. Covered stents may have the potential to decrease or eliminate the problem of occlusion caused by tumor ingrowth, but they are currently under investigation.

Unlike plastic stents that can be removed and exchanged transendoscopically or percutaneously, expandable metal stents are permanent implants. As such, revision of occluded stents consists of balloon dilation of the stent lumen, flushing out inspissated bile, removing tumor ingrowth by atherectomy, or deploying a second stent coaxially within the original stent. This second stent can be an internal metallic or plastic stent. Many inter-

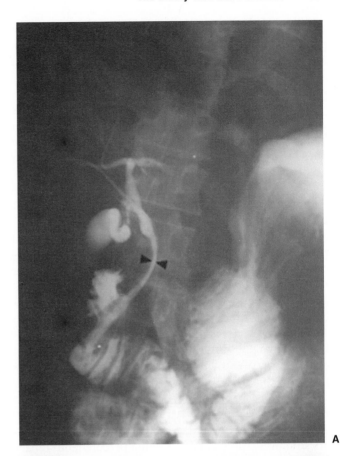

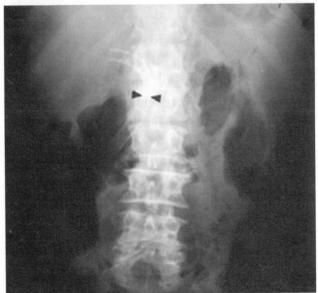

FIGURE 32-13. Self-expanding Wallstent deployed across a malignant common bile duct (CBD) obstruction. **A:** Immediately after deployment, a stent lumen within a tumor of approximately only 2 mm diameter (*black arrowheads*). **B:** Ten days after deployment, the stent within the tumor has self-dilated to approximately 7 mm diameter (*black arrowheads*).

ventional radiologists prefer to place internal-external plastic stents through the occluded metal stent from a transhepatic approach. Tumor overgrowth at the end of a stent can be treated by deploying a second stent partly overlapping the first stent.

Because metal stents are permanent implants, there is general reluctance to use them to treat nonmalignant biliary strictures, but metal stents have replaced plastic ones for treatment of malignant disease in an increasing number of interventional radiologists' practices.

Percutaneous balloon dilation of nonmalignant biliary strictures

Most nonmalignant strictures are amenable to surgical repair with good long-term results. Patients whose strictures recur after previous operative repair or are not in a favorable anatomic position for surgical repair (e.g., intrahepatic duct strictures) or patients who decline surgical repair are candidates for balloon dilatation therapy. The long-term success rate for balloon dilatation is not as high as that for surgical repair (40–55% after balloon dilatation versus 88% postsurgical revision, at 3 to 5 years postprocedure).[4,15,16]

Method

The first stage of percutaneous balloon dilatation of biliary strictures consists of establishing percutaneous biliary drainage and crossing the stricture. Usually, at least 2 days are allowed between initial percutaneous biliary drainage and the first session of biliary balloon dilatation. The patient is kept on broad-spectrum antibiotics started before the initial percutaneous biliary drainage. Balloon size is chosen based on the measured caliber of the adjacent normal duct. The first balloon dilatation usually is performed using a balloon slightly smaller than the estimated normal duct size, with progressively larger balloon diameters used on successive days until a balloon of the established duct size, or perhaps 10 to 20% larger, is used. Typically, a cycle of biliary balloon dilatation involves three different sessions with progressively increasing balloon diameters over approximately 1 week's time. Each balloon inflation lasts approximately 5 min. After completion of a balloon dilatation session, a 10Fr or 12Fr internal–external stent catheter is left across the stricture. In our practice, the stricture is stented for approximately 6 weeks after the final balloon dilatation session. There is a wide variation in the recommended duration of postprocedure stenting, however, ranging from less than a month to 12 to 13 months posttreatment.[15–17] After the stenting period, if follow-up cholangiography shows a patent duct or anastomosis (Fig. 32-14), the stent is converted to an external catheter, which is left in the bile ducts upstream of the treated area and capped for one week to provide a provocative test. If the patient does not develop symptoms of obstruction (e.g., jaundice, shaking chills, fever), the external tube is discontinued. If the cholangiogram shows a persistent stricture, the cycle of biliary balloon dilatation is repeated.

Percutaneous cholecystostomy

Percutaneous cholecystostomy, or percutaneous catheter drainage of the gallbladder, is a safe, minimally invasive interventional procedure that is useful in a number of clinical situations. The most common indication for percutaneous cholecystostomy is the treatment of acute cholecystitis in patients who are at high risk for surgical cholecystectomy for reasons of advanced age, cardiac instability, severe debilitation, or recent trauma. Percutaneous cholecystostomy is often used as a temporary measure until the patient becomes medically fit to undergo surgery, but it may constitute definitive therapy in patients who are considered to be permanently high surgical risks.

Percutaneous cholecystostomy can serve as a minimally invasive diagnostic as well as a therapeutic maneuver. In the intensive care setting, the diagnosis or exclusion of acute cholecystitis can be difficult. The classic symptom of right upper quadrant pain is frequently masked in trauma victims or otherwise severely ill patients. False-positive radionuclide gallbladder scintigraphy is common when there has been prolonged absence of oral intake. Furthermore, such patients may demonstrate sonographic evidence of gallstones or bile sludge, but they may not have acute cholecystitis, or they may have acute cholecystitis without gallstones (*acalculous cholecystitis*). In such confusing circumstances, clinical improvement (e.g., defervescence, reversal of shock, reduction in white blood count) within 24 to 48 hrs of percutaneous gallbladder drainage means that the patient almost certainly had acute cholecystitis. If no clinical improvement occurs after cholecystostomy, the gallbladder can be excluded reliably as the source of sepsis.[18,19]

Other indications for percutaneous cholecystostomy include providing access for percutaneous removal of gallstones in patients too unstable to undergo surgery, performance of diagnostic cholangiography, and as an alternate route for percutaneous biliary drainage.

Percutaneous cholecystostomy can be performed using either ultrasound or CT guidance. The advantage of ultrasound guidance is that the cholecystostomy can be performed at the bedside in patients too sick to leave their hospital bed for the radiology department, which is often the circumstance surrounding the referral for percutaneous cholecystostomy. A suitable skin site is chosen based on the ultrasound or CT evaluation of potential tracts to the gallbladder. Many practitioners prefer to make a transhepatic tract to the gallbladder under the assumption that this lessens the risk of bile leakage into the peritoneal cavity while the draining catheter is being placed, because the gallbladder wall is in close apposition to the liver at this point. Recently, however, the safety and

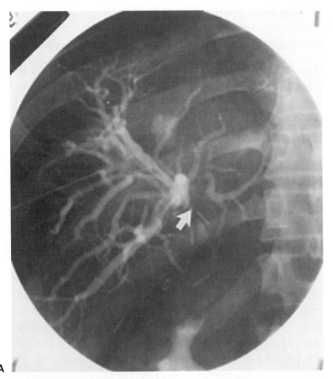

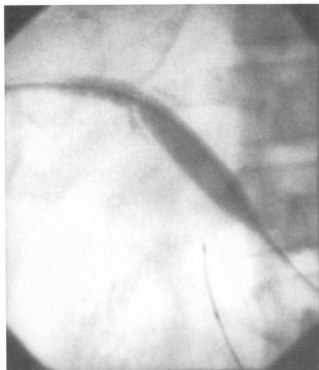

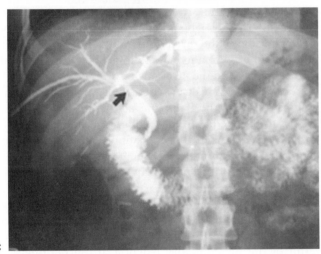

A

B

C

FIGURE 32-14. Proximal common hepatic duct (CHD) post-operative stricture (same patient as in Fig. 32-3) successfully treated by balloon dilatation. **A:** Pretreatment, percutaneous transhepatic cholangiogram (PTC) showing proximal (CHD) stricture (*white arrow*). **B:** Balloon inflated across stricture with initial "waist." **C:** Final cholangiogram after 10-mm balloon dilation and after 6 weeks of stenting with 12Fr catheter, showing elimination of stricture (*black arrow*).

feasibility of the direct transperitoneal approach to the gallbladder have been documented.[20] Thus, it is uncertain whether there is any advantage to a transheptic versus a direct transperitoneal gallbladder puncture. Lidocaine anesthesia is given from the skin along the tract to the peritoneum. Definitive access can be made by a one-step Trocar approach (drainage catheter mounted on the puncturing needle) or by the Seldinger method (i.e., the gallbladder is punctured with a skinny needle, and then the drainage catheter is advanced into the gallbladder lumen over a guidewire after suitable coaxial tract dilatation) (Fig. 32-15).

Possible complications of percutaneous cholecystos-

tomy include severe vasovagal reaction, intraperitoneal hemorrhage, bile peritonitis, and sepsis. Such major complications were reported to occur in 8.7% of patients.[21]

If the cholecystostomy catheter is to be discontinued, a mature tract must be present to decrease the risk of bile peritonitis. Contrast tract sinography over a guidewire showing no peritoneal leakage ensures a mature tract.[22]

Percutaneous extraction or dissolution of calculi in the bile ducts or the gallbladder can be performed by percutaneous access as well. Gallstone extraction can be performed using a choledochoscope introduced through the percutaneous tract,[23] which requires dilating the percutaneous tract up to 19 Fr to allow passage of the chole-

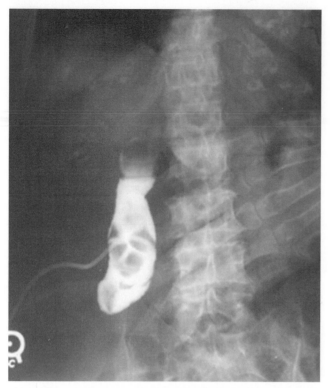

FIGURE 32-15. Percutaneous cholecystostomy. Note the multiple gallstones, including one impacted in the gallbladder neck and cystic duct demonstrated on cholecystogram.

■ The Pancreas

Pancreatitis and pancreatic pseudocysts

Pancreatitis denotes inflammation of the pancreatic exocrine glands. The most common cause is ethanol abuse, but it also can result from mechanical irritation of the distal pancreatic duct by gallstones (gallstone pancreatitis) or by iatrogenic manipulation. Iatrogenic causes include ampullary trauma from endoscopic papillotomy, edema from ampullary catheterization, and ampullary irritation from percutaneous biliary interventions. It also can result from overinjection of the pancreatic duct during ERCP and subsequent acinar extravasation. Pancreatitis can occur as a complication of surgery in the upper abdomen. Acute pancreatitis can have a spectrum of courses, from mild pancreatitis that resolves spontaneously with conservative measures, to severe pancreatitis complicated by pseudocysts, pancreatic necrosis, and abscess formation. When pancreatitis is complicated by pancreatic duct strictures, chronic pseudocysts and fistulization to various parts of the body can ensue, which, in turn, can be refractory to surgical or medical treatment. The potential for pancreatitis to progress along such a severe course is due to the extremely proteolytic nature of the pancreatic enzymes. The inflamed pancreas releases pancreatic juices into the surrounding retroperitoneal tissues in the form of peripancreatic fluid collections. About 50 to 70% of these fluid collections resolve spontaneously;[26] however, the enzymes can digest their way through contiguous spaces to the flank and abdominal wall or even track into the mediastinum or thigh, causing pancreatic enzyme collections in those locations. Grey-Turner sign and Cullen's sign are due to subcutaneous hemorrhages caused by pancreatic enzymes in the flank and paraumbilical areas, respectively.

Pseudocysts are pancreatic fluid collections that have been present for at least 3 to 4 weeks and have developed a surrounding capsule with a nonepithialized wall as the result of the inflammatory reaction at the periphery.[26] Pancreatic abscess denotes infection with suppuration evolving in a necrotic pancreas, pancreatic fluid collection, or pseudocyst. Approximately 50% of pseudocysts that arise in acute pancreatitis resolve spontaneously. The remaining 50% mostly stabilize or partly resolve, never causing clinical sequelae; however some go on to clinically relevant complications that will require intervention, as described in the following section.

Therapeutic option in the treatment of pseudocysts

Because a large percentage of pseudocysts resolve on their own, surgical or percutaneous interventions should not be undertaken in all pseudocysts. Intervention of some sort is indicated when the pseudocyst becomes in-

dochoscope. Stones can be retrieved by wire basket or treated by intracorporeal shock wave lithotripsy administered directly onto the stone by the choledochoscope; then the fragments are basketed or flushed out.

Studies have been done with solvent dissolution of gallstones. Because of the potential toxicity of the available solvents, dissolution can be attempted only in patients who have calculi obstructing the cystic duct or CBD to prevent solvent from flowing into the bowel and being absorbed. Available solvents include Monooctanoin and methyl tert-butyl ether (MTBE). Monooctanoin and MTBE work by direct infusion into the stone-bearing lumen through a percutaneous biliary drainage or cholecystostomy catheter. Monooctanoin is slow acting, usually requiring 1 to 2 weeks to work. MTBE dissolves calculi approximately 50 times faster than Monooctanoin. Both solvents work best with noncalcified cholesterol gallstones. Nonetheless, even MTBE usually requires a minimum of several hours to allow gallstone dissolution, depending on the size and number of calculi. Although success rates from 80 to 95% have been reported for solvent dissolution of gallstones,[24,25] the extreme labor intensiveness of the procedure, the risks to both patient and physician from toxic MTBE fumes, and the fact that MTBE is not FDA approved for use in patients renders this procedure of limited value at this point.

fected, enlarges progressively with the risk of rupture, causes pain, or obstructs an adjacent lumen (bowel or bile duct).

The traditional intervention has been surgical creation of a communication between the pseudocyst and the gastrointestinal tract, or marsupialization. Because some pseudocysts continue to communicate with the pancreatic duct and accumulate pancreatic juices, the iatrogenic fistula to the stomach or jejunum provides a harmless long-term outlet. Unfortunately, the mortality rate for the surgical approach is relatively high at 7.1%, because surgical pseudocyst decompression constitutes major surgery, requiring general anesthesia, and many patients in whom decompression is indicated are poor surgical risks.[27]

Percutaneous drainage is another therapeutic option. The patient with pancreatitis and suspected pseudocyst is studied with CT scanning. If pseudocyst drainage is indicated, percutaneous drainage can be performed under CT guidance.

Percutaneous drainage technique

In percutaneous pseudocyst drainage, intervening organs and major blood vessels should be avoided when possible; however, a transgastric approach can also be used (Fig. 32-16). Some reports indicate that a potential benefit of transgastric drainage is the ultimate conversion to internal stenting between the pseudocyst and stomach, in effect resulting in percutaneous marsupialization.[28]

Percutaneous CT-guided pseudocyst drainage is performed in a manner similar to any other percutaneous drainage procedure. First, a suitable tract is chosen and then anesthetized from the skin to the peritoneum with lidocaine. Definitive drainage can be accomplished either using a one-step Trocar technique or using a Seldinger approach. The advantage of the latter approach is the ability to first puncture the pseudocyst with a skinny needle and to perform a diagnostic aspiration before progressing to definitive drainage. It also allows for progressive dilation of the tract over a guidewire up to the requisite catheter size. Whereas 8Fr or 9Fr catheters are

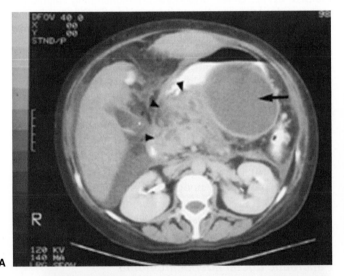

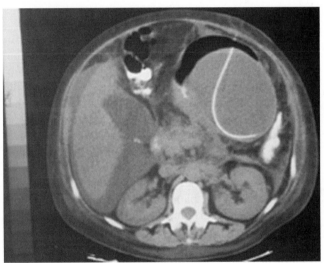

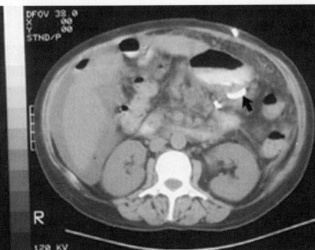

FIGURE 32-16. Percutaneous computed tomography (CT)-guided pancreatic pseudocyst drainage. **A:** Predrainage CT showing pseudocyst (*arrow*), diffusely swollen pancreas (*arrowheads*), and ascites. **B:** Percutaneous transgastric tract to pseudocyst for drainage. **C:** CT after catheter placement and pseudocyst evacuation. Catheter pigtail (*black arrow*) within collapsed pseudocyst.

sufficient to drain pseudocysts with simple fluid, 12Fr to 16Fr catheters are needed to drain abscesses, and occasionally up to 30Fr catheters are needed for extraordinarily thick collections.

After the catheter is in the pseudocyst, it is attached to external drainage in the case of simple fluid and suction in the case of an abscess. Tubes are evaluated daily for output and adequacy of drainage and are irrigated as needed. The endpoint of percutaneous drainage is the cessation of drainage, the obliteration of the pseudocyst cavity, and the obliteration of any communication between the pseudocyst cavity and pancreatic duct as ascertained by contrast cathetergram. Prolific pancreatic enzyme output from the catheter can be reduced by keeping the patient off oral feedings and on hyperalimentation and the use of somatostatin or its synthetic analog Octreotide to reduce pancreatic exocrine output.[29] It may be necessary to keep the drainage catheter in place for several weeks for a successful resolution of the pseudocyst. Success rates of approximately 90% have been reported for percutaneous pseudocyst drainage and 73% for percutaneous drainage of pancreatic abscess.[26]

Vascular complications of pancreatitis

Vascular complications of severe acute and chronic pancreatitis include arterial erosion, pseudoaneurysm formation, hemorrhage, and venous occlusion. Arterial pseudoaneurysm formation with acute hemorrhage typically involves the gastroduodenal artery, pancreaticoduodenal arcade, or splenic artery (Fig. 32-17). If the patient is hemodynamically stable, bleeding or pseudoaneurysms can be treated by selective embolotherapy with Gelfoam and/or coils.[30]

Venous thrombosis can occur in any of the portal tributaries adjacent to the pancreas. The splenic vein is most vulnerable given its proximity to the pancreas over a long distance.[30] The superior mesenteric and central portal veins are also vulnerable to thrombosis because they are in close proximity to the pancreatic head. Splenic vein thrombosis leads to gastric varices that act as collateral channels between the splenic hilar veins and coronary vein and, ultimately, the portal vein. These varices can bleed; however, unlike variceal hemorrhage secondary to sinusoidal portal hypertension, this type of hemorrhage is not amenable to portosystemic shunting. The treatment of variceal hemorrhage resulting from splenic vein thrombosis is splenectomy with or without splenic artery embolization.

Pancreatic neoplasms

Pancreatic neoplasms generally can be divided into exocrine and endocrine categories. *Exocrine tumors* are those arising from the ductal epithelium. The vast majority of exocrine tumors (> 90%) are ductal adenocarcinoma,

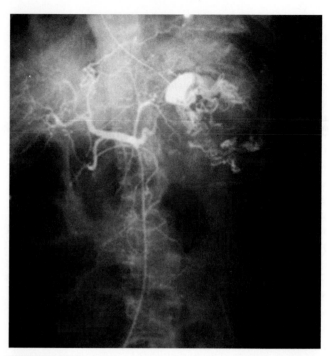

FIGURE 32-17. Celiac arteriogram demonstrating splenic artery pseudoaneurysm caused by erosion of artery by chronic pancreatitis and pseudocyst with acute hemorrhage into pseudocyst. Radiopaque strands inferior and lateral to pseudoaneurysm are surgical packing from a recent unsuccessful attempt at operative hemostasis. (Image is courtesy of Dr. Andrew Kerr, Jacobi Medical Center, Bronx, NY).

usually referred to as *carcinoma of the pancreas*.[31] Pancreatic exocrine tumors also include the uncommon benign serous cystadenoma, otherwise known as a *microcystic adenoma,* and the premalignant mucinous cyst adenoma. Endocrine pancreatic neoplasms comprise the islet cell tumors, which are rare and can be either benign or malignant. These are discussed in greater detail in Chapter 33.

Pancreatic ductal adenocarcinoma

Pancreatic ductal adenocarcinoma constitutes, by far, the most commonly encountered pancreatic neoplasm in clinical practice. Before the advent of CT scanning, angiography played a much larger role in the detection and staging of pancreatic carcinoma, along with conventional barium gastrointestinal studies. Since evolution of high-quality ultrasound, CT, and ERCP, angiography plays a more limited role.

The clinical symptoms associated with pancreatic carcinoma include anorexia, weight loss, pain, and jaundice. The pain is caused by the tumor stretching the pancreatic capsule or obstructing the pancreatic duct. Jaundice with or without pain is caused by a pancreatic head lesion compressing or invading the distal common bile duct as it passes through the pancreatic head.

Because the pancreas is a vascular organ with a rich

lymphatic network and because pancreatic carcinomas usually are not detected until they are large enough to cause symptoms by impingement on adjacent structures, few lesions are truly curable, especially those arising in the body and tail where lesions can grow to large size before manifesting symptoms. Pancreatic tumors detected in patients with jaundice tend to have a higher chance of their tumors being considered resectable (45%) compared with pancreatic carcinomas discovered in patients who are not jaundiced (10%), probably because of the greater propensity of pancreatic head lesions to obstruct the distal CBD before metastasizing or invading extrapancreatic structures (i.e., early lesions) compared with tumors elsewhere in the gland that do not cause jaundice early and therefore may elude detection until they are large enough to have disseminated or invaded other structures.[31]

Ultrasound is a valuable modality in evaluating the patient with suspected pancreatic carcinoma. It is noninvasive and relatively inexpensive and can yield information about the status of the bile ducts and liver parenchyma and the presence of ascites (also see section on ultrasound under the biliary tree); however, it does have significant limitations. A basic limitation is the deep location of the pancreas in the retroperitoneum, which necessitates the use of 3.5- to 5-MHz transducers, which yield poorer resolution. Another limitation is the presence of overlying bowel gas and, in the case of obese patients, large amounts of fat. As in any other sonographic study, the yield of the test depends heavily on the operator's skills. Nonetheless, large carcinomas can be imaged, usually appearing hypoechoic to the normal gland.

CT scanning is also valuable and can provide incremental cross-sectional views of the pancreas and its relationship to surrounding structures. CT scanning is most reliable when the gastrointestinal tract, particularly the duodenum, is well-opacified with oral contrast and major vascular structures are well-enhanced by intravenous contrast. Sections of 5-mm or thinner through the pancreas enhance the detectability of small lesions, pancreatic duct dilatation, and major vascular invasion. *Major* vascular invasion is defined as invasion of the celiac, splenic, common hepatic, or superior mesenteric arteries or the portal, superior mesenteric, or splenic veins. Involvement of any of these vessels generally precludes resection. CT findings suggestive of invasion or occlusion include complete surrounding of the vessel by tumor, direct contiguity between tumor and vessel, vessel disappearance, and the presence of varices.[32] Other CT findings that could preclude resectability include metastatic lymphadenopathy and liver metastases. CT has a high positive predictive value for tumor nonresectability but a disappointingly low positive predictive value for tumor resectability. In other words, 90% of lesions deemed unresectable by CT criteria are actually found to be so at surgery, whereas only 28% deemed resectable by CT criteria are actually

surgically resectable.[33] At present, MR has not been better than CT at preoperatively detecting or staging pancreatic carcinoma.

The role of arteriography in the preoperative evaluation of pancreatic carcinoma is confined to detecting major arterial or venous invasion and to assessing major vascular anatomy to aid in the planning of surgery. Arteriography is not useful for the detection of pancreatic carcinoma in the absence of vascular invasion, as pancreatic adenocarcinoma is usually hypovascular.

Preoperative arteriography is often requested to assist in the staging of pancreatic adenocarcinoma. Because properly performed contrast CT often can reasonably ascertain the presence or absence of major arterial or venous encasement, angiography can be used selectively.

The technique of arteriography to evaluate pancreatic adenocarcinoma is as follows. A flush aortogram is performed in the anteroposterior and lateral projections. The lateral projection is important to evaluate the origin of the superior mesenteric artery, which might be missed on selective catheterization (Fig. 32-18A). Then selective celiac and superior mesenteric arteriography is performed to assess the major peripancreatic arteries (Fig. 32-18B). The portal veins are assessed by injecting a generous quantity of contrast into the artery, usually a 5- to 6-sec-long injection with filming out to at least 18 sec (Fig. 32-18C). Superior mesenteric and portal vein visualization on cut film can be enhanced markedly by the performance of SMA injection immediately following the infusion of 30 to 60 mg of papaverine into the SMA. A slight right posterior oblique projection during superior mesenteric arteriography will desuperimpose the superior mesenteric vein off of the spine, thereby enhancing its visualization.

Pancreatic cystic neoplasms
Pancreatic cystic neoplasms constitute less than 5% of all pancreatic neoplasms. Although they may have similar clinical presentations as pancreatic adenocarcinoma, their clinical symptoms are usually more vague.

Microcystic adenomas
Microcystic adenomas are slowly expanding benign tumors. Pathologically, they consist of a mass containing a honeycomb of numerous cysts, usually small (1 mm–2 cm) and filled with clear serous fluid (hence its other name, *serous cystadenoma*). Ultrasound usually shows a microcystic adenoma to be hyperechoic to normal pancreas because of the acoustic shadowing caused by the walls of the numerous tiny cysts. Noncontrast CT scanning shows a hypodense mass that appears somewhat like ground glass. Contrast CT usually shows enhancement of the cyst walls and hence mild to moderate enhancement. The lesion sometimes contains stellate radiating bands of connective tissue that may contain calcium.

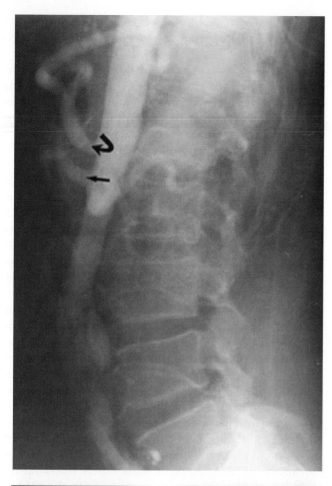

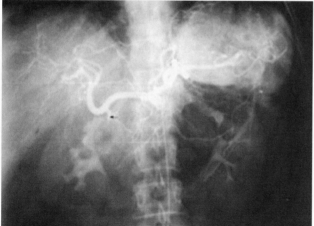

B

FIGURE 32-18. Angiographic evaluation of pancreatic carcinoma. **A:** Lateral aortogram showing patent celiac (*curved arrow*) and superior mesenteric artery (SMA) (*straight arrow*) trunks with no encasement. **B:** Celiac arteriogram demonstrating encasement and obstruction of proximal gastroduodenal artery by pancreatic head carcinoma (*black arrow*). **C:** Venous phase of another celiac arteriogram revealing encasement of splenic-portal vein junction (*long black arrow*) by pancreatic carcinoma. Note reflux into obstructed, encased central superior mesenteric vein (SMV) (*short black arrows*).

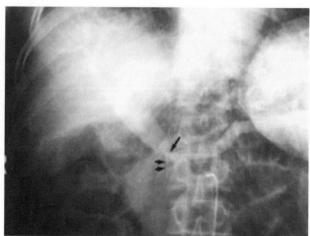

C

Microcystic adenomas almost always appear as a highly vascular tumor on angiography (celiac or superior mesenteric artery), usually manifesting as a dense blush (Fig. 32-19).

Mucinous cystoadenomas

Mucinous cystoadenomas, unlike the microcystic adenomas, are premalignant or contain malignant elements. For this reason, resection is mandatory. On ultrasound, unlike microcystic lesions, they usually appear hypoechoic, often with internal septae of large cyst compartments. Individual cysts, which are much larger than those of the microcystic adenoma, contain mucinous material (hence their name). On CT scanning, they appear as hypodense structures, often with enhancement in the septae. Angiographically, they are hypervascular but more so in the septae. There will thus be areas of hypovascularity corresponding to the unilocular or multilocular large

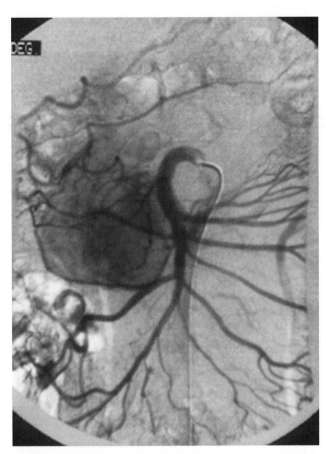

FIGURE 32-19. Pancreatic microcystic adenoma. Superior mesenteric arteriogram revealing a uniformly hypervascular tumor blush in the pancreatic head region.

cysts, as opposed to the relatively uniform blush of the microcystic adenoma.

Pancreatic endocrine neoplasms

Angiographic workup of endocrine neoplasms is discussed in Chapter 33.

■ Summary

Patients with benign and malignant disease of the pancreas and biliary tree are often a challenging, even difficult, group to manage and usually require interdisciplinary cooperation. An understanding of the roles of cross-sectional imaging and interventional radiologic techniques is essential to providing optimal patient care.

References

1. Hall-Craggs MA, Allen CM, Owens CM, et al. MR cholangiography: clinical evaluation in 40 cases. *Radiology* 1993;189:423–427.
2. Bilbao MK, Dotter CT, Lee TG, et al. Complications of endoscopic retrograde cholangiopancreatography (ERCP). *Gastroenterology* 1976;70:314–320.
3. Berk RW, Ferrucci JT, Leopold GR, Radiology of the Gallbladder and Bile Duct: Diagnosis and Intervention. Philadelphia: WB Saunders,1983:342.
4. Pitt HA, Kaufman SL, Coleman J, et al. Benign post operative biliary strictures: operate or dilate? *Ann Surg* 1989;210:417–427.
5. Joseph PK, Bizer LS, Sprayregen SS, et al. Percutaneous transhepatic biliary drainage: results and complications in 81 patients. *JAMA* 1986;255:2763–2767.
6. McPherson GAD, Benjamin IS, Hodgson HJF, et al. Pre-operative percutaneous transhepatic biliary drainage: the results of a controlled trial. *Br J Surg* 1984;71:371–375.
7. Clark CD, Picus D, Dunagan WC. Bloodstream infections after interventional procedures in the biliary tract. *Radiology* 1994; 191:495–499.
8. Carrasco CH, Zornoza J, Bechtel WJ. Malignant biliary obstruction: complications of percutaneous biliary drainage. *Radiology* 1984; 152:343–346.
9. Mitchell SE, Shuman LS, Kaufman SL, et al. Biliary catheter drainage complicated by hemobilia: treatment by balloon embolotherapy. *Radiology* 1985;157:645–652.
10. Ring EJ, Gordon RL, La Berge JM, et al. Malignant biliary obstruction complicated by ascites: transjugular insertion of an expandable metallic endoprosthesis. *Radiology* 1991;180:579.
11. Brown AS, Mueller PR, Ferrucci JT. Transhepatic removal of obstructed Carey-Coons biliary endoprosthesis. *Radiology* 1986;159: 555–556.
12. Lee MJ, Mueller PR, Saini S, et al. Occlusion of biliary endoprostheses: presentation and management. *Radiology* 1990;176:531–534.
13. Keff RM, Gilliam JH. The team approach to biliary tract intervention: current status of combined percutaneous–endoscopic techniques. *Gastrointest Endosc* 1988;34:432–434.
14. Davids PHP, Grown AK, Rauws EA, et al. Randomized trial of self expanding metal stents vs polyethylene stents for distal malignant biliary obstruction. *Lancet* 1992;340:1488–1492.
15. Trambert JJ, Bron KM, Zajko AB, et al. Percutaneous transhepatic balloon dilatation of benign biliary strictures. *AJR Am J Roentgenol* 1987;149:945–948.
16. Gallacher DJ, Kadir S, Kaufman SL, et al. Non-operative management of benign post operative biliary strictures. *Radiology* 1985; 156:625–629.
17. Mueller PR, van Sonnenberg E, Ferrucci JT, et al. Biliary stricture dilatation: multicenter review of clinical management in 73 patients. *Radiology* 1986;160:17–22.
18. Lo LD, Vogelzang RL, Braun MA, et al. Percutaneous cholecystostomy for the diagnosis and treatment of acute calculous and acalculous cholecystitis. *J Vasc Interv Radiol* 1995;6:629–634.
19. Boland BG, Lee MJ, Leung J, et al. Percutaneous cholecystostomy in critically ill patients: early response and final outcomes in 82 patients. *AJR Am J Roentgenol* 1994;163:339–342.
20. Garber SJ, Mathieson JR, Cooperberg PL, et al. Percutaneous cholecystostomy: safety of the transperitoneal route. *J Vasc Interv Radiol* 1994;5:295.
21. van Sonnenberg E, D'Agostino HB, Goodacre BW, et al. Percutaneous gallbladder puncture and cholecystostomy: results, complications, and caveats for safety. *Radiology* 1992;183:167–170.
22. D' Agostino HB, van Sonnenberg E, Sanchez RB, et al. Imaging of the percutaneous cholecystostomy tract: observations and utility. *Radiology* 1991;181:675–678.
23. Picus D. Percutaneous biliary endoscopy. *J Vasc Interv Radiol* 1995; 6:303.
24. Allen MJ, Borody TJ, Bugliosi TF, et al. Rapid dissolution of gallstones by methyl tert-butyl ether. *N Engl J Med* 1985;312:217–220.
25. van Sonnenberg E, Hofmann AF, Neoptolemus J, et al. Gallstone dissolution with methyl tert-butyl ether via percutaneous cholecystostomy: success and caveats. *AJR Am J Roentgenol* 1986;146: 865–867.

26. Balthazar EJ, Freeny PC, van Sonnenberg E. Imaging and intervention in acute pancreatitis: state of the art. *Radiology* 1994;193:297–306.

27. Adams DB, Anderson MC. Percutaneous catheter drainage compared with internal drainage in the management of pancreatic pseudocyst. *Ann Surg* 1992;215:571–578.

28. Das K, Kochhar R, Kaushik SP, et al. Double pigtail cystogastric stent in the management of pancreatic pseudocyst. *J Clin Ultrasound* 1992;20:11–17.

29. D'Agostino HB, van Sonnenberg E, Sanchez RB, et al. Treatment of pancreatic pseudocysts with percutaneous drainage and octreotide: work in progress. *Radiology* 1993;187:685–688.

30. Vujic I. Vascular complications of pancreatitis. *Radiol Clin North Am* 1989;27:81–91.

31. Moosa AR, Gamagami RA. Diagnosis and staging of pancreatic neoplasms. *Surg Clin North Am* 1995;75:871–889.

32. Freeny PC, Marks WM, Ryan JA, et al. Pancreatic ductal adenocarcinoma: diagnosis and staging with dynamic CT. *Radiology* 1988;166:125–133.

33. Megibow AJ, Zhou XH, Rotterdam H, et al. Pancreatic adenocarcinoma: CT versus MR imaging in the evaluation of resectability—report of the radiology diagnostic oncology group. *Radiology* 1995;195:327.

33

Vascular Diseases of the Lower Gastrointestinal Tract

CURTIS W. BAKAL AND SEYMOUR SPRAYREGEN

The interventional radiologist plays a critical role in the diagnosis and management of two conditions that affect the lower gastrointestinal (GI) tract: hemorrhage and ischemia, both of which can manifest as acute, life-threatening illnesses or as chronic, debilitating or episodic conditions.

■ Lower GI Bleeding

Bleeding in the lower gastrointestinal tract (distal to the ligament of Treitz) that comes to the attention of the vascular radiologist is due to diverticulosis in 50% of cases. Angiodysplasia, colon carcinoma, and benign polyps constitute most of the remaining cases. The workup of lower GI bleeding is divided into two broad categories: acute and chronic.

Acute lower GI hemorrhage

It is essential that a nuclear bleeding scan, either technetium-99 m (^{99m}Tc) red blood cells or sulfur colloid, be obtained to confirm that the patient is bleeding acutely. At our institution, a negative bleeding scan excludes the need for an emergent mesenteric angiogram, which is considerably less sensitive (0.05–0.1 mL per minute bleeding versus 0.5–1 mL per minute bleeding) (1,2). Emergency arteriography usually is performed after a positive bleeding scan because an angiogram can localize the site precisely (and sometimes the etiology) of bleeding and can be followed by catheter-directed therapy, thus avoiding urgent laparotomy. Rarely, patients are brought directly to surgery for hemicolectomy if the bleeding scan

precisely localizes a colonic bleeding site. This generally occurs in patients who have a history of multiple acute lower GI bleeds in a vascular territory with a known structural lesion, typically diverticulosis. Barium has no role in the workup of acute GI bleeding because usually it is negative and precludes performing an angiogram.

A Foley catheter should be placed in the bladder for patient comfort and so that accumulating bladder contrast does not obscure the inferior mesenteric artery (IMA) and its branches in the pelvis. Sequencing of injections depends on the likely source of bleeding; that is, if a sigmoid source is suspected, the IMA is injected first.

Chronic bleeding

Patients presenting with chronic or recurrent lower GI bleeding usually are investigated first by barium studies and colonoscopy. Angiography is performed when these studies are negative, primarily to search for angiodysplasia; occasionally, small bowel tumors that have escaped detection by other means are identified at angiography.

Transcatheter diagnosis and therapy

If the patient is actively hemorrhaging (i.e., is passing blood per rectum and has a positive bleeding scan), the "acute" workup is directed first to localizing precisely the anatomic site of hemorrhage by visualizing a point of extravasation. Angiography should be performed expeditiously. Multiple injections may be required for precise localization, and the entire vascular territory at risk must be imaged. In our view, a single negative injection is insufficient. If the bleeding scan is negative, the bleeding

has effectively ceased and the situation is managed as nonacute or "chronic." The focus of the angiogram then will be to find a structural lesion, such as an angiodysplasia; extravasation will not be demonstrated, and the angiogram should be performed electively after optimization of the patient's medical status.

It is not unusual for referring physicians to believe that a patient is actively bleeding if blood is being passed per rectum or a hematocrit decrement has occurred. In this situation, it may be tempting to forgo the bleeding scan and proceed directly to arteriography. In our view, this is usually a mistake because patients may cease bleeding spontaneously, pass residual blood per rectum, and exhibit a hematocrit drop on the basis of this most recent hemorrhage. A negative tagged red blood cell count (RBC) obviates the need for an emergent angiogram with its attendant risks to the patient. Conversely, a positive scan is more likely to demonstrate the site of active hemorrhage than is an angiogram, and thus this critical opportunity for localization may be lost if the nuclear study is omitted.[1,2]

Typically, patients with brisk, continuing lower GI bleeding are treated with intravenous vasopressin, which acts to constrict the smooth muscle of the GI tract. Intravenous vasopressin is thought to be effective for controlling variceal and left colon bleeding but less so for right colonic bleeding. If bleeding persists, nuclear scan localization and angiography are usually performed. If the arteriogram is positive, infusion of intraarterial vasopressin traditionally has been the angiographic treatment of choice. Intraarterial vasopressin is most effective in treating colonic diverticula, where it is effective in up to 90% of cases.[3] Rebleeding eventually occurs in 30% of cases, but initial control by transcatheter infusion will avoid the morbidity of emergency surgery. This agent is most often started at 0.2 units per minute via a selective catheter in the superior mesenteric artery. If a 20-min follow-up angiogram shows no further bleeding, the infusion is continued and then gradually tapered off once the hemorrhage stops. If the initial dose is unable to control bleeding, the rate can be increased to 0.4 units per minute. Repeat angiography should ensure that there is no excessive vasospasm. With intraarterial (IA) vasopressin, patients may experience abdominal pain initially from bowel contractions. Contraindications to vasopressin include the presence of severe coronary artery disease or diabetes insipidus.[3] Complications include the effects of both the agent and the indwelling catheter and occur in 5 to 9% of patients. Endoscopy has played an increasing role in diagnosis and management of acute and chronic bleeding, especially in the descending colon; it is often nondiagnostic when brisk bleeding obscures the field.

A mesenteric arteriogram performed after a positive bleeding scan may fail to demonstrate the bleeding site under the following circumstances:

1. The patient stopped bleeding between obtaining the nuclear scan and the angiogram.
2. The bleeding rate is below the threshold for detection by the angiogram.
3. The bleeding scan (or its interpreter) incorrectly localizes the bleeding; in about 15% of cases the source of acute "lower" GI bleeding is actually the duodenum.
4. There is variant anatomy: rarely, the middle colic artery arises from branches of the celiac axis.[4]

The first and second circumstances argue for prompt arteriography; the third and fourth mandate performing celiac arteriography if the superior mesenteric artery (SMA) arteriogram is negative.

Recently, the advent of 2 and 3 Fr microcatheter systems has allowed delivery of very peripheral microcoils, Gelfoam, or polyvinyl alcohol particles. Evidence suggests that this is effective and is associated with a low risk of bowel infarction,[5,6] but the concept of mesenteric embolization remains controversial because the long-term effects of permanent occlusion (e.g., the development of ischemic strictures) are not yet known. Because bleeding often is self-limited, permanent arterial blockade seems less attractive to some than a reversible infusion. Embolization may represent a cost-effective alternative to 24 to 48 hr of transcatheter infusion therapy, which requires monitoring in the intensive care unit and may put the patient at risk for iatrogenic complications related to the catheter. In many practices, embolization is now preferred over infusion.

Diverticulosis bleeds more frequently in the right colon than in the left colon. Bleeding diverticula are often transient events and may not recur. Angiography shows contrast extravasation in the diverticulum and subsequently may show extravasation into the colonic lumen (Fig. 33-1).

Arteriovenous malformations (*angiodysplasia*) of the large bowel usually occur in the cecum (*cecal ectasia*) and proximal ascending colon.[7] Endoscopy is more sensitive than angiography for localizing angiodysplasia for chronic bleeding; infrequently, an arteriovenous malformation (AVM) can be seen with contrast extravasation during the course of an acute bleed. There may be an association with aortic valvular stenosis and with Osler-Weber-Rendu syndrome. Angiographically, the most important sign of angiodysplasia is an early draining vein, visualized before 6 sec on the superior mesenteric arteriogram (Fig. 33-2). Vascular tufting or the presence of an arterial blush and persistent and dense venous opacification are less specific signs. Because of the need to visualize native arteriovenous (AV) shunting, angiograms must be performed without vasodilator enhancement. Small bowel arteriovenous malformations may also be seen. In general, AVMs should be resected, because embolization is technically difficult and involves multiple feeders. In-

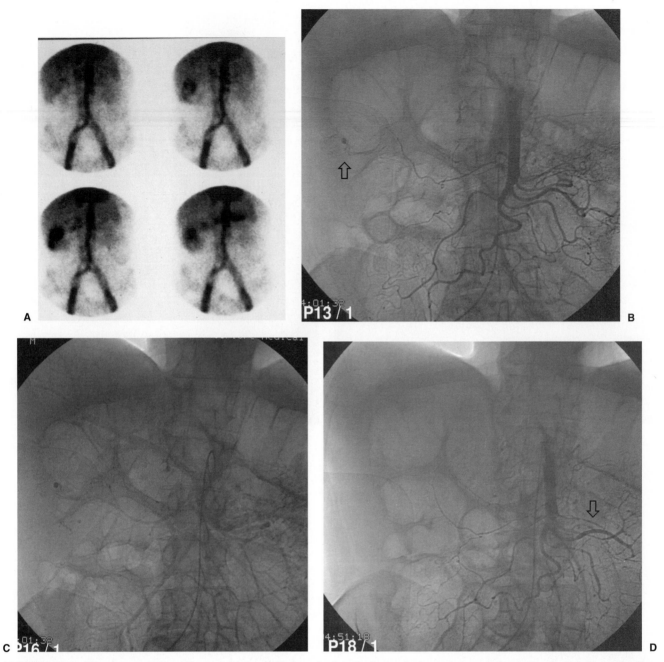

FIGURE 33-1. Bleeding scan in a 71-year-old man with known diverticulosis. **A:** Acute hemorrhage is localized to the acending colon, just proximal to the hepatic flexure. **B:** Emergency selective superior mesenteric arteriogram demonstrates punctate extravasation on the arterial phase (*arrow*), persisting into the late venous phase. **C, D:** Follow-up arteriography after transcatheter vasopressin demonstrates cessation of hemorrhage. There is moderate focal spasm in a jejeunal branch related to the vasopressin (*arrow*).

traoperative localization of a small bowel lesion such as an AVM can be quite difficult. Resection can be expedited by advancing an angiographic catheter or guidewire into the feeding artery for intraoperative palpation or injection of microcoils or methylene blue, which can be palpated or visualized on the serosal surface during laparotomy.[8,9] AVMs can be multiple.

Tumors usually present with indolent lower GI bleeding but occasionally bleed massively. Bleeding is more common in carcinomas of the left rather than right colon. There may be arterial encasement. Leiomyomas of the small bowel are usually hypervascular and present with a well-defined blush. AV shunting and early draining veins may be present (Fig. 33-3). These myomas can be

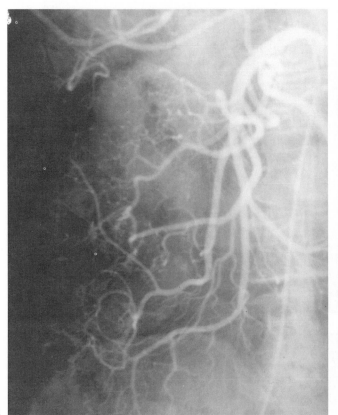

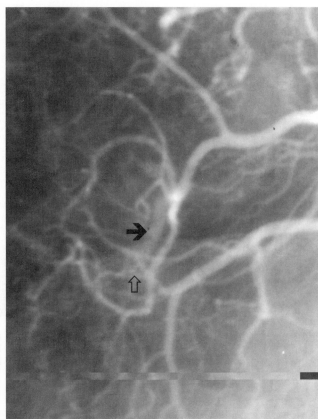

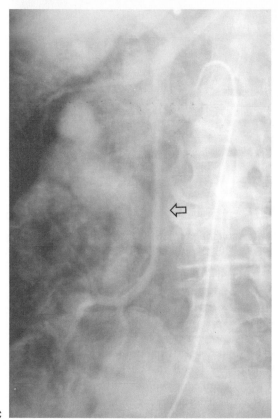

FIGURE 33-2. Angiodysplasia in proximal ascending colon in a 63-year-old woman with a history of multiple previous episodes of brisk lower gastrointestinal bleeding. **A:** There is simultaneous opacification of the ileocolic artery and vein during the arterial phase of the selective injection, consistent with an early draining vein and arteriovenous shunting. **B:** Magnification view better demonstrates the prominent, early draining vein (*black arrow*) as well as a subtle associated vascular tuft (*white arrow*), with increased tortuosity and caliber of the terminal ileocolic branch. **C:** Venous phase demonstrates marked prominence of the ileocolic vein (*arrow*).

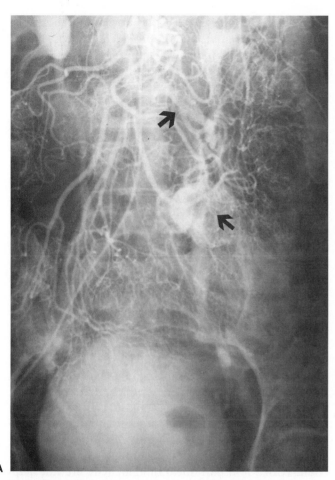
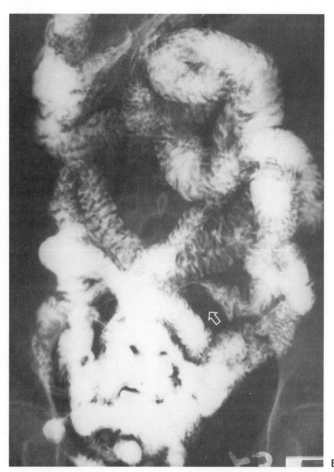

FIGURE 33-3. A 63-year-old woman with recurrent episodes of lower gastrointestinal bleeding. **A:** Hypervascular lesion in the jejeunum (*arrowhead*) with prominent draining vein (*arrow*). Because of the mass effect, this was thought to represent a tumor. **B:** Barium enema performed 1 week after angiogram demonstrates a submucosal mass (*white arrow*). At laparotomy, a schwannoma was resected.

differentiated from AV malformations by the circumscribed nature of the angiographic blush as well as the presence of mass effect. Angiography may be helpful for small bowel myomas because their extramucosal location may prevent visualization on a small bowel barium series. Arterial encasement may be seen with malignancies.

Meckel's diverticulum accounts for 1% of cases of GI bleeding and usually is seen in young patients (younger than 20 years of age), presenting as repeated episodes of brisk lower GI hemorrhage. In adults, it usually presents as slower, chronic GI bleeding. 99mTc pertechnetate abdominal scans can localize ectopic gastric mucosa and thus may be helpful in diagnosis. The scans are considered a sensitive technique for localization in children, but the sensitivity and specificity in adults are limited.[10] Angiographic localization thus can play an important role. Meckel's diverticulum is usually found in the terminal ileum, supplied by a persistent vitellointestinal artery (Fig. 33-4). Classically, this artery was described as an elongated artery without branching, having a group of

tortuous vessels at its distal aspect and arising from the distal SMA. The vitellointestinal artery also may have a number of side branches along its entire length and exhibit no appreciable tortuosity. Demonstration of a Meckel's diverticulum requires a high index of suspicion and may require the use of superselective catheterization.[11,12]

■ Mesenteric Ischemia

Ischemic diseases of the GI tract that are of interest to the vascular and interventional radiologist are caused primarily by compromise of SMA flow. Inadequate blood flow causing ischemia to all or part of the small intestine and right half of the colon can occur acutely or chronically. In the acute form, there is generally loss of viability of varying portions of the bowel supplied by the SMA, which may cause an abdominal catastrophe. Mesenteric angiography followed by transcatheter therapy or laparo-

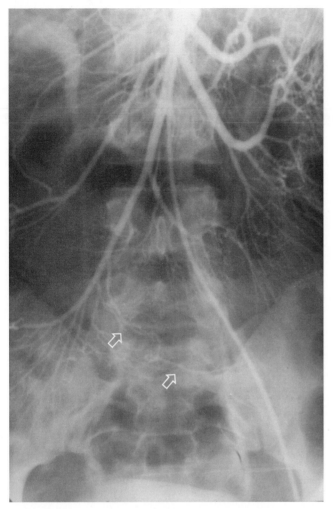

FIGURE 33-4. Meckel's diverticulum. Vitellointestinal artery supplies the diverticulum (*arrows*).

tomy needs to be performed promptly to decrease morbidity and mortality. Conversely, chronic mesenteric ischemia generally occurs without loss of tissue viability because collateral filling can compensate. The diagnosis of chronic mesenteric ischemia is often made after other entities are excluded, with angiography reserved for late in the workup.

Acute mesenteric ischemia

Acute mesenteric ischemia generally occurs in elderly patients with significant comorbidities. It has a high mortality, because it is often diagnosed too late. Patient survival requires a high clinical suspicion and an aggressive approach to both diagnosis and therapy. The occlusive forms of acute mesenteric ischemia are SMA embolus, SMA thrombosis, and superior mesenteric vein (SMV) thrombosis. Nonocclusive mesenteric ischemia (NOMI) occurs in the SMA distribution as a result of pathologic vasospasm

initiated by decreased cardiac output, typically because of myocardial infarction or pulmonary edema. Mesenteric vasoconstriction is a normal response to low cardiac output states; it can persist as pathologic vasospasm after the inciting clinical event has resolved.[13] The essentials of management include medical resuscitation, obtaining a plain film, early and liberal use of angiography and administration of transcatheter vasodilators whenever possible. In the occlusive forms of the disease, laparotomy usually is performed to revascularize the bowel. Frankly infarcted segments are resected, and questionably viable segments are left in place. These questionable segments should be evaluated (and resected if they have progressed to infarction) at a "second look" operation performed 24 hr later.

Abdominal pain is present in 75 to 90% of patients who have acute mesenteric ischemia. Classically, the pain is described as "out of proportion" to the physical findings.[14] Usually, abdominal distension and leukocytosis are present. Frank GI bleeding is unusual, although most patients have occult blood in the stool. Bowel-wall edema ensues with marked intravascular volume depletion, hemoconcentration, and shock. Fluid exudate is seen in the bowel lumen. Injury persisting less than 6 hr generally causes reversible damage, but after 12 to 24 hr, inflammation and hemorrhage intensify and usually lead to transmural infarction and gangrene. Laboratory tests for acute mesenteric ischemia, including complete blood count (CBC) and peritoneal fluid analysis, are not helpful in establishing or excluding the diagnosis of ischemia.

An obstructive series should be the initial examination in a patient with suspected acute mesenteric ischemia. The role of the plain film in suspected acute mesenteric ischemia is to exclude other causes of abdominal pain, especially a perforated viscus.[15] Plain films are normal in 26% of cases of frank intestinal infarction.[16] Nonspecific signs occur late in the course of disease and are present in one third of cases. These signs include adynamic ileus, thickened bowel wall in the SMA distribution with "pinky printing," pseudoobstruction or obstruction, and formless loops of bowel. Plain film findings that are more specific for mesenteric ischemia occur late and include pneumatosis, portal venous gas, rigid formless loops, and thickened bowel wall (*thumbprinting*). Pneumatosis although highly suggestive, is uncommon, occurring in 5% of cases. The presence of portal venous gas is associated with a 75% mortality.[17,18]

Although small bowel barium studies can determine the presence of persistent ischemic segments postoperatively or in chronic disease, barium plays no role in the workup of acute mesenteric ischemia. Computed tomography (CT) has been used increasingly as the initial study in the workup of abdominal pain. It is sensitive for intramural air and bowel-wall thickening and can be used to include or exclude alternate etiologies of pain. The role of CT in the acute workup of mesenteric ischemia is still evolving. It is currently not sufficiently sensitive enough for use in the workup of primary acute vascular insufficiency.[19] The use of relatively large amounts of intravenous contrast and the need for oral contrast agents may preclude performing an adequate arteriogram. We consider arteriography the gold standard because of its high diagnostic accuracy and because of the ability to deliver pharmacologic agents into the mesenteric artery. In patients with suspected acute mesenteric ischemia, arteriography should be performed expeditiously after the abdominal plain film.

If acute mesenteric ischemia is the leading suspected diagnosis, CT should not be performed; however, if other etiologies of abdominal pain are suspect and CT is performed, it is essential that the CT signs of mesenteric ischemia be recognized. CT findings include abrupt vascular cutoffs with nonenhancement of mesenteric vessels. Thrombosis of the SMA or SMV may be seen as an intravascular filling defect, and bowel wall enhancement may be reduced or absent. Thrombosis of the SMV usually presents with enlargement of the SMV with low-density thrombus, which is well defined by a perivascular rim (Fig. 33-5). There may be engorgement of the mesenteric veins. Bowel wall findings include intramural hemorrhage or thickening of the bowel wall, dilatation of the small intestine, and right and transverse colon (Fig. 33-6). Pneumatosis, mesenteric venous gas, and portal venous gas all are sensitively depicted by CT (Fig. 33-7). A normal CT does not rule out mesenteric ischemia.

Historically, acute mesenteric ischemia has been reported to have a 70 to 90% mortality rate. An aggressive management protocol using early angiography and transcatheter papaverine has been associated with a decreased mortality of 45%, with most survivors sustaining minimal bowel loss.[13,20] Angiography can differentiate

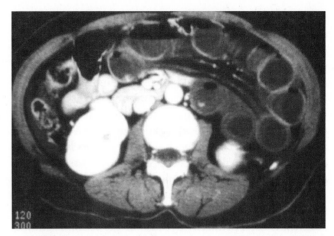

FIGURE 33-6. Dilated, thickened loops of bowel on computed tomography in a patient with acute mesenteric ischemia. (Courtesy of Ellen Wolf, M.D.)

between the occlusive and nonocclusive forms of the disease, determine the nature and site of occlusion, evaluate perfusion of the vascular bed distal to the occlusion, and be followed by intraarterial infusion of vasodilators. The presence of shock is an absolute contraindication to the use of vasodilators. If the patient is receiving vasopressors, the diagnosis of nonocclusive mesenteric ischemia cannot be made with certainty because these agents produce splanchnic vasoconstriction which mimics NOMI. Thus, shock and vasopressor infusions are relatively strong contraindications to angiography. In patients on vasopressors, diagnostic angiography may be performed if superior mesenteric artery embolus is suspected in the specific setting of acute abdominal pain and a cardiac arrhythmia.

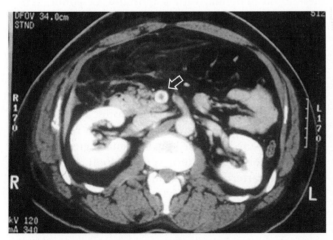

FIGURE 33-5. Superior mesenteric vein (SMV) thrombosis. Contrast-enhanced computed tomography demonstrates filling defect in the SMV with an enhanced perivascular rim (*arrow*).

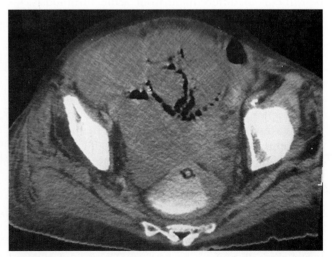

FIGURE 33-7. Intramural air seen on computed tomography in a 75-year-old man with advanced acute mesenteric ischemia. This patient died of extensive bowel necrosis. (Courtesy of Ellen Wolf, M.D.)

Acute mesenteric ischemia is a true angiographic emergency. The angiographic technique is straightforward. Lateral and anteroposterior (AP) aortography are performed to note the status of the celiac and mesenteric artery origins and arterial collateral filling patterns. Aortography is also valuable for visualizing any extramesenteric events, such as renal artery embolus, which can produce a similar clinical picture to mesenteric ischemia.[14] In addition to the occlusive and nonocclusive processes that specifically affect the SMA, aortic dissection can also cause mesenteric ischemia.

Selective superior mesenteric arteriography is performed after the aortogram is completed. Low osmolar contrast is used primarily because of the tenuous clinical condition of most of these patients. The diagnostic study should be performed without pharmacologic enhancement: administration of IA vasodilators such as papaverine (sometimes used for better delineation of the venous phase in anatomic mapping studies) could ameliorate the vasospasm seen in NOMI, precluding the diagnosis. Traditional film screen techniques are well accepted, although increasing numbers of angiographers are using high-resolution (1024 × 1024) nonsubtracted digital arteriography. It is essential to administer enough contrast and film out far enough for visualization of the venous phase (e.g., 6–8mL/sec, total volume 50–60 mL, covering 30 sec).

SMA embolus is the most frequent form of mesenteric ischemia (50% of cases). The source of the embolus is usually the left ventricle. Patients who have atrial fibrillation or who were recently cardioverted are at high risk. Angiographically, the embolus presents as a sharp, rounded filling defect and occurs most often at branch points, especially the middle colic artery (Fig. 33-8). About 18% of emboli will lodge at the SMA origin, where they can be difficult to differentiate from acute thrombosis.[21,22] Emboli lodging proximal to the ileocolic artery are considered major. Considerable vasospasm is often present, which puts the bowel at additional risk.[13,23] After making the diagnosis, a transcatheter vasodilator infusion is begun immediately in the angiography suite to ameliorate vasospasm and is continued throughout and after laparotomy (papaverine, 60-mg bolus followed by 60 mg/hr infusion). Extramesenteric emboli can occur in up to one fifth of patients with SMA embolus and should not be overlooked clinically in the course of diagnosing the patient's abdominal pain. In 10% of patients, minor emboli occur in the terminal SMA distal to the ileocolic artery origin or distally in branches of the superior mesenteric artery. If no peritonitis is present, patients may be managed with no specific therapy or with transcatheter papaverine and followed clinically without laparotomy. The role of regional thrombolysis in treating acute mesenteric artery embolus appears promising and its use is increasing; however, the use of lytic agents is not universally accepted and remains controversial. Several case reports and small series have documented the use of urokinase in selected patients.[24–29] Lysis may be effective in patients with recent onset of abdominal pain and a normal abdominal plain film and should only be continued if there is significant improvement of the angiographic signs and the clinical symptoms within the first hour of the start of the IA infusion.[24]

SMA thrombosis occurs in elderly patients with underlying atherosclerotic disease. These patients usually have a history of peripheral vascular disease or coronary or cerebrovascular comorbidity and also may have a preceding chronic course of abdominal pain (intestinal angina). Thrombosis usually occurs at the origin of the superior mesenteric artery as an extension or exacerbation of aortic atherosclerosis (Fig. 33-9). SMA thrombosis is a relatively rare cause of acute mesenteric ischemia.

NOMI typically occurs in critically ill patients in intensive care units and is frequently associated with a preceding episode of myocardial infarction of congestive heart failure. The incidence of NOMI probably has decreased with the increased use of calcium channel blockers in the intensive care unit. Unless complicated by peritonitis, surgery is contraindicated in this disease, which is treated with transcatheter papaverine for 24 to 48 hr (Fig. 33-10). The initial (nonpapaverine enhanced) arteriogram may demonstrate diffuse narrowing of the SMA trunk and branches, narrowing at branch origins, a "string of sausages" appearance of the mesenteric arterial branches, spasm of the arcades, or impaired filling of the intramural vessels (Fig. 33-11).[29]

Mesenteric venous thrombosis can be acute, subacute, or chronic and is idiopathic in 20% of cases (Fig. 33-12). Known etiologies include hypercoagulable states, neoplastic disease, peritonitis, surgery (e.g., splenectomy, pancreatectomy), and trauma. There is an association with deep venous thrombosis. Mesenteric venous thrombosis appears to have a better prognosis than arterial forms of mesenteric ischemia, with a mortality of about 32%.[30] Mortality and morbidity may be reduced even further with prompt heparinization. This disease has a more variable onset than the arterial forms of mesenteric ischemia, and extensive venous collaterals appear to prevent infarction of bowel in most cases. If no peritoneal signs are present, intravenous heparin should be given. The presence of peritoneal signs mandates a laparotomy. If only a short ischemic segment of bowel is found, it is resected and heparin is given. If a viable long ischemic segment is found and the superior mesenteric vein is patent, then heparin and an intraarterial papaverine drip are given. A "second-look operation" can be performed. In the presence of long ischemic segments and mesenteric vein occlusion, thrombectomy also is indicated. Long segments of nonviable bowel must be resected, and total parenteral nutrition may be needed. Thrombolysis for acute mesenteric venous thrombosis has been administered through the

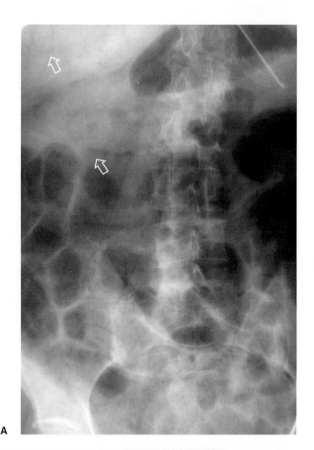

A

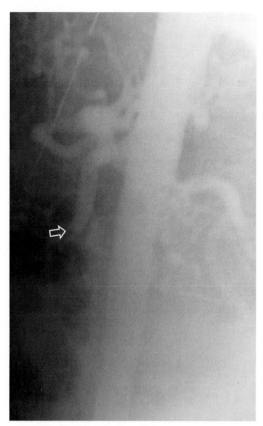

B

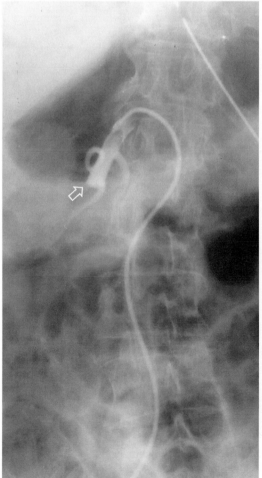

C

FIGURE 33-8. Patient with atrial fibrillation and several hours of acute abdominal pain. **A:** There are dilated bowel loops and questionable intramural and portal vein gas (*arrows.*) **B:** Lateral aortogram demonstrates cutoff of the superior mesenteric artery (SMA) trunk (*arrow*). **C:** Selective superior mesenteric arteriogram demonstrates embolus lodging in the main SMA trunk at the level of the middle colic artery, with absent distal filling (*arrow*). A papaverine infusion was begun preoperatively, but the embolus proved fatal.

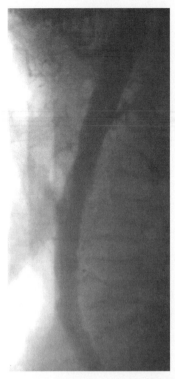

FIGURE 33-9. Lateral aortogram in an elderly patient with acute superior mesenteric artery (SMA) thrombosis.

SMA[31] and directly into the superior mesenteric vein through a transjugular, intrahepatic approach[32] in case reports; results have been promising. With the widespread use of CT, an increasing number of patients with asymptomatic, incidental mesenteric venous thrombus have been identified; the presence of such incidental cases suggests that mesenteric venous thrombosis may be associated with a very wide clinical spectrum of clinical illness.

The term *colonic ischemia* usually is reserved for a different, more benign condition than acute superior mesenteric ischemia. Colonic ischemia is generally a transient disease with low mortality, although it can be fulminant. It usually occurs in the presence of a "low flow" state and is believed to be associated with small-vessel disease in the distribution of the IMA. Plain film signs include thumb-printing in the descending colon as a result of clinical edema or hemorrhage. *Escherichia coli* 0157:H7 infection is thought to be one etiology. The diagnosis is usually confirmed by endoscopy; angiography is not indicated.

Chronic mesenteric ischemia

Chronic mesenteric ischemia or "intestinal angina" occurs when there is chronic occlusion of at least two of three celio-mesenteric arteries (Fig. 33-13).[33] The etiol-

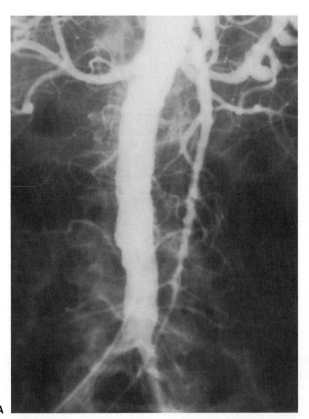

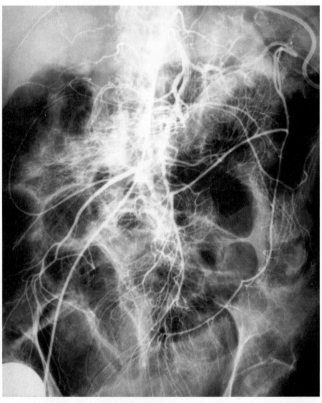

A   B

FIGURE 33-10. Nonocclusive mesenteric ischemia. **A:** There is diffuse spasm of the superior mesenteric artery (SMA) and its branches. There is poor filling of the SMA branches **B:** After an overnight transcatheter papaverine infusion, there is marked resolution with improved branch filling.

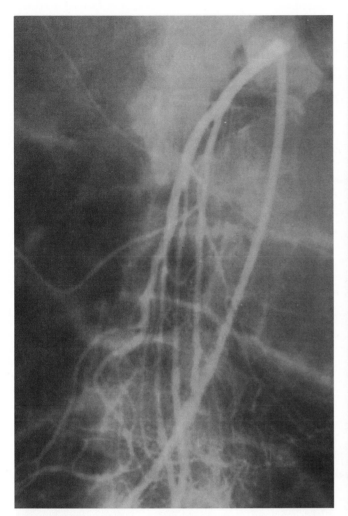

FIGURE 33-11. "String of sausages" appearance in another patient with nonocclusive mesenteric ischemia (NOMI).

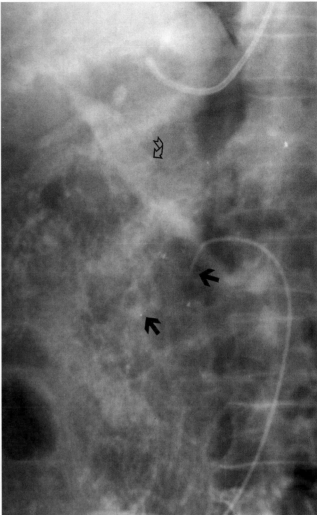

FIGURE 33-12. Patient with 2 weeks of moderate abdominal pain. There is superior mesenteric vein (SMV) thrombosis. Note absence of the superior mesenteric vein (*arrow*) and the presence of collaterals in the duodenum (*arrowhead*). There is filling of the portal vein, with nonopacified blood from the splenic vein (*curved arrow.*)

ogy is usually atherosclerotic. The chronic time course of stenosis leading to occlusion allows for extensive collateralization. (In situ thrombosis of a stenotic SMA may rarely lead to an acute exacerbation and to a clinical presentation of acute mesenteric ischemia.) Intestinal angina occurs when the metabolic demand of the bowel outstrips the ability of the compromised arteries to deliver blood and oxygen. Patients typically complain of intense abdominal pain after eating, which may lead to "food fear," with consequent marked weight loss. Malabsorbtion and abdominal bruit may develop. The diagnosis of chronic mesenteric ischemia is frequently one of exclusion, made after other possible etiologies of pain and weight loss (such as pancreatic neoplasm) are eliminated. Angiography is usually invoked late in an extensive workup and is confirmatory. The difficulty of making this diagnosis is exacerbated because two- and even three-vessel celiomesenteric arterial occlusion has been seen and reported in asymptomatic patients. Conventional therapy is surgical,

for example, aortomesenteric or iliac-mesenteric bypass. Percutaneous transluminal angioplasty (PTA) has been used for atherosclerotic SMA stenoses, with some authors reporting 80 to 90% initial success; secondary patency and a 1- to 2-year clinical success rate for SMA PTA is reported as high as 60 to 80%.[34–36] SMA stents may be important in achieving an effective result. Bypass surgery appears more durable than PTA (possibly because of the tendency to perform multiple-vessel bypasses) but most likely has a higher morbidity.[37] Thus, some recommend PTA primarily for use in candidates who are at high risk for surgery. The use of metallic stents probably increases the success rate of PTA.[38,39]

Median arcuate ligament compression (celiac compression syndrome) of the superior aspect of the celiac trunk

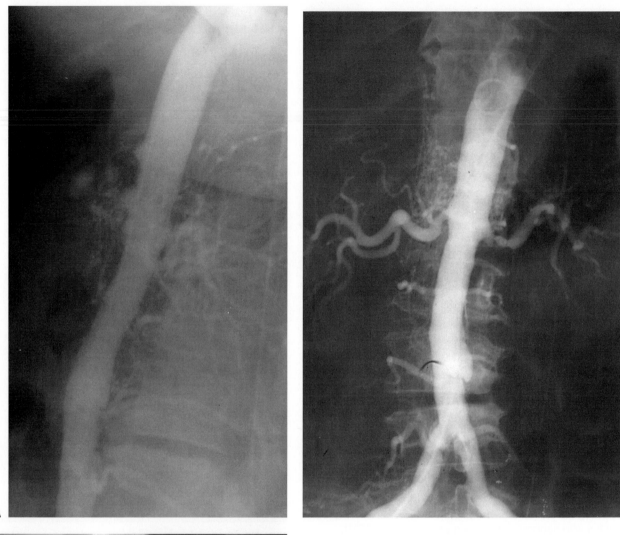

A

B

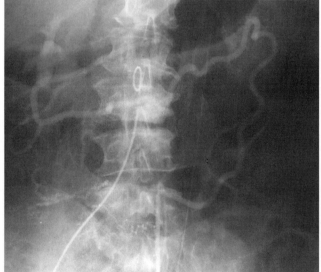

C

FIGURE 33-13. Symptomatic chronic mesenteric ischemia. Aortogram demonstrates occlusion of the celiac and mesenteric arteries in the lateral (**A**) and the frontal projections (**B**). Significant atherosclerotic plaque is seen in the aorta and left renal artery. Large collateral is responsible for mesenteric perfusion (**C**).

is usually asymptomatic and is thought to occur frequently. A bandlike superior indentation of the celiac artery is pathognomonic. PTA is not usually effective or indicated for median arcuate ligament syndrome.

■ Summary

Angiographic techniques play an important role in the diagnosis and management of lower GI hemorrhage and mesenteric ischemia. Timely and knowledgeable consultation with the interventional radiology service can make a huge impact on patient outcome.

References

1. Winzelberg GC, Froelich JW, McKusick KA, et al. Radionuclide localization of lower gastrointestinal hemorrhage. *Radiology* 1981; 139:465–469.
2. Alavi A. Detection of gastrointestinal bleeding with 99m Tc-sulfur colloid. *Semin Nucl Med* 1982;12:126–128.
3. Baum S, Nusbaum M. The control of gastrointestinal hemorrhage by selective mesenteric arterial infusion of vasopressin. *Radiology* 1971;98:497–505.
4. Kornblith PL, Boley SJ, Whitehouse BS. Anatomy of the splanchic circulation. Intestinal ischemia. *Surg Clin North Am* 1992;72:1–30.
5. Seppanen SK, Leppanen MJ, Pimenoff G, Seppanen JM. Microcatheter embolization of hemorrhages. *Cardiovasc Intervent Radiol* 1997;20:174–179.
6. Gordon RL, Ahl KL, Kerlan RK, et al. Selective arterial embolization for control of lower gastrointestinal bleeding. *Am J Surg* 1997; 174:24–28.
7. Boley SJ, Sprayregen S, Sammartano RJ, et al. The pathophysiologic basis for the angiographic signs of vascular ectasias of the colon. *Radiology* 1977;125:615–621.
8. Athanasoulis CA. Therapeutic applications of angiography. *N Engl J Med* 1980;302:117–120.
9. Schmidt SP. Boskind JF, Smith DC, Catalano RD. Angiographic localization of small bowel angiodysplasia with use of platinum coils. *J Vasc Interv Radiol* 1993;4:737–739.
10. Schwartz MJ, Lewis JH. Meckel's diverticulum: pitfalls in scintigraphic detection in the adult. *Am J Gastroenterol* 1984;79:611– 618.
11. Okazaki M, Higashihara H, Saida Y, et al. Angiographic findings of Meckel's diverticulum; the characteristic appearance of the vitellintestinal artery. *Abdom Imaging* 1993;18:15–19.
12. Mitchell AWM, Spencer J, Allison DJ, Jackson JE. Meckel's diverticulum: angiographic findings in 16 patients. *AJR Am J Roentgenol* 1998;170:329–333.
13. Boley SJ, Brandt LJ, Veith FJ. Ischemic disorders of the intestines. *Curr Probl Surg* 1978;15:1.
14. Bakal CW, Sprayregen S, Wolf EL. Radiology in intestinal ischemia: angiographic diagnosis and management. *Surg Clin North Am* 1992;72:125–142.
15. Wolf EL, Sprayregen S, Bakal CW. Radiology in intestinal ischemia—plain film, contrast, and other imaging studies. *Surg Clin North Am* 1992;72:107–124.
16. Smerud MJ, Johnson CD, Stephens DH. Diagnosis of bowel infarction: a comparison of plain films and CT scans in 23 cases. *AJR Am J Roentgenol* 1990;154:99–103.
17. Tomchik FS, Wittenberg J, Ottinger LW. The roentgenographic spectrum of bowel infarction. *Radiology* 1970;96:249.
18. Liebman PR, Patten MT, Manny J, et al. Hepatic-portal venous gas in adults; etiology, pathophysiology and clinical significance. *Ann Surg* 1978;187:281–287.
19. Taourel PG, Deneuville M, Pradel JA, et al. Acute mesenteric ischemia: diagnosis with contrast-enhanced CT. *Radiology* 1996;199: 632–636.
20. Kaleya RN, Sammartano RJ, Boley SJ. Aggressive approach to acute mesenteric ischemia. *Surg Clin North Am* 1992;72:157–182.
21. Boley SJ, Feinstein FR, Sammartano R, et al. New concepts in the management of superior mesenteric artery embolus. *Surg Gynecol Obstet* 1981;153:561.
22. Clark RA, Gallant TE. Acute mesenteric ischemia: angiographic spectrum. *AJR Am J Roentgenol* 1984;142:555.
23. Laufman H. Significance of vasospasm in vascular occlusion [thesis]. Northwestern University Medical School, Chicago, 1948.
24. Simó G, Echenagusia AJ, Camúñez F, et al. Superior mesenteric artery arterial embolism: local fibrinolytic treatment with urokinase. *Radiology* 1997;204:775–779.
25. Schoenbaum SW, Pena C, Koenisberg P, et al. Superior mesenteric artery embolism: treatment with intraarterial urokinase. *J Vasc Interv Radiol* 1992;3:485–490.
26. Gallego AM, Ramirez P, Rodriguez JM, et al. Role of urokinase in the superior mesenteric artery embolism. *Surgery* 1996 Jul;120: 111–113.
27. Fuentes FT, Muerza GS, Belda AE, et al. Successful intrarterial fragmentation and urokinase therapy in superior mesenteric artery embolism. *Surgery* 1995;117:712–714.
28. Badiola CM, Scoppetta DJ. Rapid revascularization of an embolic superior mesenteric artery occlusion using pulse-spray pharmacomechanical thrombolysis with urokinase. *AJR Am J Roentgenol* 1997;169:55–77.
29. Siegelman SS, Sprayregen S, Boley SJ. Angiographic diagnosis of mesenteric arterial vasoconstriction. *Radiology* 1974;112:533.
30. Boley SJ, Kaleya RN, Brandt LJ. Mesenteric venous thrombosis. *Surg Clin North Am* 1992;72:183–202.
31. Poplausky MR, Kaufman JA, Geller SC, et al. Mesenteric venous thrombosis treated with urokinase via the superior mesenteric artery. *Gastroenterology* 1996;110:1633–1635.
32. Rivitz M, Geller, SC, Hahn C, Waltman AC. Treatment of acute mesenteric venous thrombosis with transjugular intramesenteric urokinase infusion. *J Vasc Interv Radiol* 1995;6:219–228.
33. Cunningham CG, Reilly LM, Stoney R. Chronic visceral ischemia. *Surg Clin North Am* 1992;72:231–244.
34. Allen RC, Martin GH, Rees CH, Rivera FJ, et al. Mesenteric angioplasty in the treatment of chronic mesenteric ischemia. *J Vasc Interv Surg* 1996;24:415–421.
35. Hallisey MJ, Deschaine J, Ilescas FF, et al. Angioplasty for the relief of visceral ischemia. *J Vasc Interv Radiol* 1995;(6):785–791.
36. Matsumoto AH, Tegtmeyer CJ, Fitzcharles EK, et al. Percutaneous transluminal angioplasty of visceral arterial stenoses: results and long term clinical follow-up. *J Vasc Interv Radiol* 1995;6:165–174.
37. Rose SC, Quigley TM, Raker EJ. Revascularization for chronic mesenteric ischemia: comparison of operative arterial bypass grafting and percutaneous transluminal angioplasty. *J Vasc Interv Radiol* 1995;6:339–349.
38. Trost DW. Stents and angioplasty for relief of mesenteric ischemia. Presented at "Advances in vascular intervention and CO_2." New York City, May 30, 1997.
39. Liermann DD. The use of stents in the mesenteric arteries. Presented at "Advances in vascular intervention and CO_2." New York City, May 30, 1997.

34

Arteriography and Venous Sampling of the Parathyroid Glands, Pancreas, and Adrenal Glands

JEFFREY D. GEORGIA AND DONALD L. MILLER

All endocrine localization procedures, including arteriography and venous sampling, are used in patients with clinically evident syndromes of hormone excess. There are two indications for localization procedures: localization of otherwise occult tumors and differentiation between single and multiple gland involvement. Clinical syndromes and the invasive localization procedures that may be indicated in their workup are listed in Table 34-1. These procedures may be required for tumor localization in patients with any of these disorders. Differentiation of single and multiple gland involvement is a common problem in patients with Conn syndrome (hyperaldosteronism) and a rare problem in patients with virilizing tumors.

None of the endocrine diseases listed in Table 34-1 are common, and most are rare. It follows that the localization procedures listed in Table 34-1 also are rarely used. Except in large academic medical centers, most of these procedures are unlikely to be performed on a sufficiently regular basis that a resident or fellow in interventional radiology will become familiar with them. Nonetheless, it is useful to know when, why, and how they are performed, as well as how they are interpreted. This chapter describes the catheter-based localization procedures used for endocrine disorders of the parathyroid glands, the pancreas, and the adrenal glands. Nowadays, localization procedures are virtually never required for patients with pheochromocytoma and are needed so rarely in patients with virilizing tumors that they are not discussed here, but they are reviewed elsewhere.[1]

Arteriography and venous sampling are not used as first-line techniques in patients with endocrine disorders because of their greater risk and expense compared with noninvasive radiologic techniques. The specific order in which radiologic procedures are used varies for each organ and disease. Appropriate protocols are briefly described below in sections devoted to specific organs.

■ General Principles of Endocrine Localization

Endocrine localization procedures differ from most other radiologic studies in that their purpose is not to establish a diagnosis but rather to identify an adenoma, carcinoma, or hyperplastic gland whose existence has already been established by endocrine testing but whose location is unknown. The diagnosis of a disorder of hormone excess never requires demonstration of a tumor or enlarged gland. The most basic principle of endocrine localization efforts is "diagnosis first, localization second." These studies are certain to yield misleading results if the diagnosis is wrong.

Equally important is an understanding of the advantages and limitations of venous sampling procedures. These are physiologic studies, not imaging procedures. They do not require visualization of an abnormality to provide localization. This is both the great strength and the major weakness of this technique.

On the one hand, because it is not necessary to visualize a tumor, the sensitivity of venous sampling is independent of tumor size. It is equally good for the detection of 1-mm and 3-cm lesions. The only requirements are that the lesion secretes sufficient hormone to be detected and that the appropriate vein is sampled. Nonfunctioning adenomas and similar red herrings do not cause

TABLE 34-1. Clinical Endocrine Syndromes and Localization Procedures

Organ	Localization procedure
Pituitary	
Cushing syndrome/disease	Petrosal sinus sampling
Ectopic ACTH syndrome	
Parathyroid	
Hyperparathyroidism	Parathyroid arteriography
	Parathyroid venous sampling
Pancreas	
Zollinger-Ellison syndrome	Pancreatic arteriography
Insulinoma	Arterial stimulation and venous sampling
Adrenal	
Conn syndrome	Adrenal venous sampling
Ovary	
Virilizing tumors	Adrenal and ovarian venous sampling

ACTH, adrenocorticotropic hormone.

false-positive results with venous sampling, as they may with imaging studies.

The disadvantage of the procedure is that, because the tumor is never seen during a venous sampling procedure, it cannot be localized precisely. Instead, venous sampling permits regionalization; that is, it defines a territory drained by a specific vein or veins in which the abnormality must lie. In addition, because tumor presence is presumed based on the evidence of hormone production, the test is only accurate if all production of the hormone by normal glandular tissue is suppressed. When venous sampling procedures are performed on patients without endocrine disease, false-positive studies are virtually certain. For this reason, as already stated, a diagnosis of endocrine hyperfunction must be established before localization procedures are begun.

■ Hyperparathyroidism

Clinical review

In normal subjects, elevated serum calcium inhibits production of parathyroid hormone (PTH) through a negative feedback loop. *Primary hyperparathyroidism* is defined as excess production of PTH resulting from a loss of the normal feedback inhibition from elevated serum calcium. Increased hormone levels may result from parathyroid hyperplasia (multiple gland involvement), parathyroid adenoma (involvement of a single gland), or, rarely, parathyroid carcinoma. The elevated serum calcium concentration is caused by increased renal retention, bone resorption, and increased absorption from the gut. Patients may develop osteolysis leading to bone pain and pathologic fractures, urinary stone disease, and neuromuscular physiologic dysfunction. Symptoms may be sub-

tle, vague, and nonspecific. Increasingly, the diagnosis of abnormal parathyroid function is made through the widespread use of routine laboratory screening panels, which include calcium assays coupled with improved techniques for measurement of PTH.[2,3]

Localization

Most experienced endocrine surgeons believe that noninvasive imaging studies are not required in patients who present with primary hyperparathyroidism, because the initial neck exploration is curative in more than 90% of these patients.[4–7] No preoperative localization studies are necessary in these patients,[8–12] although some surgeons advocate their use in combination with unilateral neck exploration.[13–17] There is general agreement that patients with persistent or recurrent hypercalcemia following surgery will benefit from radiologic localization prior to reoperation, because each additional surgical exploration is more difficult, carries a alreadyhigher risk of vocal cord paralysis, and is less likely to succeed.[9]

An effective localization protocol for these patients has been devised.[9] Noninvasive studies should be performed first, because they are less expensive and less risky. The imaging studies with the greatest sensitivity at present are sestamibi scintigraphy, computed tomography (CT), magnetic resonance imaging (MRI), and ultrasound. These modalities are all operator dependent in terms of performance, interpretation, or both; their sensitivity and false-positive rates vary widely and overlap. Sestamibi scintigraphy is probably the single best noninvasive test.[18] We believe an abnormal parathyroid gland should be demonstrated by at least two of these modalities before localization is considered complete in order to avoid false-positive localizations. The order in which the various studies are performed should be based on individual institutional experience. All imaging protocols should account for the possibility of ectopic mediastinal or suprathyroid parathyroid glands, although most parathyroid glands identified at reoperation are in the neck.

At most institutions, if noninvasive studies are negative or equivocal, parathyroid arteriography is performed next.[9,19] Parathyroid arteriography will demonstrate an abnormal parathyroid gland in approximately 60% of patients in whom noninvasive studies are negative or equivocal. Parathyroid venous sampling, the final localization procedure in the workup of these patients, will permit localization to one side of the neck or to the mediastinum in 80 to 90% of the remaining few patients in whom all other studies have failed to image an abnormal gland.

Anatomy

Most people have four parathyroid glands, although as few as three and as many as eight have been reported.[20]

In the normal anatomic position, the glands adhere to the posterior surface of the thyroid gland (Fig. 34-1). They also may be ectopic and may be located anywhere from the angle of the jaw to the mediastinum (Fig. 34-2). Knowledge of the common locations of normal and ectopic glands in a prerequisite to successful localization by interventional techniques. Fortunately, most ectopic glands lie along specific, well-defined pathways of embryologic descent, either in the anterior mediastinum and thymus or in the tracheoesophageal groove and superior mediastinum.[20,21]

Each parathyroid gland usually is supplied by a single artery.[22,23] The arterial supply to parathyroid glands located in the normal anatomic position is provided by the paired superior thyroid arteries from the external carotid artery and the paired inferior thyroid arteries from the thyrocervical trunk (Fig. 34-1). Anterior mediastinal and thymic glands are supplied by branches of the internal mammary artery (Fig. 34-3). Superior mediastinal and tracheo-esophageal groove glands usually are supplied by a branch of the inferior thyroid artery. The venous anatomy of the thyroid bed is quite variable. Detailed descriptions of the venous anatomy relevant to parathyroid venous sampling have been published[24–26] and should be reviewed by the angiographer prior to attempting this study.

Venous drainage from the parathyroid glands commonly occurs through ipsilateral superior, middle, and inferior thyroid veins (Figs. 34-4 and 34-5). The superior thyroid vein drains through the facial vein into the internal jugular vein, and the middle thyroid vein drains directly into the internal jugular vein. Both inferior thyroid veins commonly drain into the left brachiocephalic vein, either separately or by a combined trunk. Less commonly, the right inferior thyroid vein drains directly into the right brachiocephalic vein (see Fig. 34-4). The left thymic vein empties into the left innominate vein; elevations of PTH in the thymic vein suggest that the abnormal parathyroid gland is located in the anterior mediastinum. The anatomy and anastomotic connections of this vein are quite variable, and mediastinal parathyroid glands often drain into the inferior thyroid veins (Fig. 34-6).[27] Analysis of the venous drainage patterns observed at arteriography is essential to permit correct interpretation of the results of venous sampling.

Arteriography

Digitally subtracted, superselective, six-vessel studies (bilateral thyrocervical trunks, internal mammary arteries, and common carotid arteries) deliver the highest yield.[28] Venous-phase images are also obtained to provide "roadmaps" and to define venous drainage patterns in cases where venous sampling proves necessary (see Fig. 34-5). If the common carotid artery injections are not clearly nega-

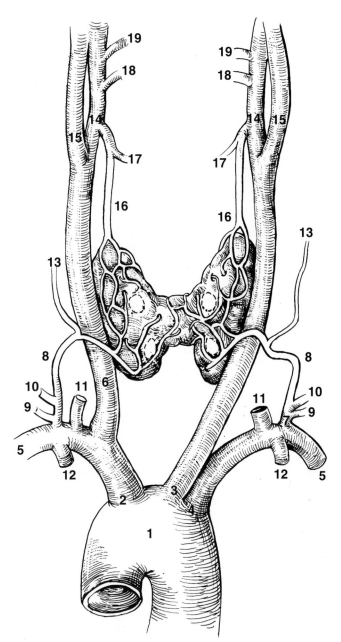

FIGURE 34-1. Arterial supply to the thyroid and parathyroid glands. The parathyroid glands are adherent to the posterior surface of the thyroid gland. The superior and inferior thyroid arteries ramify along the posterior aspect of the thyroid gland, but are shown here on the anterior surface for the purpose of clarity. The drawing displays the typical supply from the inferior and superior thyroid arteries. When ectopic parathyroid glands are located in the thymus of elsewhere in the anterior mediastinum, they are usually supplied by a branch of the internal mammary artery (see Fig. 34-3). 1, aorta; 2, brachiocephalic trunk; 3, left common carotid; 4, left subclavian; 5, subclavian; 6, right common carotid; 7, thyrocervical trunk; 8, inferior thyroid; 9, suprascapular; 10, tranverse cervical; 11, vertebral; 12, internal thoracic; 13, ascending cervical; 14, external carotid; 15, internal carotid; 16, superior thyroid; 17, superior laryngeal; 18, lingual; 19, facial.

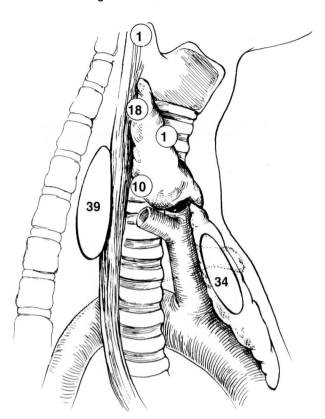

FIGURE 34-2. Location of ectopic parathyroid glands based on a series of 104 glands identified at reoperation. The numbers are percentages. Note the frequency of tracheoesophageal and thymic glands. These represent, respectively, ectopic superior and inferior glands. Tracheoesophageal groove glands typically are supplied by the inferior thyroid artery, whereas thymic glands are supplied by the internal mammary artery. (Modified from Wang C-A. Parathyroid re-exploration: a clinical and pathological study of 112 cases. *Ann Surg* 1977;186:140–145, with permission.)

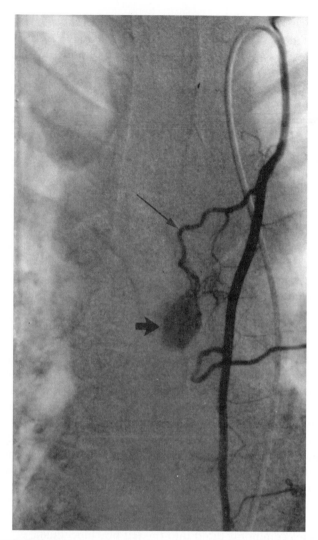

FIGURE 34-3. Parathyroid adenoma supplied by the left internal mammary artery. A single vessel from the thymic branch (*long arrow*) of the internal mammary artery supplies an oval, smooth-margined area of intense, homogeneous blush (*wide arrow*), which is typical of a parathyroid adenoma. (From Miller DL. Endocrine angiography and venous sampling. *Radiol Clin North Am* 1993;31:1051–1067, with permission.)

tive, bilateral superior thyroid artery injections may be helpful to clarify the arteriographic findings. If all else fails, an arch aortogram may reveal a thyroidea ima artery (present in approximately 6% of persons),[29] which most commonly arises from the aortic arch, the innominate artery, or the right common carotid artery and supplies variable portions of the thyroid and parathyroid glands.[29,30] This regimen demonstrates an abnormal parathyroid gland in approximately 60% of the patients in whom noninvasive imaging is negative or inconclusive.[19,31] Parathyroid arteriography has a low false-positive rate.

The aortic arch, common carotid arteries, and, if necessary, the superior thyroid arteries may be catheterized by using standard techniques and catheters; however, these are the least useful vessels for parathyroid localization. Catheterization of the thyrocervical trunk, a critical vessel

in parathyroid arteriography, is often more difficult. It may be helpful to steam a Berenstein-type catheter so that the curvature of the bend is more gradual and the angle is tighter. The internal mammary artery, which arises anteriorly or anteroinferiorly from the subclavian artery, and not directly inferiorly, should be catheterized first. After internal mammary arteriography is performed, the catheter is withdrawn slowly until it is near the orifice of the internal mammary artery. As gentle puffs of contrast material are injected, the catheter is withdrawn further and rotated anteriorly to engage the orifice of the thyrocervical trunk. The thyrocervical trunk arises from the anterior or antero-superior aspect of the subclavian artery, but it or

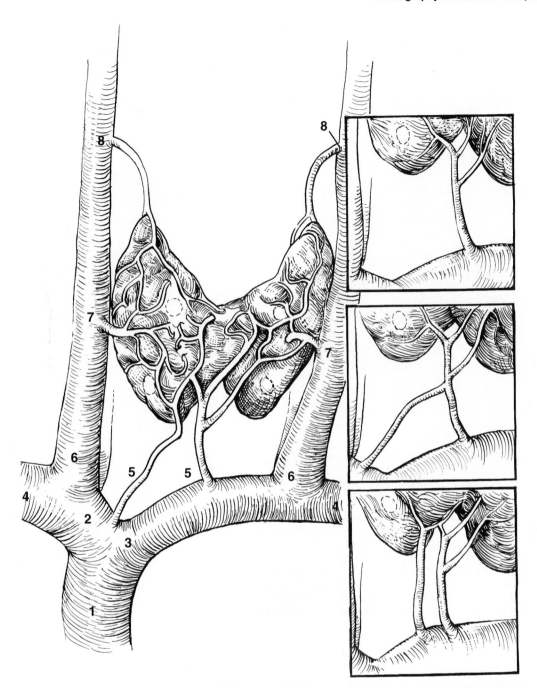

FIGURE 34-4. Anatomy of veins draining the thyroid bed and portions of the anterior mediastinum. The inferior thyroid veins, in particular, are subject to considerable variation, and both often drain into the left brachiocephalic vein, frequently as a combined trunk. The vertebral veins and thymic veins are not shown, for clarity. The vertebral veins empty in the brachiocephalic veins slightly posteromedial to the internal jugular veins and commonly have valves near their bases. The left thymic vein drains into the anteroinferior aspect of the left brachiocephalic vein in the midline. The right thymic vein drains directly into the inferior vena cava and cannot normally be catheterized. 1, superior vena cava; 2, right brachiocephalic; 3, left brachiocephalic; 4, subclavian; 5, inferior thyroid; 6, internal jugular; 7, middle thyroid; 8, superior thyroid.

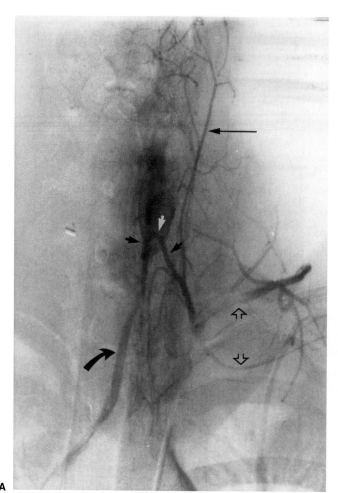
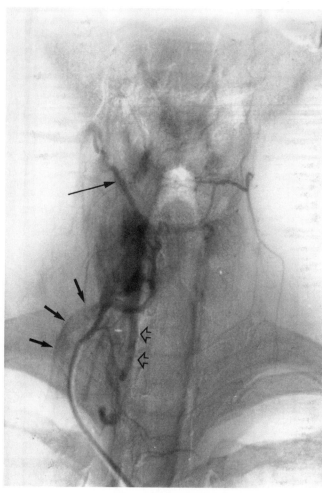

FIGURE 34-5. Thyrocervical arteriograms demonstrate arterial and venous anatomy in a patient with recurrent hyperparathyroidism following surgery. No abnormal parathyroid gland was identified on this study. **A:** A left thyrocervical trunk injection demonstrates the ascending cervical artery (*long arrow*), the transverse cervical and suprascapular arteries (*open arrows*), and the typical looping course of the inferior thyroid artery (*short arrows*). The inferiorly directed branches of the inferior thyroid artery supply portions of the esophagus and trachea. Note the excellent demonstration of the venous drainage of the left thyroid lobe into the left inferior thyroid vein (*curved arrow*). **B:** Selective injection into the right inferior thyroid artery in the same patient demonstrates venous drainage of the right thyroid lobe into the right superior thyroid vein (*long arrow*), the right inferior thyroid vein (*open arrows*), and the right vertebral vein (*short arrows*). Both arteriograms also demonstrate the normal thyroid blush.

one or more of its branches may share a common origin with the internal mammary artery.

The thyrocervical trunk can be recognized by the characteristic looping course of the inferior thyroid artery (see Figs. 34-1 and 34-5) Although the inferior thyroid artery occasionally may have been ligated at the initial surgery, failure to identify this vessel usually means that the catheter is in the costocervical trunk, not the thyrocervical trunk. The costocervical trunk arises from the posterosuperior aspect of the subclavian artery, adjacent to the thyrocervical trunk, and usually is much easier to catheterize than the thyrocervical trunk. Intentional injection of the costocervical trunk should be avoided, however, because it often supplies a major feeder to the cervical spinal cord.

At arteriography, hyperplastic and adenomatous parathyroid glands are oval or rounded areas of diffuse en-

hancement, often superimposed on thyroid tissue (see Fig. 34-3). With optimal radiographic technique and collimation, pathologic glands as small as 4 to 5 mm may be visible. Normal parathyroid glands are never visualized angiographically in these patients because their PTH production is suppressed and the glands become quite small (1–2 mm).[32]

Venous sampling

Venous sampling relies on the unilateral PTH gradients produced by hyperfunctioning parathyroid glands. Mapping the PTH concentrations in selective samples from draining veins reveals the source of elevated hormone production because the remaining normal glands are suppressed and their draining veins contain only back-

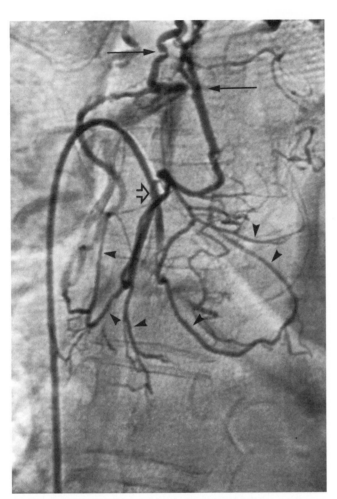

FIGURE 34-6. Thymic vein venogram. The catheter tip is in the left thymic vein (*open arrow*). Thymic vein branches (*arrowheads*) are clearly visible. In this patient, anastomoses are present between the thymic vein and both inferior thyroid veins (*long arrows*). (From Miller DL. Endocrine angiography and venous sampling. *Radiol Clin North Am* 1993;31:1051–1067, with permission.)

ground levels of PTH. Concentrations of PTH more than twice as high as the background level are generally considered diagnostic, but gradients are commonly much higher in selective samples from small veins.[33] In 80 to 90% of patients in whom angiography fails to delineate the source of abnormality, parathyroid venous sampling will be positive.[34] In a series of 86 patients with negative or equivocal noninvasive localization studies and arteriograms, parathyroid venous sampling had a sensitivity of 88% and a specificity of 86%.[34]

Because hyperplasia is often asymmetric, bilateral but usually unequal elevations in PTH above background are the most common finding in patients with primary hyperplasia. Venous sampling usually is not performed in patients with hyperplasia unless only a single gland remains occult or four glands have been identified and resected at surgery but the patient remains hypercalcemic.

The delayed venous-phase images from the parathyroid arteriogram are invaluable both for clarifying venous anatomy and for guiding interpretation of the results of venous sampling, because the venous drainage patterns of the thyroid bed are different in the postoperative neck than in the normal neck. Venous sampling usually is not performed without a preceding arteriographic study. False-positive rates for parathyroid venous sampling of 6 to 18% without arteriography drop to 0 to 4% when a preceding arteriogram is done.[9,34]

Patients who have undergone surgical exploration will invariably have undergone ligation of the middle thyroid veins (failure to do so is a mark of an inadequate exploration), and often the inferior thyroid veins have been ligated as well. Venous drainage from the thyroid bed is usually by the vertebral veins, which should always be sampled. Superior and inferior thyroid veins should be sampled bilaterally, if possible. Samples from the thymic vein may be essential to localize a thymic gland. Internal jugular vein samples are occasionally helpful. Less selective venous sampling (innominate vein, subclavian vein) generally does not produce a sufficient gradient above background to localize the abnormality. Left innominate vein samples may be particularly treacherous because this vein receives drainage from both sides of the neck as well as from the mediastinum.[33,35]

Because it is often necessary to use a number of differently shaped catheters to sample all these veins, a sheath should be placed in the femoral vein at the beginning of the procedure. The vertebral, internal jugular, and inferior thyroid veins all may be catheterized using a Berenstein or similarly shaped catheter. Difficulty advancing the guidewire past the valve at the base of the left internal jugular vein is common. Hyperextension of the neck, combined with repeatedly advancing and withdrawing of the guidewire while the patient is taking deep breaths, is usually successful.[36]

Catheterization of the superior thyroid and thymic veins is often more difficult. The original literature described the use of a tip-deflecting catheter-guidewire assembly, which is no longer manufactured. No really satisfactory substitute is available. If the brachiocephalic and internal jugular veins are large enough, a shepherd's hook, visceral hook, Mikaelsson, or inferior mesenteric catheter may be successful. It is often necessary to steam a catheter to an appropriate shape or to modify an existing catheter. Use of a tip-deflecting wire may help in catheterization of the superior thyroid veins and thymic vein. It is helpful to remember that the thymic vein originates from the anteroinferior aspect of the left brachiocephalic vein. The thymic vein is usually the most difficult vein to catheterize during parathyroid venous sampling, but it is also one of the most important, and so extensive efforts at catheterization are justified.

It is essential to obtain a sample from the femoral vein

sheath at the conclusion of the procedure. This serves as the peripheral vein sample against which all of the other, selective samples will be compared.

After each sample is obtained, and before the catheter is moved, a small amount of contrast material should be injected gently and a spot film (either conventional or digital) obtained to document the position of the catheter tip and the site from which the sample was obtained.

As each sample is obtained, the sample number and the location from which it was obtained should be recorded. At the conclusion of the procedure, this list should be included as part of the dictated report, a copy of the list attached to the patient's chart, and an additional copy included in the film jacket with the spot films. It takes several days to a week or more to get the PTH levels back from the laboratory, by which time recollection of the details of the sampling procedure may be hazy. Without the information from the spot films and the sample list, the PTH data may be meaningless.

Venous sampling is time consuming and requires careful attention to proper labeling and handling (including interim storage) of the samples; an elegant diagnostic procedure and hours of effort may come to naught by a call from the laboratory stating that the melting ice bath has caused 20 labels to be cast adrift from their parent tubes. All such preparations, including documentation of the site from which each sample was obtained, preparation of specimen tubes, and details of specimen handling and transport, should be made and reviewed in advance with the angiography suite technical staff and the hospital chemistry laboratory, particularly given the complexity and relative infrequency of the study. Delegation of sample management to an intern is not wise.

■ Pancreatic Endocrine Tumors

Clinical review

Islet cell tumors of the pancreas may produce any of a number of gastroenteropancreatic hormones. Some islet cell tumors are referred to as "clinically silent" because they overproduce hormones, such as pancreatic polypeptide, that do not result in clinical symptoms.[37] Patients with clinically silent islet cell tumors present with symptoms that result from mass effect rather than endocrine disorders; their tumors are usually larger than 5 cm and are easily identified by CT or ultrasound. Islet cell tumors that secrete excesses of other hormones, principally insulin, gastrin, and glucagon, result in well-defined endocrine syndromes. These islet cell tumors are referred to as *functioning tumors,* and tend to produce clinical symptoms while still quite small (often < 1 cm). The two functioning islet cell tumors that most commonly present difficulties in localization are insulinomas and gastrinomas.

Differences between insulinoma and gastrinoma

Whipple's triad (symptoms of hypoglycemia, demonstrated low blood glucose level, and relief of symptoms with glucose administration) is the clinical prerequisite of insulinoma. Symptoms are often due to the effects of hypoglycemia on the brain, and many patients are initially misdiagnosed as having a neurologic or psychiatric disorder. Hypoglycemia in the presence of elevated insulin levels is strong evidence of an insulinoma. (An alternative etiology is surreptitious self-administration of insulin.)

Insulinomas, the most common islet cell tumor, tend to be solitary (92%), intrapancreatic (99.5%), and benign (90%).[37] They are distributed uniformly throughout the pancreas, with 75% located to the left of the superior mesenteric artery. Accurate localization of these tumors is important because no adequate medical therapy exists and surgical resection is the definitive treatment.[38]

Gastrinoma, the second most common functioning islet cell tumor, produces elevated serum gastrin levels, which leads to hypersecretion of gastric acid and multiple peptic ulcers. These two findings, in addition to the presence of a non-beta cell islet cell tumor, constitute the Zollinger-Ellison syndrome; diarrhea is also a common feature. Unlike insulinomas, 60% of gastrinomas are malignant, 60% are multiple, and more than 30% are extrapancreatic.[37] About 75 to 90% of gastrinomas are located to the right of the superior mesenteric artery, in the pancreas, duodenum, or in the peripancreatic lymph nodes. Gastrinomas are small; duodenal tumors are typically smaller than 1 cm.

Multiple tumors are the rule in the 25% of patients with the Zollinger-Ellison syndrome who have multiple endocrine neoplasia syndrome type 1 (MEN-1), which syndrome includes tumors or hyperplasia of the pancreas, parathyroid, and pituitary. The characteristically multiple and malignant nature of gastrinomas makes their localization often more challenging than that of insulinomas. Additionally, treatment of gastrinoma is less straightforward than insulinomas because of the much higher incidence of metastatic lesions, most commonly within the liver.[38]

Localization

As with all suspected endocrine neoplasms, attempts at localization should begin only after the diagnosis has been confirmed. Preoperative imaging is undertaken initially to determine whether metastases are present. If the patient is a surgical candidate, imaging is used to locate the primary tumor. How aggressively preoperative localization should be pursued in patients with insulinoma is controversial, because these tumors usually are easily identified with the combination of intraoperative ultrasound and palpation.[37,39–45]

The four noninvasive modalities currently used to localize primary islet cell tumors and to detect liver metastases are ultrasound, CT, MRI, and somatostatin receptor scintigraphy. The first three are cross-sectional imaging studies, whereas the last is a functional study based on a physiologic property of the tumor (the presence of somatostatin receptors). Noninvasive cross-sectional studies are used primarily to evaluate for metastatic disease, but they also may reveal the primary tumor simultaneously.

If noninvasive methods have not identified a primary tumor, the patient should next undergo either arteriography with arterial stimulation and venous sampling (ASVS) or endoscopic ultrasound, depending on the availability of suitable equipment and experienced operators.[37,39–43,46,47] Some authors continue to recommend portal venous sampling as a final option, but we believe this technique has been superseded by ASVS.[37,39] Portal venous sampling is far more difficult technically and has a higher complication rate.[48]

Anatomy

The arterial anatomy of the pancreas and duodenum is described in Chapters 28 and 32. The arteries of principal concern are the celiac axis, the superior mesenteric artery, and their branches. There is considerable variability in branching patterns in the celiac and superior mesenteric arteries. The body and tail of the pancreas receive numerous branches from the splenic artery. The pancreatic head is supplied by the gastroduodenal artery. The dorsal pancreatic artery, via the transverse pancreatic artery, may supply the entire pancreas.

Pancreatic/hepatic arteriography

Arteriography has largely been replaced by newer, less invasive modalities as the initial technique for tumor detection, but it remains valuable for localization of insulinomas and in conjunction with ASVS.[1,37,42] The smallest lesion that can be visualized by arteriography is approximately 5 mm compared with at least 7 mm for CT and conventional ultrasound and 5 to 6 mm for endoscopic ultrasound.[49,50] Pancreatic endocrine tumors and their metastases appear as foci of homogeneous staining during the capillary phase (Fig. 34-7).[1,37] They are usually sharply defined, round or oval lesion with smooth margins. Neither neovascularity nor arteriovenous shunting is demonstrable in small lesions, but tumors larger than 2 cm may demonstrate abnormal vessels and prominent draining veins.[37] Arteriography is capable of demonstrating hypervascular hepatic metastases smaller than 5 mm in diameter.[51] Rare islet cell tumors may be hypovascular.[52,53]

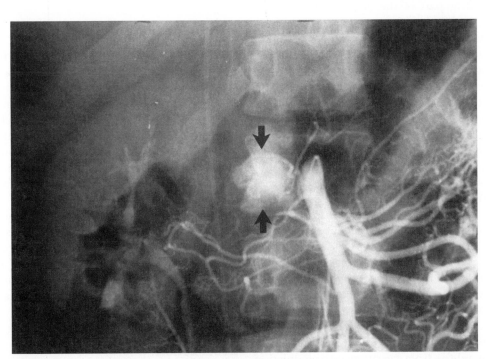

FIGURE 34-7. Arteriogram of an insulinoma. The tumor (*arrows*) is round and well defined, with a smooth margin and an intense, homogeneous blush. It is supplied by branches of the superior mesenteric artery. It is rather large for a benign insulinoma. The patient was cured following surgical resection.

Arteriography should include selective studies of the superior mesenteric, gastroduodenal, splenic, and dorsal pancreatic arteries, if technically feasible. Selective hepatic arteriography also should be performed to identify liver metastases. A variety of catheter shapes may be used for catheterization of these vessels; the choice depends on the patient's anatomy and the angiographer's personal preference.

The reported sensitivity of arteriography for localization of primary islet cell tumors has decreased in recent years.[37] Older studies report a sensitivity of approximately 65%, but more recent studies suggest that fewer than half of these tumors are detected arteriographically.[54,55] This difference is probably due in part to earlier detection and in part to referral bias. On the other hand, the false-positive rate is generally reported as less than 10%. The sensitivity of arteriography for locating primary tumors is superior to that of CT, MRI, or ultrasound when all four modalities are compared in the same patient population.[37,56–58]

Arterial stimulation and venous sampling

ASVS, also sometimes termed *selective arterial secretin injection* when used for gastrinomas, was first described as a localization procedure for patients with Zollinger-Ellison syndrome;[59] the procedure was subsequently developed and refined for localization of both gastrinomas and insulinomas.[55,60–62] It is an adjunct to arteriography and is performed as part of the arteriographic procedure.

In addition to the arteriographic catheter, a venous catheter is introduced via the femoral vein, and its tip is placed in the right hepatic vein. (A Simmons 1 catheter with one or two sideholes near the tip is ideal for this purpose.) A secretagogue is injected through the arterial catheter selectively into the hepatic artery, gastroduodenal artery, splenic artery, and superior mesenteric artery successively. The hepatic artery is studied in an effort to detect metastases that may be too small to be identify with imaging studies.[63] The dorsal pancreatic artery is not subjected to ASVS because this vessel usually supplies the entire pancreas and therefore has no localizing value. If an insulinoma or gastrinoma is present in the vascular territory supplied by one of these arteries, the injection of secretagogue will cause an increase in the insulin or gastrin concentration in the portal vein and subsequently in the hepatic vein. Hepatic vein samples are obtained before and at 20, 40, and 60 sec after the secretagogue injection.

Secretin is used as a secretagogue for gastrinomas. It stimulates gastrin release from gastrinomas by modulation of adenylate cyclase activation.[64] Current technique requires injection of 30 IU of secretin intraarterially, with 10-min intervals between injections. In the protocol developed at the National Institutes of Health (NIH), an increase in venous hormone concentration of more than 48% at 30 sec or more than 109% at 60 sec after secretin injection is a positive response.[60,63] This technique results in a sensitivity of 77 to 100%, with a false-positive rate near 0%, and it is particularly sensitive for the detection of duodenal gastrinomas.[37,55,60,65] Other protocols and criteria also may be used.[46,65]

Calcium is used as a secretagogue for the localization of insulinomas in the same fashion and is also effective.[61,62,66] Arterial injections of calcium gluconate (0.01–0.025 mEq Ca^{++}/kg), using the same protocol as used for secretin injections, yielded a sensitivity of 88% in a series of 25 patients.[62] A positive study is defined as a 100% increase in insulin level within one minute after calcium injection.

■ Hyperaldosteronism

Several endocrine syndromes caused by an excess of hormone may be caused by tumors or hyperplasia of the adrenal glands. Cushing syndrome, pheochromocytoma, and virilizing disorders may be diagnosed on the basis of endocrine studies and characterized or localized by cross-sectional imaging techniques. Adrenal venous sampling is usually employed only for primary hyperaldosteronism (Conn syndrome).

Clinical review

Primary hyperaldosteronism often presents with spontaneous (or easily provoked) hypokalemia in a hypertensive patient; It has been estimated that hyperaldosteronism is present in 1 to 2% of hypertensive patients.[67] Suggestive initial screening tests include hypokalemia in association with kaliuresis, low plasma renin activity, and a high plasma aldosterone concentration/plasma renin activity ratio. Demonstration of nonsuppressible aldosterone excretion in conjunction with normal cortisol excretion is diagnostic.

The two most common causes of primary hyperaldosteronism are a unilateral aldosterone-producing adenoma (APA; 54%) and bilateral adrenal hyperplasia (idiopathic hyperaldosteronism; 45%).[67] Thability to distinguish between these entities is a crucial part of the endocrine evaluation, because adenomas are resected, whereas hyperplasia is treated medically.

Localization

Noninvasive laboratory and imaging studies may be used to distinguish between an APA and hyperplasia with an accuracy of 70 to 80%, but most experts agree that bilateral adrenal vein sampling is the gold standard, with accuracy rates approaching 100.[68–71] In addition, several rare forms of hyperaldosteronism (e.g., unilateral primary adrenal hyperplasia) are best characterized by adrenal venous sampling because their cross-sectional imaging appearance may be confusing.[68]

Patients who have classic endocrine studies indicating an APA and a unilateral, low attenuation mass on CT may undergo adrenalectomy without the need for adrenal venous sampling. Bilateral adrenal venous sampling is indicated in patients with clinical and laboratory evidence of primary hyperaldosteronism but no clear CT or MRI demonstration of unilateral surgical disease. These patients often have bilateral adrenal abnormalities on imaging studies, but these abnormalities are frequently unrelated to the endocrine disorder. The CT diagnosis of adrenal hyperplasia is not reliable in patients with hyperaldosteronism.[69–72] In patients with apparent bilateral adrenal disease, venous sampling provides physiologic data that permit identification of the cause of the syndrome without resorting to analysis of gland morphology.

Anatomy

Adrenal venous anatomy is fairly constant (Fig. 34-8). The left adrenal vein virtually always arises from the left renal vein at the left lateral margin of the vertebral column. In the uncommon case of a retroaortic left renal vein, the adrenal vein arises either from the anomalous renal vein or, rarely, directly from the inferior vena cava (IVC). On the right side, the adrenal vein empties directly into the posterior IVC and is usually both small and quite short (5–8 mm), making selective catheterization for sampling challenging (Fig. 34-9).[68] It can be difficult to locate and is somewhat more variable in position than the left adrenal vein.

Venous sampling

The procedure consists of simultaneous sampling from a femoral vein sheath and from catheters selectively placed in the adrenal veins via ipsilateral femoral vein punctures, both before and after the intravenous administration of adrenocorticotropic hormone (ACTH). The left adrenal vein is catheterized first. A 4 or 5 Fr Weinberg or Berenstein catheter is guided into the left renal vein with the help of a tip-deflecting wire. Once in the renal vein, the catheter tip usually encounters the orifice of the left adrenal vein at the level of the left lateral margin of the vertebral column. A 4 Fr straight polyethylene catheter, shaped with the use of the steam into an S-curve, may be

used instead. Alternatively, a 5 Fr Simmons I catheter placed in the left renal vein will act as a guiding catheter to direct a microcatheter into the left adrenal vein when gentle traction is placed on the guiding catheter to direct its tip superiorly. The left inferior phrenic vein also drains into the left adrenal vein. The catheter tip should not be advanced into the inferior phrenic vein because samples from this catheter will not contain blood from the left adrenal gland.

Small, gentle hand injections of contrast material are used to verify catheter position. No attempt should be made to opacify the gland or to outline tumors. Diagnostic retrograde venography, performed commonly in the past, is no longer used, because this procedure may cause hemorrhage or infarction as a result of rupture of small adrenal venous radicals. This might seem a good way to ablate the adrenal gland, but it is not a reliable method for infarcting the gland. Ethanol should not be used for adrenal ablation either, because ethanol injection into the adrenal artery in monkeys produces immediate and severe hypertension as well as arrhythmias.[73]

The right adrenal vein is shorter than the left and trifurcates close to its orifice into the IVC. The tip of a standard Mikaelsson or Simmons catheter often occludes the trifurcation once it is adequately seated in the right adrenal vein, which prevents aspiration of right adrenal venous effluent and reduces the accuracy of the study. A single hole may be punched 3 to 4 mm from the catheter tip to permit collection of venous effluent at the point where the right adrenal vein joins the IVC.[68] Using this modified technique when necessary, collection from both adrenals is consistently possible.

After collection of baseline samples from both adrenal veins and the femoral vein sheath, ACTH is administered intravenously in the form of a 25 mcg bolus followed by an infusion of 25 mcg in 500 mL of normal saline at a rate of 150 to 200 mL/hr. (ACTH stimulates release of aldosterone as well as cortisol.) Repeat samples are obtained 15 minutes after the start of the infusion. Then the ACTH infusion is discontinued. All samples are submitted for assay of both aldosterone and cortisol.

Right adrenal vein samples will be diluted to an unknown degree by inclusion of IVC blood. To correct for this dilution, aldosterone/cortisol (A/C) ratios are used. The decrease in right adrenal aldosterone levels resulting from dilution should be equal in proportion to the decrease in cortisol levels. Cortisol production by each adrenal gland is assumed to be equal. Use of the A/C ratio corrects for any dilution and allows comparison of right and left adrenal vein samples.

Interpretation of the results is based on the physiologic suppression of aldosterone production in the adrenal gland contralateral to an APA. If an APA is present, the A/C ratio in the contralateral gland will be below back-

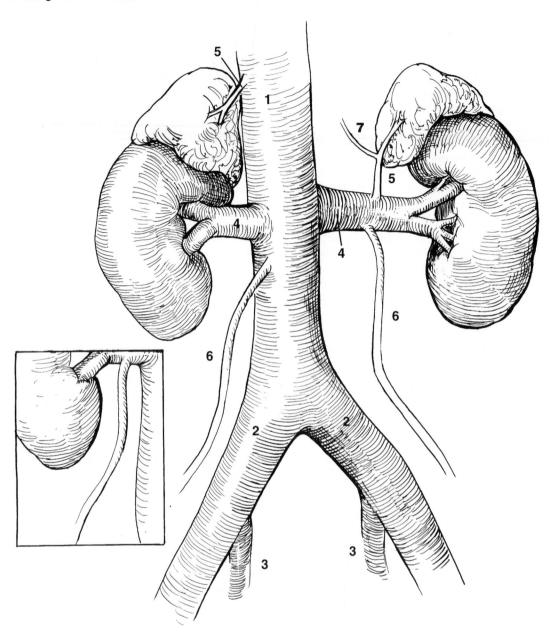

FIGURE 34-8. Anatomy of the adrenal veins. The drawing demonstrates the typical anatomy. When sampling the left adrenal vein, it is important to ensure that the catheter tip is not in the left inferior phrenic vein, or adrenal venous blood will not be obtained. 1, inferior vena cava; 2, common iliac; 3, internal iliac; 4, renal; 5, adrenal; 6, gonadal; 7, inferior phrenic.

ground levels, as indicated by the sample obtained from the femoral vein sheath, whereas the A/C ratio from the ipsilateral gland will be much greater than the background. On the other hand, in patients with bilateral hyperplasia, A/C ratios in both adrenals are comparable because neither is suppressed. The A/C ratios from both adrenal glands will be greater than that in the femoral vein sheath sample. Following ACTH stimulation in a patient with an APA, both cortisol and aldosterone levels increase significantly on the side with the adenoma, whereas there is a rise in cortisol but only a minimal increase in aldosterone in the contralateral suppressed gland. This further increases the difference in A/C ratio between the two adrenal glands. In bilateral hyperplasia, however, aldosterone and cortisol levels from both adrenal glands increase after ACTH stimulation, and the A/C ratios remain comparable between the two glands. When one gland shows suppressed aldosterone production before ACTH stimulation and a reduced aldosterone response (and normal cortisol response) following ACTH

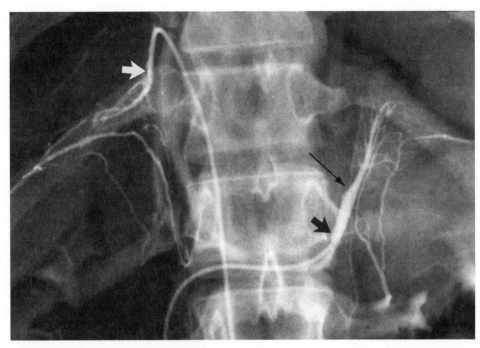

FIGURE 34-9. Bilateral adrenal vein venogram. Catheters are in place for adrenal vein sampling. Note the short course of the right adrenal vein (*white arrow*). The left adrenal vein empties into the left renal vein just to the left of the spine (*short black arrow*). Also note the point at which the left inferior phrenic vein joins the left adrenal vein (*long black arrow*). (From Miller DL. Endocrine angiography and venous sampling. *Radiol Clin North Am* 1993;31:1051–1067, with permission.)

stimulation, surgical removal of the contralateral gland produces a high cure rate.[68]

REFERENCES

1. Miller DL. Endocrine angiography and venous sampling. *Radiol Clin North Am* 1993;31:1051–1067.
2. Lee VS, Wilkinson RH Jr, Leight GS Jr, et al. Hyperparathyroidism in high-risk surgical patients: evaluation with double-phase technetium-99m sestamibi imaging. *Radiology* 1995;197:627–633.
3. Sörensen R. Selective venous sampling for parathyroid hormone excess. In: Uflacker R, Sörensen R, eds. *Percutaneous Venous Blood Sampling in Endocrine Dseases.* New York: Springer-Verlag, 1992: 125–131.
4. Bruining HA, Birkenhäger JC, Ong GL, et al. Causes of failure in operations for hyperparathyroidism. *Surgery* 1987;101:562–565.
5. Auguste L-J, Attie JN, Schnaap D. Initial failure of surgical exploration in patients with primary hyperparathyroidism. *Am J Surg* 1990; 160:333–336.
6. Summers GW. Parathyroid exploration: a review of 125 cases. *Arch Otolaryngol Head Neck Surg* 1991;117:1237–1241.
7. Shaha AR, Jaffe BM. Cervical exploration for primary hyperparathyroidism. *J Surg Oncol* 1993;52:14–17.
8. Weinberger MS, Robbins KT. Diagnostic localization studies for primary hyperparathyroidism: a suggested algorithm. *Arch Otolaryngol Head Neck Surg* 1994;120:1187–1189.
9. Miller DL. Preoperative localization and interventional treatment of parathyroid tumors: when and how? *World J Surg* 1991;15:706–715.
10. Roe SM, Burns RP, Graham LD, et al. Cost-effectiveness of preoperative localization studies in primary hyperparathyroid disease. *Ann Surg* 1994;219:582–586.
11. Serpell JW, Campbell PR, Young AE. Preoperative localization of parathyroid tumors does not reduce operating time. *Br J Surg* 1991;78:589–590.
12. Nottingham JM, Brown JJ, Bynoe RP, et al. Bilateral neck exploration for primary hyperparathyroidism. *Am Surg* 1993;53:115–119.
13. Casas AT, Burke GJ, Mansberger AR Jr, et al. Impact of technetium-99m-sestamibi localization on operative time and success of operations for primary hyperparathyroidism. *Am Surg* 1994;60:12–17.
14. Irvin GL, III, Prudhomme DL, Deriso GT, et al. A new approach to parathyroidectomy. *Ann Surg* 1994;219:574–581.
15. Russel CFJ, Laird JD, Ferguson R. Scan-directed unilateral cervical exploration for parathyroid adenomas: a legitimate approach? *World J Surg* 1990;14:406–409.
16. Wei JP, Burke GJ. Analysis of savings in operative time for primary hyperparathyroidism using localization with technetium 99m sestamibi scan. *Am J Surg* 1995;170:488–491.
17. Halvorson DJ, Burke GJ, Mansberger AR Jr, et al. Use of technetium Tc 99m sestamibi and iodine 123 radionuclide scan for preoperative localization of abnormal parathyroid glands in primary hyperparathyroidism. *South Med J* 1994;87:336–339.
18. Turton DB, Miller DL. Recent advances in parathyroid imaging. *Trends Endocrinol Metab* 1996;7:163–168.
19. Miller DL, Doppman JL, Krudy AG, et al. Localization of parathyroid adenomas in patients who have undergone surgery. Part II. Invasive procedures. *Radiology* 1987;162:138–141.
20. Wang C-A. The anatomic basis of parathyroid surgery. *Ann Surg* 1976;183:271–275.
21. Kaplan EL, Yashiro T, Salti G. Primary hyperparathyroidism in the 1990s: choice of surgical procedure for this disease. *Ann Surg* 1992;215:300–317.

22. Jander HP, Diethelm AG, Russinovich NAE. The parathyroid artery. *AJR Am J Roentgenol* 1980;135:821–828.

23. Nobori M, Saiki S, Tanaka N, et al. Blood supply of the parathyroid gland from the superior thyroid artery. *Surgery* 1994;115:417–423.

24. Doppman JL, Hammond WG. The anatomic basis of parathyroid venous sampling. *Radiology* 1970;95:603–610.

25. Shimkin PM, Doppman JL, Pearson KD, et al. Anatomic considerations in parathyroid venous sampling. *AJR Am J Roentgenol* 1973; 118:654–662.

26. Doppman JL, Melson GL, Evens RG, et al. Selective superior and inferior thyroid vein catheterization: Venographic anatomy and potential applications. *Invest Radiol* 1969;4:97–99.

27. Doppman JL, Mallette LE, Marx SJ, et al. The localization of abnormal mediastinal parathyroid glands. *Radiology* 1975;115:31–36.

28. MIller DL, Chang R, Doppman JL, et al. Localization of parathyroid adenomas: superselective arterial DSA versus superselective conventional angiography. *Radiology* 1989;170:1003–1006.

29. Lippert H, Pabst R. Arterial variations in man: classification and frequency. Munich: J.F. *Bergmann Verlag*, 1985:6.

30. Krudy AG, Doppman JL, Brennan MF. The significance of the thyroidea ima artery in arteriographic localization of parathyroid adenomas. *Radiology* 1980;136:51–55.

31. McIntyre RC Jr, Kumpe DA, Liechty RD. Reexploration and angiographic ablation for hyperparathyroidism. *Arch Surg* 1994;129:499–504.

32. Doppman JL. Parathyroid localization: arteriography and venous sampling. *Radiol Clin North Am* 1976;14:163–188.

33. Monchik JM, Doppman JL, Earll JM, et al. Localization of hyperfunctioning parathyroid tissue: radioimmunoassay of parathyroid hormone on samples from the large veins of the neck and thorax and selectively catheterized thyroid veins. *Am J Surg* 1975;129:413–420.

34. Sugg SL, Fraker DL, Alexander R, et al. Prospective evaluation of selective venous sampling for parathyroid hormone concentration in patients undergoing reoperations for primary hyperparathyroidism. *Surgery* 1993;114:1004–1011.

35. Shimkin PM, Powell D, Doppman JL, et al. Parathyroid venous sampling. *Radiology* 1972;104:571–574.

36. Miller DL, Doppman JL. Petrosal sinus sampling: technique and rationale. *Radiology* 1991;178:37–47.

37. Miller DL. Islet cell tumors of the pancreas: diagnosis and localization. In: Freeny PC, Stevenson GW, eds. *Margulis and Burhenne's Alimentary Tract Radiology*. Hanover, CV. Mosby, 1994:1167–1196.

38. Gorman B, Reading CC. Imaging of gastrointestinal neuroendocrine tumors. *Semin Ultrasound CT MR* 1995;16:331–341.

39. Miller DL, Buetow PC. Imaging procedures for the endocrine pancreas. In: Howard JM, Idezuki Y, Ihse I, et al., eds. *Surgical Diseases of the Pancreas*. Baltimore: Williams & Wilkins, 1998:703–715.

40. Hammond PJ, Jackson JA, Bloom SR. Localization of pancreatic endocrine tumours. *Clin Endocrinol* 1994;40:3–14.

41. Orbuch M, Doppman JL, Jensen RT. Localization of pancreatic endocrine tumors. *Semin Gastrointest Dis* 1995;6:90–101.

42. King CM, Reznek RH, Dacie JE, et al. Imaging islet cell tumours. *Clin Radiol* 1994;49:295–303.

43. Perry RR, Vinick AI. Diagnosis and management of functioning islet cell tumors. *J Clin Endocrinol Metab* 1995;80:2273–2278.

44. Bieligk S, Jaffe BM. Islet cell tumors of the pancreas. *Surg Clin North Am* 1995;75:1025–1040.

45. van Heerden JA, Grant CS, Czako PF, et al. Occult functioning insulinomas: which localizing studies are indicated? *Surgery* 1992; 112:1010–1015.

46. Imamura M, Takahashi K, Isobe Y, et al. Curative resection of multiple gastrinomas aided by selective arterial secretin injection test and intraoperative secretin test. *Ann Surg* 1989;210:710–718.

47. Fraker DL, Alexander HR. The surgical approach to endocrine tumors of the pancreas. *Semin Gastrointest Dis* 1995;6:102–113.

48. Miller DL, Doppman JL, Metz DC, et al. Zollinger-Ellison syndrome: technique, results, and complications of portal venous sampling. *Radiology* 1992;182:235–241.

49. Günther RW, Klose KJ, Rückert K, et al. Localization of small islet-cell tumors: preoperative and intraoperative ultrasound, computed tomography, arteriography, digital subtraction angiography, and pancreatic venous sampling. *Gastrointest Radiol* 1985;10:145–152.

50. Lightdale CJ, Botet JF, Woodruff JM, et al. Localization of endocrine tumors of the pancreas with endoscopic ultrasonography. *Cancer* 1991;68:1815–1820.

51. Anderson T, Ericksson B, Hemmingsson A, et al. Angiography, computed tomography, magnetic resonance imaging and ultrasonography in detection of liver metastases from endocrine gastrointestinal tumours. *Acta Radiol* 1987;28:535–539.

52. Fink IJ, Krudy AG, Shawker TH, et al. Demonstration of an angiographically hypovascular insulinoma with intraarterial dynamic CT. *AJR Am J Roentgenol* 1985;144:555–556.

53. Smith TR, Koenigsberg M. Low-density insulinoma on dynamic CT. *AJR Am J Roentgenol* 1990;155:995–996.

54. Doppman JL, Shawker TH, Miller DL. Localization of islet cell tumors. *Gastroenterol Clin North Am* 1989;18:793–804.

55. Doppman JL, Miller DL, Chang R, et al. Gastrinomas: localization by means of selective intraarterial injection of secretin. *Radiology* 1990;174:25–29.

56. Pisegna JR, Doppman JL, Norton JA, et al. Prospective comparative study of ability of MR imaging and other imaging modalities to localize tumors in patients with Zollinger-Ellison syndrome. *Digest Dis Sci* 1993;38:1318–1328.

57. Frucht H, Doppman JL, Norton JA, et al. Gastrinomas: comparison of MR imaging with CT, angiography, and US. *Radiology* 1989; 171:713–717.

58. Maton PN, Miller DL, Doppman JL, et al. Role of selective angiography in the management of patients with Zollinger-Ellison syndrome. *Gastroenterology* 1987;92:913–918.

59. Imamura M, Takahashi K, Adachi H, et al. Usefulness of selective arterial secretin injection test for localization of gastrinoma in the Zollinger-Ellison syndrome. *Ann Surg* 1987;205:230–239.

60. Thom AK, Norton JA, Doppman JL, et al. Prospective study of the use of intraarterial secretin injection and portal venous sampling to localize duodenal gastrinomas. *Surgery* 1992;112:1002–1009.

61. Doppman JL, Miller DL, Chang R, et al. Insulinomas: localization with selective intraarterial injection of calcium. *Radiology* 1991; 178:237–241.

62. Doppman JL, Chang R, Fraker DL, et al. Localization of insulinomas to regions of the pancreas by intra-arterial stimulation with calcium. *Ann Intern Med* 1995;123:269–273.

63. Gibril F, Doppman JL, Chang R, et al. Metastatic gastrinomas: localization with selective arterial injection of secretin. *Radiology* 1996;198:77–84.

64. Chiba T, Yamatani T, Yamaguchi A, et al. Mechanism for increase of gastrin release by secretin in Zollinger-Ellison syndrome. *Gastroenterology* 1989;96:1439–1444.

65. Imamura M, Takahashi K. Use of selective arterial secretin injection test to guide surgery in patients with Zollinger-Ellison syndrome. *World J Surg* 1993;17:433–438.

66. Doppman JL, Miller DL, Chang R, et al. Intraarterial stimulation test for detection of insulinomas. *World J Surg* 1993;17:439–443.

67. Young WF, Jr., Hogan MJ, Klee GG, et al. Primary aldosteronism: diagnosis and treatment. *Mayo Clin Proc* 1990;65:96–110.

68. Doppman JL, Gill JR, Jr. Hyperaldosteronism: sampling the adrenal veins. *Radiology* 1996;198:309–312.

69. Doppman JL, Gill JR, Jr., Miller DL, et al. Distinction between hyperaldosteronism due to bilateral hyperplasia and unilateral aldosteronoma: reliability of CT. *Radiology* 1992;184:677–682.

70. Gleason PE, Weinberger MH, Pratt JH, et al. Evaluation of diagnostic tests in the differential diagnosis of primary aldosteronism: uni-

lateral adenoma versus bilateral micronodular hyperplasia. *J Urol* 1993;150:1365–1368.

71. Tokunaga K, Nakamura H, Marukawa T, et al. Adrenal venous sampling analysis of primary aldosteronism: value of ACTH stimulation in the differentiation of adenoma and hyperplasia. *Eur Radiol* 1992;2:223–229.

72. Doppman JL. The dilemma of bilateral adrenocortical nodularity in Conn's and Cushing's syndromes. *Radiol Clin North Am* 1993; 31:1039–1050.

73. Fink IJ, Girton M, Doppman JL. Absolute ethanol injection of the adrenal artery: hypertensive reaction. *Radiology* 1985;154:357–358.

35

Central Venous Access

MATTHEW A. MAURO AND STEVEN E. BLACK

Modern medical care has rapidly expanded the need for the placement of catheters into the central venous circulation for long periods. Long-term central venous access is commonly used for hemodialysis, plasmapheresis, chemotherapy, long-term antibiotic therapy, blood drawing, parenteral nutrition, and analgesics. Outpatient dialysis centers, ambulatory chemotherapy, hospices, home health care, and other commercial enterprises have grown dramatically as an indirect result of these devices.

Broviac and Hickman described the first soft long-term right atrial silicone catheters in 1973 and 1979, respectively.[1,2] The first subcutaneous port was reported by Niederhuber in 1982.[3] Historically these devices have been placed by surgeons within an operating room. The traditional role for radiologists was to be involved in preoperative venography, catheter relocation, and intravascular catheter fragment retrieval. More recently, the interventional radiologist's role has expanded to include complex access cases and the development of an independent venous access service where they function as the primary operator in the placement and management of all long-term devices.[4,5]

Advances in vascular imaging and catheter/guidewire technology, in addition to acquired catheterization skills and a commitment to patient care, place interventional radiologists in a strong position to become an important part of this service. The development of a successful venous access service requires a knowledge of the available devices and their indications, insertion and removal techniques, and the management of complications relating to these devices.

■ Access Devices

Modern central venous access devices are available in many sizes and forms. Regardless of these differences, they all result in the positioning of a catheter in the central venous circulation: the superior vena cava (SVC), inferior vena cava (IVC), or right atrium. Early catheters were made of polyethylene and frequently were complicated by thrombosis and infection.[6] Current devices are composed of either silicone rubber or polyurethane attached to either an external connector or an implantable port. Silicone is a soft material that has a high coefficient of friction, making catheters composed of this material difficult to use with over-the-guidewire techniques when conventional stainless steel guidewires are used. Newer hydrophilic guidewires can be used with this material. Silicone catheters have been used in the central venous system since the early 1970s and are extremely biocompatible and safe. Polyurethane is a newer material that is stronger than silicone, which allows a catheter to have a larger internal diameter while maintaining the same outer diameter. Polyurethane also can be used with conventional guidewires.

Catheters have either a simple end-hole, a valved tip, or a staggered tip. Conventional end-hole catheters are the most common variety and are available with single, dual, or triple lumen. These catheters can be trimmed at the tip for proper sizing.[7] Valved-tip catheters have specially designed slits just proximal to a closed tip, allowing blood to be withdrawn and solutions to be infused but, when not in use, will not allow blood to enter the catheter. The potential advantage of these types of catheters is that they do not require routine heparinization to prevent catheter thrombosis. These devices can only be trimmed at the hub and therefore have a removable external connector.[8] Staggered-tip catheters are dual-lumen devices designed for treatments requiring simultaneous rapid aspiration and infusions (pheresis, hemodialysis) with limited admixture. These devices cannot be trimmed from either the tip or hub and therefore are available in multiple lengths to fit the individual patient's anatomy.

Central venous devices can be separated into peripherally inserted central catheters (PICC), chest-wall external catheters (nontunnelled and tunnelled), and subcutaneous ports (chest wall and extremity) (Figs. 35-1 through 35-3).

PICCs allow external access and are inserted via an upper extremity vein (see Fig. 35-1 and Table 35-1). Because they are inserted peripherally, they carry a lower procedural risk than do centrally inserted catheters and

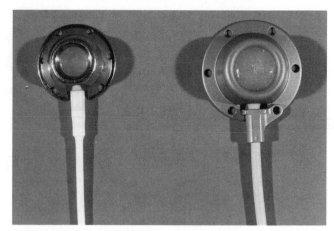

FIGURE 35-3. Photograph of subcutaneous ports: **Left:** Low profile chest-wall port used in small adults and in children; **Right:** Standard chest-wall port used in average to large adults.

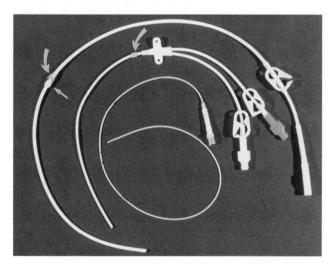

FIGURE 35-1. Photograph of external venous access devices: From top to bottom, single-lumen Hickman catheter, dual-lumen Hohn catheter, single-lumen peripherally inserted central catheter (PICC). Only the Hickman catheter has a Dacron cuff (*straight arrow*) that is placed in a subcutaneous tunnel. The Hickman and Hohn catheters have a Vita cuff (*curved arrows*) placed at the entry site

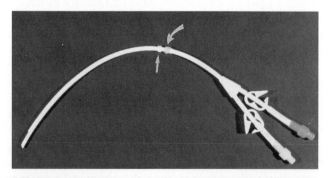

FIGURE 35-2. Photograph of dual-lumen, staggered-tip dialysis catheter. *Straight arrow:* Dacron cuff. *Curved arrow:* Vita cuff.

may be preferred by patients who dislike having catheters on their chest.[9] In many institutions, PICCs are placed at the bedside by trained nurses; however, for patients with venous occlusions from previous venipunctures and intravenous lines, blind placement of these devices is frequently unsuccessful. Ultrasound or venography often will allow successful placement by the interventional radiologists.[9–12]

Chest wall catheters

Nontunnelled

Chest-wall external catheters serve many needs. Acute-care catheters are tapered, nontunnelled catheters that are placed routinely in the units and on the floors for relatively short periods (i.e., days to weeks). In cases where access is difficult (e.g., obesity, coagulopathy, venous thromboses), the interventional radiologist may be asked to place these devices. Nontapered, nontunnelled chest wall external catheters are also available with a single or dual lumen and intended for intermediate-term care (i.e., several weeks to several months) (see Fig. 35-1).[13] Because they are nontapered and composed of silicone, they are more difficult to insert than the acute-care catheter and typically are placed near the surgeon or interventional radiologist.

Tunnelled

All tunnelled chest-wall catheters have a small-circumference Dacron cuff attached to the shaft that is positioned within the subcutaneous tunnel. Subcutaneous tunnelling provides mechanical stability and protects against infection from the skin. The Dacron cuff allows ingrowth of fibrous tissue, which secures the catheter within the tract (4–6 weeks) thus creating a long-term device (i.e., months to years).[14] Some catheters are also available with a second cuff composed of a silver-impregnated collagen

TABLE 35-1. Access Devices

Type	Sizes	Lumen	Catheter material	Indications	Conventional access site	Fixation	Duration	Advantages	Disadvantages	Comments
Peripherally inserted central catheters	3–7 Fr	S,D	Polyurethane Silicone	Chemotherapy Antibiotics Fluids Blood drawing TPN	Antecubital v. Cephalic v. Basilic v.	Suture/tape	Weeks to months	Low procedural risk Low central v. thrombosis Bedside insertion Inexpensive	Restricted flows Poor visibility Skin fixation Extremity v. thrombosis Limitation of activities Requires intact anatomy	Insertions often can be performed following bedside failure
Nontunnelled chest wall catheters: Tapered	5–13 Fr	S,D,T	Polyethylene Polyurethane Silicone	Acute care Antibiotics Fluids Blood Pheresis Dialysis	SCV/AV IJV	Suture/tape	Days to weeks	Quick bedside insertion Acute care setting Multiple indications	Complications of central insertion Hospital setting Internal fixation	
Nontapered	5–7 Fr	S,D	Silicone	Antibiotics Fluids TPN Blood	SCV/AV IJV	Suture/tape	Weeks to months	Hospital or home Atraumatic material	Complications of central insertion Skin fixation Limitation of activities	
Tunnelled chest wall external catheters	6–14 Fr	S,D,T	Polyurethane Silicone	Chemotherapy Antibiotics Fluids TPN Blood Pheresis Dialysis	SCV/AV IJV	Cuff within subcutaneous tunnel	Months to years	Full range of indications Easy access Internal fixation	Complications of central insertion Limitation of activity High maintenance	Frequent uses
Subcutaneous ports Extremity	5–7 Fr	S	Polyurethane Silicone	Chemotherapy Antibiotics Fluids TPN Blood	Antecubital v. Cephalic v. Basilic v.	Internal	Months to years	Low procedural risk Low central v. thrombosis Low maintenance Unlimited activities	Extremity v. thrombophlebitis Needle access required Small access site Difficult access	Patient and nurse preference must be considered
Chest wall	6–10 Fr	S,D	Polyurethane Silicone	Chemotherapy Antibiotics Fluids TPN Blood	SCV/AV IJV	Internal	Months to years	Large access site Easier needle access Low maintenance Unlimited activities Self access	Complications of central insertion Needle access required	Infrequent uses Cost-effective after 6 mo

Fr, French; S, single lumen; D, dual lumen; T, triple lumen; TPN, Total parenteral nutrition; SCV/AV, subclavian/axillary vein; IJV, internal jugular vein.

(VitaCuff; Vitaphore, Menlo Park, CA) that is placed at the catheter exit site to serve as an antimicrobial barrier (see Figs. 35-1 and 35-2).

Subcutaneous ports

All implantable devices have a port component buried in the subcutaneous space connected to a catheter with its tip placed in the central venous system (see Fig. 35-3).[14,15] The ports are available with single or dual chambers and are constructed of stainless steel, titanium, or plastic [magnetic resonance imaging (MRI) compatible]. The traditional reservoir port is accessed by the use of a non-coring needle that enters the port via a compressed silicone disc. Subcutaneous ports are now available in a wide range of sizes that can better accommodate the patient's size and amount of subcutaneous tissue (see Fig. 35-3). Small ports are also available for extremity placement in the forearm or upper arm.[9,16]

■ Device Selection

The appropriate choice of a device depends on multiple factors: frequency, length, and type of therapy and use and personal preference (e.g., physician, nurse, home health care personnel, patient). Frequent access (daily) will favor the choice of an external catheter, whereas infrequent use (weekly, monthly) favors a port. Ports are significantly more expensive than external catheters, but they require significantly less maintenance when not in use. Therefore, when the devices are used infrequently, ports become more cost efficient when in place approximately 6 months or longer. Because of the different diameters and thicknesses of the port septum in chest wall (standard size) and extremity ports, the chest-wall ports will accept twice as many needle punctures.

Multiple-lumen catheters have a higher infection rate compared with single-lumen devices. Therefore, the device with the fewest lumens required should be selected. A single-lumen device should be selected for single use or nonsimultaneous multiple uses, whereas a multilumen device will be needed for multiple simultaneous uses. Often, the type of therapy will affect the device choice.[4] If blood drawing will be needed, devices larger than 3 or 4 Fr will be helpful. If a triple-lumen device is required, a port or PICC is not a possibility. If high flow rates are required (pheresis, hemodialysis) staggered tip external catheters will be needed.

Finally, the personal preference of the physician may be a factor but should not be the overriding consideration. A device must be selected that will accomplish the treatment plan. Physician preference is the least important factor. The interventional radiologist should be able to place all types of devices. It is much more important to consider the opinions and experience of the health care personnel that will be accessing and managing the device over the long term as well as the feelings of the patient. If a variety of options exist, they should be discussed with the patient before the procedure.

■ Placement Techniques

Percutaneous placement of long-term central venous access devices requires three basic procedural steps: (a) venous access, (b) formation of a subcutaneous tunnel or pocket, and (c) placement of the catheter into the central venous circulation.

Venous access

Conventional access sites include the subclavian vein (SCV), axillary vein, internal and external jugular veins, and the cephalic and basilic veins of the upper extremity. The choice of access site depends on the device to be placed, venous patency, existing access, and patient preference. Nontunnelled and tunnelled catheters as well as chest wall ports are routinely placed via SCV or axillary access.[7,15] The internal jugular (IJV) vein is preferred for the placement of dialysis catheters to avoid injury to the SCV and complications following upper-extremity shunt or fistula placement.[17] The right IJV also is preferred to minimize catheter malposition when fluoroscopic guidance is unavailable because of its direct relationship to the SVC and right atrium. PICC are routinely placed through the antecubital veins or the basilic and cephalic veins in the upper arm.[10]

A routine ultrasound examination of the conventional access sites is performed to determine venous patency. When all conventional access sites are occluded, a variety of unconventional sites are considered, including the inferior vena cava (via translumbar or transhepatic approaches), hepatic vein, collateral channels, and occluded venous segments.[18] A patient with an existing catheter usually will have a new site chosen for the device to minimize the risk of infection. In cases of difficult or limited access sites, the existing site may be used. Indwelling tunnelled catheters also can be exchanged for new catheters using conventional guidewire exchange techniques, particularly when the tunnel has matured.

Most patients prefer to have the device placed on the nondominant side if possible. Previous surgery (e.g., mastectomy) or radiation therapy will dictate contralateral access.

Subclavian/axillary vein

Access techniques to the subclavian vein include (a) standard percutaneous insertion using bony landmarks, (b) fluoroscopic guidance with or without venography, and (c) ultrasound guidance. The standard "blind" technique describes advancing the entry needle along a horizontal plane under the medial two thirds of the clavicle toward the suprasternal notch. Entry into the SCV is quite medial.

Direct puncture of the axillary or SCV can be made under direct fluoroscopic vision during contrast administration via an extremity vein or placement of a guidewire via an antecubital or transfemoral approach (Fig. 35-4).[19] When contrast is being used, a preliminary injection is performed to document patency and to select an appropriate skin site. Following preparation, a second contrast injection is performed, and when the vein is opacified, the needle is advanced at an oblique angle (45 degrees) with a tightly collimated field. The vein will be indented initially by the needle and then entered. Safe entry into the SCV also can be accomplished by using the first rib as a fluoroscopic marker.[20] A skin nick is made at the lateral margin of the second rib, and the 21-gauge needle is obliquely inserted to hit the anterior lateral first rib immediately caudal to the most lateral extent of that rib. With the most lateral aspect of the first rib 90 degrees from vertical, the SCV will cross the first rib between 85 and 104 degrees in 82% of patients.[20] This technique has proved to be an alternative to contrast administration or ultrasonography.

Ultrasound guidance using a 5- or 7.5-MHz linear transducer is our preferred guidance method for venous access (Fig. 35-5). Ultrasound guidance confirms venous patency, allows a more peripheral entry and reduces the risk of pneumothorax and inadvertent arterial puncture.[4,21] It is absolutely critical to enter the vein lateral to the first rib–clavicle junction to prevent the "pinch-off" syndrome.[22,23] When punctures are made more medial, the catheter will traverse the costoclavicular ligament and the tendon of the subclavius muscle. Subsequent arm motion will compress the catheter and lead to fracture and an intravascular foreign body. The SCV/axillary venous segment can be imaged in either the transverse or longitudinal plane (see Fig. 35-5). Longitudinal imaging allows constant identification of the needle tip, whereas transverse imaging allows simultaneous imaging of the vein and adjacent artery.[24] Venous entry should be located between the lateral margins of the first and second ribs. The needle is advanced until the vein is indented. A short thrust is then necessary to puncture the wall. Blood should be freely aspirated before guidewire insertion. Contrast confirmation can be performed but is not necessary with ultrasound guidance. The course of the 0.018-inch guidewire should be observed to ensure that it enters the right atrium and not the aorta and left ventricle (indicating an inadvertent arterial puncture). Note that pulsatile blood (signifying arterial entry) will not occur when a 21-gauge needle enters an artery. The needle should not be advanced farther beyond the vein (avoiding a pneumothorax) but partially withdrawn and redirected when venous entry is not successful. Following placement of the mandril guidewire, a transition catheter is placed into the venous system.

Internal jugular vein

IJV access can be accomplished by using standard or ultrasonography-guided techniques. The most common standard approach to the IJV consists of retracting the carotid artery medially while the needle is inserted at a point midway between the angle of the mandible and clavicle directed toward the ipsilateral nipple. The IJV and immediately adjacent carotid artery are easily imaged with ultrasonography. Displayed in the transverse orientation, the IJV and carotid artery will be side by side, or the vein will lie anterior to the artery (Fig. 35-6). With ultrasound guidance, a rather low site is selected between the two heads of the sternocleidomastoid muscle. Ordinarily, this low approach increases the risk of a pneumothorax when standard techniques are used, but this is not a concern with ultrasonography guidance.[24] A short (4 cm) 21- or 18-gauge needle is used and directly inserted into the IJC. A short, brisk thrust is needed to enter the vein. The appropriate guidewire is then advanced to the right atrium.

Extremity veins

Access for the radiological placement of PICC and extremity ports is most commonly by the cephalic or basilic veins in the upper arm. These devices also can be placed following access of the antecubital veins. Venous access for the upper arm veins is accomplished by either fluoroscopic guidance during contrast administration or by ultrasound (Fig. 35-7). Entry usually is made halfway be-

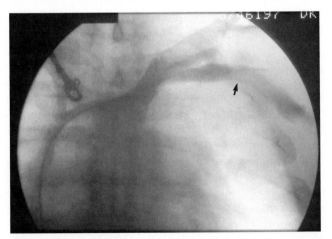

FIGURE 35-4. Venogram of the axillary/subclavian venous segment for venous access. Location where venous entry should be made, lateral to the first rib/clavicle junction (*arrow*).

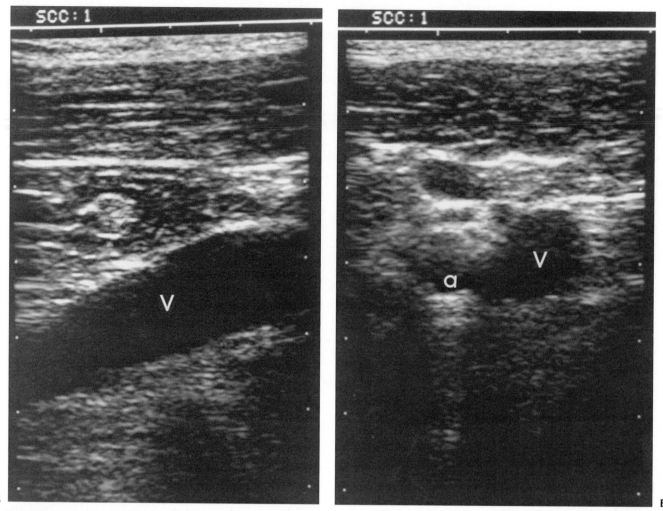

FIGURE 35-5. Subclavian/axillary ultrasound for venous access. **A:** Longitudinal view of large axillary vein (V). **B:** Transverse view of axillary artery (a) and vein (V). The vein is located just inferior to the artery in this location. Safe access requires image guidance.

tween the elbow and axilla. When the fluoroscopic method is used, an intravenous line is started in the antecubital fossa or more distally in the arm.[25,26] A venogram is initially performed to identify an appropriate vein to enter. The vein should be of adequate size (at least 3 to 4 mm in diameter) and should lead directly to the central circulation. Following preparation of the upper arm, a contrast injection is repeated to select the specific site of entry. A local anesthetic is placed and a small dermatotome created. During another contrast injection, a 7-cm, 21-gauge needle is inserted into the vein followed by the 0.018-inch guidewire. If venospasm is present, intravenous nitroglycerin should be administered in small aliquots of 100 to 200 μg.

Veins in the upper extremity also can be imaged by using ultrasound.[24] The veins are imaged in the transverse plane, and the needle is guided directly into the vein. Following free return of blood, a contrast injection should be performed to confirm a continuous path to the heart. The contrast injection can be performed following the placement of a small (3 Fr) dilator.

Unconventional venous access

When conventional sites are occluded, successful catheter placement still can be accomplished by using unconventional sites. The IVC can be accessed via a translumbar approach similar to translumbar aortography (Fig. 35-8). If the common femoral veins are patent, a guidewire can be easily placed into the IVC to serve as a fluoroscopic marker. The chosen skin site is just superior to the iliac crest to allow a 45-degree medial and slight cephalad angulation. Oblique fluoroscopy is used to direct the 21-gauge diamond-tipped needle to the target. If a guidewire was not inserted, the needle is directed to the L-3 vertebral body. Once bony contact is made, the needle is

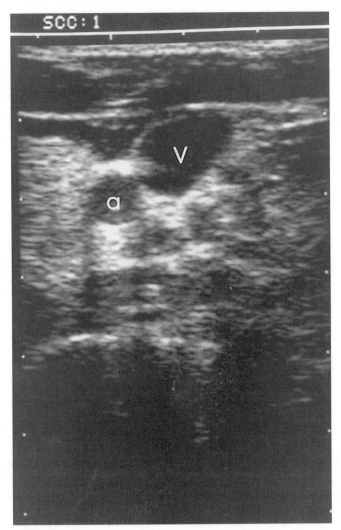

FIGURE 35-6. Transverse ultrasound of the internal jugular vein (V) and carotid artery (a). Access is easily accomplished using transverse imaging.

withdrawn slightly and redirected anteriorly. The stylet is removed, and aspiration is performed as the needle is withdrawn until blood is returned. The 0.018-inch mandril guidewire then is inserted, followed by a transition dilator.[27–31]

If the infrarenal IVC is occluded, the suprarenal IVC can be accessed either by a direct transhepatic approach or through a hepatic vein.[32] We prefer to access the IVC via a peripheral hepatic vein to maximize intravascular catheter length and to facilitate subsequent manipulation. Hepatic vein access usually is accomplished by either a subcostal or intercostal approach using ultrasound guidance. The middle hepatic vein is most suitable for ultrasound targeting because of its anterior course. The hepatic veins also can be accessed using fluoroscopic guidance in which percutaneous transhepatic cholangiography (PTC)-like passes are made through the liver

with a 21- or 22-gauge needle and withdrawn during aspiration. When blood is returned, contrast is injected to confirm hepatic vein entry. Hepatic-vein access has been most useful in children with short-gut syndrome in whom all other sites have become occluded.

Collateral channels develop around chronic venous occlusions. These channels can be identified with either ultrasonography or during venography and directly accessed. With the use of hydrophilic and steerable catheters and guidewires, these collateral channels may be able to be catheterized with eventual central access. Exchange-length hydrophilic guidewires then can be used to insert catheters into the central circulation. The newer polyurethane materials are preferable to silicone because they have small outer diameters and they track over guidewires more easily.[18,33] Catheterization of the dominant collateral can result in extremity edema if subsequent thrombosis occurs, but if it must be done, the patient should be given a low dose of coumadin (1 mg/day) to help prevent thrombosis.

■ Device Insertion (Table 35-2)

PICC

Immediately following access, an appropriately sized peel-away sheath is inserted. A more exact measurement can be obtained by advancing the guidewire to the final location of the catheter tip and clamping the guidewire at the hub of the dilator. An additional length often is added to allow the catheter to be coiled so that the hub is directed toward the axilla (for upper arm placement).[10–12, 26]

Nontunnelled, centrally placed catheters: Hohn catheter

The nontapered catheter often can be inserted into the venous system directly over the 0.018-inch guidewire. In obese patients, a transition dilator, followed by an 8 Fr peel-away sheath, can be inserted, followed by the Hohn catheter. The peel-away sheath is removed following placement.[4,13]

Tunnelled catheters (Figs. 35-9 and 35-10)

Following venous access, a transition dilator is placed into the right atrium, and an intravascular guidewire measurement is made. The tip of the guidewire is placed at the desired location of the catheter tip, and the guidewire then is kinked at the hub. The guidewire is withdrawn until the tip is at the venous access site, at which time a hemostat is clamped to the guidewire. The distance from the clamp and kink represents the length of catheter required from the venous access site to final tip location.

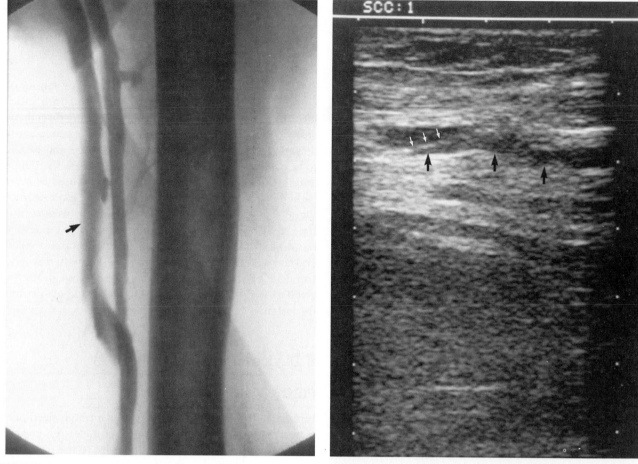

FIGURE 35-7. Extremity vein access. **A:** Venogram of upper extremity demonstrating continuity of flow to the heart and localizing site of venous entry (*arrow*). **B:** Longitudinal ultrasound of basilic vein (*black arrows*) showing guide wire (*white arrows*) within vein.

Typically, catheter tips are located in the distal SVC or proximal right atrium.[4,5,7,34]

The exit site in the skin for tunnelled catheters placed through the SCV/axillary vein is typically adjacent to the inferior aspect of the sternum. For IVC catheters, the exit site is usually in the lateral aspect of the upper abdominal or lower chest wall.[18,31]

For end-hole catheters, a blunt tunnelling tool (supplied in a kit) is negotiated from the catheter exit site to the venous access site. Then the catheter is connected to the tail of the tunnelling tool and brought through the tunnel. The Dacron cuff is situated approximately 1 to 2 cm from the exit site. The catheter is trimmed using the intravascular guidewire measurement. For valved-tipped catheters, the tunnel is created in the reverse direction: from venous access site to skin exit site. Valved-tipped catheters should not be cut at the tip but should instead be trimmed from the hub end following placement of the tip into the venous system and the proximal end through the subcutaneous tunnel.[8]

After the end-hole catheter has been trimmed to the correct length, a 0.038-inch guidewire is inserted through the transition dilator and exchanged for the appropriately sized peel-away sheath (supplied in a kit). The patient must be carefully instructed and reminded to suspend respirations during this period to avoid air embolism. Alternatively, the patient can be instructed to hum, or if the patient is unable to cooperate, the sheath can be pinched between the fingers to help avoid air embolism.[35] The catheter is inserted and its position is intermittently checked until its final location is satisfactory, at which time the sheath is removed.

Occasionally, the catheter will enter the IJV (from an SCV access) or the contralateral brachiocephalic vein.[36–38] Rotation of the beveled catheter tip, deep inspirations, placement of a long sheath or a forceful saline injection will often correct the situation.[4,36] When these maneuvers fail, a hydrophilic guidewire steered into the SVC will solve the problem. Kinking of the sheath will not allow passage of the catheter and may occur at the site of venous entry

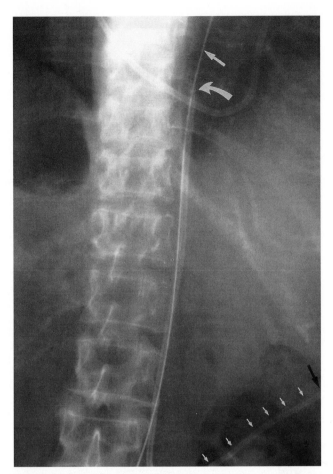

FIGURE 35-8. Translumbar Hickman catheter placement. Because of occlusion of all chest access sites, a Hickman catheter was placed into the central venous system via a translumbar approach. *Large straight white arrow:* guidewire placed transfemorally to mark the location of the IVC. *Curved white arrow:* tip of catheter at right atrium (RA) *Small white arrows:* course of catheter through retoperitoneum. *Black arrow:* skin site for venous access. Patient is prone.

TABLE 35-2. Device Insertion

Device	Insertion steps
Peripherally inserted central catheter	Access vein
	GW to RA, insert sheath
	GW measurement, trim catheter
	Insert catheter
Nontunnelled chest wall catheter	Access vein
	GW to RA
	Dilate
	Insert catheter
Tunnelled chest-wall catheter "Hickman type"	Access vein
	Place temporary catheter
	GW measurement
	Create tunnel
	Bring catheter through tunnel and trim length
	Insert sheath
	Insert catheter
Subcutaneous port: chest wall "pre-attached"	Access vein
	Place temporary catheter
	GW measurement
	Create pocket and tunnel
	Bring catheter through tunnel and seat port into pocket
	Secure port to deep fascia
	Access port and flush
	Close incision
	Trim catheter to length
	Insert sheath
	Insert catheter
Extremity "attachable"	Access vein
	Insert sheath
	Insert catheter and flush
	Create pocket and tunnel (if needed)
	Bring catheter through tunnel and trim to length
	Attach catheter to port and flush
	Seat port into pocket
	Close incision

US, ultrasound; GW, Guidewire; RA, Right atrium.

(e.g., in obese patients in whom a vertical-needle approach is used) or at the acute angle formed by the SCV and right brachiocephalic vein. This can often be avoided by a peripheral and oblique needle insertion. If kinking occurs at the brachiocephalic vein, the sheath is withdrawn as forward pressure is maintained on the catheter. The catheter will eventually pass when the sheath is withdrawn proximal to the acute junction. Kinking at the vein must be overcome by external pressure applied to the soft tissues in an effort to reduce the kink.

After venous placement is completed, the catheter is secured with sutures (3-0 or 4-0) placed at the venous access and catheter exit sites. The suture placed at the catheter exit site is also wrapped around the catheter for additional stability. The catheter then is heparinized, and an external dressing is applied.

Subcutaneous ports

Chest wall ports (Figs. 35-11 and 35-12)

In addition to the standard materials for venous entry, a surgical cut-down tray containing the appropriate scalpels, scissors, and other instruments will be needed. Formation of the subcutaneous pocket will follow the initial venous access. A site on the upper chest wall inferior to the clavicle with ample subcutaneous tissue is chosen. The pocket should avoid breast tissue and the axilla. Following local anesthesia of xylocaine with epinephrine, a horizontal 5-cm skin incision is made with a no. 15 blade. Vertical incisions can be made but are not preferred. The pocket may be situated either superior or inferior to the incision. The relationship of the pocket to the incision is based on physician preference. The following discussion assumes that the incision has been placed inferior to the pocket.[4,14,15]

The pocket is formed using blunt dissection and should be just large enough to accommodate the device

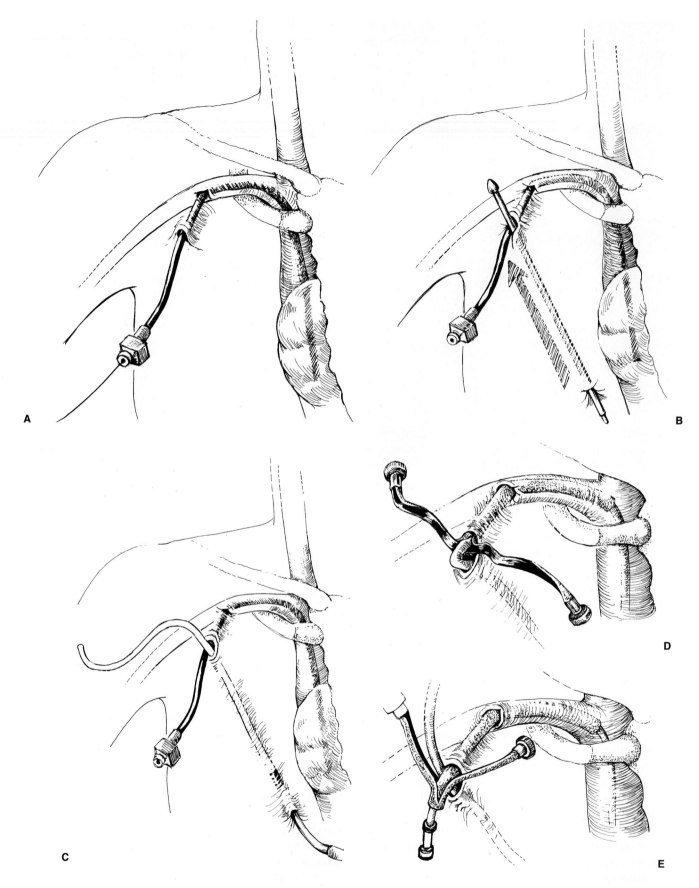

A

B

C

D

E

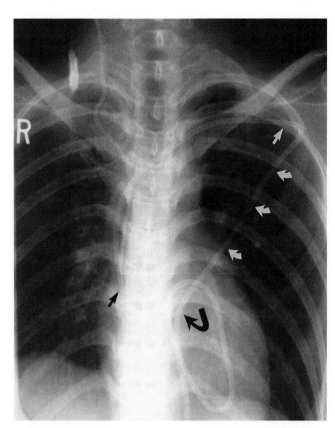

FIGURE 35-10. Postinsertion radiograph of a Hickman catheter. *Straight black arrow:* Catheter tip at right atrium (RA)/superior vena cava (SVC) junction. *Curved black arrow:* Catheter exit site at parasternal border. *Straight white arrow:* Venous access site. *Curved white arrows:* Catheter within subcutaneous tunnel.

needle connected to tubing. The port and catheter are flushed with normal saline. The pocket is closed in a two-layer fashion using deep interrupted, inverted subcuticular stitches with 3-0 or 4-0 absorbable sutures and interrupted skin sutures using 3-0 or 4-0 monofilament nonabsorbable suture. This wound closure method is the technique used at the University of North Carolina. Another popular closure technique is a running subcuticular stitch with absorbable suture and Steristrips (3M Health Corp., St. Paul, MN) applied at the skin level.

Following closure of the subcutaneous pocket, the catheter is cut to a length based on the intravascular guidewire measurement obtained during placement of the transition dilator. The appropriately sized peel-away sheath is placed. While the patient suspends respirations (having the patient hum is also useful), the guidewire and dilator are removed and the catheter is placed through the peel-away sheath into the proper location confirmed by fluoroscopy. The peel-away sheath is removed. Blood is aspirated from the port through the indwelling needle and flushed first with saline and then with heparin (according to manufacturer's recommendations). A single nonabsorbable suture is placed in the original venous access dermatotom. Then all incisions are dressed.

When a valved type catheter or a detached end-hole catheter has been chosen, the subcutaneous pocket is placed inferior to the incision. After the pocket is created, the catheter is placed into the venous system via its peel-away sheath and is properly positioned. The peel-away sheath is removed, and a tunnel is created from the venous access dermatotom to the incision. The back end of the catheter is brought through the tunnel, trimmed to the correct length, and connected to the port. Blood is aspirated from the port and flushed with saline. The port is placed in the pocket and secured to the deep fascia. All incisions are closed. The port is finally accessed through the skin with a noncoring needle to confirm a functioning port. Then the port is heparinized.

Extremity ports

Following venous access into the basilic or cephalic veins, a peel-away sheath is placed in the venous system. The pocket is created by making a transverse incision, which may include the initial access site. Alternatively, the in-

without excessive tension on the apposed margins of the incision. A pocket that is too large may allow port torsion to occur. The port is placed into the pocket, checking for size and position. If these are suitable, the pocket is inspected visually to ensure that no bleeding is present. At this time, a tunnel is created to connect the upper outer portion of the subcutaneous pocket to the original venous access site. If a preattached port (catheter and port connected in the factory) was chosen, the catheter is brought through the tunnel and the port positioned into the pocket. The port then is sutured to the deep fascia using 3-0 absorbable suture. At this time, the port is accessed through the skin with a special noncoring

FIGURE 35-9. Hickman catheter insertion. **A:** Following venous entry, a transition dilator is placed into the subclavian axillary vein (SVC). Note entry lateral to first rib/clavicle junction. **B:** The subcutaneous tunnel then is created by using a blunt tunneling tool passed within the subcutaneous space from the catheter exit site (adjacent to the lower aspect of the sternum) to the venous access skin site. **C:** The catheter is attached to the rear of the tunneling tool and dragged through the tunnel such that the Dacron cuff lies 1 to 2 cm from the catheter exit site. The catheter tip then is trimmed to length based on the intravascular guidewire measurement obtained earlier in the procedure. **D:** The transition dilator is exchanged over a guidewire for the peel-away sheath. While the patient suspends respirations, the inner dilator and guidewire are removed and the Hickman catheter is placed through the sheath to its final location. The peel-away sheath is removed, the catheter is flushed and heparinized, incisions are closed, and the catheter is dressed. **E:** The peel-away sheath is removed while maintaining portion of indwelling catheter.

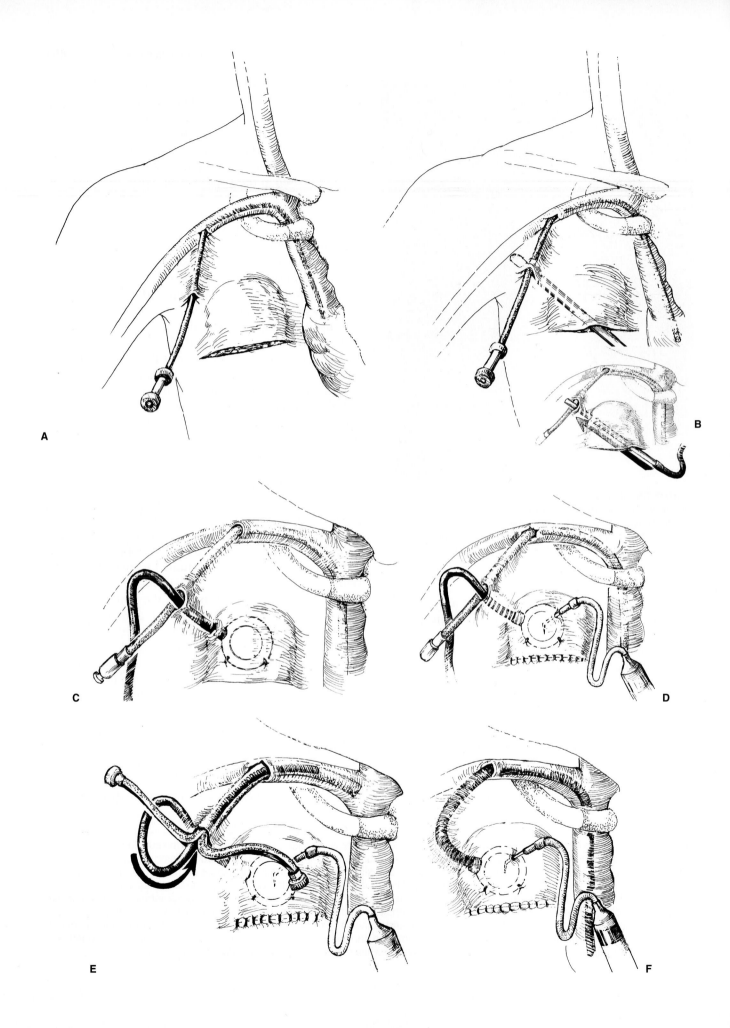

A

B

C

D

E

F

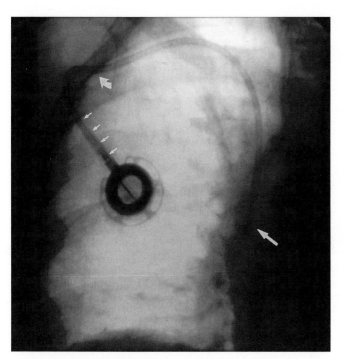

FIGURE 35-12. Postinsertion radiography of a subcutaneous port: *Large straight arrow:* Tip of catheter at right atrium (RA)/subclavian axillary vein (SVC) junction. *Curved arrow:* venous access site. *Small straight arrows:* portion of catheter in subcutaneous tunnel connecting pocket to the venous access site.

Dialysis catheters (Fig. 35-13)

Most dialysis catheters are dual-lumen, staggered-tipped catheters that are capable of high (> 250 mL/min) flow rates. They are available in cuffed (long-term catheters requiring a subcutaneous tunnel) or noncuffed (temporary, short-term catheters without a tunnel) designs. Dialysis catheters are placed via the large central veins because of their relatively large size. The IJV is preferred, but the risk of subclavian vein stenosis is avoided because it may complicate upper-extremity shunt placement.

Noncuffed tapered dialysis catheters are designed for short-term use and are placed using standard Seldinger techniques.[4] The cuffed dialysis catheters have a non-tapered tip and are available in a number of fixed lengths. These catheters cannot be trimmed. Following venous access, an intravascular guidewire measurement is made from the projected position of the distal tip (usually in the proximal RA) to the venous access site. Using this measurement, the appropriate catheter is chosen so that the cuff will lie in the proximal portion of the tunnel. The tunnel may be created in a supraclavicular or infraclavicular location. The tunnel is created from the catheter exit site to the venous access site, and the catheter is brought through it. The large peel-away sheath is placed in the vein and the catheter is placed in the venous system after the guidewire and dilator is removed while the patient suspends respirations,[4,42] which is critically important, because if the patient inspires while the large sheath is not occluded, an air embolism will occur. The peel-away sheath is removed, and each lumen is heparinized according to manufacturer's recommendations, which vary with the length of the catheter.

An alternative to the standard dual-lumen catheter is two single-lumen catheters. The Tesio twin-catheter system entails two 10 Fr catheters, each with a large end hole and multiple side holes that are placed via adjacent internal jugular vein punctures. The two catheters serve as the "venous" and "arterial" lumen, respectively. The venous catheter is positioned 2 to 4 cm distal to the arterial catheter.[43–45] Following placement, twin parallel tunnels are created from the access site to the catheter exit site, which is commonly positioned adjacent to the sternum inferior to the clavicle. The back ends of these catheters can be trimmed because of their removable hubs.

cision for the pocket can be placed distal to the venous access site, in which case a short tunnel connecting the two sites will be required. Once an adequate pocket is made, the catheter is inserted into the venous system through the peel-away sheath and placed at the SVC/right atrium (RA) junction confirmed by fluoroscopy. The sheath is removed, and the back end of the catheter is brought through the tunnel (if needed) to exit at the incision. The catheter is trimmed and connected to the port, which then is flushed with saline. The port then is placed in the pocket and secured with absorbable sutures. The incision is closed by using either interrupted subcuticular plus skin suture or a running subcuticular stitch with Steri-strips at the skin. The port is finally accessed through the skin and heparinized.[16,39–41]

←

FIGURE 35-11. Subcutaneous port insertion: **A:** Following venous access and the placement of a temporary catheter into the superior vena cava (SVC) a horizontal incision is made with a no. 15 blade and the subcutaneous pocket is created with blunt dissection. In this diagram, a preattached port will be placed which allows the pocket to be created superior to the incision. **B:** Following the creation of an adequately sized pocket, a tunnel is made from the upper outer aspect of the pocket to the venous access site. **C:** The tip of the catheter is attached to the tunneling tool and brought through the tunnel, and the port is placed into the pocket. Two sutures usually are placed, fixating the port to the deep fascia, and the catheter is cut to length. **D:** The port is accessed with a special noncoring needle and flushed with heparinized saline. The incision then is closed. **E:** The temporary catheter is exchanged over a guide for the peel-away sheath, and the catheter is inserted into the venous system as the patient suspends respirations. **F:** The peel-away sheath is removed, and the port is flushed and heparinized.

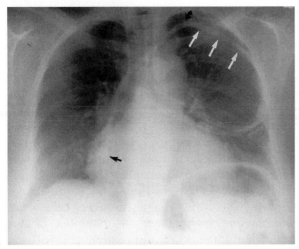
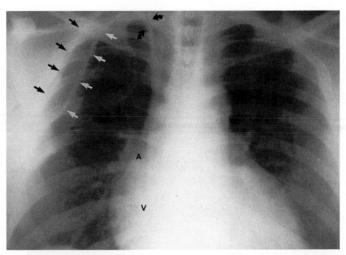

A   B

FIGURE 35-13. Dialysis catheters. **A:** Radiograph of a dual-lumen dialysis catheter placed via the left internal jugular vein (IJV) and tunneled over the clavicle onto the chest wall. *Straight black arrow:* tip of catheter in RA. *Curved black arrow:* access site in left IJV. *Straight white arrows:* catheter within subcutaneous tunnel on the chest wall. **B:** Radiograph of the dual Tesio dialysis catheter system placed via the right IJV and tunneled onto the chest wall. A, tip of arterial catheter at RA/SVC junction V, tip of venous catheter 4 cm lower in the right atrium. *Curved arrows:* sites of right IJV access. *Straight arrows:* parallel tunnels onto the chest wall.

■ Catheter Management and Removal

In addition to device selection and insertion, the interventional radiologist must become familiar with postprocedural catheter care, patient follow-up, diagnosis, and management of catheter-related complications and, finally, device removal. A specialized nursing team for patient education and supervision of routine catheter care will help in significantly reducing the frequency of catheter-related thrombosis and infections.[46] Adherence to strict sterile techniques while accessing these devices, routine dressing changes, and proper catheter heparinization cannot be overemphasized. Nurses who are specialized in infusion management also are trained in catheter repair using commercially available repair kits. Radiologists involved in this service should have these kits available and become familiar with their use.

Device removal is the responsibility of the service that initially places that device. Nontunnelled catheters are simply removed following release of the tape or sutures. Before a tunnelled catheter is removed, the catheter and tunnel are thoroughly prepared and draped. The skin site and the area around the cuff are infiltrated with a local anesthetic. Gentle blunt dissection is performed around the cuff using a hemostat. The catheter then is removed with steady traction. The cuff usually is dislodged from the subcutaneous tissues along with the catheter. If the cuff is not dissected free, it may be left behind. The retained cuff could be a continued nidus of infection in cases of sepsis or a tunnel infection. In these cases, the cuff should be removed. When the cuff is initially positioned within 1 to 2 cm from the exit site (as is our standard practice), it usually can be dissected free and removed with the cathe-

ter. When the cuff is located some distance from the exit site and requires removal, a separate incision over the cuff parallel to the tunnel is required for its removal.

Removal of a subcutaneous port requires a sterile site preparation analogous to its insertion. A surgical cutdown also is used to provide the adequate tools. For removal, the skin incision is made overlying the prior incision. Following dissection, a white sheath is identified surrounding the device and catheter, which will need to be incised and dissected free. The port will easily slide from this pocket. External pressure is applied for hemostasis. A two-layer closure is preferred. When needed, additional deep sutures should be placed to eliminate only any dead space that could lead to subsequent hematoma or seroma formation and an increased risk of infection.

■ Complications

Procedural complications

Access failure and catheter malposition constitute minor procedural complications. Blinded percutaneous access failure occurs in 5 to 8.9% of cases compared with less than 2% when radiologic guidance techniques are used.[8,15,16,21,47] Similarly, blind placement results in a 1.2 to 2.5% incidence of catheter malposition immediately following placement.[21,47,48] With radiologic guidance, catheter malposition is immediately detected and corrected. A patient should not leave the suite with a malpositioned catheter.

Major procedural complications include hematomas, pneumothorax, air embolism, and nerve injury.[35] Hematomas typically result from an inadvertent arterial needle puncture or bleeding within the subcutaneous tunnel or pocket. The use of a 21-gauge needle, image guidance (ultrasound, fluoroscopy), and a peripheral puncture has virtually eliminated a significant hematoma resulting from an inadvertent arterial puncture.[8,15,21] Contrast injection or careful observation of the 0.018-inch guidewire will always confirm venous entry. Tunnel and subcutaneous pocket hematomas occur more commonly in patients with a coagulopathy. Any coagulation and platelet abnormality should be corrected before tunneled or buried devices are placed. If necessary, a temporary nontunneled device may be placed until the patient's coagulation status is normalized.

Image guidance also has reduced the pneumothorax rate to less than 1%.[8,15,21] In addition, the pneumothorax secondary to a 21-gauge needle is typically small and will resolve spontaneously. If not, it is easy to place a small catheter percutaneously in the apex through the second anterior intercostal space and to place it to an underwater seal.

An air embolism may occur if the patient inspires when the peel-away is open to the atmosphere. In a study of percutaneously placed large-bore hemodialysis catheters, air embolism occurred in 0.8% of cases, with no sequelae.[42] The air accumulates in the pulmonary outflow tract and main pulmonary artery. Oxygen should be administered, and the patient should be observed. The air will dissipate in several minutes.

Long-term complications

Long-term or delayed complications include mechanical, thrombotic, and infectious complications. The interventional radiologist must be familiar with the detection and management of these complications.

Mechanical complications

Delayed catheter migration into the internal jugular vein, azygous vein, or contralateral innominate vein is caused by head or arm motion and a short catheter. A forceful injection of saline or placement of a guidewire or a transfemoral relocation can correct the malposition.[36–38] If catheter migration recurs, the device should be exchanged for a longer catheter.

Catheter fragmentation is caused by the mechanical stress on the catheter when it pierces the subclavius muscle and the costoclavicular ligament as it courses through the clavicle/first rib space ("pinch-off" syndrome).[22,23,49] The fragment may lie anywhere from the subclavian vein to the pulmonary arteries. The average time between insertion and fragmentation is 6.5 months.[23] When fragmentation is discovered, the remaining device is removed and the free fragment is retrieved by using conventional intravascular foreign-body retrieval techniques. This potential complication can be eliminated with venous entry lateral to the clavicle/first rib space.

The repeated use of external catheters may cause fatigue and fracture of the hubs and external tubing. Repair kits are commercially available for their repair. A severely damaged device must be replaced.

Thrombotic complications

Catheter-related thrombosis is a general term that may include thrombus within the catheter lumen and thrombus within the vein and the fibrin sheath that surrounds the catheter. The reported incidence varies greatly, depending on whether the diagnosis is made clinically or by some diagnostic test. The incidence of catheter-related thrombus varies from 3 to 70%.[50–52] Patients who have malignancies or who are in hypercoagulable states and those that are receiving caustic solutions (chemotherapy, hyperalimentation) are particularly susceptible to thrombotic complications. Clinical signs and symptoms of catheter-related thrombosis include ipsilateral swelling of the neck and arm, venous distention, and nonspecific pain in the neck and anterior chest wall.

The inability to aspirate blood is often the first indication of problems relating to thrombus or a fibrin sheath. A fibrin sleeve develops around all catheters in place for longer than a week.[50] When the sleeve reaches the tip of the catheter, it will cause dysfunction. Contrast injection will show a stream of contrast that tracks back along the catheter and even extravasate from the venous entry site. Passing a guidewire through the catheter breaking the fibrin sleeve at the tip may restore function. Fibrin stripping using a transfemorally placed loop snare has been used successfully in maintaining catheter function.[53,54] The snare is placed over the catheter, tightened, and pulled down, stripping the sleeve. Simple catheter exchange over a guidewire through the same tunnel (for tunnelled catheters) also will restore function and will avoid a new puncture; the patient will be able to leave immediately after the procedure. The relationships of this fibrin sleeve and catheter thrombosis and infection are not well understood. Inability to aspirate blood can also occur when the catheter tip is against the vein wall, a problem often corrected by a change in head or arm position or a Valsalva maneuver.

Treatment of luminal or vein thrombosis involves combinations of intracatheter thrombolytic therapy, anticoagulation, venous thrombolysis, and catheter removal. Luminal thrombotic occlusion is treated with a low-dose thrombolytic regimen. A bolus is injected into the catheter and aspirated after a 30-min dwell time. If this is unsuccessful, an infusion may be used for 6 to 12 hr.[5,42] Patency is restored in more than 95% of cases. Treatment of venous thrombosis depends on the severity of symptoms, the need for access, and the availability of other sites. In patients with long-term need and limited access, heparinization followed by coumadin is used with the catheter left in place. For particularly symptomatic patients, venous thrombolytic therapy with urokinase also will be used.[50,55,56] Symptomatic patients with long-term need but with other available sites simply may be treated with catheter removal, new catheter placement, and anticoagulation. Signs of septic thrombophlebitis require immediate catheter removal and appropriate antibiotic treatment. Long-term low-dose (1 mg daily) coumadin and even full anticoagulation have been used to prevent thrombosis.[57]

Infectious complications

Catheter-related infections occur at the catheter exit site, within the subcutaneous tunnel or pocket or systemically as catheter related bacteremia (or sepsis).[58-60] Exit-site infections often present with erythema and tenderness at the exit site in addition to an exudate. A tunnel or subcutaneous pocket infection is more serious and is characterized by erythema and tenderness along the tunnel or over the pocket. Pus may be expressed from the tunnel by "milking" the tract. Catheter-related bacteremias present with fever and a leukocytosis and often are used as a diagnosis of exclusion in a patient with no other apparent source of sepsis. Clinical evidence implicating the catheter as a source of sepsis includes (a) an exit-site or tunnel infection caused by the same organism isolated from the blood, (b) clinical sepsis refractory to antibiotics but resolves following catheter removal, (c) positive quantitative catheter culture with isolation of the same organism from bloodstream, and (d) a differential quantitative blood culture greater than 10-fold colony count of organisms isolated from blood obtained through the catheter and from blood obtained from a peripheral site.[58,61] Catheter-related infections arise from contamination at the skin insertion site, colonization of the catheter hub, hematogenous seeding of the catheter, and infusate contamination.[58-60] Catheter-related infections occur in 10 to 30% of patients with a rate of 0.2 episodes per 100 days at risk.[42,59,60] This rate compares favorably to surgical reports.

Local (exit site or subcutaneous) infections must be detected early and aggressively treated to save the device. Gram stain and culture of any drainage should be performed. Most (50–70%) of these infections are caused by skin flora. Gram-positive organisms are effectively treated with a 10- to 14-day course of intracath vancomycin hydrochloride.[42,50] Early erythema with drainage may be treated with oral antibiotics. If the condition does not improve or worsens on therapy, the device is removed immediately and new cultures are obtained. Even with treatment, the device is salvaged in only 25% of patients with tunnel infections and 70% with exit site infections.[50,59]

Catheter-related bacteremias are treated with intravenous antibiotics according to culture and sensitivity studies. If, however, no improvement has occurred in 48 to 72 hr, the device must be removed. Even when the device is salvaged, there is a 20% chance the bacteremia will recur compared with a 3% risk of recurrence if the device is removed.[58]

■ Conclusion

The need for central venous access is expanding rapidly. This service can be provided economically and expeditiously by an interventional radiologist. Most cases can be completed within 45 to 60 min. The devices can be placed safely, and the late infectious and thrombotic complications seen with these procedures are comparable to those seen when the devices are placed within an operating room. The skills and technology available to interventional radiologists place them in a unique position to deliver this service.

REFERENCES

1. Broviac JW, Cole JJ, Scribner BH. A silicone rubber atrial catheter for prolonged parenteral alimentation. *Surg Gynecol Obstet* 1973; 136:602–606.
2. Hickman RO, Buckner CD, Clift RA, et al. A modified right atrial catheter for access to the venous system in marrow transplant recipients. *Surg Gynecol Obstet* 1979;148:871–875.
3. Niederhuber JE, Ensminger W, Gyves J, et al. Totally implanted venous and arterial access system to replace external catheters in cancer treatment. *Surgery* 1982;92:706–712.
4. Mauro MA, Jaques PF. Radiological placement of long-term central venous catheters: a review. *J Vasc Interv Radiol* 1993;4:127–137.
5. Denny DF. Placement and management of long-term central venous access catheters and ports. *AJR Am J Roentgenol* 1993;161: 385–393.
6. Denny DF. Venous access: techniques and management. In: SCVIR Program. San Diego: Society of Cardiovascular and Interventional *Radiology* 1994:210–218.
7. Robertson LJ, Mauro MA, Jaques PF. Radiologic placement of Hickman catheters. *Radiology* 1989;170:1007–1009.
8. Hull JE, Hunter CS, Luiken GA. The groshong catheter: initial experience and early results of imaging-guided placement. *Radiology* 1992;185:803–807.
9. Braun MA. Image-guided peripheral venous access catheters and implantable ports. *Semin Interv Radiol* 1994;2,358–365.
10. Cardella JF, Fox PS, Lawler JB. Interventional radiological placement of peripherally inserted central catheters. *J Vasc Interv Radiol* 1993;4:653–660.
11. Andrews JC, Marx MV, Williams DM, et al. The upper arm approach for placement of peripherally inserted central catheters for protracted venous access. *AJR Am J Roentgenol* 1992;158:427–429.
12. Hovsepian DM, Bonn J, Eschelman DJ. Techniques for peripheral insertion of central venous catheters. *J Vasc Interv Radiol* 1993;4: 795–803.
13. Openshaw KL, Picus D, Hicks ME, et al. Interventional radiologic placement of Hohn central venous catheters: results and complications in 100 consecutive patients. *J Vasc Interv Radiol* 1994;5:111–115.

14. Campbell WE, Mauro MA, Jaques PF. Radiological insertion of long-term venous access devices. *Semin Interv Radiol* 1994;2:366–376.

15. Morris SL, Jaques PF, Mauro MA. Radiology-assisted placement of implantable subcutaneous infusion ports for long-term venous access. *Radiology* 1992;184:149–151.

16. Kahn MO, Barboza RB, Kling GA, et al. Initial experience with percutaneous placement of the P.A.S. port implantable venous access device. *J Vasc Interv Radiol* 1992;3:459–461.

17. Stalter KA, Stevens GF, Sterling WA. Late stenosis of the subclavian vein after hemodialysis catheter injury. *Surgery* 1986;100:924–927.

18. Kazanjian SA, Kaufman JA. Strategies for central venous catheter placement in patients with limited access. *Semin Interv Radiol* 1994;2:377–387.

19. Selby JB, Tegtmeyer CJ, Amodeo C. Insertion of subclavian hemodialysis catheters in difficult cases: value of fluoroscopy and angiographic techniques. *AJR Am J Roentgenol* 1989;152:641–643.

20. Jaques PF, Campbell WE, Dumbleton S, et al. The first rib as a fluoroscopic marker for subclavian vein access. *J Vasc Interv Radiol* 1995;6:619–622.

21. Lameris JS, Post PJM, Zonderland HM, et al. Percutaneous placement of Hickman catheters: comparison of sonographically guided and blind techniques. *AJR Am J Roentgenol* 1990;155:1097–1099.

22. Hinke DH, Zandt-Stastny DA, Goodman LR, et al. Pinch-off syndrome: a complication of implantable subclavian venous access devices. *Radiology* 1990;177:353–356.

23. Lafrenirre R. Indwelling subclavian catheters and a visit with the "pinch-off" syndrome. *J Surg Oncol* 1991;47:261–264.

24. Jaques PF, Mauro MA, Keefe B. Ultrasonographic guidance for vascular access. *J Vasc Interv Radiol* 1992;3:427–430.

25. Andrews JC, Walker-Andrews SC, William DE. Long-term central venous access with a peripherally placed subcutaneous infusion port: initial results. *Radiology* 1990;176:45–47.

26. Bonn J. Venous access: peripherally inserted central catheters, SCVIR Program. San Diego: Society of Cardiovascular and Interventional Radiology, 1994:204–210.

27. Denny DF, Dorfman GS, Greenwood LH, et al. Translumbar inferior vena cava Hickman catheter placement for total parenteral nutrition. *AJR Am J Roentgenol* 1987;148:621–622.

28. Denny DF, Greenwood LH, Morse SS, et al. Inferior vena cava: translumbar catheterization for central venous access. *Radiology* 1989;170:1013–1014.

29. Kaufman JA, Greenfield AJ, Fitzpatrick GF. Transhepatic cannulation of the inferior vena cava. *J Vasc Interv Radiol* 1991;2:321–334.

30. Robertson LJ, Jaques PF, Mauro MA, et al. Percutaneous inferior vena cava placement of tunnelled Silastic catheters for prolonged vascular access in infants. *J Pediatr Surg* 1990;25:596–598.

31. Lund GB, Lieberman RP, Haire WD, et al. Translumbar inferior vena cava catheters for long-term venous access. *Radiology* 1990; 174:31–35.

32. Azizkhan RG, Taylor LA, Jaques PF, et al. Percutaneous translumbar and transhepatic inferior vena cava catheters for prolonged vascular access in children. *J Pediatr Surg* 1992;27:165–169.

33. Andrews JC. Percutaneous placement of a Hickman catheter with use of an intercostal vein for access. *J Vasc Interv Radiol* 1994;5:859–861.

34. Dick L, Mauro MA, Jaques PF, et al. Radiologic insertion of Hickman catheters in HIV-positive patients: infectious complications. *J Vasc Interv Radiol* 1991;2:327–329.

35. Lund GB. Complications from long-term tunnelled venous access catheters: a review. *Semin Interv Radiol* 1994;2:340–348.

36. Carasco CH, Richli WR, Chusilp C, et al. Technical note: repositioning misplaced central venous catheters. *Cardiovasc Interv Radiol* 1987;10:234–236.

37. Lois JF, Gomes AS, Pussey R. Non-surgical repositioning of central venous catheters. *Radiology* 1987;165:329–333.

38. Olcott EW, Gordon RL, Ring EJ. The injection technique for repositioning central venous catheters: technical note. *Cardiovasc Interv Radiol* 1989;12:292–293.

39. Andrews JC, Marx MV, Williams DM, et al. The upper arm approach for placement of peripherally inserted central catheters for protracted venous access. *AJR Am J Roentgenol* 1992;158:427–429.

40. Brant-Zawadzki M, Anthony M, Mercer EC. Implantation of P.A.S. port venous access device in the forearm under fluoroscopic guidance. *AJR Am J Roentgenol* 1993;160:1127–1128.

41. Foley MJ. Radiologic placement of long-term central venous peripheral access system ports (PAS port): results in 150 patients. *J Vasc Interv Radiol* 1995;6:255–262.

42. Lund GB, Trerotola SO, Scheel PF, et al. Outcome of tunneled hemodialysis catheters placed by radiologists. *Radiology* 1996;198:467–472.

43. Tesio F, De Baz H, Panarello G, et al. Double catheterization of the internal jugular vein for hemodialysis: indication, techniques, and clinical results. *Artif Organs* 1993;18:301–304.

44. Ganaud B, Beraud JJ, Joyeux H, et al. Internal jugular vein cannulation using 2 silastic catheters: a new, simple and safe long-term vascular access for extracorporeal treatment. *Nephron* 1986;43:133–138.

45. Canaud B, Beraud JJ, Joyeux H, et al. Internal jugular cannulation with two silicone rubber catheters: a new and safe temporary vascular access for hemodialysis: thirty months' experience. *Artif Organs* 1986;10:397–403.

46. Keohane PP, Attrill H, Northover J. Effect of catheter tunnelling and a nutrition nurse on catheter sepsis during parenteral nutrition. *Lancet* 1983;17:1388–1390.

47. Takasugi JK, O'Connell TX. Prevention of complications in permanent central venous catheters. *Surg Gynecol Obstet* 1988;167:6–11.

48. Delmore JE, Horbelt DV. Jack BI, et al. Experience with the groshong long-term central venous catheter. *Gynecol Oncol* 1989; 34:215–218.

49. Rubenstein RB, Alberty RE, Michels LG, et al. Hickman catheter separation. *JPEN* 1985;9:754–757.

50. Lowell JA, Bothe A Jr. Venous access preoperative, operative, and postoperative dilemmas. *Surg Clin North Am* 1991;71:1231–1246.

51. Haire WD, Lieberman RP, Lund GB, et al. Thrombotic complications of silicone rubber catheters during autologous marrow and peripheral stem cell transplantation: prospective comparison of Hickman and groshong catheters. *Bone Marrow Transplant* 1991;7:57–59.

52. Anderson AJ, Krasnow SH, Boyer MW, et al. Thrombosis: the major Hickman catheter complication in patients with solid tumor. *Chest* 1989;95:71–75.

53. Crain MR, Mewissen MW, Ostrowski GJ, et al. Fibrin sleeve stripping for salvage of failing hemodialysis catheters: technique and initial results. *Radiology* 1996;198:41–44.

54. Hosal VL, Ause RG, Hoskins PA. Fibrin sleeve formation on indwelling subclavian central venous catheters. *Arch Surg* 1971;102:353–358.

55. Moss JF, Wagman LD, Riihimaki DU, et al. Central venous thrombosis related to the silastic Hickman-Broviac catheters in an oncologic population. *J Parenter Enteral Nutr* 1989;13:397–400.

56. Gray WJ, Bell WR. Fibrinolytic agents in the treatment of thrombotic disorder. *Semin Oncol* 1990;17:228–237.

57. Bern MM, Lokich JJ, Wallach SR, et al. Very low doses of warfarin can prevent thrombosis in central venous catheters. *Ann Intern Med* 1990;112:423–428.

58. Raad II, Bodey GP. Infectious complications of indwelling vascular catheters. *Clin Infect Dis* 1992;15:197–210.

59. Clarke DE, Raffin TA. Infectious complications of indwelling long-term central venous access catheters. *Chest* 1990;96:966–972.

60. Press OW, Ramsey PG, Larson EB, et al. Hickman catheter infections in patients with malignancies. *Medicine* 1984;63:189–200.

61. Weightman NC, Simpson EM, Speller DCE, et al. Bacteremia related to indwelling central venous catheters: prevention, diagnosis, and treatment. *Eur J Clin Microbiol Infect Dis* 1988;7:125–129.

36

Hemodialysis Access Management

ANNE C. ROBERTS AND JAMES E. SILBERZWEIG

Dialysis is defined as the removal of blood elements by diffusion through a semipermeable membrane. The purpose of dialysis is to remove metabolic waste products and maintain fluid and electrolyte balance. The hemodialysis machine functions as an "artificial kidney." Blood is drawn from the patient at a rate of 300 to 500 mL per minute, passed through the dialysis machine, and then returned to the patient. Patients with end-stage renal disease typically require hemodialysis three times per week for 3 to 4 hours. The rapid circulation of blood between patient and hemodialysis machine requires a conduit that is durable, has a low infection rate, and is easily accessible. Peritoneal dialysis is an alternative form of dialysis in which dialysate is instilled into the peritoneal cavity, periodically drained, and replaced with fresh solution via a catheter. The peritoneal membrane acts as the dialyzing surface in peritoneal dialysis.

Alternatives for access to the patient's blood circulation for hemodialysis include the use of a central venous catheter, a surgically created arteriovenous fistula, or a prosthetic graft interposed between an artery and vein. Central venous catheters have one lumen for drawing blood from the patient into the hemodialysis machine (*arterial*) and one lumen for blood return to the patient from the hemodialysis machine (*venous*). Access to a prosthetic graft or the venous outflow of a surgically created fistula is made with two 14- to 16-gauge needles.

Renal transplantation is the treatment of choice for many patients with end-stage-renal disease. Because of limited organ availability, however, dialysis is the primary therapy for most of these patients. More than 280,000 persons in the United States require chronic dialysis.[1] For these patients, functioning dialysis access is their "lifeline," and maintenance of this access is critical. Hemodialysis access maintenance represents one of the most challenging problems for interventional radiologists. Thrombosis is the most common cause of hemodialysis access graft loss and usually is related to stenoses in the venous outflow. The goal of hemodialysis access maintenance is to detect and treat access dysfunction prior to access thrombosis and to salvage thrombosed grafts.

■ Arteriovenous Graft

Most patients requiring chronic hemodialysis have an upper-extremity arteriovenous graft (AVG) constructed of 6-mm-diameter polytetrafluoroethylene (PTFE) tubular graft material. Typical upper-extremity grafts include a *loop graft* with anastomoses at the brachial artery and basilic vein or cephalic vein and a *straight graft* with anastomoses at the distal radial artery and the basilic or cephalic vein near the antecubital fossa. The graft is tunneled subcutaneously and is easily accessible by percutaneous needle puncture. A lower-extremity loop graft extending from the common or superficial femoral artery to the saphenous vein is constructed when upper-extremity veins are no longer usable for graft construction. The most common complication associated with PTFE hemodialysis access grafts is the development of stenosis at the venous anastomosis or venous outflow of the graft resulting in graft thrombosis. Patency rates at 1 year range from 55 to 75%,[2,4,5] and the life span of the average graft is estimated to be less than 2 years.[6]

■ Brescia–Cimino Fistula

The preferred access for hemodialysis is an endogenous arteriovenous fistula because it provides the greatest chance for long-term function. A Brescia–Cimino arteriovenous fistula is usually constructed with a side-to-side anastomosis of the cephalic vein and radial artery at the wrist. A fistula also can be placed at the antecubital fossa with an anastomosis of the brachial artery and cephalic vein. Brescia–Cimino fistulas are less likely to thrombose than a PTFE graft because a fistula has a single anastomosis with multiple potential areas of venous outflow.

After an arteriovenous fistula is created, the patient cannot undergo dialysis using this access until fistula maturation occurs. Maturation involves vein-wall thickening and dilatation, which facilitates vein puncture with large-bore needles and accommodates arterial blood flow required for dialysis. The maturation process typically takes 1 to 4 months. Fistulas are ideally placed several months prior to anticipated use to ensure adequate maturation.

Unfortunately, Brescia–Cimino fistulas have a high early failure rate, usually as a result of inadequate venous size or runoff. When the fistula is established and used successfully for hemodialysis, late failure is rare. In about 20 to 30% of cases, the fistula will never mature.[2–4]

■ Causes of Graft Dysfunction

Thrombosis is the most common cause of hemodialysis access graft loss and usually is related to stenoses in the venous outflow. If thrombosis occurs in the first few weeks after placing the access, there is often a technical problem related to the graft. Technical problems include graft kinking, narrow arterial or venous anastomoses, or pre-existing arterial inflow or venous outflow disease (Fig. 36-1).[7] Occasionally, there is rapid development of venous outflow stenosis after graft insertion.[8] Thrombosis that occurs after 2 to 3 months is usually due to the development of stenosis in the venous outflow. Arterial inflow stenosis may occur, but it is a much less frequent

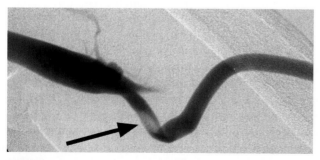

FIGURE 36-1. Kinking of this newly placed hemodialysis graft near the venous anastomosis (*arrow*) required surgical revision.

problem.[9] Occasionally, no underlying anatomic lesion can be found. It has been postulated that these grafts may have thrombosed due to excessive postdialysis graft compression at the needle puncture sites, hypotension, hypovolemia, compression of the graft due to sleeping position, or a hypercoagulable state.[10]

The development of venous stenoses appears to be caused by neointimal hyperplasia. The cause of this hyperplasia is not well understood. A variety of theories have been proposed to explain the development of neointimal hyperplasia. One mechanism of hyperplasia is a response to turbulent blood flow and vibration resulting from placement of the graft.[11] Other factors such as the transition between the relatively noncompliant graft material and the compliant vein,[12] or angulation and stretching of the vein at the anastomosis,[13] may be important. Whatever the cause, these stenoses inevitably recur after intervention because the underlying pathophysiology is unchanged. This is the cause for the ongoing requirement for repeated angioplasty and thrombolysis of the dialysis grafts. Until the pathophysiology of intimal hyperplasia is understood and techniques are developed to prevent intimal hyperplasia, there will be a need for the mechanical treatment of venous stenoses.

■ Treatment of the Poorly Functioning Graft

The sites available for hemodialysis access are limited; therefore, it is important to extend the life of each access for as long as possible. Treatment of grafts prior to thrombosis is more cost- and time-effective than treatment of thrombosed grafts. Long-term patency of grafts is improved if stenoses are treated prior to thrombosis as opposed to undertaking angioplasty or surgical revision after thrombosis has occurred; however, this requires identifying functioning grafts that are at risk for thrombosis. If the developing stenosis can be identified and treated with angioplasty, the risk and cost of thrombolysis can be avoided.

A number of signs may identify developing graft stenoses, including elevated venous pressure,[8,14] difficulty with needle placement, increased bleeding following needle removal, extremity edema, dilatation of collateral veins over the upper extremity or chest,[15] and conversion of the normal graft thrill to a pulse.[16,17] *Venous pressure* refers to the pressure measured by the dialysis machine as blood is returned to the patient. Venous return pressure greater than 150 mm Hg at a blood flow of 200 mL per minute is indicative of a venous outflow stenosis.[18] Recent studies showed that Doppler ultrasound may be useful in the evaluation for stenoses.[19,20]

Angiographic evaluation of a hemodialysis access graft should include the arterial anastomosis, graft, venous anastomosis, and the entire venous outflow. This can be done easily by using a dialysis needle, which can be left in place following a dialysis session or using standard Seldinger technique. If a stenosis is identified, angioplasty can be performed immediately and the patient discharged following completion of the procedure (Fig. 36-2).

Early correction of venous stenoses prolongs access viability. A recent study followed up on 106 grafts suspected on clinical examination to have a venous stenosis.[21] The grafts were studied angiographically, and any venous stenosis was treated with balloon angioplasty. The technical success for angioplasty was 98%. The primary patency at 1 year was 23% for PTFE grafts. Repeated angioplasty improved the patency rate to 68% at 1 year and 51% at 2 years (primary assisted patency rate). A combination of thrombolysis and repeated angioplasty improved patency further, with secondary patency rates at 1 year of 82% and at 2 years of 65%.[21]

Recurrence of stenoses should not be considered a failure of the procedure but rather an expression of the underlying pathophysiology. Redilatations allow easy and safe maintenance for months and even years.[17] Gaining added months of patency through redilatations could be of great value for dialysis patients. In contrast to a surgical graft revision, loss of central veins does not occur with angioplasty. Because angioplasty and surgical techniques may have similar secondary patency, the loss of future access sites becomes an important issue.

The treatment of a poorly functioning Brescia–Cimino fistula is less likely to involve thrombolysis and more likely to require angioplasty of a venous stenosis. In patients with Brescia–Cimino fistulas, most stenoses occur in the anastomotic and postanastomotic area before the puncture area for dialysis.[22] These fistulas are difficult to evaluate because of the number of outflow veins that become opacified with angiographic evaluation. This is particularly apparent when a stenosis in the main outflow and development of collateral veins occur. The collateral veins may overlie and obscure the venous stenosis, and angiography in multiple projections may be required to demonstrate an abnormality.

■ The Thrombosed Graft

The traditional therapy for failing hemodialysis access has been surgical thrombectomy with or without revision of the venous anastomosis. Thrombectomy alone is usually not successful because thrombectomy does not address the cause of graft failure, and replacement is not a realistic option because the possible access sites would be exhausted rapidly.

During the past 10 to 15 years, percutaneous techniques have become widely used for dialysis access salvage. Graft thrombolysis and balloon angioplasty of stenoses are the essence of percutaneous therapy for clotted hemodialysis access grafts. The thrombolysis portion of the procedure can be performed by several methods, including a combination of clot-dissolving medications and mechanical "declotting" devices.

A hemodialysis graft has unique characteristics that make it particularly amenable to percutaneous therapy. The graft is easy to access percutaneously, contains fresh clot responsive to thrombolytic agents, and is a closed system with only a single inflow and outflow, keeping the thrombolytic agent from diffusing into the systemic circulation.

The percutaneous approach to a thrombosed dialysis graft allows not only for thrombolysis but also for angiographic evaluation of the graft. The entire graft, including the arterial inflow and the complete venous outflow, can be evaluated easily. The venous anastomotic stenosis that is often encountered can be treated with balloon angioplasty.

The percutaneous graft declotting and angioplasty procedure is performed in a single session and usually is performed on an outpatient basis. Following the conclusion of the procedure, the patient can be discharged to a dialysis unit or home. The graft is functional for dialysis immediately following percutaneous therapy, unlike after surgical revision or new graft insertion. This is crucial because successful percutaneous therapy obviates the need for the insertion of a temporary central venous hemodialysis catheter. Avoidance of the use of temporary

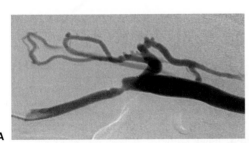

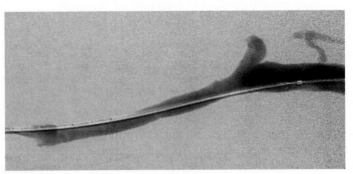

A   **B**

FIGURE 36-2. Arteriovenous shunt stenosis. Venous anastomotic stenosis. **(A).** Before the 7-mm balloon angioplasty. **(B).** After angioplasty.

jugular or femoral central venous dialysis catheters decreases expenses and eliminates the risk of complications from these catheters, such as central venous stenosis and infection.

■ Patient Selection

Usually, thrombosis of a recently (within a few weeks) constructed graft is due to a surgical technical problem. Sometimes thrombolysis is performed to identify the cause of the problem, which may allow a focused surgical repair. There is some increased risk of bleeding from recent anastomotic sites; however, if this does occur, it is usually controlled easily with manual pressure. Balloon angioplasty of the anastomosis of a recently placed graft, however, is at increased risk for rupture and should be avoided.

Some patients should not undergo thrombolysis. Criteria that would exclude a patient with a thrombosed dialysis graft are the same for other thrombolytic procedures. Absolute contraindications to thrombolysis are active gastrointestinal bleeding and recent neurologic processes, including intracranial bleeding, stroke, or neurologic surgery. Relative contraindications include major surgery or organ biopsy within 2 weeks; recent serious trauma; preexisting coagulation defects; uncontrolled, severe hypertension; pregnancy or the immediate postpartum period. The use of a mechanical thrombectomy device may be ideal for patients at increased risk for bleeding.

A contraindication to percutaneous graft thrombolysis is the presence of a graft infection. Lysis of infected clot may precipitate bacteremia and lethal sepsis.[23] Also an infected clot is relatively resistant to thrombolysis. Determining the presence of infection in a graft is often difficult. The classic signs of infection, such as redness, tenderness, warmth, swelling, and fever, are often blunted in patients with uremia. Purulent discharge or skin breakdown around the graft are obvious signs of infection, but these sign are uncommon. Needle aspiration of the graft clot for Gram stain and culture or of perigraft fluid collections found on ultrasound evaluation may be helpful in diagnosing graft infections.[24] Infection of the graft mandates treatment with antibiotics and referral for surgical removal of the graft.

Grafts that have undergone attempts at access just prior to the thrombolytic procedure are more likely to develop bleeding from the puncture sites during the thrombolytic procedure. It is worthwhile to develop a policy with the referring dialysis center so that if a patient presents with a pulseless graft, no attempts will be made to cannulate the graft, and the patient is immediately referred for percutaneous recanalization. Bleeding occasionally develops from puncture sites that are several days old, particularly if the puncture was traumatic. Usually

bleeding is not a serious problem. Bleeding can be managed by manual compression over the site and by rapid relief of the outflow stenosis by angioplasty that will decrease the pressure within the graft. On occasion, it is not possible to control the bleeding site while continuing to recanalize the graft. In this situation, surgical therapy may be required.

■ Graft Recanalization Technique

Graft access

The crossed-catheter technique is the basis of the approach to the thrombosed graft (Fig. 36-3 and Table 36-1).[25–27] This approach allows access to both the arterial and venous ends of the graft simultaneously. A standard single-wall entry needle or a Micropuncture Introducer set (Cook, Bloomington, IN, U.S.A.) is used to access the graft. The first puncture is made in the graft at the junction of the proximal and middle third of the graft (the arterial end of the graft) directed toward the venous end of the graft. The graft can be accessed most successfully if it is fixed between the thumb and index finger and held firmly while the puncture is being made. As the graft wall is punctured, there is a "popping" sensation. This sensa-

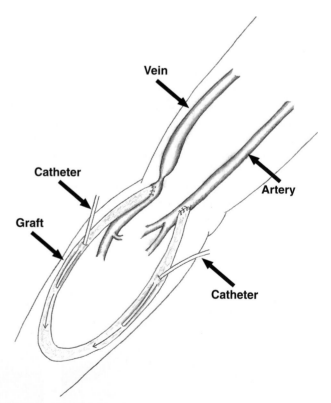

FIGURE 36-3. Initial catheter access for declotting of an upper-extremity hemodialysis loop graft using the crossed catheter technique.

TABLE 36-1. Hemodialysis Graft Declotting Procedure

1. Obtain antegrade access to the graft near the arterial anastomosis.
2. Cross the venous anastomosis with diagnostic catheter.
3. Obtain pullback venogram of central veins and graft outflow.
4. Angioplasty/stent central venous stenosis/occlusion.
5. Obtain retrograde access to the graft near the venous anastomosis.
6. Insert infusion catheters and inject thrombolytic agent or perform mechanical thrombectomy.
7. Angioplasty venous anastomotic stenosis/occlusion.
8. Remove residual clot at the arterial anastomosis by passing a deflated Fogarty or occlusion balloon catheter through the graft into the inflow artery. Inflate the balloon with contrast and pull back into the graft.
9. Macerate residual clot with the angioplasty balloon.
10. Perform completion angiogram of the inflow artery, graft, and outflow veins.
11. Exchange vascular sheaths for temporary hemodialysis catheters and transfer patient to hemodialysis unit.
12. Remove catheters after hemodialysis.

tion can be blunted in an older graft because scar tissue builds up around the graft after many punctures. The graft is thrombosed; thus, there will be no pulse within the graft and usually no return of blood when the lumen is entered. When the graft is entered, the guidewire usually passes easily through the lumen, even in the presence of clot. In some cases, a small amount of dark blood returns through the needle.

If the wire does not pass easily and coils in the soft tissues, as seen on fluoroscopy, the needle should be repositioned until it is within the graft lumen. If the patient complains of pain when the wire is advanced, this is an indication that the guidewire is not within the graft. On the other hand, the patient may not complain of pain when the wire is in the soft tissues, and so fluoroscopy and "feel" are extremely important. When the puncture is difficult, it is tempting to inject contrast to determine whether the graft has been entered. This temptation should be resisted. If the needle is not in the graft and contrast is injected into the soft tissues, the appearance may be misleading. At first, it may appear that the graft has been entered, as the injection continues, it will become evident that the contrast is not within the graft. At this point, however, the graft is often obscured and will remain obscured for the remainder of the procedure. Although it can be difficult to do so, it is best to rely on observing the wire following the course of the graft as evidence of correct placement of the needle within the graft.

After the guidewire has been placed correctly into the graft, a vascular sheath is placed over the guidewire, which then must be passed through the venous anastomosis and into the venous outflow. If difficulty is encountered in passing the venous anastomosis or the stenosis that is often in the same vicinity, an angled Glidewire (Terumo,

Boston Scientific, Natick, MA, U.S.A.) may be useful. It is crucial to confirm passage of the wire into the venous outflow before proceeding. If the venous outflow stenosis cannot be passed, thrombolysis should not be performed. If venous outflow is not reestablished and blood flow is reestablished, bleeding will occur from previous puncture sites or from around the catheters. If the venous anastomosis cannot be crossed, surgical thrombectomy and revision of the venous anastomosis are the most appropriate therapy.

When the guidewire can be passed beyond the venous anastomosis, a catheter is placed into the outflow vein. An outflow venogram then is performed to evaluate for any central venous stenosis and the presence of thrombus within the outflow vein.

The second vascular sheath in the cross-catheter technique is placed by puncturing the graft at the junction of the middle one third and the distal one third of the graft (the venous end of the graft). The guidewire is directed toward the arterial end of the graft. The catheter and wire manipulations at the arterial end of the graft should be done gently. Vigorous movement of the wire or forceful contrast injections can cause embolization of clot from the arterial anastomosis into the artery (Fig. 36-4).

■ Thrombolysis/Thrombectomy

Thrombolysis

The tissue plasminogen activator (tPA) (Activase, Genentech, South San Fransisco, CA, USA; Retauase, Centoeor, Malvern, PA, USA) has become the thrombolytic agent of choice following the recall of Urokinase in 1999.

Several methods to deliver the thrombolytic agent are available, including endhole, coaxial, and multi-sidehole catheter infusions and forced intrathrombic injections (pulse-spray) with use of tip-occluded multi-sidehole and multislit-type catheters. Prolonged thrombolytic infusion,

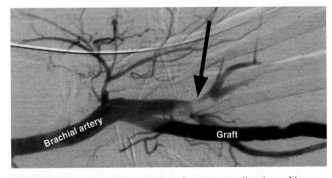

FIGURE 36-4. Arterial embolus. A rare complication of hemodialysis declotting is arterial embolization. The embolus to the bifurcation of the brachial artery (*arrow*) was successfully removed with the use of a Fogarty balloon catheter.

as often performed for native artery or arterial bypass graft occlusions, is no longer performed for hemodialysis access grafts because the procedure would take hours to days to dissolve the thrombus.

Pulse-spray thrombolysis

Pulse-spray thrombolysis is the technique most commonly used for administration of thrombolytic agent into a thrombosed AVG. This technique is characterized by the high-pressure delivery of small aliquots of highly concentrated thrombolytic agents via a multi-sidehole catheter. It allows for the homogeneous and simultaneous distribution of concentrated thrombolytic agent throughout the entire length of the occluded graft. This type of distribution enhances the diffusion of the thrombolytic agent in the clot and produces some mechanical disruption of the clot matrix, increasing the surface area exposed to the thrombolytic agent. Although the thrombolytic agent lyses most of the graft thrombus, residual thrombus is often within the graft. Removal of the residual graft thrombus requires additional maneuvers, including balloon maceration of the thrombus or balloon thrombectomy.

A number of commercially available catheter systems are suitable for pulse-spray procedures. The catheters used most often are the multi-sidehole infusion catheter (Cook Inc.) and the multislit catheter (Angiodynamics, Queensbury, NY, U.S.A.). These catheters have multiple sideholes or slits over a length of 4 to 30 cm. A tip-occluding guidewire is used to allow the thrombolytic agent to spray out the sideholes rather than primarily exiting the larger endhole. A hemostatic Touhy-Borst (Y adapter) allows injections around the guidewire. Injections of the 0.2 mL aliquots of urokinase are performed every 20 to 30 seconds. If the length of sideholes on the catheter is shorter than the clot being treated, after about half of the urokinase has been administered, the catheter is repositioned to treat the remainder of the clot.

Lyse and wait

One variation of the thrombolytic infusion technique is known as "lyse and wait." This technique was originally described as injection of 250,000 U of urokinase mixed with 5000 U of heparin through a standard intravenous catheter inserted within the venous limb of the graft. The graft was then manually compressed at the arterial and venous anastomoses while the urokinase–heparin mixture was infused over 1 minute into the graft. This portion of the procedure can be performed in a holding area outside the interventional radiology suite. After at least 30 minutes, the patient was transferred to the interventional radiology suite, and the declotting procedure was continued. Introducing the urokinase–heparin mixture into the graft before bringing the patient into the interventional radiology suite resulted in the declotting portion of the

procedure using little or no room time and avoided the added expense of an infusion catheter.[28] The "lyse and wait" technique has recently been reported with the use of tPA.[29]

Mechanical thrombectomy

Percutaneous mechanical thrombectomy (PMT) is becoming an established means of restoring flow to thrombosed hemodialysis access grafts. The term *percutaneous mechanical thrombectomy* refers to the use of mechanical energy to clear thrombus percutaneously with the use of any combination of mechanical dissolution, fragmentation, and aspiration. Compared with other thrombolytic techniques, mechanical thrombolysis with a device offers the potential for more efficient clot removal. The following devices and techniques have been used for dialysis graft declotting.

Pulse-spray with heparin

One clinical study suggested that pulse-spray intrathrombic injection of heparinized saline without thrombolytic agent is as effective for AVG declotting as pulse-spray injection of urokinase, indicating that mechanical effects are primarily responsible for clot lysis.[30] Two in vitro studies, however, concluded that forced intrathrombic injection of urokinase produce faster and more thrombolysis compared with intrathrombic injections of saline.[31,32]

Percutaneous aspiration thrombectomy (thromboaspiration)

Percutaneous aspiration thrombectomy involves the removal of thrombus by manual suction through a large-lumen aspiration catheter such as a vascular sheath or a 7 to 8 French angled guiding catheter. One recent study using manual thromboaspiration for thrombosed hemodialysis access grafts showed a high technical success rate; however, the mean procedure time was nearly 2 hours.[33]

Balloon-assisted thrombectomy

Percutaneous balloon mechanical thrombectomy without administration of a thrombolytic agent has been reported to be feasible for treatment of occluded dialysis access grafts.[34] Using this technique, all the clots are pushed into the pulmonary circulation. The major potential drawback of this technique is the risk of symptomatic and potentially fatal pulmonary embolism.[35]

Recirculation mechanical thrombectomy

During recirculation mechanical thrombectomy, thrombus is pulverized into microscopic fragments by using devices that generate a hydrodynamic vortex. The Amplatz Thrombectomy Device (Microvena, White Bear Lake, MN) uses a rotating impeller blade at the tip of the catheter that pulverizes the clot. The high rotation speed of the impeller generates a strong recirculation vortex. The clot enters the endhole at the tip of the device, becomes fragmented by the rotating blades, and recirculates out from three sideholes.[36] One drawback of this system is that the device is not steerable.

The AngioJet catheter (Possis, Minneapolis, MN, U.S.A.) uses a saline jet and aspiration system to create a Venturi effect. High-speed retrograde fluid jets create an area of low pressure (Venturi effect), resulting in a zone of hydrodynamic recirculation that pulls and fragments thrombus. The AngioJet is a 5 Fr catheter that can track over a guidewire.[37]

Nonrecirculation mechanical thrombectomy

Thrombus is macerated with the use of mechanical fragmentation. The Arrow-Trerotola percutaneous thrombolytic device (PTD) consists of a rotating nitinol basket driven by a hand-held electric motor (Fig. 36-5). The rotating basket strips thrombus from the walls of the graft and macerates the thrombus into small fragments. The resulting fragments are aspirated from the side port of the vascular sheath.[38]

The MTI thrombolytic brush catheter (Micro Therapeutics, San Clemente, CA, U.S.A.) consists of a 6 Fr infusion catheter housing a coaxial nylon brush with a diameter of 6 mm and a length of 10 mm. The brush is coaxially rotated by a hand-held electric motor used with simultaneous infusion of thrombolytic agent through the catheter, which results in both mechanical fragmentation of the clot and increased clot surface area exposed to the thrombolytic agent.[37]

The Gelbfish Endo-vac system is a mechanical thrombectomy device that both fragments and aspirates thrombus. A "clot-spoon" is manually reciprocated through a 6 Fr sheath to fragment the clot. The clot fragments are

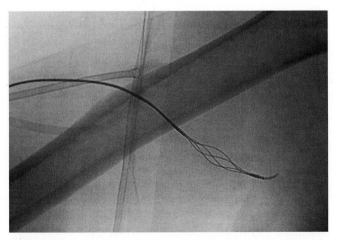

FIGURE 36-5. Fluoroscopic image of the Arrow-Trerotola percutaneous thrombolytic device within a thrombosed hemodialysis graft.

mobilized by saline irrigation through the sheath and removed by aspiration through the sidearm of the sheath.[37]

Treatment of venous stenoses

When the thrombolytic agent is administered or mechanical thrombectomy is performed, it is not necessary at this point for the graft to be completely free of clot. The most crucial aspect of thrombolysis is the reestablishment of flow through the thrombosed segment. It is common to find a significant degree of clot lysis and yet still have slow flow in the graft. Attention should be directed toward determining why the flow is not normal. The most common reason is a venous stenosis limiting outflow from the graft. Other possibilities include resistant thrombus at the arterial anastomosis, incomplete administration of urokinase to the entire clot, insufficient heparinization, or infected thrombus that is resistant to lysis. Injection of contrast and visual evaluation of the graft should allow determination of the venous stenosis or the residual clot at the arterial anastomosis.

The first intervention, after administration of a thrombolytic agent or use of a mechanical thrombectomy device, is treatment of venous stenosis, which is present in 90% of thrombosed grafts.[10,27,39] Resistant clot at the arterial inflow may also be present, but treatment of that clot should follow the venous intervention. The venous stenosis is treated with balloon angioplasty. Relieving the stenosis will allow outflow from the graft and minimize bleeding from around the catheter or previous dialysis needle-puncture sites. Residual clot within the graft then can be macerated with the same angioplasty balloon.

At times, it may be difficult to visualize the venous stenosis because of the overlapping outflow veins. If necessary, multiple views of the proximal venous outflow should be obtained so that the stenosis can be identified. When the stenosis is found, it should be dilated with an appropriately sized angioplasty balloon. The balloon diameter is determined by the diameter of the PTFE graft and the size of the draining vein. Usually a 6-mm balloon is used, but sizes from 5 mm to 8 mm may be more appropriate in some situations. Angioplasty with a high-pressure balloon is often helpful because these stenoses are often somewhat resistant to dilatation. In some cases, the stenosis may not respond to the first dilatation, and multiple prolonged inflations may be necessary to expand the balloon and thus efface the stenosis completely. In some cases, the balloon may inflate completely but the stenosis is still present. This situation represents elastic recoil that usually can be treated by using a larger angioplasty balloon. In some cases, insertion of a stent may be necessary to overcome the elastic recoil (Fig. 36-6).[40,41] Directional atherectomy also has been described for treatment of balloon-resistant lesions,[42] but no study has demonstrated superior results for venous lesions following atherectomy compared with angioplasty.[43]

Treatment of arterial plug

Residual thrombus at the arterial anastomosis is a common finding. This lysis-resistant plug is present at the arterial anastomosis in up to 60% of patients.[39] The arterial plug is removed by a "balloon thrombectomy" procedure (Fig. 36-7). Thrombectomy is performed using a standard Fogarty embolectomy balloon catheter (Baxter, Irvine, CA, U.S.A.), an 8.5-mm occlusion balloon catheter (Meditech, Inc., Watertown, MA, U.S.A.), or an "over-the-wire" Fogarty balloon catheter (Baxter). A guidewire is carefully positioned past the residual clot and into the native artery. The occlusion balloon catheter then is placed over the wire and situated just past the clot. Using dilute contrast, the balloon is inflated and the catheter pulled back, displacing the clot into the graft. This procedure is performed using fluoroscopy to avoid arterial injury and overinflation of the balloon in the native artery. As the balloon is pulled back next to the clot, it is often necessary to expand the balloon slightly to dislodge the clot. Several passes of the balloon may be necessary

to dislodge the clot from the side of the graft. After the plug is dislodged, it may become trapped in the graft, usually at the site of the crossed catheters. If this occurs, the angioplasty balloon is used to macerate the clot, which is now safely within the graft.

Unlike conventional angioplasty balloon catheters, the compliant nature of the Fogarty balloon allows relatively atraumatic manipulation within the inflow artery and arterial anastomosis of hemodialysis grafts. Use of a noncompliant angioplasty balloon to pull adherent clot from the arterial anastomosis of a hemodialysis graft may cause excessive shear stress within the graft or native artery and increase the risk of vascular injury. The thrombectomy procedure is similar to surgical thrombectomy. Compared with the blind surgical procedure, however, the angiographic procedure has the advantage of fluoroscopic guidance; a wire can be placed beyond the clot serving as a guide for the catheter and immediate angiographic evaluation.

Completion study

Following thrombolysis, balloon dilatation of the venous outflow stenosis, and removal of the arterial plug, the

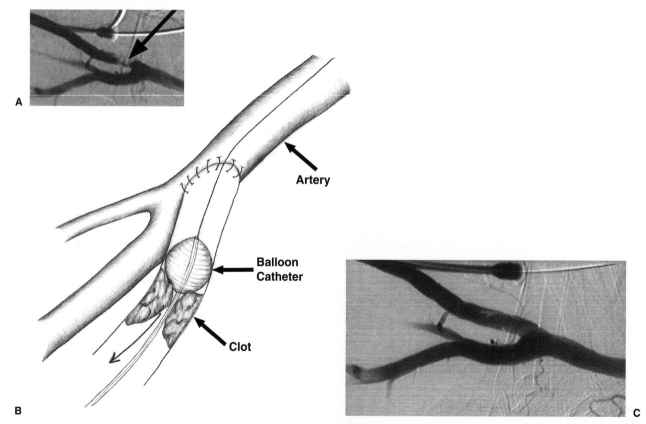

FIGURE 36-6. Lysis-resistant plug near arterial anastomosis. **(A).** A persistent narrowing near the arterial graft anastomosis (*arrow*) is the lysis-resistant plug frequently encountered during hemodialysis graft declotting. (B). The plug was mobilized with the use of a Fogarty balloon catheter. (C). Restoration of a patent graft lumen.

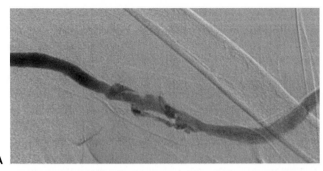
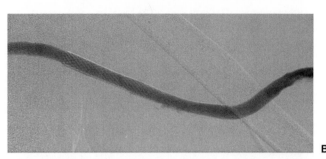

A   B

FIGURE 36-7. Stent insertion for venous outflow stenosis. **(A).** A stenosis in the basilic vein beyond the venous anastomosis was treated with a 7-mm balloon angioplasty. There was significant elastic recoil despite complete inflation of the angioplasty balloon. **(B).** The residual narrowing was treated with insertion of an 8-mm diameter Wallstent.

entire graft should be evaluated. The arterial inflow, the body of the graft, and the venous outflow to the superior vena cava should be assessed for residual thrombus or stenoses. Intragraft pressure measurement can be used to assess the adequacy of the intervention. A drop from arterial pressure to venous pressure is expected throughout the length of the graft. An intragraft systolic pressure of 40% of systolic arterial blood pressure can be considered borderline between normal function and dysfunction.[44] A graft pressure greater than 40% of systolic pressure is suggestive of venous outflow stenosis.

If dialysis is to follow the declotting procedure immediately, the vascular sheaths can be exchanged for dialysis sheaths (Angiodynamics, Glen Falls, NY, U.S.A.). These sheaths come as a set; one catheter is red and directed toward the arterial inflow, and the other is blue and placed with the tip directed toward the venous outflow. Placement of these catheters helps to speed the procedure because access site compression is not required and spares the patient reaccessing the graft in the dialysis center. Recently, vascular sheaths (Micro Therapeutics) have become commercially available through which both the declotting procedure and hemodialysis can be performed.

■ Other causes of graft thrombosis

Other causes of thrombosis are much less common than perianastomotic venous stenoses. Arterial stenosis is a contributing factor in fewer than 15% of treated grafts.[10,39,45] Visualization of the artery is performed best by placing a catheter just at the arterial anastomosis. Manual compression of the graft, inflation of a blood pressure cuff or placement of a tourniquet above the graft, or inflation of a Fogarty balloon catheter within the venous limb of the graft can be used to allow reflux of contrast into the arterial inflow. Multiple angiographic projections may be needed to assess the arterial anastomosis.

If an arterial anastomotic stenosis is identified, it may be possible to place a wire from the graft, through the

anastomosis, and into the artery and to perform an angioplasty. If an angioplasty balloon cannot be manipulated across the stenosis from a graft approach, direct puncture of the artery can be used to access the stenosis. Angioplasty at the arterial anastomosis should be performed cautiously. The artery is not as forgiving as the vein and may represent a significant blood supply to the fingers. The size of the angioplasty balloon catheter must be chosen carefully, and the catheterization should be performed cautiously. In some cases, the arterial anastomosis may appear narrowed because of a surgically tapered anastomosis. Overdilatation may result in anastomotic rupture.

Stenoses within the graft are uncommon. The cause of such stenoses is not understood. They may be caused by mural thrombus, or they may represent hypertrophy of the neointima that develops on the luminal surface of the graft.[46]

Central venous stenoses are another uncommon cause of thrombosis. In the setting of graft thrombosis, there is usually a simultaneous peripheral stenosis that is more likely to have been the inciting cause of thrombosis. The subclavian vein is the most common central vein to be involved as a result of venous injury from previous dialysis access catheters.[47,48] Patients with previous internal jugular vein catheters have a 0 to 10% incidence of significant central vein stenosis compared with a previous subclavian catheter, where the incidence is 42 to 50% (Fig. 36-8).[49,50] Stenoses in any portion of the outflow probably should be treated because they may contribute to the potential for graft thrombosis. The consequences of central vein stenoses include the potential for compromise of future dialysis access and significant upper-extremity swelling. The initial treatment for central venous stenoses is balloon angioplasty. Elastic recoil after angioplasty is characteristic of central venous lesions. The results of balloon angioplasty are poor, with a 6-month cumulative primary patency of only 28.9% in one study.[6] One recent study of central venous stenting reported promising short-term patency results.[51]

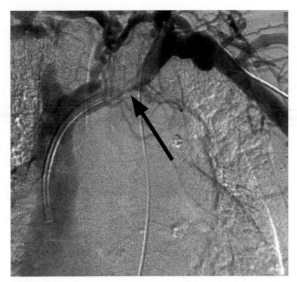

FIGURE 36-8. Central venous stenosis. The left brachiocephalic vein stenosis probably was related to the presence of the indwelling hemodialysis catheter (*arrow*).

■ Complications of Thrombolysis

Complications associated with pulsed-spray thrombolysis are uncommon. Bleeding is infrequent. Occasionally, bleeding from previous puncture sites occurs, usually developing when graft flow has been reestablished but the venous stenosis has not yet been dilated. The best treatment is gentle compression over the bleeding site and angioplasty of the venous outflow. Severe bleeding requiring termination of the procedure or other therapy has occurred in fewer than 1% of patients undergoing pulse-spray thrombolysis.[39]

Embolization into the arterial system is also uncommon. If it occurs, it usually can be treated with additional thrombolytic agent, administered by placing a catheter into the affected artery and positioning the catheter at the clot. Alternatively, an occlusion balloon catheter or Fogarty embolectomy catheter can be placed into the artery beyond the clot, and the clot is pulled back into the graft. Aspiration thrombectomy is an additional maneuver that can be used to remove arterial emboli. The best treatment is prevention; careful guidewire and catheter manipulations at the arterial anastomosis will minimize the risk of embolization.

■ Results

The immediate technical results of pulse-spray thrombolysis have been excellent. Time for lysis has been decreased from several hours to fewer than 20 minutes, at which time flow has been reestablished and angioplasty can be performed.[10,39] Total procedure times are less than 2 hours and not uncommonly are only slightly more than 1 hour. Most importantly, successful lysis can be achieved in 96% of cases with a clinical success rate of 92%.

Long-term primary patency of thrombosed dialysis grafts is relatively poor; however, this is true with both percutaneous and surgical approaches to thrombosed dialysis grafts. Primary patency at 1 year is 11 to 26%,[27,51,52] and secondary patency at 1 year is 51 to 69%.[26,53] Studies directly comparing surgical thrombectomy with thrombolysis demonstrate similar patency rates.[54,55]

■ Conclusion

Hemodialysis access failure is a major cause of morbidity for patients undergoing hemodialysis. Prevention and treatment of dialysis graft thrombosis are important but frustrating clinical problems. The National Kidney Foundation recently formulated *Clinical Practice Guidelines for Vascular Access* in an effort to reduce patient morbidity and improve patient survival and quality of life. Two primary goals of these guidelines are to encourage the placement of native arteriovenous fistulae and the detection of access dysfunction prior to access thrombosis.[56]

Significant progress has been achieved in the therapy for thrombosed dialysis grafts. The procedure of graft declotting has been refined so it takes less time and less thrombolytic agent, and results in fewer complications. The pathophysiology underlying venous stenoses is beginning to be understood, and there has been an improvement in the early detection and treatment of the stenoses. Prevention of the development of neointimal hyperplasia remains to be solved.

REFERENCES

1. US Renal Data System: *USRDS 1998 Annual Data Report.* Bethesda, MD: The National Institutes of Health, National Institute of Diabetes and Digestive and Kidney Diseases; 1998.
2. Ballard JL, Bunt TJ, Malone JM. Major complications of angioaccess surgery. *Am J Surg* 1992;164:229–232.
3. Windus DW, Audrain J, Vanderson R, et al. Optimization of high-efficiency hemodialysis by detection and correction of fistula dysfunction. *Kidney Int* 1990;38:337–341.
4. Palder S, Kirkman R, Whittemore A, et al. Vascular access for hemodialysis. *Ann Surg* 1985;202:235–239.
5. Beathard G. Percutaneous transvenous angioplasty in the treatment of vascular access stenosis. *Kidney Int* 1992;42:1390–1397.
6. Schwartz C, McBrayer C, Sloan J, et al. Thrombosed dialysis grafts: comparison of treatment with transluminal angioplasty and surgical revision. *Radiology* 1995;194:337–341.
7. Glanz S, Bashist B, Gordon DH, et al. Angiography of upper extremity access fistulas for dialysis. *Radiology* 1982;143:45–52.
8. Zeit RM. The problems and management of hemodialysis accesses. In: Castaneda-Zuniga W, Tadavarthy S, eds. *Interventional Radiology.* Baltimore: Williams & Wilkins; 1992:422–437.
9. Roberts A, Valji K, Bookstein J, et al. Pulse-spray pharmacomechani-

cal thrombolysis for treatment of thrombosed dialysis access grafts. *Am J Surg* 1993;16:221–226.

10. Fan PY, Schwab SJ. Vascular access: concepts for the 1990s [editorial]. *J Am Soc Nephrol* 1992;3:1–11.

11. Fillinger M, Reinitz E, Schwartz R, et al. Graft geometry and venous intimal-medial hyperplasia in arteriovenous loop grafts. *J Vasc Surg* 1990;11:556–566.

12. Windus DW. Permanent vascular access: a nephrologist's view. *Am J Kidney Dis* 1993;21:457–471.

13. Malchesky P, Koshino I, Pennza P, et al. Analysis of the segmental venous stenosis in blood access. *Trans Am Soc Artif Int Organs* 1975; 21:310–319.

14. Schwab SJ, Raymond JR, Saeed M, et al. Prevention of hemodialysis fistula thrombosis: early detection of venous stenoses. *Kidney Int* 1989;36:707–711.

15. Schwab SJ, Quarles D, Middleton JP, et al. Hemodialysis-associated subclavian vein stenosis. *Kidney Int* 1988;33:1156–1159.

16. Ziegler TW, Safa A, Amarillis K, et al. Prolonging the life of difficult hemodialysis access using thrombolysis, angiography and angioplasty. *Adv Ren Replace Ther* 1995;2:52–59.

17. Beathard GA. Physical examination of AV grafts. *Semin Dial* 1992; 5:74.

18. Besarab A, Sullivan KL, Ross RP, et al. Utility of intra-access pressure monitoring in detecting and correcting venous outlet stenoses prior to thrombosis. *Kidney Int* 1995;47:1364–1373.

19. Gadallah MF, Paulson WD, Vickers B, et al. Accuracy of Doppler ultrasound in diagnosing anatomic stenosis of hemodialysis arteriovenous access as compared with fistulography. *Am J Kidney Dis* 1998;32:273–277.

20. Robbin ML, Oser RF, Allon M, et al. Hemodialysis access graft stenosis: US detection. *Radiology* 1998;208:655–661.

21. Safa A, Valji K, Roberts A, et al. Detection and treatment of dysfunctional hemodialysis access grafts: effect of a surveillance program on graft patency and the incidence of thrombosis. *Radiology* 1996; 199:653–657.

22. Turmel-Rodrigues L, Pengloan J, Blanchier D, et al. Insufficient dialysis shunts: improved long-term patency rates with close hemodynamic monitoring, repeated percutaneous balloon angioplasty and stent placement. *Radiology* 1993;187:273–278.

23. Davis G, Dowd C, Bookstein J, et al. Thrombosed dialysis grafts: efficacy of intrathrombic deposition of concentrated urokinase, clot maceration, and angioplasty. *AJR Am J Roentgenol* 1987;149: 177–182.

24. Valji K, Roberts A, Bookstein J. Thrombosed hemodialysis access grafts: management with pulse-spray thrombolysis and balloon angioplasty. In: Strandness D, Van Breda A, eds. *Vascular Diseases: Surgical and Interventional Therapy.* Vol 2. New York: Churchill Livingstone; 1994:1087–1095.

25. Bookstein J, Fellmeth B, Roberts A, et al. Pulsed-spray pharmacomechanical thrombolysis: preliminary clinical results. *AJR Am J Roentgenol* 1989;152:1097–1100.

26. Roberts A, Bookstein J. Dialysis fistula occlusion: treatment by thrombolysis. In: Kadir S, ed. *Current Practice of Interventional Radiology.* Philadelphia: B C Decker; 1991:291–294.

27. Valji K, Bookstein JJ, Roberts AC, et al. Pharmacomechanical thrombolysis and angioplasty in the management of clotted hemodialysis grafts: early and late clinical results. *Radiology* 1991;178:243–247.

28. Cynamon J, Lakritz PS, Wahl SI, et al. Hemodialysis graft declotting: description of the "lyse and wait" technique. *J Vasc Interv Radiol* 1997;8:825–829.

29. Falk A, Mitty H, Guller J, et al. Thrombolysis of clotted hemodialysis grafts with tissue–type plasminogen activator. *J Vasc Interv Radiol* 2001;12:305–311.

30. Beathard GA, Welch BR, Maidment HJ. Mechanical thrombolysis for the treatment of thrombosed hemodialysis access grafts. *Radiology* 1996;200:711–716.

31. Khilnani NM, Winchester PA, Zanzonico P, et al. In vitro evaluation of the relative thrombolytic efficiency of forced intrathrombic injections: saline versus urokinase. *J Vasc Interv Radiol* 1998;9: 786–792.

32. Froelich JJ, Freymann C, Hoppe M, et al. Local intraarterial thrombolysis: in vitro comparison between automatic and manual pulse-spray infusion. *Cardiovasc Interv Radiol* 1996;19:423–427.

33. Turmel-Rodrigues L, Sapoval M, Pengloan J, et al. Manual thromboaspiration and dilation of thrombosed dialysis access: mid-term results of a simple concept. *J Vasc Interv Radiol* 1997;8:813–824.

34. Trerotola S, Lund G, Scheel P, et al. Thrombosed dialysis access grafts: percutaneous mechanical declotting without urokinase. *Radiology* 1994;191:721–726.

35. Swan TL, Smyth SH, Ruffenach SJ, et al. Pulmonary embolism following hemodialysis access thrombolysis/thrombectomy. *J Vasc Interv Radiol* 1995;6:683–686.

36. Uflacker R, Rajagopalan PR, Vujic I, et al. Treatment of thrombosed dialysis access grafts: randomized trial of surgical thrombectomy versus mechanical thrombectomy with the Amplatz device. *J Vasc Interv Radiol* 1996;7:185–192.

37. Sharafuddin MJA, Hicks ME. Current status of percutaneous mechanical thrombectomy, II: Devices and mechanisms of action. *J Vasc Interv Radiol* 1998;9:15–31.

38. Trerotola SO, Vesely TM, Lund GB, et al. Treatment of thrombosed hemodialysis access grafts: Arrow-Trerotola percutaneous thrombolytic device versus pulse-spray thrombolysis. *Radiology* 1998;206: 403–414.

39. Valji K. Transcatheter treatment of thrombosed hemodialysis access grafts. *AJR Am J Roentgenol* 1995;164:823–829.

40. Kovalik EC, Newman GE, Suchocki P, et al. Correction of central venous stenoses: use of angioplasty and vascular Wallstents. *Kidney Int* 1994;45:1177–1181.

41. Patel RI, Peck SH, Cooper SG, et al. *Radiology* 1998;209:365–370.

42. Zemel G, Katzen BT, Dake MD, et al. Directional atherectomy in the treatment of stenotic dialysis access fistulas. *Nephrol Dial Transplant* 1991;6:5–10.

43. Gray RJ. Percutaneous intervention for permanent hemodialysis access: a review. *J Vasc Intery Radiol* 1997;8:313–327.

44. Sullivan KL, Besarab A, Dorrell S, et al. Relationship between dialysis graft pressure and stenosis. *Invest Radiol* 1992;27:352–355.

45. Saeed M, Newman GE, McCann RL, et al. Stenoses in dialysis fistulas: treatment with percutaneous angioplasty. *Radiology* 1987; 164:693–697.

46. Puckett J, Lindsay S. Midgraft curettage as a routine adjunct to savage operations for thrombosed polytetrafluoroethylene hemodialysis access grafts. *Am J Surg* 1988;156:139.

47. Okadome K, Komori K, Fukumitsu T, et al. The potential risk for subclavian vein occlusion in patients on haemodialysis. *Eur J Vasc Surg* 1992;6:602–606.

48. Kerstein K. End-stage renal disease with venous occlusion in both upper extremities. *South Med J* 1993;86:1229–1232.

49. Schillinger F, Schillinger D, Montagnac R, et al. Post catheterization vein stenosis in hemodialysis: comparative angiographic study of 50 subclavian and 50 internal jugular accesses. *Nephrol Dial Transplant* 1991;6:722–724.

50. Cimochowski GE, Worley E, Rutherford WE, et al. Superiority of the internal jugular over the subclavian access for temporary dialysis. *Nephron* 1990;54:154–161.

51. Gray RJ, Horton KM, Dolmatch BL, et al. Use of Wallstents for hemodialysis access-related venous stenoses and occlusions untreatable with balloon angioplasty. *Radiology* 1995;195:479–484.

52. Sands JJ, Patel S, Plaviak D, et al. Pharmacomechanical thrombolysis with urokinase for treatment of thrombosed hemodialysis access grafts: a comparison with surgical thrombectomy. *ASAIO J* 1994;40:M886–M888.

53. Cohen MAH, Kumpe DA, Durham JD, et al. Improved treatment of

thrombosed hemodialysis access sites with thrombolysis and angioplasty. *Kidney Int* 1994;46:1375–1380.

54. Summers S, Drazan K, Gomes A, et al. Urokinase therapy for thrombosed hemodialysis access grafts. *Surg Gynecol Obstet* 1993;176:534–538.

55. Schuman E, Quinn S, Standage B, et al. Thrombolysis versus throm-bectomy for occluded hemodialysis grafts. *Am J Surg* 1994;167:473–476.

56. Schwab S, Besarab A, Beathard G, et al. NKF-DOQI clinical practice guidelines for vascular access. *Am J Kidney Dis* 1997;30 (suppl 3): 150–191.

Index